THE HEALTHCARE QUALITY BOOK

VISION, STRATEGY, AND TOOLS

THIRD EDITION

THE HEALTHCARE QUALITY BOOK

VISION, STRATEGY, AND TOOLS

THIRD EDITION

Maulik S. Joshi, Elizabeth R. Ransom, David B. Nash, Scott B. Ransom, Editors

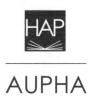

AUPHA

Health Administration Press, Chicago, Illinois

Association of University Programs in Health Administration, Arlington, Virginia

Library of Congress Cataloging-in-Publication Data

The healthcare quality book : vision, strategy, and tools / Maulik S. Joshi, Elizabeth R. Ransom, David B. Nash, and Scott B. Ransom, editors. -- Third edition.
    pages cm
  Includes index.
  ISBN 978-1-56793-590-5 (alk. paper)
  1. Medical care--United States--Quality control. 2. Health services administration--United States--Quality control. 3. Total quality management--United States. I. Joshi, Maulik, editor of compilation. II. Ransom, Elizabeth R., editor of compilation. III. Nash, David B., editor of compilation. IV. Ransom, Scott B., editor of compilation.
  RA399.A3H433 2014
  362.1068--dc23
                    2013031975

Acquisitions editor: Tulie O'Connor; Project manager: Andrew Baumann; Cover designer: Marisa Jackson; Layout: Cepheus Edmondson

Found an error or a typo? We want to know! Please e-mail it to hapbooks@ache.org, and put "Book Error" in the subject line.

For photocopying and copyright information, please contact Copyright Clearance Center at www.copyright.com or at (978) 750–8400.

Health Administration Press
A division of the Foundation of the American
   College of Healthcare Executives
One North Franklin Street, Suite 1700
Chicago, IL 60606–3529
(312) 424–2800

Association of University Programs
   in Health Administration
2000 North 14th Street
Suite 780
Arlington, VA 22201
(703) 894–0940

BRIEF CONTENTS

DETAILED CONTENTS

FOREWORD

Improving care outcomes is "job number one" for healthcare organizations in the United States. As we watch national healthcare reform unfold in Washington, DC, we know that real reform will take place in our local communities and that it will take coordination of care and collaboration between physicians and healthcare systems to advance quality.

The quality imperative will be advanced only when it becomes part of the strategy of an organization and when the results produce healthier communities and reductions in hospital admissions and readmissions. Alignment of the many parts of the industry around this focus as well as engagement and participation by payers and consumers will lift the quality of care and service to new heights and create a healthier America.

The third edition of *The Healthcare Quality Book* provides the practical tools necessary for measuring and improving healthcare performance and promotes transparency of clinical pathways and outcomes. This easy-to-read guide offers clinicians and nonclinicians numerous insights and proven strategies for unlocking and managing performance improvement.

This edition has arrived at the right time, as healthcare transforms from vertical care to coordinated care. Each chapter adds to the value equation that must drive healthcare: quality, safety, service, and cost. It is a mind-opening book and a must-read for healthcare leaders.

Douglas D. Hawthorne, FACHE
Chief Executive Officer
Texas Health Resources
Arlington, Texas

PREFACE

The US healthcare system is undergoing a transformation. While much has changed since the previous edition of this book, many of the challenges the US healthcare system faces remain the same, including high costs, lack of access to care, inconsistent quality, and disparities in care. In 2010, President Barack Obama signed the Affordable Care Act (ACA) into law—the largest healthcare reform effort since the creation of Medicare and Medicaid in 1965. The ACA seeks to expand coverage, control costs, improve quality, and transform care delivery. While it creates unique opportunities for learning and improvement across the US healthcare system, it also presents many uncertainties and challenges with regard to implementation. Despite these many uncertainties, one thing is assured: Healthcare quality is paramount. Ensuring healthcare that is safe, effective, efficient, equitable, patient centered, and timely is fundamental to all current and future healthcare reform plans, whether big, small, global, national, or regional.

This textbook provides a framework, a context, strategies, and practical tactics to help all stakeholders understand, learn, teach, and lead healthcare improvement. We have assembled an internationally prominent group of contributors to bring to this book the best, most current thinking and practices from each of their disciplines.

The third edition includes new case studies, up-to-date content, new study questions, and three new chapters. Despite these changes, the framework of the book remains the same. Chapters 1 through 4 discuss foundational healthcare quality principles. Chapters 5 through 17 discuss critical quality issues at the organizational and microsystem levels. Chapters 18 through 21 detail the influence of the environment and emerging trends on the organizations, teams, and individuals delivering healthcare services and products.

In Chapter 1, Maulik Joshi and Donald Berwick focus on the patient and articulate key findings from sentinel national reports of healthcare quality published over the past 14 years. In Chapter 2, Leon Wyszewianski discusses the fundamental concepts of quality. In Chapter 3, David Ballard and colleagues discuss medical practice variation and provide an updated case study. In Chapter 4, Kevin Warren describes the latest quality improvement tools and programs.

In Chapter 5, John Byrnes discusses measurement as a building block in quality assessment and improvement. Stephen Schmaltz and colleagues describe statistical tools for quality improvement in Chapter 6, and David Nash and colleagues detail a physician profiling system in Chapter 7. In Chapter 8—a new chapter—Quint Studer describes the importance of culture to providing consistent quality, and in Chapter 9, Susan Edgman-Levitan tackles an often discussed but less understood area of patient satisfaction—experiences and perspectives of care—and includes an update on the latest surveys. In Chapter 10, Michael Pugh aggregates data into management tools known as *scorecards* and *dashboards*. Frances Griffin in Chapter 11 and Edward Walker in Chapter 12 dive deeper into two evolving subjects essential to driving performance improvement—patient safety and a culture of reliability, respectively. In Chapter 13, Ferdinand Velasco describes the many implications of information technology for healthcare quality.

In Chapters 14 through 16, James Reinertsen, A. Al-Assaf, and Scott Ransom and colleagues provide a triad of keys for change in organizations seeking to become high performers by addressing leadership, infrastructure, and strategies for quality improvement. Chapter 17 by Valerie Weber and Jaan Sidorov is a compilation of strategies and tactics for changing staff behavior.

Chapter 18 by Kimberly Acquaviva and Jean Johnson provides examples of many of the recent national quality improvement initiatives and an overview of the quality improvement landscape. In Chapter 19, Diane Storer Brown and Kevin Park summarize the work of the two major accrediting bodies in healthcare—the National Committee for Quality Assurance and The Joint Commission—and cover the latest changes in the accreditation process. Chapter 20 by François de Brantes describes the power of the purchaser to select and pay for quality services and provides updated information on pay for performance. The final chapter, a new chapter by Steffanie Bristol and Maulik Joshi, brings the latest developments in healthcare to the forefront and paves a path to healthcare transformation.

Several of these chapters could stand independently. Each is an important contribution to our understanding of the environment and the patient-centered organizations that deliver healthcare services. The science and knowledge of quality measurement are rapidly expanding and evolving. This book provides a timely analysis of the most current tools and techniques.

Who should read this book? The editors believe all current stakeholders would benefit from the information included in it, but its primary audiences are undergraduate and graduate students in healthcare and business administration, public health, nursing, allied health, and medical programs. As leadership development and continuing education programs proliferate, this text also is a resource for executives and practitioners at the front line.

We hope this book will break down the educational silos that prevent stakeholders from sharing their understanding of patient-centered organizational systems and the environment of healthcare quality.

We are extremely fortunate to have an all-star list of contributors. These authors have incredible experience and expertise in healthcare, from which our readers benefit greatly.

We also want to thank Natalie Erb, who was instrumental to this book's success. Natalie contributed to the textbook in so many ways, including development of all instructor materials, and lent tireless support to the final work.

This textbook and the accompanying instructor manual are designed to facilitate discussion and learning. The instructor manual contains teaching aids for each chapter, including answers to the end-of-chapter study questions, PowerPoint presentations, and a test bank. To access these resources, e-mail hapbooks@ache.org.

Please contact us at mjoshi@aha.org. Your feedback, teaching, learning, and leadership are essential to transforming healthcare. Thank you.

Maulik S. Joshi
Elizabeth R. Ransom
David B. Nash
Scott B. Ransom

THE FOUNDATION OF HEALTHCARE QUALITY

HEALTHCARE QUALITY AND THE PATIENT

Maulik S. Joshi and Donald Berwick

Quality in the US healthcare system is not what it should be. Even before evidence was available, people had long been aware of the numerous failings of the healthcare system from personal stories and anecdotes. At the end of the twentieth century, many reports revealed strong evidence of widespread quality deficiencies and highlighted a need for substantial change to ensure high-quality care for all patients. The major reports highlighting the imperative for quality improvement included the following:

- "The Urgent Need to Improve Health Care Quality" by the Institute of Medicine (IOM) National Roundtable on Health Care Quality (Chassin and Galvin 1998)
- IOM's *To Err Is Human: Building a Safer Health System* (Kohn, Corrigan, and Donaldson 2000)
- IOM's *Crossing the Quality Chasm: A New Health System for the 21st Century* (IOM 2001)
- *National Healthcare Quality Report*, published annually by the Agency for Healthcare Research and Quality (AHRQ) since 2003
- *National Priorities and Goals: Aligning Our Efforts to Transform America's Healthcare* by the National Priorities Partnership (NPP 2008)

More than a decade since some of them were first published, these reports continue to make a tremendous statement. They draw attention to current gaps in care, call for action, and identify opportunities to significantly improve the quality of care in the United States.

Before we discuss these reports, let us first define quality and describe its evolution and implications for our work as healthcare professionals.

Avedis Donabedian, a pioneer in the field of quality assurance, discussed in detail the various definitions of quality as it relates to perspective. One of Donabedian's conceptual constructs of quality rang particularly true: "The balance of health benefits and harm is the essential core of a definition of quality" (Donabedian 1980). Balance between benefits and harm is essential in medicine: It is one part science and one part art (Donabedian 2001).

The IOM Committee to Design a Strategy for Quality Review and Assurance in Medicare has developed an often-cited definition of quality (Lohr 1990):

> Quality of care is the degree to which health services for individuals and populations increase the likelihood of desired health outcomes and are consistent with current professional knowledge. . . . How care is provided should reflect appropriate use of the most current knowledge about scientific, clinical, technical, interpersonal, manual, cognitive, and organization and management elements of health care.

In 2001, IOM's *Crossing the Quality Chasm* stated powerfully and simply that healthcare should embrace six dimensions: It should be safe, effective, efficient, timely, patient centered, and equitable. This six-dimensional aim, discussed later in this chapter, is the best known and most goal-oriented definition (or at least conceptualization) of the components of quality today.

Important Reports

"The Urgent Need to Improve Health Care Quality"

Published in 1998, the IOM's National Roundtable report "The Urgent Need to Improve Health Care Quality" included two notable contributions. The first was an assessment of the state of quality: "Serious and widespread quality problems exist throughout American medicine. These problems . . . occur in small and large communities alike, in all parts of the country, and with approximately equal frequency in managed care and fee-for-service systems of care. Very large numbers of Americans are harmed" (Chassin and Galvin 1998). The second contribution was the categorization of quality defects into three broad categories: underuse, overuse, and misuse. This classification scheme has become a common nosology for quality defects:

- *Underuse* is evidenced by the fact that many scientifically sound practices are not used as often as they should be. For example, biannual mammography screening in women aged 50 to 75 has been proven to be beneficial, yet fewer than 75 percent of women report receiving a mammogram in the past two years (CDC 2012). That is, nearly one in four women does not receive treatment consistent with evidence-based guidelines.
- *Overuse* occurs when treatments and practices are used to a greater extent than evidence deems appropriate. Examples of overuse include imaging studies for diagnosis of acute asymptomatic low-back pain and

the prescription of antibiotics when not indicated (e.g., for viral upper respiratory infections).

- *Misuse* occurs when clinical care processes are not executed properly—for example, when the wrong drug is prescribed or the correct drug is prescribed but incorrectly administered.

Many reports have identified and quantified the gap between current and optimal healthcare practice. Findings range from evidence that specific processes are falling short of the standard (e.g., children are not receiving all their immunizations by age 2) to overall performance gaps (e.g., fivefold variation of risk-adjusted mortality rates in hospitals) (McGlynn et al. 2003).

To Err Is Human: Building a Safer Health System

Although the healthcare community had been cognizant of these many quality challenges for years, the 2000 publication of the IOM report *To Err Is Human* exposed the severity and prevalence of these problems in a way that captured the attention of a large variety of key stakeholders for the first time.

The executive summary of *To Err Is Human* begins with these headlines (Kohn, Corrigan, and Donaldson 2000):

> The knowledgeable health reporter for the *Boston Globe*, Betsy Lehman, died from an overdose during chemotherapy. . . . Ben Kolb was eight years old when he died during "minor" surgery due to a drug mix-up. . . .
>
> [A]t least 44,000 Americans die each year as a result of medical errors. . . . [T]he number may be as high as 98,000. . . .
>
> Total national costs . . . of preventable adverse events . . . are estimated to be between $17 billion and $29 billion, of which health care costs represent over one-half.

These headlines focus on patient safety and medical errors as perhaps the most urgent forms of quality defects. Although many had spoken about improving healthcare in the past, this report focused on the negative in an unprecedented way. It framed the problem in a manner that was accessible to the public and defined the status quo as unacceptable. One of the foundations of this report was the Harvard Medical Practice Study I conducted more than ten years earlier, which revealed that approximately 4 percent of all hospitalized patients experience an in-hospital adverse event and nearly 30 percent of these adverse events occur as a result of negligent care (Brennan et al. 1991). For the first time, patient safety (i.e., ensuring safe care and preventing mistakes) became a unifying cause for policymakers, regulators, providers, and consumers.

Crossing the Quality Chasm: A New Health System for the 21st Century

In March 2001, soon after the release of *To Err Is Human*, IOM released *Crossing the Quality Chasm*, a more comprehensive report that offered a new framework for a redesigned US healthcare system. *Crossing the Quality Chasm* provides a blueprint for the future that classifies and unifies the components of quality through six aims for improvement. These aims, also viewed as six dimensions of quality, provide healthcare professionals and policymakers with simple rules for redesigning healthcare (Berwick 2002):

1. *Safe:* Care should be as safe for patients in healthcare facilities as in their homes.
2. *Effective:* The science and evidence behind healthcare should be applied and serve as standards in the delivery of care.
3. *Efficient:* Care and service should be cost-effective, and waste should be removed from the system.
4. *Timely:* Patients should experience no waits or delays when receiving care and service.
5. *Patient centered:* The system of care should revolve around the patient, respect patient preferences, and put the patient in control.
6. *Equitable:* Unequal treatment should be a fact of the past; disparities in care should be eradicated.

The six aims for improvement can be translated into respective outcome measures and goals. The following points are examples of the types of global measures that can be used to track IOM's six aims:

1. *Safe* care may be measured by overall mortality rates or the percentage of patients experiencing adverse events or harm.
2. *Effective* care may be measured by how well evidenced-based practices are followed, such as the percentage of time that patients with diabetes receive all recommended care at each doctor visit. Effective care may also be measured through indicators of harm, such as the percentage of patients who contract hospital-acquired infections and the percentage of patients who develop pressure ulcers (bed sores) while in a nursing home.
3. *Efficient* care may be measured by analyzing the costs of care by patient, by organization, by provider, or by community.
4. *Timely* care may be measured by wait times to receive needed care, services, and test results.
5. *Patient-centered* care may include measures such as patient or family satisfaction with care and service.

6. *Equitable* care may be assessed by examining differences in quality measures (e.g., measures of effectiveness and safety) by race, gender, income, or other population-based demographic and socioeconomic factors.

The healthcare system comprises four levels, each of which requires change for the healthcare system to achieve the IOM's six aims for improvement. *Level A* is the patient's experience. *Level B* is the microsystem where care is delivered by small provider teams. *Level C* is the organizational level—the macrosystem or aggregation of microsystems and supporting functions. *Level D* is the external environment, which includes payment mechanisms, policy, and regulatory factors. Exhibit 1.1 illustrates these four levels. The environment affects how organizations operate, operations affect the microsystems housed within organizations, and microsystems affect the patient. True North in the model lies at Level A, in the experience of patients, their loved ones, and the communities in which they live (Berwick 2002).

National Healthcare Quality Report

Since 2003, AHRQ has published the *National Healthcare Quality Report*. Mandated by the US Congress to focus on "national trends in the quality of health care provided to the American people" (42 U.S.C. 299b-2(b)(2)), the report highlights progress that has been made toward improving healthcare quality and identifies opportunities for improvement. This report is developed in combination with the *National Healthcare Disparities Report*. Recognizing that alleviating healthcare disparities is integral to achieving quality

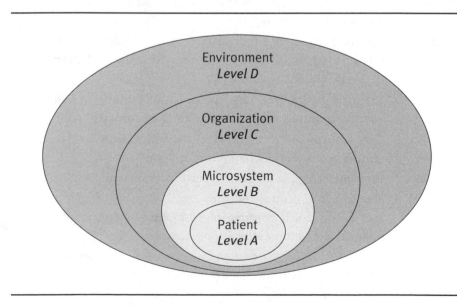

EXHIBIT 1.1
The Four Levels of the Healthcare System

Source: Ferlie and Shortell (2001). Used with permission.

goals, Congress further mandated that this report focus on "prevailing disparities in health care delivery as it relates to racial factors and socioeconomic factors in priority populations" (42 U.S.C. 299a-1(a)(6)). The combined report is fundamental to ensuring that improvement efforts simultaneously advance quality in general and work toward eliminating inequitable gaps in care.

The report uses national quality measures to track the state of healthcare quality and addresses three questions:

1. What is the status of healthcare quality and disparities in the United States?
2. How have healthcare quality and disparities changed over time?
3. Where is the need to improve healthcare quality and reduce disparities greatest?

In 2010, for the first time the report centered on national priorities identified by the US Department of Health and Human Services' National Strategy for Quality Improvement in Health Care. Thus, the report is now organized into nine chapters that are closely aligned with IOM's six dimensions of care. These chapters and examples of national metrics include the following:

Chapter 1. Introduction and Methods

Chapter 2. Effectiveness of Care (e.g., inpatient deaths per 1,000 adult hospital admissions following a heart attack)

Chapter 3. Patient Safety (e.g., rate of hospital-acquired infections per 1,000 central-line days)

Chapter 4. Timeliness (e.g., number of adults who required immediate care in the past 12 months but only sometimes or never received immediate care)

Chapter 5. Patient Centeredness (e.g., percentage of adults and children who reported poor communication at the doctor's office)

Chapter 6. Care Coordination (e.g., percentage of patients who received adequate hospital discharge information)

Chapter 7. Efficiency (e.g., average cost per inpatient stay)

Chapter 8. Health System Infrastructure (e.g., indicators of adoption and use of health information technology; percentage of the population living in a health professional shortage area)

Chapter 9. Access to Health Care (e.g., percentage of the population under age 65 with health insurance)

To further demonstrate alignment, numerous chapters or segments of chapters are aligned with the National Quality Strategy priority areas (see Exhibit 1.2).

Each report also features spotlights on care received by one of AHRQ's priority populations: women, children, persons with disabilities, low-income individuals, and the elderly. Recent reports also include examples and case studies of initiatives and strategies to improve quality and reduce disparities to further accelerate transformation of the delivery system.

National Priorities and Goals: Aligning Our Efforts to Transform America's Healthcare

The National Priorities Partnership (NPP), convened by the National Quality Forum, comprises 28 leading national healthcare organizations and a variety of key stakeholders, including healthcare professionals, patients, payers, community members, suppliers, government entities, and others. In 2008, NPP released its landmark report *National Priorities and Goals* to further underscore the pressing need to develop, implement, and assess change initiatives. The report focuses on national performance improvement efforts that address four major challenges: eliminating harm, eradicating disparities, reducing disease burden, and removing waste. It stresses that bringing together a wide variety of perspectives to create a shared vision is critical to achieving widespread transformation across public and

National Quality Report Chapter	National Quality Strategy Priority Area
Chapter 3: Patient Safety	Making care safer
Chapter 5: Patient Centeredness	Ensuring person- and family-centered care
Chapter 6: Care Coordination	Promoting effective communication and care coordination
Chapter 2: Effectiveness of Care (cardiovascular disease)	Promoting effective prevention and treatment of leading causes of mortality (beginning with cardiovascular disease)
Chapter 2: Effectiveness of Care (lifestyle modification)	Working with communities to promote wide use of best practices to enable healthy living
Chapter 7: Efficiency Chapter 9: Access to Health Care	Making quality care more affordable

EXHIBIT 1.2
National Quality Report Chapter and Corresponding National Quality Strategy Priority Area

private entities. A shared vision is fundamental to successful improvement efforts.

NPP identifies six priority areas:

1. Engaging patients and families in managing their health and making decisions about their care
2. Improving the health of the population
3. Improving the safety and reliability of America's healthcare system
4. Ensuring patients receive well-coordinated care within and across all healthcare organizations, settings, and levels of care
5. Guaranteeing appropriate and compassionate care for patients with life-limiting illness
6. Eliminating overuse while ensuring the delivery of appropriate care

The report further highlights the primary strategies that drive improvement in care: performance measurement, public reporting, payment systems, research and knowledge dissemination, professional development, and system capacity development. Yet the *National Priorities and Goals* report is only a first step toward achieving the shared aim of transforming US healthcare to a well-functioning, high-performing industry. While it provides a multidisciplinary framework for improvement, ongoing assessment and implementation will be essential to accomplishing the outlined goals in communities across the United States.

A Focus on the Patient

All healthcare professionals and organizations exist to serve their patients. Technically, medicine has never had more potential to help patients than it does today. The number of efficacious therapies and life-prolonging pharmaceutical regimens has exploded. Yet the system falls short of its technical potential. Patients are dissatisfied and frustrated with the care they receive, providers are overburdened and uninspired by a system that asks too much and makes their work more difficult, and attempts to reform payment models and implement regulations too often add unwarranted complexity and chaos to the system.

Demands for a fundamental redesign of the US healthcare system are ever increasing. IOM has proposed that a laser-like focus on the patient must sit at the center of efforts to improve and restructure healthcare. Patient-centered care is the proper future of medicine, and the current focus on quality and safety is a step on the path to excellence.

Patients' perception of the quality of our healthcare system is not favorable. In the context of healthcare, *quality* is a household word that evokes great emotion, including the following:

- *Frustration and despair* among patients who experience healthcare services firsthand or family members who observe the care of their loved ones
- *Anxiety* over the ever-increasing costs and complexities of care
- *Tension* between individuals' need for care and the difficulty and inconvenience of obtaining care
- *Alienation* from a care system that seems to have little time for understanding, much less meeting, patients' needs

To illustrate these issues, later in this chapter we examine the insights and experiences of a patient who has lived with chronic back pain for more than 50 years. We use this case study to demonstrate the inadequacies of the current delivery system and highlight the potential for improvement.

Lessons Learned in Quality Improvement

We have noted the chasm in healthcare as it relates to quality. This chasm is wide, and the changes to the system are challenging to implement. But changes are being made, and patient and community health outcomes are improving in many instances. Let us take this opportunity to highlight examples of improvement projects and the progress that has been made.

Improvement Project: Reducing Surgery-Related Mortality and Complications

One improvement project success story comes from the University of Washington Medical Center. The project was part of a larger patient safety effort that has spread both across Washington State and to numerous countries around the world. The University of Washington Medical Center, a 450-bed academic medical center in Seattle, is part of the greater University of Washington Health System. Approximately 7,200 inpatient surgeries and 8,000 outpatient surgeries are performed annually in the facility's 24 operating rooms.

Leaders at the hospital and in the division of general surgery are highly engaged in quality improvement initiatives. In 2005, high variation in surgical quality across and within institutions prompted an investigation of innovative strategies to reduce mortality and prevent complications that arise from a high degree of variability in care. They also found that a dearth of data on surgery and outcomes hindered improvement efforts.

Dr. E. Patchen Dellinger, chief of the division of general surgery, began participating in the World Health Organization's (WHO) Safe Surgery Saves Lives campaign—an international initiative to develop and implement a surgical safety checklist—in 2005 after attending a presentation by Johns Hopkins Hospital clinicians. The clinicians had described the potential for improvements in surgical outcomes from developing and using standard-ized surgical team briefings and debriefings before and after each surgical procedure.

The WHO Surgical Safety Checklist includes three primary time frames: (1) before induction of anesthesia, (2) before skin incision, and (3) before the patient's departure from the operating room (see Exhibit 1.3). Dr. Dellinger led the implementation of the checklist at the University of Washington.

After the development of the initial checklist, the University of Washington Medical Center served as one of the eight WHO Surgical Safety Checklist international pilot sites. The checklist includes four major steps:

1. Team member introductions and initial discussion
2. Confirmation of patient identity, procedure, and surgical site
3. Pre-incision and role-specific review of necessary preparations
4. Debriefing after the surgical procedure

While Dr. Dellinger and the project implementation team initially encountered resistance to the checklist from physicians and nurses, most clinicians were highly supportive of the checklist after implementation. One general surgeon stated, "At first the checklist seemed somewhat burdensome due to its length. It now takes me about one minute to run through the list, which I don't think is at all excessive." A nurse reflected, "I was probably one of the most negative nurses at the start of this project because I thought it was just one more piece of paper to fill out. But now I find it very helpful, especially if the surgeon takes the lead and actively requests the participation of everyone in the room."

Qualitative surveys found that nine in ten respondents "indicated that they would want the checklist-guided process used if they were undergoing surgery" and that "surgeons, anesthesiology teams, and surgical nurses believe the program improved team communication and coordination, their impressions of patient safety, and their comfort level in reporting safety concerns to colleagues."

Dr. Dellinger, who donated his time to the program's development, spearheaded numerous strategies that largely influenced the program's success at the medical center, including the following:

EXHIBIT 1.3
WHO Surgical
Safety Checklist

Surgical Safety Checklist

World Health Organization | Patient Safety
A World Alliance for Safer Health Care

Before induction of anaesthesia

(with at least nurse and anaesthetist)

Has the patient confirmed his/her identity, site, procedure, and consent?
☐ Yes

Is the site marked?
☐ Yes
☐ Not applicable

Is the anaesthesia machine and medication check complete?
☐ Yes

Is the pulse oximeter on the patient and functioning?
☐ Yes

Does the patient have a:

Known allergy?
☐ No
☐ Yes

Difficult airway or aspiration risk?
☐ No
☐ Yes, and equipment/assistance available

Risk of >500ml blood loss (7ml/kg in children)?
☐ No
☐ Yes, and two IVs/central access and fluids planned

Before skin incision

(with nurse, anaesthetist and surgeon)

Confirm all team members have introduced themselves by name and role.

Confirm the patient's name, procedure, and where the incision will be made.

Has antibiotic prophylaxis been given within the last 60 minutes?
☐ Yes
☐ Not applicable

Anticipated Critical Events

To Surgeon:
☐ What are the critical or non-routine steps?
☐ How long will the case take?
☐ What is the anticipated blood loss?

To Anaesthetist:
☐ Are there any patient-specific concerns?

To Nursing Team:
☐ Has sterility (including indicator results) been confirmed?
☐ Are there equipment issues or any concerns?

Is essential imaging displayed?
☐ Yes
☐ Not applicable

Before patient leaves operating room

(with nurse, anaesthetist and surgeon)

Nurse Verbally Confirms:
☐ The name of the procedure
☐ Completion of instrument, sponge and needle counts
☐ Specimen labelling (read specimen labels aloud, including patient name)
☐ Whether there are any equipment problems to be addressed

To Surgeon, Anaesthetist and Nurse:
☐ What are the key concerns for recovery and management of this patient?

This checklist is not intended to be comprehensive. Additions and modifications to fit local practice are encouraged.

Revised 1 / 2009   © WHO, 2009

Source: WHO (2009). Used with permission.

- Securing leadership support
- Obtaining clinician buy-in
- Recruiting surgeon and nurse champions
- Engaging all relevant clinicians, including surgeons, nurses, and anesthesiologists, in process development
- Creating and displaying checklist posters in all operating rooms
- Pilot testing the project and then spreading it across the hospital
- Incorporating new processes into the current workflow
- Amending the checklist as necessary for specific surgical cases

Results from the project indicated that the surgical checklist decreased length of stay, reduced surgery-related mortality, reduced surgical-site infections and unplanned operations, and improved adherence to evidence-based care steps. Among colectomy patients, improvements included the following:

- The percentage of colectomy patients requiring a reoperation decreased from 7.8 percent to 3.4 percent.
- The percentage of colectomy patients requiring postoperative antibiotics or wound opening decreased from 22 percent to 9 percent.
- Use of deep vein thrombosis prophylaxis, a nationally recommended treatment, increased from nearly 50 percent to 80 percent among all patients.
- Use of anastomosis testing, also a recommended treatment, increased from 11 percent to 94 percent among eligible patients.

As a result of the success at the University of Washington Medical Center, the checklist was expanded to more than 50 hospitals in the state of Washington in 2008 through the Surgical Care and Outcomes Assessment Program (SCOAP). SCOAP is a voluntary hospital collaborative that aims to reduce variability and improve quality and outcomes in surgical care across the state. SCOAP enhanced the checklist by adding items that were inconsistently applied across its member hospitals and enlisted the aid of the Washington State Hospital Association and other third parties to promote checklist adoption. The latest version of the checklist is featured in Exhibit 1.4.

Other hospitals that adopted the checklist experienced results similar to those of the University of Washington Medical Center, such as a decline in length of stay from 8.5 days to 7.5 days for colon resections and 3 days to 2 days for gastric bypass surgery and a reduction in the percentage of colorectal surgery patients requiring a second surgery from 7 percent to less than 4 percent. Results from the WHO Surgical Safety Checklist pilot, a program that was implemented in sites around the world, suggest similar improvements,

EXHIBIT 1.4
SCOAP
Surgical Safety
Checklist,
Version 3.4

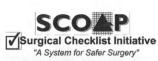

SCO▲P
☑ Surgical Checklist Initiative
"A System for Safer Surgery"

Version 3.4

Step 1: Operative Preparation (Nursing and Anesthesia)

With Patient Confirm: ❑ Identity ❑ Site and site marked (or N/A) ❑ Procedure ❑ Consent ❑ Allergies
Anesthesia Confirms: ❑ Anesthesia Machine Ready
                           ❑ Patient Position
                           ❑ Airway/aspiration risk assessment completed
                              ❑ If increased risk, needed equipment available, plan described
For Clean-Contaminated Cases ❑ Confirm that skin prep is with chlorhexidine unless contraindicated

Step 2: Briefing—Prior to Skin Incision (All Team Members)

❑ Team members introduce themselves by name and role
❑ Surgeon, Anesthesia, Nursing/Surgical Tech Team: Confirm Patient (at least 2 identifiers), Site, Procedure
❑ Personnel exchanges discussed (timing of and plan for announcing exchanges)

Anesthesia Team Reviews

❑ Concerns (airway, special meds [beta blockers], relevant allergies, conditions affecting recovery, etc)

Surgeon Reviews

❑ Brief description of procedure and anticipated difficulties
❑ Expected duration of procedure
❑ Expected blood loss
❑ Need for instruments/supplies/IV access beyond those normally used for the procedure

Nursing/Surgical Tech Team Reviews

❑ Equipment issues (e.g., instruments ready and trained on, requested implants available, gas tanks full)
❑ Sharps management plan reviewed
❑ Other patient concerns

Step 3: Process Control—Prior to Skin Incision (Surgeon Leads)

❑ Essential imaging displayed, right and left confirmed   ❑ N/A
❑ Antibiotic prophylaxis given in last 60 minutes   ❑ N/A
❑ Active warming in place   ❑ N/A

Case expected to be less than 1 hour?

❑ Yes (proceed with operation)

❑ No (follow arrow to right)

➡

CASE EXPECTED TO BE ≥ 1 HOUR:

❑ Glucose checked for diabetics
  ❑ Insulin protocol initiated if needed
❑ DVT/PE chemoprophylaxis plan in place
❑ If patient on beta blocker, post-op plan formulated
❑ Re-dosing plan for antibiotics
❑ Specialty-specific checklist

Step 4: Debriefing—At Completion of Case (All Team Members)

❑ (Surgeon and Nursing) Before closure: Are instrument, sponge, and needle counts correct?
❑ (Surgeon and Nursing) If specimen, confirm label & instructions (e.g., orientation,12-lymph nodes for colon CA)
❑ (All) Confirm name of procedure
❑ (All) Equipment issues to be addressed?   ❑ No ❑ Yes, and response plan formulated (Who/When)
❑ (All) What could have been better? ❑ Nothing ❑ Something, with plan to address (Who/When)
❑ (Surgeon and Anesthesia) Key concerns for recovery (e.g., plan for pain management, nausea/vomiting)

✦ Adapted from the WHO "Safe Surgery Saves Lives" campaign ✦
SCOAP is a program of the Foundation for Health Care Quality
www.scoapchecklist.org   rev 2/11/2010

Source: SCOAP (2010). Used with permission.

such as a decrease in surgery-related mortality rate from 1.5 percent to 0.8 percent among the eight international pilot sites (see Exhibit 1.5).

Furthermore, the WHO pilot sites realized stark reductions in surgery-related complication rates, from 11 percent to 7 percent (see Exhibit 1.6).

EXHIBIT 1.5

Changes in
Mortality Rate
Before and After
Implementation
of the WHO
Surgical Safety
Checklist at
Eight Pilot
Sites*

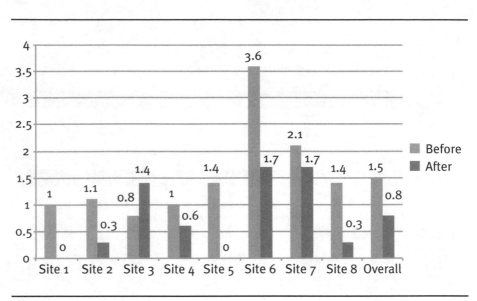

*Percentage of all eligible surgical patients.
Source: Data from Haynes et al. (2009).

Surgical-site infection dropped from 6.2 percent to 3.4 percent (see Exhibit 1.7). Finally, unplanned reoperations fell from 2.4 percent to 1.8 percent among surgical patients (see Exhibit 1.8).

One of the key lessons learned from the WHO and SCOAP efforts is that continuous emphasis on patient safety is critical. To those who were hesitant about the project, Dr. Dellinger posed the following question: "How

EXHIBIT 1.6

Changes in
Surgery-Related
Complication
Rates Before
and After
Implementation
of the WHO
Surgical Safety
Checklist at
Eight Pilot
Sites*

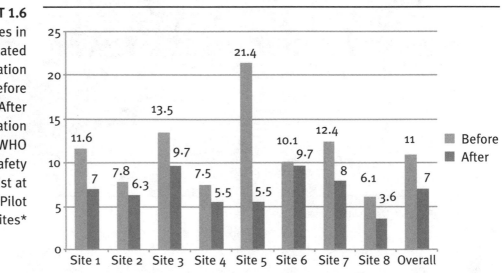

*Percentage of all eligible surgical patients.
Source: Data from Haynes et al. (2009).

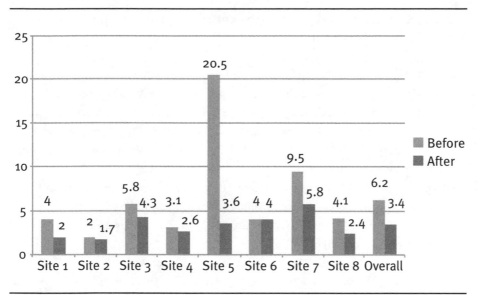

EXHIBIT 1.7

Changes in Surgical-Site Infection Rate Before and After Implementation of the WHO Surgical Safety Checklist at Eight Pilot Sites*

*Percentage of all eligible surgical patients.
Source: Data from Haynes et al. (2009).

many of you sitting here would be willing to board an airplane knowing that the pilot was not going to go through his checklist before takeoff?" There were no volunteers. He then asked, "How many of you think that having an operation is safer than flying in an airplane?" Dr. Dellinger quickly gained the support of those who initially resisted, and the program continues to

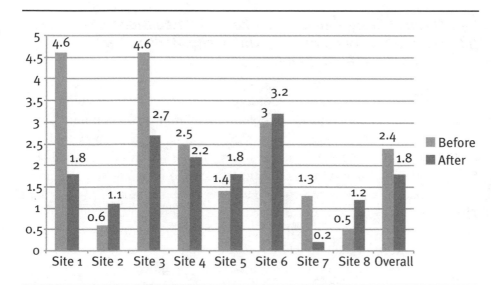

EXHIBIT 1.8

Changes in Unplanned Returns to the Operating Room Before and After Implementation of the WHO Surgical Safety Checklist at Eight Pilot Sites*

*Percentage of all eligible surgical patients.
Source: Data from Haynes et al. (2009).

serve as a landmark quality improvement success story at the University of Washington Medical Center.

Sources

AHRQ Health Care Innovations Exchange. 2010. "Checklist-Guided Process Reduces Surgery-Related Mortality and Complications." Agency for Healthcare Research and Quality, US Department of Health & Human Services. Published June 9; updated August 29, 2012. www.innovations.ahrq.gov/content.aspx?id=2748.

Dellinger, E. P. 2009. "Washington Patient Safety Coalition & Surgical Public Health: Surgical Quality in Washington State, Surgical Safety, and the Introduction of the WHO/SCOAP Surgical Checklist." www.wapatientsafety.org/downloads/Dellinger.pdf.

Haynes, A. B., T. G. Weiser, W. R. Berry, S. R. Lipsitz, A. H. Breizat, E. P. Dellinger, T. Herbosa, S. Joseph, P. L. Kibatala, M. C. Lapitan, A. F. Merry, K. Moorthy, R. K. Reznick, B. Taylor, A. A. Gawande; Safe Surgery Saves Lives Study Group. 2009. "A Surgical Safety Checklist to Reduce Morbidity and Mortality in a Global Population." *New England Journal of Medicine* 360 (5): 491–99.

Surgical Care and Outcomes Assessment Program (SCOAP). 2010. "SCOAP Surgical Checklist Initiative, Version 3.4." Foundation for Health Care Quality. Revised February 11. www.scoap.org/downloads/SCOAP-Surgical-Checklist_v3_4.pdf.

World Health Organization (WHO). 2009. *Surgical Safety Checklist.* http://whqlibdoc.who.int/publications/2009/9789241598590_eng_Checklist.pdf.

Improvement Story: Stopping Catheter-Related Blood Stream Line Infections at the Johns Hopkins University Medical Center and Hospitals Across the United States

A second improvement story derives from growing evidence that medical errors result in part from the lack of a patient safety culture—a culture that encourages detection of quality problems—and from poor communication and teamwork in addressing quality problems. In response to these findings, in 2001 a team of researchers at the Johns Hopkins University Quality and Safety Research Group developed an innovative, comprehensive program to improve patient safety at the Johns Hopkins Hospital. The Johns Hopkins Hospital, a 1,015-bed tertiary care facility, treats more than 268,000 patients annually from across the United States and around the world.

The efforts of the Johns Hopkins team led to the creation of the Comprehensive Unit-based Safety Program (CUSP), designed to

- be implemented sequentially in work units,

- improve the culture of safety,
- enable staff to focus safety efforts on unit-specific problems, and
- include rigorous data collection through which tangible improvements in patient safety are empirically derived to educate and improve awareness about eliminating central line–associated bloodstream infections (CLABSI).

CUSP is a continuous measurement, feedback, and improvement program. It engages frontline staff and uses a combination of tools and compliance reports to achieve improvement goals. Implementation of CUSP consists of five major steps:

1. Train staff in the science of safety (e.g., basic strategies for safe design, including standardized processes and independent checklists for key processes).
2. Engage staff in identifying defects (e.g., ask staff how the next patient could be harmed on their unit).
3. Perform senior executive partnership/safety rounds (i.e., hospital executives interact and discuss safety issues with staff on hospital units).
4. Continue to learn from defects by answering four questions:
   a. What happened?
   b. Why did it happen?
   c. What was done to reduce risk?
   d. How do we know that risk was actually reduced?
5. Implement tools for improvement (e.g., morning briefs, daily goals checklists, operating room debriefings).

A detailed flowchart of CUSP is provided in Exhibit 1.9.

The program was first piloted in two Johns Hopkins Hospital surgical intensive care units (ICUs). Errors are more common in ICUs because of the severity of patients' conditions. Furthermore, significant adverse outcomes may occur in the event of errors among this high-risk patient population.

To implement the program, at least one physician and one nurse from each unit are required to participate. These individuals should be able to dedicate four to eight hours per week to implement CUSP and serve on the improvement team. Program expenses are the costs associated with CUSP team members' time.

Upon initial investigation of the work, researchers uncovered stark findings:

EXHIBIT 1.9
Comprehensive
Unit-Based
Safety
Program (CUSP)
Flowchart

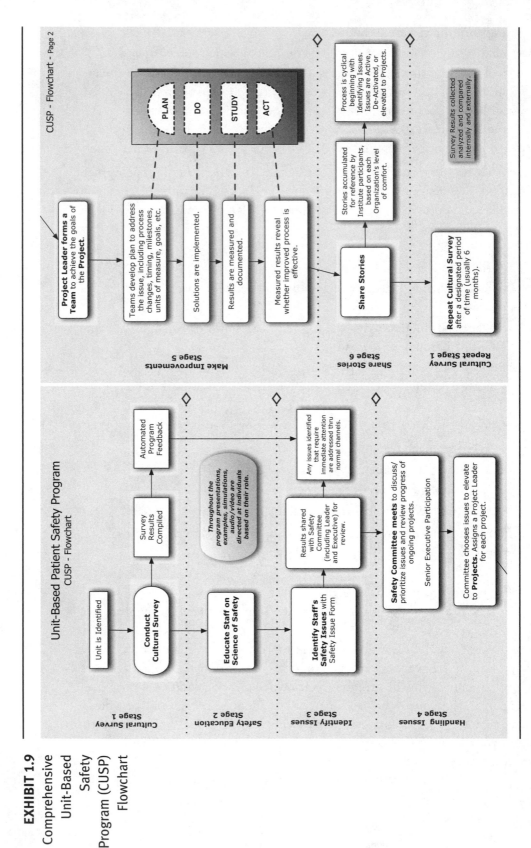

Source: Published with permission of Johns Hopkins HealthCare LLC.

- *Length of stay (LOS):* LOS decreased from 2 days to 1 day in one unit and from 3 days to 2.3 days in the other unit.
- *Medication errors:* The medication error rate dropped from 94 percent to 0 percent in one unit and from 40 percent to 0 percent in the other unit.
- *Nursing turnover:* The nurse turnover rate decreased from 9 percent to 2 percent in one unit and from 8 percent to 2 percent in the other unit.
- *Safety culture:* The percentage of staff who self-reported a positive safety climate increased from 35 percent to 52 percent in one unit and from 35 percent to 68 percent in the other unit.

Due to the considerable success of the pilot program, CUSP was implemented in approximately 170 clinical areas across the Johns Hopkins Hospital. Subsequently, CUSP was implemented at hospitals across the state of Michigan in collaboration with the Michigan Health and Hospital Association's Center for Patient Safety and Quality.

A total of 108 ICUs initially participated in the Michigan program. The program brought about dramatic decreases in CLABSI rates in Michigan hospitals, from a mean of 2.7 infections per 1,000 catheter days to 0 infections per 1,000 catheter days 18 months after implementation.

The success of the program did not go unnoticed. AHRQ awarded the Health Research & Educational Trust (HRET), a nonprofit research and educational affiliate of the American Hospital Association, an $18 million contract to spread CUSP to hospitals across the United States to reduce CLABSI. The new program—On the CUSP: Stop BSI—was implemented in 44 states as well as throughout Spain and England. More than 1,000 hospitals and 1,800 hospital units across the 44 states, the District of Columbia, and Puerto Rico have collectively reduced the national CLABSI rate from a baseline of 1.915 infections per 1,000 line days to 1.133 infections, a relative reduction of 41 percent (see Exhibit 1.10).

The percentage of participating units with a 0 percent CLABSI rate also increased drastically, from 30 percent to 68 percent of all units (see Exhibit 1.11). Additionally, the percentage of units reporting a CLABSI rate of less than one per 1,000 line days increased over time from 45 percent to 71 percent.

Building on the success of the On the CUSP: Stop BSI program, HRET also led the implementation of a neonatal CLABSI prevention program in partnership with the Perinatal Quality Collaborative of North Carolina (PQCNC). This effort resulted in a decrease in CLABSI rates from 2.043 at baseline in August 2011 to 0.855 in August 2012, a 58 percent relative reduction.

EXHIBIT 1.10

Average
CLABSI Rates
(infections per
1,000 catheter
days) per Unit

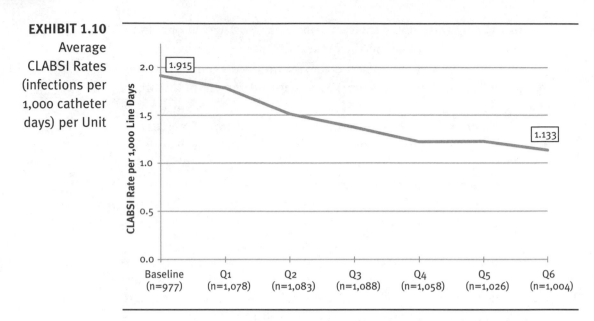

Source: AHRQ (2013). Used with permission.

In addition to the expansion of the CUSP program to reduce CLABSI in numerous care settings, the CUSP toolkit is now being applied to address other hospital-acquired infections, most notably catheter-associated urinary tract infections (CAUTI). HRET is working with numerous partners on the On the CUSP: Stop CAUTI project to reduce CAUTI rates by 25 percent over 18 months.

EXHIBIT 1.11

Percentage of
Reporting Units
with CLABSI
Rate of 0/1,000
or Less than
1/1,000 Central
Line Days

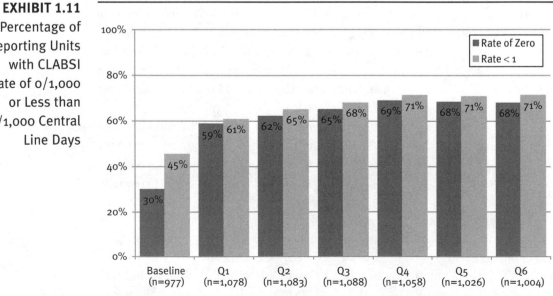

Source: AHRQ (2013). Used with permission.

The path to improvement has not been simple; it has required collaboration between many multidisciplinary stakeholders. The perseverance of clinical leaders and organizations across the United States continue to make the On the CUSP: Stop BSI program and its many successive iterations a notable success.

Sources

Agency for Healthcare Research and Quality (AHRQ). 2013. *Eliminating CLABSI, A National Patient Safety Imperative: Final Report: Final Report on the National* On the CUSP: Stop BSI *Project*. Published in January. www.ahrq.gov/professionals/quality-patient-safety/cusp/clabsi-final/index.html.

AHRQ Health Care Innovations Exchange. 2008. "Unit-Based Safety Program Improves Safety Culture, Reduces Medication Errors and Length of Stay." Agency for Healthcare Research and Quality, US Department of Health & Human Services. Published November 24. www.innovations.ahrq.gov/content.aspx?id=1769.

Health Research & Educational Trust, Johns Hopkins University Quality and Safety Research Group, and Michigan Health & Hospital Association Keystone Center for Patient Safety & Quality. 2011. *Eliminating CLABSI: A National Patient Safety Imperative. Second Progress Report on the National On the CUSP: Stop BSI Project*. AHRQ Publication No: 11-0037-1-EF. Published in September. www.ahrq.gov/professionals/quality-patient-safety/cusp/clabsi-update/clabsi-update.pdf.

Johns Hopkins Center for Innovation in Quality Patient Care. 2013. "The Comprehensive Unit-Based Safety Program (CUSP)." www.hopkinsmedicine.org/innovation_quality_patient_care/areas_expertise/improve_patient_safety/cusp/.

Patient Safety Group. 2013. "Introduction—eCUSP." www.patientsafetygroup.org/program/index.cfm.

Pronovost, P., D. Needham, S. Berenholtz, D. Sinopoli, H. Chu, S. Cosgrove, B. Sexton, R. Hyzy, R. Welsh, G. Roth, J. Bander, J. Kepros, and C. Goeschel. 2006. "An Intervention to Decrease Catheter-Related Bloodstream Infections in the ICU." *New England Journal of Medicine* 355 (26): 2725–32.

Case Study: Mr. Roberts and the US Healthcare System[1]

Mr. Roberts is a 77-year-old gentleman who is retired and living in Florida with his wife. A child of the Depression, he grew up to become an accomplished, affluent person. At age 13, he began working as a longshoreman and barracks builder. He started to experience back pain in his early 20s. At that time, he did not receive particularly good medical advice and did not pursue alternative therapies. World War II, 25 years in Asia, and life as a busy executive took priority, and the pain became a constant but secondary companion.

At age 50, the pain became unbearable. He returned to New York and spent the better part of a year "on his back." In 1980 he underwent the first of four major spine surgeries. Since then, he has had multiple intervertebral discs partially or completely removed. Despite these operations, his pain has been worsening over the past two to three years and his functional status has been decreasing.

It is hard to live with pain, and Mr. Roberts is not sure he deals with it very well. He does not want to take narcotics because they interfere with his ability to stay sharp and active, and his stomach problems prohibit the use of many non-narcotic medications. Most of the time he experiences only mild or temporary relief of his pain.

Despite the pain, Mr. Roberts is active and gets out as much as he can. Although it has become more difficult, he still takes his wife dancing on Saturday nights. The pain is exhausting and limits his ability to do what he wants. The worst part about the pain is that it is changing—worsening—and he is uncertain of its future trajectory. As the pain increases, how will he survive? What are the possibilities that he will remain active and independent?

Mr. Roberts states that he has had "reasonably good" doctors. He feels he is privileged because he has connections and advocates for himself. These assets have enabled him to expand his healthcare options and seek the best providers and institutions. He is also well informed and assertive and has been an active participant in his healthcare. Although his overall experience in the healthcare system has been favorable, many instances of care have been less than ideal.

Communication Deficits and Lack of a Team Approach

Mr. Roberts has observed that the lack of communication between providers is a huge problem. He has multiple specialists who care for different parts of his body; however, no one person is mindful of how these systems interact to create the whole person or illness. He is never sure whether one physician knows what the other is doing or how one physician's prescriptions might interfere or interact with another's. The physicians never seem inclined to "dig deeply" or communicate as team members treating one person. On many occasions, physicians have recommended therapies that have already been tried and failed. On other occasions, they disagree on an approach to his problem and leave Mr. Roberts to decide which advice to follow. No system is in place to encourage teamwork. "Unless the physician is extremely intelligent, on the ball, or energetic, it just doesn't happen," he says.

Seldom do physicians listen to his full story or elicit his thoughts before jumping to conclusions. Mr. Roberts suggests that physicians should carefully analyze their therapeutic personalities. They cannot assume that all patients are alike or that they will react similarly to a given intervention. Each patient needs to be treated as an individual, and service needs to be respectful of individual choice.

Record keeping and transfer of information are also faulty. Despite the fact that physicians take copious notes, the information is not put to use. Mr. Roberts has expended a great deal of time and energy ensuring that his medical records are sent to a new consultant's office, only to find within a few minutes of the encounter that the consultant has not reviewed the chart or absorbed the information. This realization has affected how he uses care. For instance, at one point Mr. Roberts's stomach problems were worsening. His gastroenterologist was away on vacation for four weeks, and there was no covering physician. The thought of amassing his patient records for transfer to another physician (who likely would not review them and would suggest the same tests and therapies) was so unpleasant that he chose to go without care.

Removing the Question Mark from Patient–Provider Interactions

Mr. Roberts is particularly concerned with patients' inability to know the true qualifications of their physicians or judge their prescriptions. At one point, he was experiencing severe arm and finger pain. Assuming these symptoms were related to his spine, he sought the advice of a highly recommended chief of neurosurgery at a premier academic center. After eliciting a brief history and performing a short examination, the chief admitted him to the hospital.

The following day, an anesthesiologist came into the room to obtain his consent for surgery. Mr. Roberts had not been told that surgery was under consideration. He asked to speak to the neurosurgeon and insisted on additional consultations. Three days later, a hand surgeon reassured him that his problem was likely self-limiting tendonitis and prescribed conservative therapy. Within a few weeks, his pain had resolved. Mr. Roberts was grateful that he had followed his instinct but was concerned for other patients who might not have asserted themselves in this manner.

Mismatch Between Supply and Demand

Mr. Roberts also stated that there is a profound disconnect between supply and demand in the healthcare system. In 1992 his pain had become particularly disabling, and his mobility was extremely restricted. His physicians suggested that he see the only neurosurgeon in the county. Despite his health emergency, he was not able to make an appointment to see this neurosurgeon for more than ten weeks. No other solutions were offered. In pain and unable to walk because of progressively worsening foot drop and muscle weakness, he sought the help of a physician friend.

This friend referred him to a "brash, iconoclastic" Harvard-trained neurologist, who in turn referred him to a virtuoso neurosurgeon at a county hospital 100 miles away. After only 20 minutes with this neurosurgeon, he was rushed to the operating room and underwent a nine-hour emergency procedure. Apparently, he had severe spinal cord impingement and swelling. The neurosurgeon later told him that he would have been a paraplegic or died had he not undergone surgery that day.

He subsequently had a series of three more spinal operations. Postoperative care was suboptimal; he had to travel 100 miles to see the surgeon for follow-up. Eventually, this surgeon chose to travel to a more centralized location twice per month to accommodate his patients in outlying areas.

Mr. Roberts states that we need to "overcome petty bureaucracies" that do not allow matching of supply with demand. The ready availability of quality care should be patient driven and closely monitored by a third party that does not have a vested interest in the market.

Knowledge-Based Care

Mr. Roberts is concerned about the status of continuing medical education. He guesses that it is probably easy for physicians in large, urban teaching hospitals to keep abreast of the latest diagnostic and therapeutic advances. However, the majority of physicians may not have similar opportunities. The system does not necessarily encourage physicians to keep up to date. This lack of current, in-depth knowledge is particularly important as issues of supply and demand force consumers to seek care in "instant med clinics." For example, Mr. Roberts believes emergency care to be an oxymoron. On many occasions, he has gone to the emergency department and has had to wait four to five hours before being treated. This experience is unpleasant and forces people to seek alternative facilities that may not provide the best care for complex, chronically ill patients.

Mr. Roberts also feels that we need to learn from our errors as well as from our successes. We should require that groups of physicians regularly review cases and learn how to deliver care in a better way. This analysis needs to occur internally within institutions as well as externally across institutions. Ideally, the analysis would directly involve patients and families to gain their perspectives. In addition, the learning should be contextual; we should not only learn how to do better the next time but also know whether what we are doing makes sense within our overall economic, epidemiological, and societal context.

Mr. Roberts believes that quality healthcare is knowledge based. This knowledge comes not only from science but also from analysis of mistakes that occur in the process of delivering care. Patients should be involved in the collection and synthesis of these data. The transfer of knowledge among patients, scientists, and practitioners must be emphasized and simplified.

Nonphysician/Nonhospital Care

Mr. Roberts has been impressed with the quality of the care he has received from nonphysician clinicians, and he believes the growth of alternative healthcare provider models has been a definite advance in the system. As an example, Mr. Roberts cites the effectiveness of his physical therapists as healthcare providers; they are alert, patient conscious, conscientious, and respectful. Mr. Roberts believes that their interventions "guide people to better life," and his functional status has improved as a result of their assistance. In addition, these providers are careful to maintain close communication with physicians. They function as members of a team.

Postoperative care also has improved. At the time of his first surgery more than two decades ago, Mr. Roberts spent two weeks in the hospital. Now, after three days he is discharged to a rehabilitation facility that is better equipped to help him recuperate and regain full function.

Mr. Roberts knows how crucial his family and friends are to his medical care. Without their support, recommendations, constant questioning, and advocacy, his condition would be more precarious. The system needs to acknowledge patients' other caregivers and involve them in shared decision making and knowledge transfer.

Conclusion

The previous sections provide brief insight into some successful improvement projects. We could also find many examples of failed improvement projects and the lessons learned from them. Although the gaps between current practice and best practice can be daunting, improvement is occurring, albeit in pockets. We must continue to make quality a necessity, not just a nicety, in healthcare. Pervasive quality challenges played a critical role in the passage of recent healthcare reform legislation, which is encouraging the transformation of healthcare from a quantity-driven industry to a value-driven industry.

Improvement does not develop from viewing healthcare through one lens; disparate silos must be bridged to provide high-quality care. As depicted by the improvement projects featured in this chapter, widespread quality improvement necessitates the sharing of successful efforts among institutions, and national leadership must work to spread and appropriately adapt these strategies to institutions across the United States.

The aim of this textbook is to provide a comprehensive overview of the critical components of the healthcare quality landscape. Numerous case studies highlight the complex interactions between multiple systems and stakeholders that are necessary for success in quality improvement efforts. We will need to improve these systems at every level—from the patient to the external environment—to truly transform healthcare. You, as readers and leaders, should use this text as a resource and framework for understanding the connectivity of multiple aspects of healthcare quality from the bases of science, patient perspective, organizational implications, and environmental effects. This chapter sets the stage by highlighting the following:

- The current state of healthcare quality
- The importance of the patient in goals and results
- Promising evidence of the great capacity for significant improvement in systems of care
- Examples of breakthrough improvements
- A call to action for all healthcare stakeholders to continue to rethink and redesign our systems to achieve better health for all

Study Questions

1. Identify five ways in which patients can gain more control over their care.
2. Think of an experience you, a family member, or a friend has had with healthcare. Gauge the experience against IOM's six aims, and identify any opportunities for improvement.
3. You are the CEO of a hospital, and the local newspaper has just run a story on "how bad healthcare is." How do you respond to the reporter asking you to comment on the situation? How do you respond to your employees?

Note

1. This patient story was edited by Matthew Fitzgerald, center director, Center for Health Data Analysis at Social & Scientific Systems, and was originally composed by Heidi Louise Behforouz, MD, assistant professor of medicine, Harvard Medical School; associate physician in the Division of Global Health Equity at Brigham and Women's Hospital; and medical and executive director of the Prevention and Access to Care and Treatment Project.

References

Berwick, D. M. 2002. "A User's Manual for the IOM's 'Quality Chasm' Report." *Health Affairs (Millwood)* 21 (3): 80–90.

Brennan, T. A., L. L. Leape, N. M. Laird, L. Hebert, A. R. Localio, A. G. Lawthers, J. P. Newhouse, P. C. Weiler, and H. H. Hiatt. 1991. "Incidence of Adverse Events and Negligence in Hospitalized Patients—Results of the Harvard Medical Practice Study I." *New England Journal of Medicine* 324 (6): 370–76.

Centers for Disease Control and Prevention (CDC). 2012. "Cancer Screening—United States, 2010." *Morbidity and Mortality Weekly Report* 61 (3): 41–45.

Chassin, M. R., and R. H. Galvin. 1998. "The Urgent Need to Improve Health Care Quality. Institute of Medicine National Roundtable on Health Care Quality." *Journal of the American Medical Association* 280 (11): 1000–1005.

Donabedian, A. 2001. "A Founder of Quality Assessment Encounters a Troubled System Firsthand." Interview by Fitzhugh Mullan. *Health Affairs (Millwood)* 20 (1): 137–41.

———. 1980. *The Definition of Quality and Approaches to Its Assessment, Volume I: Explorations in Quality Assessment and Monitoring.* Chicago: Health Administration Press.

Ferlie, E., and S. M. Shortell. 2001. "Improving the Quality of Healthcare in the United Kingdom and the United States: A Framework for Change." *Milbank Quarterly* 79 (2): 281–316.

Institute of Medicine (IOM). 2001. *Crossing the Quality Chasm: A New Health System for the 21st Century.* Washington, DC: National Academies Press.

Kohn, L. T., J. M. Corrigan, and M. S. Donaldson (eds.). 2000. *To Err Is Human: Building a Safer Health System.* Washington, DC: National Academies Press.

Lohr, K. N. (ed.). 1990. *Medicare: A Strategy for Quality Assurance, Volume I.* Washington, DC: National Academies Press.

McGlynn, E. A., S. M. Asch, J. Adams, J. Keesey, J. Hicks, A. DeCristofaro, and E. A. Kerr. 2003. "The Quality of Health Care Delivered to Adults in the United States." *New England Journal of Medicine* 348 (26): 2635–45.

National Priorities Partnership (NPP). 2008. *National Priorities and Goals: Aligning Our Efforts to Transform America's Healthcare.* Washington, DC: National Quality Forum.

BASIC CONCEPTS OF HEALTHCARE QUALITY

Leon Wyszewianski

People perceive the quality of healthcare services in different ways. Consider these two cases:

1. In one rural community, Medicare served notice that it would stop doing business with several of the area's physicians. According to Medicare officials, the physicians had a pattern of providing unnecessary and even harmful care to Medicare patients, such as prescribing medications more likely to harm rather than help patients with a heart condition. The residents of the community were stunned. The physicians were highly respected and well loved by their patients and had practiced in the community for 20 to 40 years. Their willingness to travel to remote locations without regard to time of day or weather was legendary, as was their generosity toward patients who had fallen on hard times and were unable to pay their medical bills.
2. An expert panel of trauma care specialists surveyed and rated hospital emergency departments in a major metropolitan area. The results surprised many of the area's residents. The emergency department rated number one by the panel was known mostly for its crowded conditions, long waits, and harried and often brusque staff.

Several concepts can help one make sense of these and similar apparent contradictions and inconsistencies. This chapter focuses on the ways in which the definition and measurement of quality and the relationship between quality and cost shape people's perceptions of care and contribute to these differences.

Definition-Related Concepts

A number of attributes can characterize the quality of healthcare services (Campbell, Roland, and Buetow 2000; Donabedian 2003). Different groups involved in healthcare, such as physicians, patients, and health insurers, attach different levels of importance to particular attributes and define *quality of care* differently as a result (Bodenheimer and Grumbach 2009; Harteloh 2004). Exhibit 2.1 captures these stereotypical differences.

The Definitional Attributes

Attributes relevant to the definition of quality of care include

- technical performance,
- patient centeredness,
- amenities,
- access,
- equity,
- efficiency, and
- cost-effectiveness.

Technical Performance

Quality of *technical performance* refers to the degree to which current scientific medical knowledge and technology are applied in a given situation. Assessments of technical performance typically focus on the timeliness and accuracy of diagnoses, the appropriateness of therapies, the skill with which procedures and other medical interventions are performed, and the absence of accidental injuries (Donabedian 1988a, 1980). These criteria correspond to three of the six key "aims for improvement" identified in the Institute of Medicine's pathbreaking report *Crossing the Quality Chasm*: safety, effectiveness, and timeliness (IOM 2001).

Patient Centeredness

The concept of *patient centeredness*, originally formulated by Gerteis and colleagues (1993), is characterized in *Crossing the Quality Chasm* as encompassing "qualities of compassion, empathy, and responsiveness to the needs, values, and expressed preferences of the individual patient" and rooted in the idea that "health care should cure when possible, but always help to relieve suffering" (IOM 2001). The report states that the goal of patient centeredness is "to modify the care to respond to the person, not the person to the care" (IOM 2001).

Patient centeredness is valued for its intrinsic qualities and for its potential effects on other aspects of healthcare quality, such as technical performance. For example, in a patient-centered setting, a clinician is more likely to establish with patients the kind of rapport that elicits a complete and accurate medical history (especially with respect to potentially sensitive topics such as the use of illicit drugs) and as a result is more likely to make a timely, accurate diagnosis, thereby enhancing technical performance.

EXHIBIT 2.1
Stereotypical
Differences in
Importance
of Selected
Aspects of
Care to Key
Stakeholders'
Definitions of
Quality

Stakeholder	Technical Performance	Patient Centeredness	Amenities	Access	Equity	Efficiency	Cost-Effectiveness
Clinician	+++	+	+	+	+	+	—
Patient	++	+++	+++	++	+	+	—
Payer	+	+	+	+	+	+++	+++
Manager	++	+	+++	+++	++	+++	+++
Society	+++	+	+	+++	+++	+++	+++

Reprinted from: *Clinics in Family Practice*, Volume 5 (4), Wyszewianski, L. "Defining, Measuring, and Improving Quality of Care." 807–825, 2003. Used with permission from Elsevier.

Amenities

The quality of the *amenities* of care is determined by the characteristics of the setting in which the patient–clinician encounter takes place—for example, comfort, convenience, and privacy (Donabedian 1980). Amenities such as ample and convenient parking, good directional signs, comfortable waiting rooms, and tasty hospital food are all valued by patients and their visitors. Much like patient centeredness, amenities are valued both in their own right and for their potential effect on other aspects of healthcare quality. For example, in a comfortable, private setting that puts patients at ease, good relationships between patients and clinicians are more easily established and patients are more likely to fully express their needs and preferences as a result.

Access

The quality of *access* to care refers to the "degree to which individuals and groups are able to obtain needed services" (IOM 1993). The ease with which people obtain services depends on the extent to which their characteristics and expectations match those of providers. For example, cost becomes an impediment to access when the amount the provider charges exceeds what the patient is able or willing to pay. Other factors that may impede individuals' access to care include remote provider location, limited means of transportation, conflict between providers' and patients' schedules, and clashes between patients' and providers' cultures (McLaughlin and Wyszewianski 2002; Penchansky and Thomas 1981).

Equity

Findings that the amount, type, or quality of healthcare provided can relate systematically to an individual's characteristics—particularly race and ethnicity—rather than to the individual's need for care or healthcare preferences have heightened concern about *equity* in health services delivery (IOM 2002; Wyszewianski and Donabedian 1981). But the inclusion of equity as an element of healthcare quality is not a novel idea. Many decades ago, Lee and Jones (1933) asserted that "good medical care implies the application of all the necessary services of modern, scientific medicine to the needs of all the people. . . . No matter what the perfection of technique in the treatment of one individual case, medicine does not fulfill its function adequately until the same perfection is within the reach of all individuals."

Efficiency

Efficiency refers to how well resources are used to achieve a given result. Efficiency improves whenever fewer resources are used to produce an output. Although economists typically treat efficiency and quality as separate concepts, a case can be made for including efficiency as an attribute of healthcare quality. Because inefficient care uses more resources than necessary, it is wasteful care, and care that involves waste is deficient—and therefore of lower quality—no matter how good it may be in other respects. "Wasteful care is either directly harmful to health or is harmful by displacing more useful care" (Donabedian 1988a).

Cost-Effectiveness

The *cost-effectiveness* of a given healthcare intervention is determined by comparing the benefit, typically measured in terms of improvement in health status, an intervention yields with the cost of the intervention (Drummond et al. 2005; Gold et al. 1996). As discussed in greater detail in a later section, as the amounts spent on services in a given case grow, past a certain point each unit of expenditure yields ever-smaller benefits until no further benefit accrues from additional expenditures on care (Donabedian, Wheeler, and Wyszewianski 1982).

Different Definitions

Virtually everyone can be expected to value the attributes of quality just described, but as discussed earlier, clinicians, patients, payers, managers, and society attach different levels of importance to individual attributes of care and define quality of care differently as a result.

Clinicians

Clinicians, especially physicians, tend to perceive the quality of care foremost in terms of technical performance. Their concerns focus on aspects highlighted in IOM's (1990) often-quoted definition of quality:

> Quality is the degree to which health services for individuals and populations increase the likelihood of desired health outcomes and are consistent with current professional knowledge.

Reference to "current professional knowledge" draws attention to the changing nature of what constitutes good clinical care. Because medical knowledge advances rapidly, clinicians strongly believe that assessing care provided in 2010 on the basis of knowledge acquired in 2013 is neither meaningful nor appropriate. Similarly, "likelihood of desired health outcomes" aligns with clinicians' widely held view that no matter how good their technical performance is, predictions about the ultimate outcome of care can be expressed only as a probability due to the presence of influences beyond clinicians' control, such as a patient's inherent physiological resilience.

Patients

Although patients care deeply about technical performance, it plays a relatively small role in shaping their view of healthcare quality. To the dismay of clinicians, many patients see technical performance strictly in terms of the outcomes of care; if the patient did not improve, the physician's technical competence is called into question (Muir Gray 2009). Additionally, many patients recognize that they do not possess the wherewithal to evaluate technical elements of care and defer to others on most matters of technical quality, especially to organizations presumed to have the requisite expertise, such as accrediting bodies, state licensing agencies, and medical specialty boards (Donabedian 1980). Patients therefore tend to form their opinions about the quality of care on the basis of their assessment of aspects of care they are most readily able to evaluate, chiefly patient centeredness and amenities (Cleary and McNeil 1988; Sofaer and Firminger 2005).

Payers

Third-party payers—health insurance companies, government programs such as Medicare, and others who pay on behalf of patients—tend to assess the quality of care on the basis of costs. From their perspective, inefficient care is poor-quality care. Because payers typically manage a finite pool of resources, they also tend to be concerned about cost-effectiveness—that is, whether a potential outcome justifies the associated costs.

Clinicians and their patients consider cost-effectiveness to be antithetical to high-quality care. Both see clinicians as duty bound to do everything possible to help their patients, including advocating for high-cost interventions, even if those interventions have a small but positive probability of benefiting the patient (Donabedian 1988b; Strech et al. 2009). Third-party payers—especially governmental units that must make multiple trade-offs when allocating resources—are more apt to view the spending of large sums in instances where the odds of a positive result are small not as high-quality care but rather as a misuse of finite resources, especially given the public's growing unwillingness to pay the higher premiums or taxes needed to provide patients with all care that is available and potentially beneficial.

Managers

The primary concern of managers responsible for the operations of hospitals, clinics, and other healthcare delivery organizations is the quality of the nonclinical aspects of care over which they have the most control—primarily amenities and access to care. Managers' perspective on quality can differ from that of clinicians and patients with respect to efficiency, cost-effectiveness, and equity. Because of managers' role in ensuring that resources are spent where they will do the most good, efficiency and cost-effectiveness are of central concern to them, as is the equitable distribution of resources.

Society

At a collective, or societal, level, the definition of quality of care reflects concerns about efficiency and cost-effectiveness similar to those of governmental third-party payers and managers, and much for the same reasons. In addition, technical aspects of quality loom large at the societal level, where many believe care can be assessed and safeguarded more effectively than it can be at the level of individuals. Similarly, access to care and equity are important to society-level concepts of quality to the extent that society is seen as responsible for ensuring access to care for everyone, particularly disenfranchised groups.

Are the Five Definitions Irreconcilable?

Different though they may seem, the five definitions—those of the clinician, the patient, the payer, the manager, and society—have a great deal in common. Although each definition emphasizes different attributes, none of the other attributes is typically excluded (see Exhibit 2.1). The definitions directly conflict only in relation to cost-effectiveness. Cost-effectiveness is often central to how payers, managers, and society define quality of care, whereas physicians and patients typically do not recognize cost-effectiveness as a legitimate consideration in defining quality.

Strong disagreements do arise, however, among the five parties' definitions, even outside the realm of cost-effectiveness. Conflicts typically emerge when one party holds that a particular practitioner or clinic is a high-quality provider by virtue of having high ratings on a single aspect of care, such as patient centeredness. Those objecting to this conclusion point out that just because a provider rates highly on patient centeredness does not necessarily mean that it rates equally highly on technical performance, amenities, efficiency, and other aspects of care (Wyszewianski 1988). Physicians who relate well to their patients and thus score high on patient centeredness nevertheless may have failed to keep up with medical advances and as a result provide care deficient in technical terms. This discrepancy apparently was present in the case involving Medicare and the rural physicians described at the start of this chapter.

Conversely, practitioners who are highly skilled in trauma and other emergency care but have a distant, even brusque, manner and work in crowded conditions may rate low on patient centeredness and amenity aspects of care even though, as in the second case described at the start of this chapter, the facility receives top marks from a team of expert clinicians whose primary focus is technical performance.

Summary

When clinicians, patients, payers, managers, society, and other involved parties refer to quality of care, they each tend to focus on the quality of specific aspects of care, sometimes to the apparent exclusion of other aspects important to other parties. The aspects a party overlooks, however, are seldom in direct conflict with that party's own overall concept of quality.

Measurement-Related Concepts

Just as definition-related concepts are useful for advancing one's understanding of quality of care, so are measurement-related concepts, particularly with respect to technical care. Consider the following two cases:

1. At the urging of one state's nurses' association, legislators passed a law specifying minimum nurse staffing levels in hospitals. The nurses' association had argued that nurse staffing cutbacks around the state had affected the quality of care to the point of endangering patient safety. Critics of the law charged that the legislators passed the law without first proving that the cutbacks had indeed compromised safety. In the critics' view, the law had more to do with the nurses' fear of losing their jobs than with documented quality-of-care problems.
2. Several health plans are competing to be among those offered to the employees of one of the area's newest and largest employers. One of the plans, HealthBest, claims that the quality of care it provides is higher than that provided by its competitors. Among the data cited by HealthBest to back its claim are statistics showing that the rate of mammogram screening for breast cancer among its female members aged 52 to 69 is 10 to 20 percent higher than the rates among members of the other plans. One competitor, PrimeHealth, argues that the percentage of women screened through mammography is not a good indicator of the quality of care; detection of breast cancer at an early stage is a better criterion. On that measure, PrimeHealth claims to do better than HealthBest and the other plans.

The following section introduces several concepts that can help one make sense of these two cases and similar situations involving measurement of the quality of care.

Structure, Process, and Outcome
As Donabedian first noted in 1966, all evaluations of the quality of care can be classified in terms of one of three measures: structure, process, or outcome.

Structure
In the context of measuring the quality of care, *structure* refers to characteristics of the individuals who provide care and of the settings where the care

is delivered. These characteristics include the education, training, and certification of professionals who provide care and the adequacy of the facility's staffing, equipment, and overall organization.

Evaluations of quality based on structural elements assume that well-qualified people working in well-appointed and well-organized settings provide high-quality care. However, although good structure makes good quality more likely to ensue, it does not guarantee it (Donabedian 2003). Structure-focused assessments are therefore most revealing when deficiencies are found; good quality is unlikely, if not impossible, if the individuals who provide care are unqualified or if necessary equipment is missing or in disrepair. Licensing and accrediting bodies have relied heavily on structural measures of quality not only because the measures are relatively stable and thus easier to capture but also because they reliably identify providers who lack the means to deliver high-quality care.

Process

Process—the series of events that takes place during the delivery of care—also can be a basis for evaluating the quality of care. The quality of the process can vary on three aspects: (1) appropriateness—whether the right actions were taken, (2) skill—the proficiency with which actions were carried out, and (3) the timeliness of the care.

Ordering the correct diagnostic procedure for a patient is an example of an *appropriate* action, but to fully evaluate the process in which this particular action is embedded, we also need to know how promptly the procedure was ordered and how skillfully it was carried out. Similarly, successful completion of a surgical operation and a good recovery are not enough evidence to conclude that the process of care was high quality; they only indicate that the procedure was performed skillfully. For the entire process of care to be judged as high quality, one also must ascertain that the operation was indicated (i.e., appropriate) for the patient and that it was carried out in time. Finally, as was the case for structural measures, the use of process measures for assessing the quality of care rests on a key assumption—that if the right things are done and are done right, good results (i.e., good outcomes of care) are more likely to be achieved.

Outcome

Outcome measures capture whether healthcare goals were achieved. Because the goals of care can be defined broadly, outcome measures have come to include the costs of care as well as patients' satisfaction with their care (Iezzoni 2013). In formulations that stress the technical aspects of care, however, outcomes typically refer to indicators of health status, such as whether a patient's pain subsided or condition cleared up or whether the patient regained full function (Donabedian 1980).

Clinicians tend to be leery of outcome measures of quality. As mentioned earlier, clinicians are aware that many factors that determine clinical outcomes—including genetic and environmental factors—are not under their control. At best, they control the process, and a good process only increases the likelihood of good outcomes; it does not guarantee them. Some patients do not improve in spite of the best treatment that medicine can offer, whereas other patients regain full health even though they received inappropriate and potentially harmful care. However, the relationship between process and outcome is not completely random and unpredictable. In particular, the likelihood that a specific set of clinical activities—a given process—will result in a desirable outcome depends on how efficacious the process is.

Efficacy

A clinical intervention is *efficacious* if it has been shown to produce a given outcome reliably when other potentially confounding factors are held constant. Formal clinical trials or similarly systematic, controlled studies typically establish the efficacy of a clinical intervention. Knowledge about efficacy is crucial to making valid judgments about the quality of care when process or outcome measures are used. If a given clinical intervention was undertaken in circumstances that match those under which the intervention has been shown to be efficacious, one can be confident that the care was appropriate and, to that extent, of good quality. Conversely, if the outcome of a particular episode of care was poor, one can find out whether it resulted from an inappropriate clinical intervention by determining whether the circumstances under which it took place conformed to those under which the intervention's efficacy has been demonstrated.

Which Is Best?

Of structure, process, and outcome, which is the best measure of the quality of care? The answer—that none of them is inherently better and it all depends on the circumstances (Donabedian 2003)—often does not satisfy those who are inclined to believe that outcome measures are superior to the others. After all, they reason, the outcome addresses the ultimate purpose, the bottom line, of all caregiving: Was the condition cured? Did the patient improve?

As previously mentioned, however, it is possible to experience a good outcome even when the care (i.e., process) was clearly deficient. The reverse is also possible: Although the care was excellent, the outcome may not be good due to a number of factors not within clinicians' control—such as a patient's frailty. To assess outcomes meaningfully across providers, one must account for such non-care factors by performing complicated risk adjustment calculations (Goode at al. 2011; Iezzoni 2013).

What a particular outcome ultimately denotes about the quality of care crucially depends on whether the outcome can be attributed to the care provided. In other words, one has to examine the link between the outcome and the antecedent process and determine—on the basis of efficacy—whether the care was appropriate and provided skillfully. Outcomes are therefore useful for identifying possible problems of quality ("fingering the suspects") but not for ascertaining whether poor care was actually provided ("determining guilt"). The latter determination requires delving into the antecedent process of care to establish whether the care provided was the likely cause of the observed outcome.

Criteria and Standards

To assess quality using structure, process, or outcome measures, one needs to establish criteria and standards to know what constitutes a good structure, a good process, and a good outcome.

Definitions

Criteria refer to specific attributes that are the basis for assessing quality. *Standards* quantitatively express the level the attributes must reach to satisfy preexisting expectations about quality.

An example unrelated to healthcare may help clarify the difference between criteria and standards. Universities often evaluate applicants for admission on the basis of standardized test scores. The scores are thus one of the criteria by which programs judge the quality of their applicants. However, although two programs may use the same criterion—scores on a specific standardized examination—to evaluate applicants, the programs may differ markedly on standards: One program may consider applicants acceptable if they have scores above the 50th percentile, whereas scores above the 90th percentile may be the standard of acceptability for the other program. Exhibit 2.2 provides examples of criteria and standards for structure, process, and outcome measures in healthcare.

Sources

The way healthcare criteria and standards are derived is changing. Before the 1970s, formally derived criteria and standards for quality-of-care evaluations relied on consensus among groups of clinicians selected for their clinical knowledge and experience and the respect they commanded among their colleagues (Donabedian 1982). This approach to formulating criteria took for granted that the experts would incorporate in their deliberations the latest scientific knowledge relevant to the topic under consideration, but formal requirements that they do so seldom existed.

EXHIBIT 2.2
Examples of
Criteria and
Standards
for Structure,
Process, and
Outcome
Measures in
Healthcare

Type of Measure	Focus of Assessment	Criterion	Standard
Structure	Nurse staffing in nursing homes	Hours of nursing care per resident day	At least four hours of nursing care per resident day
Process	Patients undergoing surgical repair of hip fracture	Percentage of patients who received prophylactic antibiotics on day of surgery	100% receive antibiotic on day of surgery
Outcome	Hospitalized patients	Rate of falls per 1,000 patient days	Fewer than five falls per 1,000 patient days

In the 1970s, however, the importance of scientific literature to the evaluation of healthcare quality gained new visibility through the work of Cochrane (1973), Williamson (1977), and others. At about the same time, Brook and colleagues (1977) at RAND began to use systematic reviews and evaluations of scientific literature as the starting point for the deliberations of panels charged with defining criteria and standards for studies of quality. The evidence-based medicine movement of the 1990s, which advocated medical practice guided by the best evidence about efficacy, reinforced the focus on the literature and stressed consideration of the soundness of study design and validity (Evidence-Based Medicine Working Group 1992; Straus et al. 2005). As a result, derivation of criteria and standards has come to revolve more around the strength and validity of scientific evidence than around the unaided consensus of experts (Eddy 2005, 1996).

Levels

When standards are being formulated, a critical decision is the level at which the standards should be set: minimal, optimal, achievable, or something in between (Muir Gray 2009). *Minimal* standards specify the level that must be met for quality to be considered acceptable; if care does not meet the minimal standard, remedial action is called for. *Optimal* standards denote the level of quality that can be reached under the best conditions—typically conditions similar to those under which efficacy is determined. Optimal standards are useful as a reference point for setting *achievable* standards, the level of performance that everyone being evaluated should meet or exceed. One way to define achievable standards is in terms of the performance of the top quartile of providers of care; if the top quartile can perform at that level, the argument goes, the other three quartiles should be able to reach it (Muir

Gray 2009). Other approaches to setting standards have been proposed for evaluating, for example, access to care (Bower et al. 2003). Because there is no a priori level at which a particular standard should be set, a sensible and frequently adopted approach is to choose the level according to the goals of the underlying evaluation effort.

Utility of Measurement-Related Concepts

How does understanding structure, process, outcome, efficacy, criteria, and standards provide insight into quality-of-care measurement issues? The two cases cited at the beginning of this section illustrate the concepts' potential utility.

The first case specified minimum standards of quality in terms of nurse staffing levels, a structural measure of quality. The critics were not questioning the choice of that measure, nor should they have; structural measures are well suited to detecting a lack of capacity to deliver care of acceptable quality. In this case, hospitals that did not meet minimum staffing levels were presumed to be unable to deliver care of acceptable quality (safe care). However, the critics contended that the law's standards for minimum staffing levels were not evidence based but instead were set at levels intended to reverse or minimize job losses among members of the state nurses' association; no evidence was provided to support the law's staffing standards. To be persuasive, evidence would have to come from properly controlled studies showing that care cannot be considered safe when nurse staffing ratios fall below a specific level, holding all else constant. In other words, the evidence ideally would come from the kind of studies on which efficacy determinations are based.

In the second case, both measures under discussion were process measures. However, mammograms belong to a subset of process measures that represent a "resting point" along a continuum of activities that constitute a process of care. Like outcomes, these resting points are discrete events that are easily counted; Donabedian (1980) labels them *procedural endpoints*. PrimeHealth argued that mammograms are not an outcome—that is, they are not an end in themselves but rather a means for achieving a different outcome: early detection of breast cancer.

Because performing mammograms is certainly the right thing to do for the target population, appropriateness is not in question. However, PrimeHealth's argument reminds us that the skill with which the mammograms are performed matters just as much as the number performed. If mammograms are performed incorrectly because of skill deficiencies and thus interpreted incorrectly, or if they are performed correctly but interpreted incorrectly, the mammograms may fail as a means for early detection of breast cancer. Therefore, early detection of breast cancer is a better measure of quality because it indicates not just whether mammograms were performed when indicated (appropriateness) but also how well they were performed and interpreted (skill).

Summary

The main insight that can be drawn from a deeper understanding of concepts related to the measurement of healthcare quality is that the type of measure used—structure, process, or outcome—matters less than the measure's relationship to the others. Structural measures are only as good and useful as the strength of their link to desired processes and outcomes. Similarly, process and outcome measures must relate to each other in measurable and reproducible ways—as demonstrated by efficacy studies—to be truly valid measures of quality.

Criteria and standards are essential to evaluating structure, process, and outcome. Whereas the formulation of criteria is typically expected to be evidence driven—and thus based on efficacy—the setting of standards is not necessarily tied to the scientific literature. Instead, the decision to set standards at a minimal, ideal, or achievable level is most meaningful if driven by the goals behind the specific quality-of-care evaluation for which the standards are to be used.

Concepts Pertinent to the Quality–Cost Relationship

Discussion now turns to the relationship between the quality and costs of healthcare. Consider the following two quotes written within a few months of each other:

1. Every country in the world is battling the rising cost of health care. No community anywhere has demonstrably lowered its health-care costs (not just slowed their rate of increase) by improving medical services. They've lowered costs only by cutting or rationing them. To many people, the problem of health-care costs is best encapsulated in a basic third-grade lesson: you can't have it all. You want higher wages, lower taxes, less debt? Then cut health care services. People like Jeff Brenner are saying that we can have it all. . . . The new health-reform law—Obamacare—is betting big on the Brenners of the world. It says that we can afford to subsidize insurance for millions, remove the ability of private and public insurers to cut high-cost patients from their rolls, and improve the quality of care (Gawande 2011).

2. Our own experience in trying to talk about the kind of wholesale reforms we think necessary for medicine's future is that people are far more concerned about what it will mean for themselves and their families than for something as general and abstract as the health care system. Their heads tell them that

rationing and limits will probably be necessary, but they reject these ideas if it means that a loved one might not have what is needed to be kept alive, even if in a bad or terminal state. Unhappily, however, some rationing and limit setting will be necessary. There is no way the Medicare program can survive unless it both sharply cuts benefits and raises taxes (Callahan and Nuland 2011).

Theoretical Relationship Between Quality and Costs

The theoretical relationship between quality of care (however it may be defined and measured) and healthcare costs (i.e., the resources that went into providing care) has been represented by graphs similar to Exhibit 2.3 (Bodenheimer and Grumbach 2009; Donabedian, Wheeler, and Wyszewianski 1982).

The curve in Exhibit 2.3 represents the level of quality that the most efficient provider of healthcare can attain—based on current knowledge and technology—at any given level of costs incurred. The curve is S shaped, reflecting that, as long as the costs incurred are relatively low, the level of quality achieved is low and may even be hard to detect. Overall, however, the slope of the curve is either increasing or constant, indicating that the higher the costs incurred, the higher the quality achieved. However, at the point where the slope of the curve begins to decrease, the amount of quality achieved for each additional unit of cost gradually becomes smaller until quality cannot be improved, no matter how large the increase in costs.

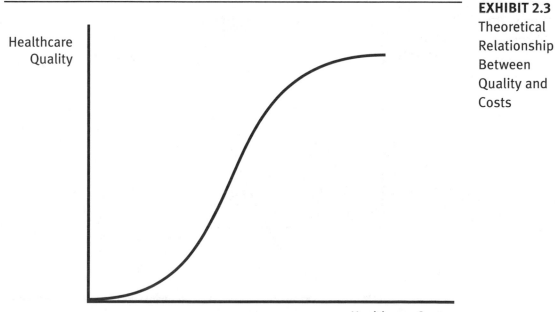

EXHIBIT 2.3
Theoretical Relationship Between Quality and Costs

Healthcare Quality

Healthcare Costs

Donabedian (1986) encapsulated the relationship between quality and costs into three aphorisms:

1. *Quality costs money.* As Exhibit 2.3 illustrates, costs must be incurred to achieve any level of quality.
2. *Money does not necessarily buy quality.* Although higher costs generally are associated with higher quality, this relationship does not necessarily hold, as illustrated by points A and B in Exhibit 2.4.
3. *Some improvements in quality are not worth the added cost.* Consider the increase in quality from A to B in Exhibit 2.5. Costs nearly doubled to achieve it, but the improvement in quality is much smaller. In this kind of situation, some would argue that the large increase in costs is not justified, given the disproportionately small improvement in quality.

This theoretical representation of the relationship between quality and costs provides further insight into two concepts discussed earlier: efficiency and cost-effectiveness.

Efficiency

Because the curve in Exhibit 2.3 represents the levels of quality that the most efficient provider of healthcare can attain, it is unlikely that the typical

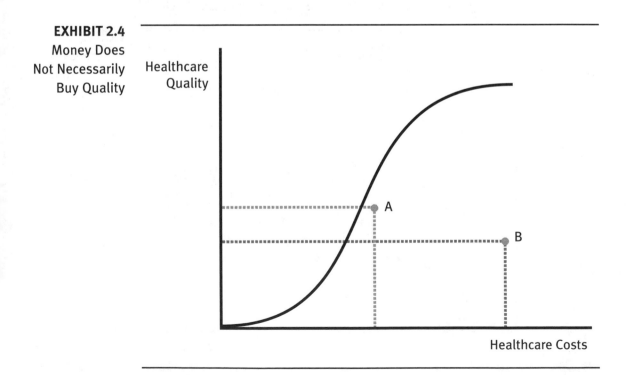

EXHIBIT 2.4
Money Does
Not Necessarily
Buy Quality

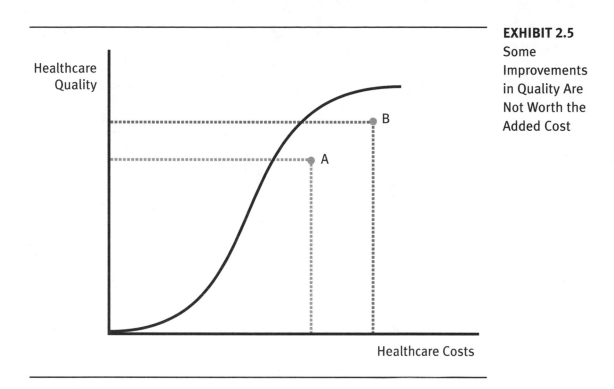

EXHIBIT 2.5
Some Improvements in Quality Are Not Worth the Added Cost

provider of care operates on the curve (i.e., is maximally efficient). More likely, the great majority of providers operate below the curve. Therefore, by improving efficiency, such providers are able to both improve quality and reduce costs (see Exhibit 2.6).

At the one extreme, a provider at point A in Exhibit 2.6 can move to B by increasing efficiency—improving quality while incurring no additional costs. At the other extreme, if the provider increases efficiency so as to move to C, costs decrease while quality remains the same. Providers can do some of both—reduce costs and increase quality—by moving to any point in the shaded area delimited by A, B, and C.

Cost-Effectiveness

Cost-effectiveness—the benefit derived from a particular level of expenditures—is the core concept behind Donabedian's third aphorism: Some improvements in quality are not worth the added cost.

Consider, for the sake of clarity, the most efficient provider, the one operating on the curve. For that provider, the quality—the benefit—derived from each additional unit of cost begins to gradually decrease at point A in Exhibit 2.7, until at point B quality cannot be further improved, no matter what additional costs are incurred. The distinction between point B and other points on the curve corresponds to two different definitions of quality: maximized and optimized (Donabedian 2003).

EXHIBIT 2.6
Range for
Increasing
Efficiency
and Quality
Simultaneously

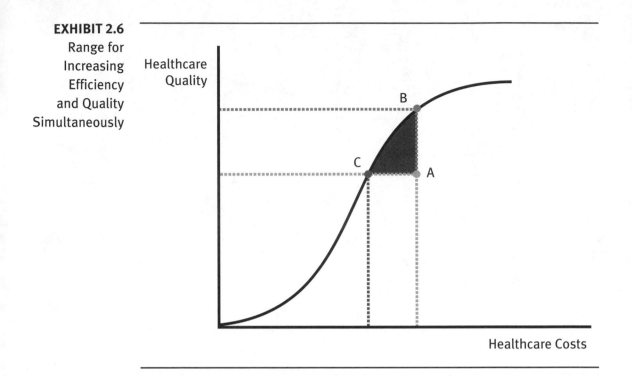

Maximized quality refers to the highest level of quality achievable given current knowledge and technology and unconstrained by cost; it corresponds to point B in Exhibit 2.7. Maximized quality is achieved by expending resources as long as a positive benefit can result, no matter how small. *Optimized quality* is the level of quality a given stakeholder considers optimal in terms of cost versus benefits. In other words, optimized quality is reached when, according to the stakeholder, benefits are too small to justify any additional costs.

Points at or around A in Exhibit 2.7 have been suggested as good candidates for representing optimized quality because in that range, the relatively small improvement in quality from A to, say, B is insufficient to justify almost doubled costs. However, different stakeholders may consider different points to be optimal. In particular, as discussed earlier, neither patients nor providers are inclined to consider cost-effectiveness when defining quality. For them, the notion of optimized quality is not relevant, leaving maximized quality—which doesn't take cost-effectiveness into consideration—as the only option.

Utility of Concepts Pertinent to the Quality–Cost Relationship

The two quotations cited at the beginning of this section help illustrate the potential utility of the concepts pertinent to the quality–cost relationship. In the first quotation, Jeff Brenner's claim that "we can have it all" can be translated as "we can improve quality and at the same time reduce costs." As

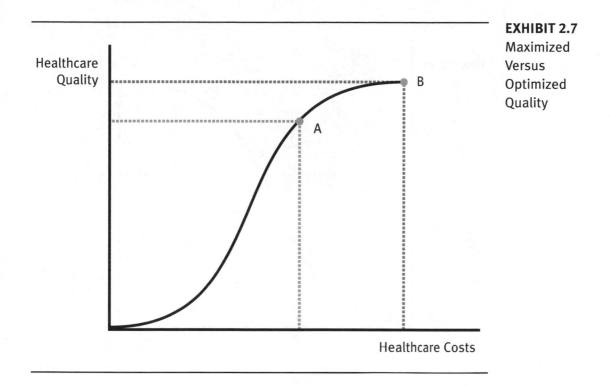

EXHIBIT 2.7
Maximized
Versus
Optimized
Quality

Healthcare
Quality

A

B

Healthcare Costs

discussed in connection with Exhibit 2.6, it is indeed possible for providers operating below the curve (i.e., those less than maximally efficient) to do so within a defined range.

However, the authors of the second quotation remind us that, in general, individuals expect—at least for themselves and their loved ones—maximized quality, but as Exhibit 2.8 illustrates, achieving maximized quality by improving efficiency and quality is not always possible. Assume that the current situation—high costs and inefficient, low-quality care—is represented by point A in Exhibit 2.8. Even if a provider improves both efficiency and quality as much as current technology and knowledge allow, it still ends up at point B, short of maximized quality (point C).

If we start at point A, the only way to reach maximized quality (point C) is to incur additional costs, which is not consistent with Brenner's claim that we can simultaneously reduce costs and improve quality. If incurring higher costs is not an option, the best a provider can do is reach a point around B. But B is not maximized quality; at point B, a provider is denying the patient potentially beneficial care, thus engaging in what is typically described as *rationing*.

On the other hand, if the starting point is D, where the costs incurred are higher than the amount required to provide maximized quality, then indeed it is possible to reach point C by improving quality and reducing costs. More generally, if current expenditures are equal to or exceed the cost

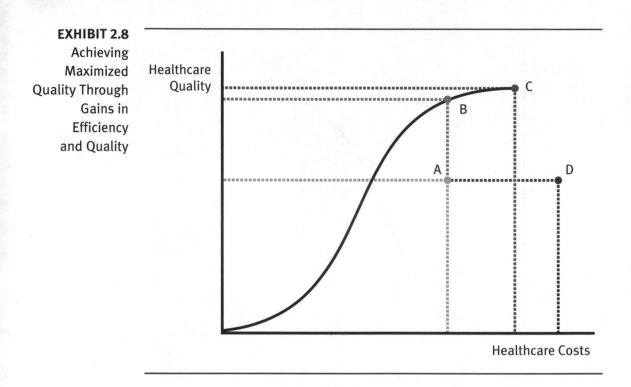

EXHIBIT 2.8
Achieving
Maximized
Quality Through
Gains in
Efficiency
and Quality

of providing maximized quality—as is the case at point D—then, and only then, is Brenner's claim that "we can have it all" correct.

Summary

Concepts pertinent to the quality–cost relationship are useful for gaining a deeper understanding of efficiency and cost-effectiveness. They also provide useful insight into the much debated issue of whether rationing care is an unavoidable consequence of any effort to reduce healthcare costs.

Study Questions

1. Because of possible complications at delivery, Mrs. T. is told by her doctor that she will have to give birth at South General Hospital. When Mrs. T. tells her friends what her doctor said, they are appalled and urge her to do all she can to go to Community Hospital instead.

    The friends draw sharp contrasts between the two hospitals. Community has quiet birthing rooms and was recently redecorated, and each patient is assigned a specific nurse. Because the nurses work 12-hour shifts, most women who deliver at the hospital have just one or two nurses attending to them. At South General, deliveries take place in ordinary, noisy hospital rooms. Staff tend to be busy and are not especially friendly, and women in labor are typically under the care of multiple nurses.

Who is right? Is South General a bad place to have a baby? Should Mrs. T. go to Community instead? Explain the reasoning behind your answer.

2. Describe three instances in which outcomes would not be a good measure of healthcare quality, and explain why.

3. Do you agree that care can be both high quality and inefficient? Why or why not?

4. Your friend Alicia is puzzled by an observation she read in a newspaper column:

Research by John Wennberg and colleagues at Dartmouth Medical School suggests that if everyone in America went to Mayo Clinic for care, our annual healthcare bill would be 25 percent lower (more than $500 billion in savings!) and the average quality of care would improve.

It makes sense to Alicia that, given Mayo's reputation, the average quality of care would improve if everyone received care of the caliber Mayo provides. The part she doesn't understand is how providing Mayo Clinic–level care could possibly reduce annual expenditures on healthcare by 25 percent. Wouldn't it cost more to provide better care? If anything, Alicia believes, providing everyone Mayo Clinic–level care would increase expenditures by 25 percent. Did the columnist get the facts wrong? Address Alicia's puzzlement with a clear, complete explanation.

References

Bodenheimer, T. S., and K. Grumbach. 2009. *Understanding Health Policy: A Clinical Approach*, fifth edition. New York: Lange Medical Books.

Bower, P., M. Roland, J. Campbell, and N. Mead. 2003. "Setting Standards Based on Patients' Views on Access and Continuity." *British Medical Journal* 326: 258–62.

Brook, R. H., A. Davies-Avery, S. Greenfield, L. J. Harris, T. Lelah, N. E. Solomon, and J. E. Ware Jr. 1977. "Assessing the Quality of Medical Care Using Outcome Measures: An Overview of the Method." *Medical Care* 15 (9 suppl.): 1–165.

Callahan, D., and S. B. Nuland. 2011. "The Quagmire: How American Medicine Is Destroying Itself." *New Republic* 242 (8): 16–18.

Campbell, S. M., M. O. Roland, and S. A. Buetow. 2000. "Defining Quality of Care." *Social Science and Medicine* 51 (11): 1611–25.

Cleary, P. D., and B. J. McNeil. 1988. "Patient Satisfaction as an Indicator of Quality Care." *Inquiry* 25 (1): 25–36.

Cochrane, A. L. 1973. *Effectiveness and Efficiency: Random Reflections on Health Services.* London: Nuffield Provincial Hospitals Trust.

Donabedian, A. 2003. *An Introduction to Quality Assurance in Health Care.* New York: Oxford University Press.

———. 1988a. "The Quality of Care: How Can It Be Assessed?" *Journal of the American Medical Association* 260 (12): 1743–48.

———. 1988b. "Quality and Cost: Choices and Responsibilities." *Inquiry* 25 (1): 90–99.

———. 1986. "The Price of Quality and the Perplexities of Care." 1986 Michael M. Davis Lecture. Chicago: Center for Health Administration Studies, University of Chicago.

———. 1982. *Explorations in Quality Assessment and Monitoring. Volume II: The Criteria and Standards of Quality.* Chicago: Health Administration Press.

———. 1980. *Explorations in Quality Assessment and Monitoring. Volume I: The Definition of Quality and Approaches to Its Assessment.* Chicago: Health Administration Press.

———. 1966. "Evaluating the Quality of Medical Care." *Milbank Memorial Fund Quarterly* 44 (3): 166–206.

Donabedian, A., J. R. C. Wheeler, and L. Wyszewianski. 1982. "Quality, Cost, and Health: An Integrative Model." *Medical Care* 20 (10): 975–92.

Drummond, M. F., M. J. Sculpher, G. W. Torrance, B. J. O'Brien, and G. L. Stoddart. 2005. *Methods for the Economic Evaluation of Health Care Programs,* third edition. New York: Oxford University Press.

Eddy, D. M. 2005. "Evidence-Based Medicine: A Unified Approach." *Health Affairs* 24 (1): 9–17.

———. 1996. *Clinical Decision Making: From Theory to Practice.* Sudbury, MA: Jones and Bartlett.

Evidence-Based Medicine Working Group. 1992. "Evidence-Based Medicine. A New Approach to Teaching the Practice of Medicine." *Journal of the American Medical Association* 268 (17): 2420–25.

Gawande, A. 2011. "The Hot Spotters: Can We Lower Medical Costs by Giving the Neediest Patients Better Care?" *New Yorker* January 24.

Gerteis, M., S. Edgman-Levitan, J. Daley, and T. L. Delbanco (eds.). 1993. *Through the Patient's Eyes: Understanding and Promoting Patient-Centered Care.* San Francisco: Jossey-Bass.

Gold, M. R., J. E. Siegel, L. B. Russell, and M. C. Weinstein (eds.). 1996. *Cost-Effectiveness in Health and Medicine.* New York: Oxford University Press.

Goode, A. P., C. Cook, J. B. Gill, S. Tackett, C. Brown, and W. Richardson. 2011. "The Risk of Risk-Adjustment Measures for Perioperative Spine Infection After Spinal Surgery." *Spine* 36 (9): 752–58.

Harteloh, P. P. M. 2004. "Understanding the Quality Concept in Health Care." *Accreditation and Quality Assurance* 9: 92–95.

Iezzoni, L. I. (ed.). 2013. *Risk Adjustment for Measuring Health Care Outcomes*, fourth edition. Chicago: Health Administration Press.

Institute of Medicine (IOM). 2002. *Unequal Treatment: Confronting Racial and Ethnic Disparities in Healthcare.* Washington, DC: National Academies Press.

———. 2001. *Crossing the Quality Chasm: A New Health System for the 21st Century.* Washington, DC: National Academies Press.

———. 1993. *Access to Health Care in America.* Washington, DC: National Academies Press.

———. 1990. *Medicare: A Strategy for Quality Assurance.* Washington, DC: National Academies Press.

Lee, R. I., and L. W. Jones. 1933. "The Fundamentals of Good Medical Care." *Publications of the Committee on the Costs of Medical Care*, no. 22. Chicago: University of Chicago Press.

McLaughlin, C. G., and L. Wyszewianski. 2002. "Access to Care: Remembering Old Lessons." *Health Services Research* 37 (6): 1441–43.

Muir Gray, J. A. 2009. *Evidence-Based Healthcare: How to Make Decisions About Health Services and Public Health*, third edition. Edinburgh, UK: Churchill Livingstone.

Penchansky, R., and J. W. Thomas. 1981. "The Concept of Access: Definition and Relationship to Consumer Satisfaction." *Medical Care* 19 (2): 127–40.

Sofaer, S., and K. Firminger. 2005. "Patient Perceptions of the Quality of Health Services." *Annual Review of Public Health* 26: 513–59.

Straus, S. E., W. S. Richardson, P. Glasziou, and R. B. Haynes. 2005. *Evidence-Based Medicine: How to Practice and Teach EBM*, third edition. Edinburgh, UK: Churchill Livingstone.

Strech, D., G. Persad, G. Marckmann, and M. Danis. 2009. "Are Physicians Willing to Ration Health Care? Conflicting Findings in a Systematic Review of Survey Research." *Health Policy* 90 (2–3): 113–24.

Williamson, J. W. 1977. *Improving Medical Practice and Health Care: A Bibliographic Guide to Information Management in Quality Assurance and Continuing Education.* Cambridge, MA: Ballinger.

Wyszewianski, L. 1988. "Quality of Care: Past Achievements and Future Challenges." *Inquiry* 25 (1): 13–22.

Wyszewianski, L., and A. Donabedian. 1981. "Equity in the Distribution of Quality of Care." *Medical Care* 19 (12 suppl.): 28–56.

VARIATION IN MEDICAL PRACTICE AND IMPLICATIONS FOR QUALITY

David J. Ballard, Briget da Graca,
Robert S. Hopkins III, and David Nicewander

Despite the growing interest in and use of evidence-based medicine, the art of medical practice remains empirical and is subject to considerable differences in process and outcome, even among the finest healthcare delivery organizations (Reinertsen 2003). In examining the top 50 hospitals noted for their "compassionate geriatric and palliative care," the Dartmouth Atlas of Health Care Project found in 1999 that the percentage of patients admitted one or more times to an intensive care unit during the last six months of life differed widely by region, from 23 percent to 45 percent (Wennberg 2002; Wennberg and Cooper 1999). The 2008 update to the Dartmouth Atlas again found that, for the period 2003–2007, end-of-life care for Medicare beneficiaries with chronic illnesses varied widely between academic medical centers—and that while most of the academic medical centers changed the intensity of the care they provided during this period, they varied in the direction of that change; some moved toward more aggressive treatment while others shifted toward more conservative approaches (Goodman et al. 2011). Such disagreements about care across even this elite group of providers continue to raise questions about the adequacy of evidence-based medicine with respect to both the evidence and the implementation.

It is tempting to suggest that such variation in healthcare indicates inconsistencies in the quality of care provided to different populations of patients. However, such a conclusion presumes that variation is undesirable and results largely from some providers following "best practices" in medical treatment while others do not. More in-depth examination of variation in clinical practice suggests that the situation is far more complex, with multiple contributing influences and outcomes.

This chapter discusses the application of several distinct types of variation to studies of medical processes and outcomes. Variation can be just as illuminating for what it offers in terms of innovation and improvement as it is instructive in its revelation of irregularity and incompatibility (Wheeler 2000).

Background and Terminology

Statisticians, medical researchers and practitioners, and hospital administrators use and understand variation in ways that are not always compatible. Each definition is valuable in its particular application, so none should be considered correct at the expense of another. Measurement of variation in healthcare and its application to quality improvement must begin with the identification and articulation of what is to be measured and the standard against which it is to be compared—a process based on extensive research, trial and error, and collaborative discussion.

Random Versus Assignable Variation

Variation can be either random or assignable (Wheeler 2000). *Random variation* is a physical attribute of an event or process, adheres to the laws of probability, and cannot be traced to a root cause. Traditionally, it is considered "background noise," or "expected" or "common-cause" variation, and it is usually not worth studying in detail. *Assignable variation* (or "special-cause" variation) arises from a single or small set of causes that are not part of the event or process and can be traced and identified and then implemented or eliminated. Such variation is therefore of greater interest and use to healthcare quality researchers. Researchers trained in statistics (or collaborating with statisticians) generally can measure assignable variation easily because of the breadth of tests and criteria available for determining whether variation is assignable or random and because of the increasing sensitivity and power of numerical analysis. Statistical expertise is, however, essential in the measurement of assignable variation because the complexity of study design and the difficulty of distinguishing true variation from artifacts or statistical errors raise the risk of misinterpretation (Powell, Davies, and Thomson 2003; Samsa et al. 2002).

Process Variation

Process variation is one category of variation in medical practice. It refers to different usage of a therapeutic or diagnostic procedure in an organization, geographic area, or other grouping of healthcare providers. In addition to variation in use versus nonuse of a particular procedure, variation may arise when multiple procedures can be used to achieve approximately the same ends. For example, in the case of screening for colorectal cancer, the same purpose (screening) may be served by fecal occult blood testing, sigmoidoscopy, colonoscopy, or some combination of these options. Process variation should not be confused with *technique*, which refers to the multitude of ways in which a particular procedure can be performed within the realm of acceptable medical practice (Mottur-Pilson, Snow, and Bartlett 2001).

Outcome Variation

Another category is *outcome variation*, which occurs when different results follow from a single process. Healthcare quality researchers and medical practitioners often focus on this measure and seek to identify the process that yields optimal results (Samsa et al. 2002). When the results of a particular process can be observed in relatively short order or when procedural changes can be made in a timely fashion, the optimal process is easily determined. Unfortunately, genuine outcome studies often require extensive follow-up periods—often years or decades—making it difficult to determine in real-time whether the process being applied is, in fact, yielding optimal results.

Performance Variation

Performance variation—the difference between any given result and the optimal result—is arguably the most important category of variation applicable to healthcare quality improvement (Ballard 2003). Logically, it may relate to both choice of process and application of that process to achieve the optimal result. This best practice is the standard against which other practices are compared to determine the variation—although some key analytical tools, such as statistical process control, do not directly address performance relative to a standard. As Steinberg (2003) noted, with respect to quality of care, "the variation that is the greatest cause for concern is that between actual practice and evidence-based 'best practice.'" The measurement of performance variation—and its application to quality improvement work—assumes, however, that a best practice has been identified. In such a scenario, performance variation tells us where we are and how far we are from where want to be and suggests ways to achieve the desired goal. However, a recurring theme in the discussion of variation in medical practice is the role of uncertainty, including uncertainty about what the best practice is in a given situation.

Variation in Medical Practice

Variation in medical practice has excited interest since 1938, when Dr. J. Allison Glover (1938) published his classic study on the incidence of tonsillectomy in school children in England and Wales, uncovering geographic variation that defied any explanation other than variation in medical opinion on the indications for surgery. Subsequent studies have revealed similar variation internationally and across a variety of medical conditions and procedures, including prostatectomy, knee replacement, arteriovenous fistula dialysis, and invasive cardiac procedures (Katz et al. 1996; Lu-Yao and Greenberg 1994; McPherson et al. 1982; Rayner 2011; Sejr et al. 1991; Wennberg et al. 1996). Interestingly, similar degrees of practice variation are found in countries with quite different absolute rates of use of procedures (Wennberg, Barnes, and Zubkoff 1982; Westert et al. 2004) and variability in supply of healthcare services (e.g., the United States, where supply varies widely, and the Netherlands, where until recently the healthcare system was centrally planned and controlled to ensure consistent supply nationwide) (Westert and Faber 2011) as well as in diverse systems of healthcare organization and financing (e.g., health maintenance organizations, fee-for-service, and national universal healthcare systems) (Wennberg, Barnes, and Zubkoff 1982).

The degree of variation seen in utilization of a particular procedure (although not the absolute rate of use) is more related to the characteristics of that procedure than to the country or healthcare system in which it is being performed—although there are some exceptions (McPherson et al. 1982). For example, Canadian government health insurance restricts coverage for endovascular abdominal aortic aneurysm repair (EVAR) to high-surgical-risk patients. This restriction not only keeps the absolute rate of EVAR use in Canada to less than half that in the United States (where there is no such restriction on insurance coverage), but it also eliminates the variation stemming from patient or physician preference in the lower-risk population of patients needing abdominal aortic aneurysm repair (Ballard et al. 2012).

Important procedural characteristics include the degree of professional uncertainty about the diagnosis and treatment of the condition the procedure addresses, the availability of alternative treatments, and controversy versus consensus regarding the appropriate use of the procedure. Differences among physicians in diagnosis style and in belief in the efficacy of a treatment contribute substantially to variation (McPherson et al. 1982).

The first important distinction to make when considering variation in medical practice is the difference between *warranted variation*, which is based on differences in patient preferences, disease prevalence, or other patient-related factors, and *unwarranted variation*, which cannot be explained by patient preference or condition or evidence-based medicine (Gauld et al. 2011). While the former is a necessary part of providing appropriate and personalized evidence-based patient care, the latter is typically regarded as a quality-of-care concern by hospitals and healthcare systems (Gauld et al. 2011). The effects of unwarranted variation include inefficient care (i.e., underutilization of effective procedures and/or overutilization of procedures with limited or no benefit) and related cost implications as well as disparities in care between geographic regions or healthcare providers (Gauld et al. 2011).

John Wennberg, a leading scholar in the area of unwarranted clinical practice variation and founding editor of the Dartmouth Atlas of Health Care, defines three categories of care in which unwarranted variation indicates different possible problems:

1. *Effective care* (15 percent of healthcare) is care for which the evidence has established that its benefits outweigh its risks and the "right rate" of use is 100 percent of the patients defined by evidence-based guidelines as needing such care. In this category, variation in the rate of use within a defined patient population indicates areas of underuse (Smith 2011; Wennberg 2011).

2. *Preference-sensitive care* (25 percent of healthcare) includes areas of care in which there is more than one generally accepted treatment available for the condition being addressed, so the "right rate" should depend on patient preference (Smith 2011; Wennberg 2011). A challenge posed by this type of care is the uncertainty of whether patient preferences can be accurately measured using current methods—and if they can, whether measurement methods are so resource intensive that inclusion of patient preference is impracticable in large population-based studies (Mercuri and Gafni 2011).

3. *Supply-sensitive care* (60 percent of healthcare) is care whose frequency of use relates to the capacity of the local healthcare system. Studies have repeatedly shown that regions with high use of supply-sensitive care do not perform better on mortality or quality-of-life indicators than do regions with low use, so variation in this area of healthcare services can provide evidence of overuse (Smith 2011; Wennberg 2011).

The objective for quality improvement researchers is not simply to identify variation but also to determine its value. If variation reveals a sub-optimal process, the task is to identify how the variation can be reduced or eliminated. If the variation is good or desirable, understanding how it can be applied across an organization to improve quality broadly is essential. The quality improvement goals in each of Wennberg's categories of care are different. For effective care, the goal is to achieve 100 percent utilization in the relevant patient population; as such, variation can indicate areas of underuse (Wennberg 2011). For preference-sensitive care, the goal is a rate of utilization of each alternative that is consistent with patient preference; this goal can be achieved through active engagement of patients in decision making (Greer et al. 2002; O'Connor, Llewellyn-Thomas, and Flood 2004; Wennberg 2011). Use of decision aids to increase patient involvement appears to decrease the demand for invasive treatments, which suggests that the "right rate" based on preference may be lower than that seen when physicians dominate the decision-making process (O'Connor et al. 2009). For supply-sensitive care, the goal is twofold: (1) to acquire the evidence (through comparative effectiveness research) necessary to move procedures currently in the supply-sensitive care category to either the effective care or preference-sensitive care category and (2) to adopt a pattern of use that achieves the best value (O'Connor et al. 2009; Ham 2011).

Sources of Unwarranted Variation in Medical Practice

A critical aspect of achieving the quality-of-care improvements indicated by observations of unwarranted variation is understanding the factors contributing to the variation. Frameworks for investigating unwarranted variation should provide (Mercuri and Gafni 2011)

1. a scientific basis for including or excluding each influencing factor and for determining when the factor is applicable and not applicable;
2. a clear definition and explanation of each factor suggested as a cause; and
3. an explanation of how the factor is operationalized, measured, and integrated with other factors.

Existing frameworks' definitions of unwarranted variation vary, ranging from variation that is unexplained by type or severity of illness or patient preference, to variation not explained by population difference, to differences in care that exist despite evidence of agreement on what constitutes evidence-based best practice, to variation that—as a matter of judgment—is unacceptable (Bojakowski 2010; Chalkidou 2009; Goodman 2009; Mercuri and Gafni 2011; Wennberg 2002). They similarly identify different causes of unwarranted variation, including inadequate patient involvement in decision making, inequitable access to resources, poor communication, role confusion, and misinterpretation or misapplication of relevant clinical evidence (Sepucha, Ozanne, and Mulley 2006; Wennberg 2011).

Other views are that variation is driven by clinician uncertainty (in defining disease, making a diagnosis, selecting a procedure, observing outcomes, assessing probabilities, and assigning preferences) and/or by physicians' economic incentives (Davis et al. 2000; Eddy 1984). Under the uncertainty hypothesis, the exercise of clinical judgment produces unwarranted variation because physicians develop individual practice styles, while under the economic incentives or "supply" hypothesis, physicians take advantage of their dual role as seller of a service and agent for the buyer (patient) to influence demand for a service, and marginal/deviant physician behavior is the most important regulatory focus in addressing quality-of-care deficits (Davis et al. 2000; Wennberg, Barnes, and Zubkoff 1982). The latter hypothesis has strongly influenced public policy in the past but has been criticized as being neither generally in operation nor able to establish a rational medical market because it misinterprets physician behavior by underestimating the market implications of uncertainty in diagnosing and treating disease (Wennberg, Barnes, and Zubkoff 1982). Rather, the variation in demand among

communities for specific procedures ("demand shift") is better characterized as the impact on consumption rates by the different belief sets held by
individual physicians (Wennberg, Barnes, and Zubkoff 1982). These belief
sets are sometimes divided into endogenous (e.g., education and ability)
and exogenous (e.g., reimbursement structures, role models, organizational
policies, patients' economic constraints) sources of variation. Exogenous
forces are able to overcome endogenous forces, bringing about conformity
with local practice (Long 2002). From this viewpoint, the physician resource
demand model suggests that physicians demand resources consistent with
patients' clinical needs but modified by local exogenous influences, including
patient–agency constraints (e.g., patients' financial resources and access to
care), organizational constraints (e.g., policies and protocols), and environmental constraints (e.g., surgeons, hospital beds, other facilities per capita)
(Long 2002). These exogenous factors might influence physician behavior
in multiple ways, and the resulting behavior may contribute to local variation. For example, physicians might choose to practice in a particular area or
organization to be able to exercise their aggressive/nonaggressive intervention style, or they might adapt to the style of the community where they
settle. Physicians might also adapt their practices to local patient expectations
and demands or adapt to local market forces to maintain their income (e.g.,
shortening patient follow-up intervals when practicing in an area with a large
number of physicians per capita to keep a full schedule) (Sirovich et al. 2008).

Hospitals and physician practices might similarly be influenced by
exogenous factors compelling them to comply with a local standard. For
example, those in high-spending, high-healthcare-density areas might be
subject to greater competitive stresses and might pressure physicians to order
profitable services, while less availability of such services in low-spending
areas could dissuade physicians from ordering them (Sirovich et al. 2008).
Certainly, overall practice intensity is strongly correlated with local healthcare
spending; physicians in all areas are equally likely to recommend guideline-
supported interventions, but those in high-spending areas see patients more
frequently, recommend more tests of uncertain benefit, and opt for more
resource-intensive interventions without achieving improved patient outcomes (Fisher et al. 2003; Sirovich et al. 2008).

Applying Evidence of Unwarranted Variation to Quality Improvement

Unlike patient safety and "appropriate use" studies, practice variation studies compare utilization rates in a given setting or by a given provider to an
average utilization rate rather than impose a rate based on expert opinion
of best practices (Parente, Phelps, and O'Connor 2008). Policymakers
and managers can use these data-driven studies to pinpoint areas of care in
which best practices may need to be identified or—if they have already been

identified—implemented (Parente, Phelps, and O'Connor 2008). Appropriate use and patient safety studies constitute the next level of analysis once best practices have been established and serve as ongoing performance management tools (Parente, Phelps, and O'Connor 2008).

Where best practices have been identified (i.e., effective care), a common approach to decreasing unwarranted variation/increasing the quality of care is the development of clinical guidelines (Timmermans and Mauck 2005). However, the development and availability of clinical guidelines are often insufficient to align practice with scientific standards due to numerous factors, including physician inertia, uncertainty regarding the knowledge base for the guidelines, the perception that guidelines "deskill" physicians through the introduction of "cookbook medicine," and physicians' common perception that their practice is already consistent with best practices (Kennedy, Leathley, and Hughes 2010; Timmermans and Mauck 2005). Moreover, the "evidence-based bandwagon" has become so popular and so many guidelines have been produced by individuals, organizations, and insurers that the benefits of consistency may disappear under the confusion of overlapping, poorly constructed practice standards (Timmermans and Mauck 2005).

Other strategies hospitals have used to reduce unwarranted variation in effective care include benchmarking and report cards, academic detailing, and pay-for-performance programs (Gauld et al. 2011). Additional recommendations for tackling underuse include establishing the necessary infrastructure for systemic implementation of evidence-based clinical guidelines and regionalization of care for procedures for which higher use by hospitals and physicians is associated with better outcomes (e.g., complex cardiovascular or thoracic surgeries such as esophagectomy, open descending thoracic aortic aneurysm repair, aortic root replacement, and open and endovascular abdominal aortic aneurysm repair) (Allareddy and Konety 2007; Brooke et al. 2008; Hughes et al. 2013; Schermerhorn et al. 2008; Wennberg 2004). However, the ability to monitor variation patterns and relate them to outcomes is limited to hospital systems that have the infrastructure (e.g., electronic health records [EHRs] and data analysts) necessary to collect and analyze these data on an ongoing basis (Gauld et al. 2011).

Where unwarranted variation is identified in preference-sensitive care, improvement calls for comparative effectiveness research to elucidate differences between available treatment options and thus enable selection of the option that best addresses the patient's concerns and priorities; this research needs to be complemented by increased involvement of patients in treatment choices (Ham 2011). To date, much of the research related to unwarranted variation has focused on physician/hospital/healthcare system behavior, treating the patient as inert; however, hospitals report including initiatives to increase patient engagement and education in their quality improvement strategies focused on unwarranted variation (Gauld et al. 2011; Greer et al. 2002). Ironically, while informed patient involvement decreases unwarranted variation in preference-sensitive care (bringing utilization rates into line with patient preferences), it might increase total variation because the preferences of patients coming from varied backgrounds and contexts might be more diverse than those of their physicians, who generally have similar educational backgrounds and training (Greer et al. 2002).

With respect to unwarranted variation in supply-sensitive care, quality improvement strategies need to target the issue of overuse—for example, eliminating inappropriate use of percutaneous coronary intervention (Ballard and Leonard 2011). Thus, two types of research are needed to propel meaningful quality improvement: (1) outcomes research to determine whether the observed unwarranted variation represents inappropriate rationing of particular resources in low-utilization regions or overuse in high-utilization regions and (2) effectiveness or comparative effectiveness research that provides the evidence base needed to convert supply-sensitive care into effective or preference-sensitive care (O'Connor et al. 2009). To achieve the latter goal, basic mechanisms must be put in place to ensure the orderly evaluation of new technologies and clinical theories (Wennberg 2004). Other necessary reforms include integrating primary and specialty care in organized systems that coordinate care, rationalizing clinical pathways for managing chronic illnesses, and adjusting capacity to reflect efficient use of resources (i.e., reducing acute care capacity toward the population benchmarks of efficient providers—an action that current reimbursement systems are not designed to reward) (Wennberg 2011, 2004). Overuse research is needed to support these efforts. To date, such research has been scarce because it faces the quadruple challenge of

1. requiring detailed and historical clinical data to estimate overuse;
2. lacking national guidelines for appropriate use of many procedures;
3. confronting physician skepticism and hostility based on the mistaken impression that such research contains an implicit suggestion that overuse results primarily from physicians' self-interest in generating income; and
4. surmounting political barriers, such as the lobbying efforts of the North American Spine Society (NASS) in response to guidelines and underlying research recommending nonsurgical approaches in the initial management of acute back problems (perceived as threatening NASS's scope or practice), which led to zero-funding—and the functional demise—of the Agency for Healthcare Research and Quality's predecessor in 1996 (Keyhani and Siu 2008).

Policy reforms will also be needed to alleviate political pressure from special interest groups on the Centers for Medicare & Medicaid Services (CMS) to reimburse for tests and treatments of unclear benefit, which contribute to the unnecessary use—and expense—of health services (Keyhani and Siu 2008).

Scope and Use of Variation in Healthcare

Quality researchers use a variety of indicators to measure improvements and detect variation in the quality of care, including fiscal, service, and clinical indicators. Hospital-based clinical indicators, for example, include the process and outcome measures for acute myocardial infarction (AMI), community-acquired pneumonia, congestive heart failure, and surgical care improvement projects publicly reported on the US Department of Health and Human Services' Hospital Compare website (HHS 2013). Organizations can define thresholds for such measures that indicate satisfactory compliance with acceptable standards of care (Ballard 2003). For example, one process-of-care measure for AMI is the administration of beta-blockers within 24 hours of admission; if the threshold is set at 90 percent of admitted AMI patients, hospitals that fall below it are effectively "on notice" to improve the quality of AMI care. Beyond compliance with such condition-specific standards of care, the Institute of Medicine (2001) has established six aims for healthcare improvement to ensure that medical care is safe, timely, effective, efficient, equitable, and patient centered. Quality indicators that address these domains span several clinical areas that must be aggregated to assess a hospital's time-dependent quality of care.

Variability plays an obvious role in identifying, measuring, and reporting these quality indicators (Goldberg et al. 1994). For example, even within a single hospital system, differences in patient mix between facilities may create the appearance of variation in performance between hospitals if adjustment for patient mix is inadequate. The same may be true for a single facility over time. Consequently, some healthcare services administrators are reluctant to use quality indicators, perceiving them as biased toward large academic medical centers or large healthcare organizations, which are less subject to changes in underlying factors such as patient mix (Miller et al. 2001). However, analytical techniques and appropriate indicators that are sensitive only to unwarranted variation can be successfully applied to small organizations and practices, including single-physician practices, facilitating their efforts to maintain or improve the quality of care they provide (Geyman 1998; Miller et al. 2001).

An important issue to keep in mind is that the vantage point from which healthcare managers and quality improvement staff view and seek to use data regarding variation in healthcare processes is different from that of health services researchers (Neuhauser, Provost, and Bergman 2011). Where practical, real-time quality improvement is the goal, variation itself needs to be examined in real time to answer the questions (1) are we getting better? and (2) where can we improve? Thus, "just-in-time" performance data are essential to the effective use of variation data, and the focus is on creating stable processes and learning from *special-cause variation*—variation that stems from causes external to the core processes of the work (Neuhauser, Provost, and Bergman 2011). In contrast, health services researchers pose the question, does A cause B (other things being equal)?, often taking the long view to examine several years' worth of data and seeking to eliminate special-cause variation and test for significance (Neuhauser, Provost, and Bergman 2011).

These different perspectives can lead healthcare managers and health services researchers to look at the same set of results and reach very different conclusions about their significance and the actions that should be taken in response. For example, if research showed that age and sex predict patient outcomes following hip surgery and, in particular, explain 10 percent of the variation seen in early ambulation, a health services researcher might conclude that more variables need to be measured so that more variation can be explained and a better understanding of what influences this postsurgical outcome can be gained. Meanwhile, the healthcare manager focused on real-time quality improvement might note that the 90 percent unexplained variation could be *common-cause variation*—the expected random variation seen in all healthcare processes—and conclude that the process is sound and under control (Neuhauser, Provost, and Bergman 2011).

Clinical and Operational Issues

Implementing best practices, establishing clinical indicators, and measuring and interpreting variation are not enough; a healthcare organization must also direct considerable effort toward creating and maintaining an environment conducive to sustaining these quality improvement efforts, and an organization's size and complexity create functional, geographic, and other systemic constraints to success. The ability to collect appropriate and accurate data that can be rigorously analyzed depends on diligent planning (Ballard 2003). Patient demographics and case mix affect the data to be studied and can arbitrarily skew study conclusions. These factors need to be accounted for when one is monitoring or comparing performance on the chosen quality indicators to ensure that quality improvement efforts are targeting unwarranted variation in the quality of care provided and not reacting to underlying changes in the patient population.

Organizational Size

The size of an organization affects its ability to disseminate best practices. One group of physicians in a large healthcare delivery system may have developed an effective method to achieve high levels of colorectal cancer screening, but an initiative to describe, champion, and implement such process redesign across dozens of other groups within the system is challenging and typically requires incremental resource commitment (Stroud, Felton, and Spreadbury 2003). Large organizations tend to have rigid frameworks or bureaucracies; change is slow and requires perseverance and the ability to make clear to skeptics as well as enthusiasts the value of the new procedure in their group and across the system. Small practices bring their own challenges to effective change, especially if their small group of decision makers is unwilling or uninterested in pursuing quality improvements.

Large organizations have both the potential and the need for multiple layers of quality assessment. For example, an integrated delivery system that includes acute care hospitals, rehabilitation facilities, and ambulatory care physician practices must evaluate the quality of care at these different levels as well as quality related to communication and movement between these levels. Different quality indicators and quality improvement efforts are needed to capture relevant information and effect necessary changes in these different settings.

Organizational Commitment

An organization's capacity for quality monitoring and improvement depends on its size and infrastructure. As value-based purchasing comes increasingly into play, an organization's survival will depend on its ability to monitor and improve its quality of care and resulting patient outcomes. Even prior to mandated minimum standards of quality in reimbursement schemes, a number of hospitals and delivery systems chose to apply quality threshold levels because of the compelling business case to do so: Satisfied patients return for additional care or recommend that friends and relatives use the same services (Ballard 2003; Holtz and de Vol 2013; Stroud, Felton and Spreadbury 2003).

Planning the collection and analysis of suitable data for quality measures requires significant forethought to minimize the indicators' sensitivity to warranted variation and ensures that changes detected truly relate to the quality of care provided. This planning includes selecting appropriate measures, controlling for case mix and other variables, minimizing chance variability, and collecting high-quality data (Powell, Davies, and Thomson 2003).

The importance of careful planning is demonstrated by a study that compared generalists' and endocrinologists' treatment of patients with diabetes. The initial results showed what most people would expect—that specialists provided better care. However, following adjustment for patient case mix and clustering (physician-level variation), there was no significant difference between generalists' and endocrinologists' treatment of diabetes patients. Such quality assessment studies must be designed with sufficient power and sophistication to account for a variety of confounding factors; one necessity is inclusion of sufficient numbers of physicians and patients per physician to prevent the distortion of differences in quality that can arise when the group of study subjects is small (Greenfield et al. 2002).

Strength of Data

The data used for any quality assessment must be a representative sample. Clinicians and administrators will be reluctant to accept results as valid and requiring quality improvement action if they consider them to be based on data suffering from selection bias, collection errors, or other inaccuracies. For example, despite the impartiality of external record abstractors in gathering data from patient medical charts, critics may claim that these independent abstractors lack an insider's understanding or that they select data to fit an agenda, affecting the results unpredictably. Patient socioeconomic status, age, gender, and ethnicity also influence physician profiles in medical practice variation and analysis efforts (Franks and Fiscella 2002).

Keys to Successful Implementation and Lessons Learned from Failures

Despite the appeal of quality improvement projects, considerable barriers and limitations can impede successful implementation. These barriers are subject to or the result of variation in culture, infrastructure, and economic influences across an organization, and overcoming them requires a stable infrastructure, sustained funding, and the testing of sequential hypotheses on how to improve care.

Administrative and Physician Views

Quality improvement efforts must consider organizational mind-set, administrative and physician worldviews, and patient knowledge and expectations. Their pace is subject to considerable variability in an organization's propensity to change. One example from a primary care setting demonstrated that screening for colorectal cancer improved steadily from 47 to 86 percent over a two-year period (Stroud, Felton, and Spreadbury 2003). This relatively rapid change was possible because it was collaborative, simple, and made good business sense and because the intervention in question was not dependent on scheduled annual patient visits or preventive care visits.

Successful conversion of daily practice requires patience and a long-term vision. Many decision makers expect immediate and significant results and are sensitive to short-term variation that suggests the improvements may be fleeting or not cost-effective. A monthly drop in screening rates, for example, could be viewed as an indication that the screening protocol is not working and should be modified or abandoned altogether to conserve resources. The observed decrease also could be random variation and no cause for alarm or change (Wheeler 2000). Cultural tolerance to variation and change is critical to the successful implementation of quality improvement efforts and can be cultivated by systemic adjustments and educational and motivational interventions (Donabedian and Bashur 2003; Palmer, Donabedian, and Povar 1991).

Physicians often think in terms of treating disease on an individual basis rather than in terms of population-based preventive care. Cultural change is thus required to reduce undesired variation or create new and successful preventive systems of clinical care and achieve physician buy-in to the new model (Stroud, Felton, and Spreadbury 2003). One method of achieving this change that has proven successful is training physician champions who then serve as models, mentors, and motivators to other physicians, thereby reducing the risk of alienating these key players in quality improvement efforts. Physicians' failure—or refusal—to follow best practices is often inextricably linked to the presence—or absence—of role models who have both the subject matter expertise and professional respect of their peers (Mottur-Pilson, Snow, and Bartlett 2001).

Organizational Mind-Set

Organizational infrastructure is an essential component in minimizing unwarranted variation, disseminating best practices, and supporting a research agenda associated with quality improvements. EHRs, computerized provider order entry systems, and clinical decision support tools may reduce errors, allow specific best practices to be shared across large organizations, and enable widespread automated collection of data to support quality improvement research (Bates and Gawande 2003; Casalino et al. 2003; Dutton and Dukatz 2011; Garg et al. 2005). Healthcare organizations therefore are addressing the challenge to articulate and implement a long-term strategy to employ EHR resources. Unfortunately, the economic implications of both short- and long-term infrastructure investments undermine these efforts. Working in an environment that embraces short-term financial gain (in the form of either the quarterly report to stockholders or the report to the chairman of the board), physicians and hospital administrators "often face an outright disincentive to invest in an infrastructure that will improve compliance with best practices" (Leatherman et al. 2003).

However, those same economic incentives may effectively address variation in healthcare by awarding financial bonuses to physicians and administrators who meet quality targets or by withholding bonuses from those who do not. This approach communicates that future success within an organization is dependent on participating in quality improvement efforts, reducing undesirable variation in processes of care, and cultivating an environment conducive to quality research and improvement. The goals of such incentives are to help people understand that their organization is serious about implementing quality changes and minimizing unwanted variation to ensure alignment with national standards and directions in quality of care as well as to encourage them to use an organization's resources to achieve this alignment (Casalino et al. 2003). Moreover, with the introduction of the CMS value-based purchasing scheme—under which hospitals receive incentive payments (or not) based on their performance/improvement on 12 clinical process measures and 9 patient experience measures—successful quality improvement becomes critical to the survival of the hospital as a whole, not just to the individual's success in the organization (Shoemaker 2011).

Examples of Quality Improvement Efforts Applying Variation

Hospitals and healthcare systems as well as health services researchers are using variation data in a variety of ways and across many clinical fields to identify, implement, and evaluate quality improvement efforts. For example, examination of coronary angiography data from 691 US hospitals in the CathPCI Registry revealed that the rate of finding obstructive coronary artery disease (CAD) varied between hospitals, from a low of 23 percent to a high of 100 percent (Douglas et al. 2011). Upon further investigation, the researchers discovered that this variation was not random but rather was associated with the hospitals' patient selection and preprocedural assessment strategies. This discovery revealed opportunities to reduce the number of unnecessary procedures prescribed (which place patients at unnecessary, if minimal, risk and incur unnecessary costs for the healthcare system) (Douglas et al. 2011). Specifically, if the "low-finding" centers implemented referral strategies used by the "high-finding" centers such that the median rate of obstructive CAD finding reached 70 percent, the number of patients undergoing cardiac angiography that does not find obstructive CAD could be reduced from approximately 280,000 to 85,000. Even with the less ambitious target of raising the finding rates for hospitals in the two lowest quartiles to the national median (45 percent), the number of coronary angiographies without a finding of obstructive CAD would drop by 23 percent.

In other words, between one-quarter and one-third of cardiac angiographies performed may be unnecessary, and their elimination could improve the safety and efficiency of care (Douglas et al. 2011).

A second example of research revealing opportunities for improvement based on variation is the Florida Initiative for Quality Cancer Care's finding of highly variable rates of documentation of key variables in the medical charts of 622 breast cancer patients (Gray et al. 2011). While the performance rates of these key variables (e.g., sentinel node biopsy) may well be more consistent than the documentation, accurate and complete documentation is necessary for good quality care—and for accurate measurement of the quality of care provided (Gray et al. 2011).

In other cases, opportunities for improvement have not merely been identified; the relevant healthcare organization has also taken steps to address the unwarranted variation observed. For example, following observation of wide variation in specialist referrals between primary care physicians (PCPs), primary care practices partnered with specialist consultants in the Gwent Healthcare National Health Service Trust in the United Kingdom to examine the quality of the referrals and implement strategies to improve PCPs' referral practices (Evans, Aiking, and Edwards 2011). The referral management strategy they designed incorporated peer review/audit of referrals (supported by feedback from the specialists) and provided clear referral criteria and evidence-based guidelines. At the practice level, the result of this strategy was a decrease in the median referral rate from 5.5 per 1,000 patients per quarter to 4.3 per 1,000 patients per quarter and a reduction in variability from 2.6–7.7 per 1,000 patients per quarter to 3.0–6.5 per 1,000 patients per quarter (Evans, Aiking, and Edwards 2011). General surgery referrals decreased by 5 percent; ophthalmology, dermatology, and orthopedic referrals decreased by 11 to 13 percent each; and neurology referrals decreased by 16 percent. Anomalously, ear/nose/throat referrals increased by 26 percent (Evans, Aiking, and Edwards 2011). The PCPs' own assessment of the quality of their referrals was that they had improved: The proportion of referrals for which they agreed that complete information was provided in the referral letter increased from 89 to 95 percent, and the proportion for which they agreed that the appropriate work-up was completed before referral increased from 86 to 94 percent (Evans, Aiking, and Edwards 2011).

Intermountain Healthcare (IHC), a large healthcare delivery system in Utah, has effectively used variation data to identify and address opportunities for quality improvement. The quality improvement team started by looking at practice variation in common care processes, revealed by chart review. While the team found no evidence that one physician's patients demonstrated higher degrees of severity or complexity than did other physicians' patients, it saw "massive" variation in physician practices (James and Savitz

2011). Specifically, when the team examined patients with similar admissions and good outcomes, the highest rates of use of common care processes examined were 1.6 to 5.6 times higher than the lowest rates of use, and hospital costs per case (other than physician payment) varied twofold (James and Savitz 2011). To address this variation, IHC focused on the processes underlying the particular treatments (rather than on the physicians exercising them), implementing tools such as a guideline for treatment of respiratory distress embedded in checklists, order sets, and clinical flow sheets to help standardize practices (James and Savitz 2011). Following initial implementation, the quality improvement team examined variation again, this time looking at the adaptations clinicians had made to the guideline in applying it to their patients. These data were fed back to the patient care team, which led in some cases to modification of the guideline to more accurately reflect the realities of care and in others to modification of clinician practice. This method, which IHC refers to as "shared baselines," achieved a reduction in guideline variance from 59 to 6 percent in four months, with an accompanying increase in survival in the subcategory of patients seriously ill with acute respiratory distress from 9.5 to 44 percent and a 25 percent decrease in the total cost of care (James and Savitz 2011). A similar process was used to successfully reduce variation in clinicians' use of elective inductions of labor; the proportion of elective inductions that did not meet strong indications for clinical appropriateness decreased from 28 percent to less than 2 percent (James and Savitz 2011).

Baylor Health Care System Case Study

According to 2005–2008 National Health and Nutrition Examination Survey data, an estimated 5.7 million American adults have heart failure (HF), and it is estimated that by 2030 this number could rise to 10 million (Roger et al. 2012). There is substantial evidence that HF mortality and morbidity can be reduced through angiotensin-converting enzyme inhibitor (ACEI) or angiotensin receptor blocker (ARB) therapy, beta-blocker therapy, and other treatment modalities (CIBIS-II Investigators and Committees 1999; CONSENSUS Trial Study Group 1987; Fonarow et al. 2004; Hjalmarson et al. 2000; SOLVD Investigators 1991), and clinical practice guidelines strongly recommend such therapies as part of the standard care for HF (Hunt et al. 2009). Yet these evidence-based therapies were inconsistently used at the turn of the twenty-first century; specifically, they were underutilized in HF patients who did not have contraindications against these therapies (Fonarow 2002; Masoudi et al. 2004). For example, studies on HF patients who required hospitalization showed that only 60 to 80 percent of eligible patients were prescribed ACEIs and beta-blockers at discharge, 24 to 55 percent received discharge instructions, 86 to 88 percent underwent left ventricular function assessment, and 43 to 72 percent received smoking cessation counseling (Ahmed et al. 2002; Fonarow et al. 2007, 2004; Fonarow, Yancy, and Heywood 2005; Jencks, Huff, and Cuerdon 2003; Williams et al. 2005); and in 2005, only 57.3 percent of HF patients treated in nonfederal US hospitals received all process-of-care measures for which they were eligible (Vogeli et al. 2009).

At Baylor Health Care System (BHCS), an integrated healthcare delivery system in North Texas, compliance with treatment recommendations as well as mortality and costs of care for adult pneumonia patients improved following widespread adoption of a standardized pneumonia order set (Ballard et al. 2008; Fleming, Masica, and McCarthy 2013; Fleming, Ogola, and Ballard 2009). When routine monitoring of quality-of-care indicators showed inconsistent use of evidence-based HF therapies despite relatively constant characteristics of the HF patient population, BHCS developed and implemented a standardized order set for HF care across its eight acute care and two specialty heart hospitals as part of a system-wide improvement initiative focused on HF (Ballard et al. 2010). This intervention and its impact on HF mortality, readmissions, lengths of stay, and costs of care have been detailed elsewhere (Ballard et al. 2010; Fleming, Masica, and McCarthy 2013). The impact of the order set on compliance with evidence-based recommendations for HF care was measured in terms of administration of an "all-or-none bundle," calculated as the proportion of HF patients who received all HF measures for which they were eligible as identified in the *Specifications Manual for National Hospital Quality Measures* (used for public reporting of quality data on the Hospital Compare website), including discharge instructions, evaluation of left ventricular function, ACEI or ARB for left ventricular systolic dysfunction, and smoking cessation counseling (QualityNet 2012). The findings showed a reduction in in-hospital mortality and hospital costs that, if applied nationally, would have translated into annual savings of 15,147 lives and $1.9 billion dollars (Ballard et al. 2010).

The BHCS standardized HF order set was developed internally but based on the prevailing American College of Cardiology/American Heart Association clinical practice guidelines, and the order set was deployed system-wide via the intranet physician portal in December 2007 (Ballard et al. 2010). By June 2008, physicians were using the order set for approximately 50 percent of eligible patients; a patient was not eligible if (1) the diagnosis of HF was made after admission orders were written by the attending physician (not the emergency department physician), (2) both HF and pneumonia were present on admission and the physician used the BHCS pneumonia order set, or (3) the patient was admitted for an elective implantable cardioverter defibrillator placement and other order sets were in place for the specific procedure (Ballard et al. 2010).

Variability in system-wide performance on administration of the HF all-or-none bundle was assessed using a statistical process control p-chart (see Exhibit 3.1). Central tendency and upper and lower control limits were calculated separately for 18-month periods before and after implementation of the HF order set. The p-chart shows that the overall proportion of HF patients receiving all indicated services for the 18-month period preceding order set implementation (July 2006 through December 2007) was 0.85. More noteworthy, though, is the highly variable nature of the measure during this period, as evidenced by the sharp month-to-month variability as well as two points that fall outside the control limits (September 2006 and November 2007) (Hart and Hart 2001). During the period following deployment of the HF order set, the chart shows not only higher mean compliance (0.92) but also less variation in compliance with administration of the all-or-none bundle, as indicated by the narrower control limits, the lack of points falling outside the control limits, and a smoother line. The sharpness observed in the first few months of the postimplementation period can be somewhat explained by the fact that 50 percent usage of the order set was not achieved until May 2008. Both the decreased variability and the change in mean provide evidence of improved compliance with administration of the HF all-or-none bundle (and thus, presumptively, improvement in the quality of care provided) following order set deployment.

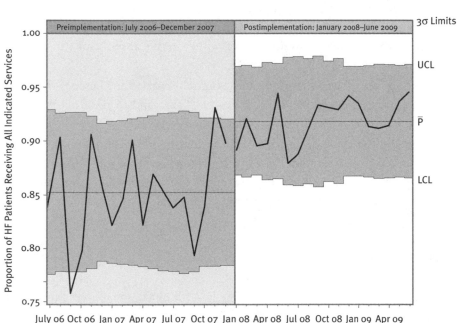

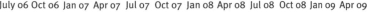

EXHIBIT 3.1
p-Chart Showing the Proportion of HF Patients Receiving All Evidence-Based HF Processes of Care for Which They Were Eligible Before and After Deployment of the BHCS Standardized HF Order Set

Note: UCL = upper control limit; LCL = lower control limit.

Conclusion

Contemporary industrial and commercial quality improvement methods (e.g., Six Sigma) emphasize the need to minimize variation, if not eliminate it altogether. Although appropriate in a setting characterized by repetitive manufacturing of mass quantities of identical products, these tools may unnecessarily mask variation in the healthcare environment and consequently obscure opportunities to change or improve essential processes of care. The keys to successful management—rather than elimination—of variation in pursuit of quality healthcare are the ability to identify variation; distinguish between random and assignable variation; determine the meaning, importance, or value of the observed variation relative to some standard (i.e., distinguish between warranted and unwarranted variation); and implement methods that will take advantage of or rectify what the variation reveals. Ultimately, variation tells us what is working and what is not, and how far from optimal our healthcare processes are. Rather than avoid variation in pursuit of quality healthcare, we should embrace it as a useful guide on our pathway to success.

Study Questions

1. While exploring opportunities to improve processes of care for a group practice, you find no variability in compliance with the US Preventive Services Task Force's recommendations for colorectal cancer screening across the practice's physicians over time. Is this absence of variation optimal? Why or why not?
2. Distinguish between random and assignable variation. Discuss the relevance of each to measuring quality of care and to the design and evaluation of quality improvement initiatives.
3. Describe the three categories of care identified by Wennberg (2011), the possible opportunities for improvement unwarranted variation might indicate in each of these categories, and the goals of health services research and quality improvement initiatives in each category.

References

Ahmed, A., R. M. Allman, J. F. DeLong, E. V. Bodner, and G. Howard. 2002. "Age-Related Underutilization of Angiotensin-Converting Enzyme Inhibitors in Older Hospitalized Heart Failure Patients." *Southern Medical Journal* 95 (7): 703–10.

Allareddy, V., and B. R. Konety. 2007. "Specificity of Procedure Volume and In-Hospital Mortality Association." *Annals of Surgery* 246 (1): 135–39.

Ballard, D. J. 2003. "Indicators to Improve Clinical Quality Across an Integrated Health Care System." *International Journal for Quality in Health Care* 15 (Suppl. 1): i13–23.

Ballard, D. J., G. Filardo, B. da Graca, and J. T. Powell. 2012. "Clinical Practice Change Requires More Than Comparative Effectiveness Evidence: Abdominal Aortic Aneurysm Management in the USA." *Journal of Comparative Effectiveness Research* 1 (1): 31–44.

Ballard, D. J., and B. M. Leonard. 2011. "National Priorities Partnership Focus on Eliminating Overuse: Applications to Cardiac Revascularization." *American Journal of Medical Quality* 26 (6): 485–90.

Ballard, D. J., G. Ogola, N. S. Fleming, D. Heck, J. Gunderson, R. Mehta, R. Khetan, and J. D. Kerr. 2008. "The Impact of Standardized Order Sets on Quality and Financial Outcomes." *Advances in Patient Safety: New Directions and Alternative Approaches*, vols. 1–4. Rockville, MD: Agency for Healthcare Research and Quality.

Ballard, D. J., G. Ogola, N. S. Fleming, B. D. Stauffer, B. M. Leonard, R. Khetan, and C. W. Yancy. 2010. "Impact of a Standardized Heart Failure Order Set on Mortality, Readmission, and Quality and Costs of Care." *International Journal for Quality in Health Care* 22 (6): 437–44.

Bates, D. W., and A. A. Gawande. 2003. "Improving Safety with Information Technology." *New England Journal of Medicine* 348 (25): 2526–34.

Bojakowski, S. 2010. "Managing the Paradox Between Equality and Diversity in Healthcare: Unwarranted vs. Warranted Variations." *Journal of Management & Marketing Healthcare* 3 (4): 241–47.

Brooke, B. S., B. A. Perler, F. Dominici, M. A. Makary, and P. J. Pronovost. 2008. "Reduction of In-Hospital Mortality Among California Hospitals Meeting Leapfrog Evidence-Based Standards for Abdominal Aortic Aneurysm Repair." *Journal of Vascular Surgery* 47 (6): 1155–56; discussion 1163–64.

Casalino, L., R. R. Gillies, S. M. Shortell, J. A. Schmittdiel, T. Bodenheimer, J. C. Robinson, T. Rundall, N. Oswald, H. Schauffler, and M. C. Wang. 2003. "External Incentives, Information Technology, and Organized Processes to Improve Health Care Quality for Patients with Chronic Diseases." *Journal of the American Medical Association* 289 (4): 434–41.

Chalkidou, K. 2009. *Comparative Effectiveness Review Within the U.K.'s National Institute for Health and Clinical Excellence.* Issue brief. Pub. 1296, vol. 59. New York: The Commonwealth Fund.

CIBIS-II Investigators and Committees. 1999. "The Cardiac Insufficiency Bisoprolol Study II (CIBIS-II): A Randomised Trial." *Lancet* 353 (9146): 9–13.

CONSENSUS Trial Study Group. 1987. "Effects of Enalapril on Mortality in Severe Congestive Heart Failure. Results of the Cooperative North Scandinavian

Enalapril Survival Study (CONSENSUS)." *New England Journal of Medicine* 316 (23): 1429–35.

Davis, P., B. Gribben, A. Scott, and R. Lay-Yee. 2000. "The 'Supply Hypothesis' and Medical Practice Variation in Primary Care: Testing Economic and Clinical Models of Inter-Practitioner Variation." *Social Science & Medicine* 50 (3): 407–18.

Donabedian, A., and R. Bashur (eds.). 2003. *An Introduction to Quality Assurance in Health Care.* New York: Oxford University Press.

Douglas, P. S., M. R. Patel, S. R. Bailey, D. Dai, L. Kaltenbach, R. G. Brindis, J. Messenger, and E. D. Peterson. 2011. "Hospital Variability in the Rate of Finding Obstructive Coronary Artery Disease at Elective, Diagnostic Coronary Angiography." *Journal of the American College of Cardiology* 58 (8): 801–9.

Dutton, R. P., and A. Dukatz. 2011. "Quality Improvement Using Automated Data Sources: The Anesthesia Quality Institute." *Anesthesiology Clinics* 29 (3): 439–54.

Eddy, D. M. 1984. "Variations in Physician Practice: The Role of Uncertainty." *Health Affairs (Millwood)* 3 (2): 74–89.

Evans, E., H. Aiking, and A. Edwards. 2011. "Reducing Variation in General Practitioner Referral Rates Through Clinical Engagement and Peer Review of Referrals: A Service Improvement Project." *Quality in Primary Care* 19 (4): 263–72.

Fisher, E. S., D. E. Wennberg, T. A. Stukel, D. J. Gottlieb, F. L. Lucas, and E. L. Pinder. 2003. "The Implications of Regional Variations in Medicare Spending. Part 2: Health Outcomes and Satisfaction with Care." *Annals of Internal Medicine* 138 (4): 288–98.

Fleming, N. S., A. Masica, and I. McCarthy. 2013. "Evaluation of Clinical, Economic, and Financial Outcomes." In *Achieving STEEEP Health Care*, edited by D. J. Ballard, N. S. Fleming, J. T. Allison, P. B. Convery, and R. Luquire, 85–92. Boca Raton, FL: CRC Press.

Fleming, N. S., G. Ogola, and D. J. Ballard. 2009. "Implementing a Standardized Order Set for Community Acquired Pneumonia: Impact on Mortality and Cost." *Joint Commission Journal on Quality and Patient Safety* 35 (8): 414–21.

Fonarow, G. C. 2002. "The Role of In-Hospital Initiation of Cardioprotective Therapies to Improve Treatment Rates and Clinical Outcomes." *Reviews in Cardiovascular Medicine* 3 (Suppl. 3): S2–S10.

Fonarow, G. C., W. T. Abraham, N. M. Albert, W. Gattis Stough, M. Gheorghiade, B. H. Greenberg, C. M. O'Connor, K. Pieper, J. L. Sun, C. W. Yancy, and J. B. Young; OPTIMIZE-HF Investigators and Hospitals. 2007. "Influence of a Performance-Improvement Initiative on Quality of Care for Patients Hospitalized with Heart Failure: Results of the Organized Program to Initiate Lifesaving Treatment in Hospitalized Patients with Heart Failure (OPTIMIZE-HF)." *Archives of Internal Medicine* 167 (14): 1493–502.

Fonarow, G. C., W. T. Abraham, N. M. Albert, W. A. Gattis, M. Gheorghiade, B. Greenberg, C. M. O'Connor, C. W. Yancy, and J. Young. 2004. "Organized Program to Initiate Lifesaving Treatment in Hospitalized Patients with Heart Failure (OPTIMIZE-HF): Rationale and Design." *American Heart Journal* 148 (1): 43–51.

Fonarow, G. C., C. W. Yancy, and J. T. Heywood. 2005. "Adherence to Heart Failure Quality-of-Care Indicators in US Hospitals: Analysis of the ADHERE Registry." *Archives of Internal Medicine* 165 (13): 1469–77.

Franks, P., and K. Fiscella. 2002. "Effect of Patient Socioeconomic Status on Physician Profiles for Prevention, Disease Management, and Diagnostic Testing Costs." *Medical Care* 40 (8): 717–24.

Garg, A. X., N. K. Adhikari, H. McDonald, M. P. Rosas-Arellano, P. J. Devereaux, J. Beyene, J. Sam, and R. B. Haynes. 2005. "Effects of Computerized Clinical Decision Support Systems on Practitioner Performance and Patient Outcomes: A Systematic Review." *Journal of the American Medical Association* 293 (10): 1223–38.

Gauld, R., J. Horwitt, S. Williams, and A. B. Cohen. 2011. "What Strategies Do US Hospitals Employ to Reduce Unwarranted Clinical Practice Variations?" *American Journal of Medical Quality* 26 (2): 120–26.

Geyman, J. P. 1998. "Evidence-Based Medicine in Primary Care: An Overview." *Journal of the American Board of Family Practice* 11 (1): 46–56.

Glover, J. A. 1938. "The Incidence of Tonsillectomy in School Children (Section of Epidemiology and State Medicine)." *Proceedings of the Royal Society of Medicine* 31 (10): 1219–36.

Goldberg, H. I., M. A. Cummings, E. P. Steinberg, E. M. Ricci, T. Shannon, S. B. Soumerai, B. S. Mittman, J. Eisenberg, D. A. Heck, S. Kaplan, J. E. Kenzora, A. M. Vargus, A. G. Mulley, and B. K. Rimer. 1994. "Deliberations on the Dissemination of PORT Products: Translating Research Findings into Improved Patient Outcomes." *Medical Care* 32 (7 Suppl.): JS90–110.

Goodman, D. C. 2009. "Unwarranted Variation in Pediatric Medical Care." *Pediatric Clinics of North America* 56 (4): 745–55.

Goodman, D. C., A. R. Esty, E. S. Fisher, and C.-H. Chang. 2011. *Trends and Variation in End-of-Life Care for Medicare Beneficiaries with Severe Chronic Illness.* Lebanon, NH: Dartmouth Institute for Health Policy & Clinical Practice.

Gray, J. E., C. Laronga, E. M. Siegel, J-H. Lee, W. J. Fulp, M. Fletcher, F. Schreiber, R. Brown, R. Levine, T. Cartwright, G. Abesada-Terk Jr., G. Kim, C. Alemany, D. Faig, P. Sharp, M-J. Markham, D. Shibata, M. Malafa, and P. B. Jacobsen. 2011. "Degree of Variability in Performance on Breast Cancer Quality Indicators: Findings from the Florida Initiative for Quality Cancer Care." *Journal of Oncology Practice* 7 (4): 247–51.

Greenfield, S., S. H. Kaplan, R. Kahn, J. Ninomiya, and J. L. Griffith. 2002. "Profiling Care Provided by Different Groups of Physicians: Effects of Patient

Case-Mix (Bias) and Physician-Level Clustering on Quality Assessment Results." *Annals of Internal Medicine* 136 (2): 111–21.

Greer, A. L., J. S. Goodwin, J. L. Freeman, and Z. H. Wu. 2002. "Bringing the Patient Back In. Guidelines, Practice Variations, and the Social Context of Medical Practice." *International Journal of Technology Assessment in Health Care* 18 (4): 747–61.

Ham, C. 2011. "A Roadmap for Health System Reform." *British Medical Journal* 342: d1757.

Hart, M. K., and R. E. Hart. 2001. *Statistical Process Control for Health Care.* St. Paul, MN: Brooks/Cole Publishing Co.

Hjalmarson, A., S. Goldstein, B. Fagerberg, H. Wedel, F. Waagstein, J. Kjekshus, J. Wikstrand, D. El Allaf, J. Vítovec, J. Aldershvile, M. Halinen, R. Dietz, K. L. Neuhaus, A. Jánosi, G. Thorgeirsson, P. H. Dunselman, L. Gullestad, J. Kuch, J. Herlitz, P. Rickenbacher, S. Ball, S. Gottlieb, and P. Deedwania. 2000. "Effects of Controlled-Release Metoprolol on Total Mortality, Hospitalizations, and Well-Being in Patients with Heart Failure: The Metoprolol CR/XL Randomized Intervention Trial in Congestive Heart Failure (MERIT-HF). MERIT-HF Study Group." *Journal of the American Medical Association* 283 (10): 1295–302.

Holtz, K., and E. de Vol. 2013. "Alignment, Goal Setting, and Incentives." In *Achieving STEEEP Health Care,* edited by D. J. Ballard, N. S. Fleming, J. T. Allison, P. B. Convery, and R. Luquire, 23–28. Boca Raton, FL: CRC Press.

Hughes, G. C., Y. Zhao, J. S. Rankin, J. E. Scarborough, S. O'Brien, J. E. Bavaria, W. G. Wolfe, J. G. Gaca, J. S. Gammie, D. M. Shahian, and P. K. Smith. 2013. "Effects of Institutional Volumes on Operative Outcomes for Aortic Root Replacement in North America." *Journal of Thoracic and Cardiovascular Surgery* 145 (1): 166–70.

Hunt, S. A., W. T. Abraham, M. H. Chin, A. M. Feldman, G. S. Francis, T. G. Ganiats, M. Jessup, M. A. Konstam, D. M. Mancini, K. Michl, J. A. Oates, P. S. Rahko, M. A. Silver, L. W. Stevenson, and C. W. Yancy; American College of Cardiology Foundation; American Heart Association. 2009. "Focused Update Incorporated into the ACC/AHA 2005 Guidelines for the Diagnosis and Management of Heart Failure in Adults: A Report of the American College of Cardiology Foundation/American Heart Association Task Force on Practice Guidelines Developed in Collaboration with the International Society for Heart and Lung Transplantation." *Journal of the American College of Cardiology* 53 (15): e1–e90.

Institute of Medicine. 2001. *Crossing the Quality Chasm. A New Health System for the 21st Century.* Washington, DC: National Academies Press.

James, B. C., and L. A. Savitz. 2011. "How Intermountain Trimmed Health Care Costs Through Robust Quality Improvement Efforts." *Health Affairs (Millwood)* 30 (6): 1185–91.

Jencks, S. F., E. D. Huff, and T. Cuerdon. 2003. "Change in the Quality of Care Delivered to Medicare Beneficiaries, 1998–1999 to 2000–2001." *Journal of the American Medical Association* 289 (3): 305–12.

Katz, B. P., D. A. Freund, D. A. Heck, R. S. Dittus, J. E. Paul, J. Wright, P. Coyte, E. Holleman, and G. Hawker. 1996. "Demographic Variation in the Rate of Knee Replacement: A Multi-Year Analysis." *Health Services Research* 31 (2): 125–40.

Kennedy, P. J., C. M. Leathley, and C. F. Hughes. 2010. "Clinical Practice Variation." *Medical Journal of Australia* 193 (8 Suppl.): S97–99.

Keyhani, S., and A. L. Siu. 2008. "The Underuse of Overuse Research." *Health Services Research* 43 (6): 1923–30.

Leatherman, S., D. Berwick, D. Iles, L. S. Lewin, F. Davidoff, T. Nolan, and M. Bisognano. 2003. "The Business Case for Quality: Case Studies and an Analysis." *Health Affairs (Millwood)* 22 (2): 17–30.

Long, M. J. 2002. "An Explanatory Model of Medical Practice Variation: A Physician Resource Demand Perspective." *Journal of Evaluation in Clinical Practice* 8 (2): 167–74.

Lu-Yao, G. L., and E. R. Greenberg. 1994. "Changes in Prostate Cancer Incidence and Treatment in USA." *Lancet* 343 (8892): 251–54.

Masoudi, F. A., S. S. Rathore, Y. Wang, E. P. Havranek, J. P. Curtis, J. M. Foody, and H. M. Krumholz. 2004. "National Patterns of Use and Effectiveness of Angiotensin-Converting Enzyme Inhibitors in Older Patients with Heart Failure and Left Ventricular Systolic Dysfunction." *Circulation* 110 (6): 724–31.

McPherson, K., J. E. Wennberg, O. B. Hovind, and P. Clifford. 1982. "Small-Area Variations in the Use of Common Surgical Procedures: An International Comparison of New England, England, and Norway." *New England Journal of Medicine* 307 (21): 1310–14.

Mercuri, M., and A. Gafni. 2011. "Medical Practice Variations: What the Literature Tells Us (or Does Not) About What Are Warranted and Unwarranted Variations." *Journal of Evaluation in Clinical Practice* 17 (4): 671–77.

Miller, W. L., R. R. McDaniel Jr., B. F. Crabtree, and K. C. Stange. 2001. "Practice Jazz: Understanding Variation in Family Practices Using Complexity Science." *Journal of Family Practice* 50 (10): 872–78.

Mottur-Pilson, C., V. Snow, and K. Bartlett. 2001. "Physician Explanations for Failing to Comply with 'Best Practices.'" *Effective Clinical Practice* 4 (5): 207–13.

Neuhauser, D., L. Provost, and B. Bergman. 2011. "The Meaning of Variation to Healthcare Managers, Clinical and Health-Services Researchers, and Individual Patients." *BMJ Quality & Safety* 20 (Suppl. 1): i36–40.

O'Connor, A. M., C. L. Bennett, D. Stacey, M. Barry, N. F. Col, K. B. Eden, V. A. Entwistle, V. Fiset, M. Holmes-Rovner, S. Khangura, H. Llewellyn-Thomas, and D. Rovner. 2009. "Decision Aids for People Facing Health Treatment or Screening Decisions." *Cochrane Database of Systematic Reviews* 3: CD001431.

O'Connor, A. M., H. A. Llewellyn-Thomas, and A. B. Flood. 2004. "Modifying Unwarranted Variations in Health Care: Shared Decision Making Using Patient Decision Aids." *Health Affairs (Millwood)* Suppl Variation: VAR63–72.

Palmer, R. H., A. Donabedian, and G. J. Povar. 1991. *Striving for Quality in Health Care: An Inquiry into Practice and Policy.* Chicago: Health Administration Press.

Parente, S. T., C. E. Phelps, and P. J. O'Connor. 2008. "Economic Analysis of Medical Practice Variation Between 1991 and 2000: The Impact of Patient Outcomes Research Teams (PORTs)." *International Journal of Technology Assessment in Health Care* 24 (3): 282–93.

Powell, A. E., H. T. Davies, and R. G. Thomson. 2003. "Using Routine Comparative Data to Assess the Quality of Health Care: Understanding and Avoiding Common Pitfalls." *Quality & Safety in Health Care* 12 (2): 122–28.

QualityNet. 2012. *Specifications Manual for National Hospital Quality Measures.* Accessed March 20. www.qualitynet.org/dcs/ContentServer?c=Page&pagename=QnetPublic%2FPage%2FQnetTier2&cid=1141662756099.

Rayner, H. C. 2011. "Tackling Practice Variation. Lessons from Variation Can Help Change Health Policy." *British Medical Journal* 342: d2271.

Reinertsen, J. L. 2003. "Zen and the Art of Physician Autonomy Maintenance." *Annals of Internal Medicine* 138 (12): 992–95.

Roger, V. L., A. S. Go, D. M. Lloyd-Jones, E. J. Benjamin, J. D. Berry, W. B. Borden, D. M. Bravata, S. Dai, E. S. Ford, C. S. Fox, H. J. Fullerton, C. Gillespie, S. M. Hailpern, J. A. Heit, V. J. Howard, B. M. Kissela, S. J. Kittner, D. T. Lackland, J. H. Lichtman, L. D. Lisabeth, D. M. Makuc, G. M. Marcus, A. Marelli, D. B. Matchar, C. S. Moy, D. Mozaffarian, M. E. Mussolino, G. Nichol, N. P. Paynter, E. Z. Soliman, P. D. Sorlie, N. Sotoodehnia, T. N. Turan, S. S. Virani, N. D. Wong, D. Woo, and M. B. Turner; American Heart Association Statistics Committee and Stroke Statistics Subcommittee. 2012. "Heart Disease and Stroke Statistics—2012 Update: A Report from the American Heart Association." *Circulation* 125 (1): e2–e220.

Samsa, G., E. Z. Oddone, R. Horner, J. Daley, W. Henderson, and D. B. Matchar. 2002. "To What Extent Should Quality of Care Decisions Be Based on Health Outcomes Data? Application to Carotid Endarterectomy." *Stroke* 33 (12): 2944–49.

Schermerhorn, M. L., K. A. Giles, A. D. Hamdan, S. E. Dalhberg, R. Hagberg, and F. Pomposelli. 2008. "Population-Based Outcomes of Open Descending Thoracic Aortic Aneurysm Repair." *Journal of Vascular Surgery* 48 (4): 821–27.

Sejr, T., T. F. Andersen, M. Madsen, C. Roepstorff, T. Bilde, H. Bay-Nielsen, R. Blais, and E. Holst. 1991. "Prostatectomy in Denmark. Regional Variation and the Diffusion of Medical Technology 1977–1985." *Scandinavian Journal of Urology and Nephrology* 25 (2): 101–6.

Sepucha, K., E. Ozanne, and A. G. Mulley Jr. 2006. "Doing the Right Thing: Systems Support for Decision Quality in Cancer Care." *Annals of Behavioral Medicine* 32 (3): 172–78.

Shoemaker, P. 2011. "What Value-Based Purchasing Means to Your Hospital." *Healthcare Financial Management* 65 (8): 60–68.

Sirovich, B., P. M. Gallagher, D. E. Wennberg, and E. S. Fisher. 2008. "Discretionary Decision Making by Primary Care Physicians and the Cost of U.S. Health Care." *Health Affairs (Millwood)* 27 (3): 813–23.

Smith, R. 2011. "Dartmouth Atlas of Health Care." *British Medical Journal* 342: d1756.

SOLVD Investigators. 1991. "Effect of Enalapril on Survival in Patients with Reduced Left Ventricular Ejection Fractions and Congestive Heart Failure." *New England Journal of Medicine* 325 (5): 293–302.

Steinberg, E. P. 2003. "Improving the Quality of Care—Can We Practice What We Preach?" *New England Journal of Medicine* 348 (26): 2681–83.

Stroud, J., C. Felton, and B. Spreadbury. 2003. "Collaborative Colorectal Cancer Screening: A Successful Quality Improvement Initiative." *Proceedings (Baylor University Medical Center)* 16 (3): 341–44.

Timmermans, S., and A. Mauck. 2005. "The Promises and Pitfalls of Evidence-Based Medicine." *Health Affairs (Millwood)* 24 (1): 18–28.

US Department of Health and Human Services (HHS). 2013. "Measures Displayed on Hospital Compare." Accessed October 17. www.medicare.gov/hospitalcompare/Data/Measures-Displayed.html.

Vogeli, C., R. Kang, M. B. Landrum, R. Hasnain-Wynia, and J. S. Weissman. 2009. "Quality of Care Provided to Individual Patients in US Hospitals: Results from an Analysis of National Hospital Quality Alliance Data." *Medical Care* 47 (5): 591–99.

Wennberg, D. E., M. A. Kellett, J. D. Dickens, D. J. Malenka, L. M. Keilson, and R. B. Keller. 1996. "The Association Between Local Diagnostic Testing Intensity and Invasive Cardiac Procedures." *Journal of the American Medical Association* 275 (15): 1161–64.

Wennberg, J. E. 2011. "Time to Tackle Unwarranted Variations in Practice." *British Medical Journal* 342: d1513.

———. 2004. "Practice Variations and Health Care Reform: Connecting the Dots." *Health Affairs (Millwood)* Suppl Variation: VAR140–44.

———. 2002. "Unwarranted Variations in Healthcare Delivery: Implications for Academic Medical Centres." *British Medical Journal* 325 (7370): 961–64.

Wennberg, J. E., B. A. Barnes, and M. Zubkoff. 1982. "Professional Uncertainty and the Problem of Supplier-Induced Demand." *Social Science & Medicine* 16 (7): 811–24.

Wennberg, J. E., and M. M. Cooper (eds.). 1999. *The Quality of Medical Care in the United States: A Report on the Medicare Program. The Dartmouth Atlas of Health Care*. Chicago: American Hospital Association Press.

Westert, G. P., and M. Faber. 2011. "Commentary: The Dutch Approach to Unwarranted Medical Practice Variation." *British Medical Journal* 342: d1429.

Westert, G. P., P. P. Groenewegen, H. C. Boshuizen, P. M. Spreeuwenberg, and M. P. Steultjens. 2004. "Medical Practice Variations in Hospital Care; Time Trends of a Spatial Phenomenon." *Health & Place* 10 (3): 215–20.

Wheeler, D. J. 2000. *Understanding Variation: The Key to Managing Chaos*, second edition. Knoxville, TN: SPC Press.

Williams, S. C., S. P. Schmaltz, D. J. Morton, R. G. Koss, and J. M. Loeb. 2005. "Quality of Care in U.S. Hospitals as Reflected by Standardized Measures, 2002–2004." *New England Journal of Medicine* 353 (3): 255–64.

QUALITY IMPROVEMENT: FOUNDATION, PROCESSES, TOOLS, AND KNOWLEDGE TRANSFER TECHNIQUES

Kevin Warren

This chapter describes some of the tools and methods that can be used to improve the quality of healthcare and provides a case study example of some knowledge transfer concepts that promote adoption and sustainability. Included are a number of different approaches to quality improvement. Although they may have different names and belong to different categories, it is important to recognize their core commonalities.

The Quality Foundation

The strength, principles, and foundation of a product, belief, or concept can ultimately determine the sustainability of that product, belief, or concept. To better understand and appreciate quality improvement systems and theories used today, you should be familiar with their origins and the influences that have shaped them.

This chapter first introduces thought leaders who have contributed to quality improvement systems and theories focused on producing sustainable results at highly productive levels. These leaders include

- Walter A. Shewhart,
- W. Edwards Deming,
- Joseph M. Juran,
- Taiichi Ohno,
- Kaoru Ishikawa,
- Armand V. Feigenbaum, and
- Philip B. Crosby.

Walter A. Shewhart (1891–1967)
Dr. Walter A. Shewhart earned his doctorate in physics from the University of Illinois and the University of California. Shewhart used his understanding

of statistics to design tools to respond to variation. Following his arrival at Western Electric Co. in 1924, Shewhart introduced the concepts of common-cause variation, special-cause variation, and statistical process control (SPC). He designed these concepts to assist Bell Telephone in its efforts to improve reliability and reduce the frequency of repairs in its transmission systems (Cutler 2001). Before Shewhart introduced these concepts, workers reacted to each new data point to improve future output. This tampering actually made matters worse.

Shewhart felt that his most important contribution was not the control chart but rather his work on operational definitions, which ensured that people used common language to define what they measured (Kilian 1988). In his book *Economic Control of Quality of Manufactured Product*, Shewhart introduced the concept of SPC, which has since become the cornerstone for process control in industry (Cutler 2001). These efforts and Shewhart's emphasis on the importance of precise measurement were part of the founding principles that ultimately led to Motorola's development of the Six Sigma approach in the mid-1980s.

W. Edwards Deming (1900–1993)

Many consider Dr. W. Edwards Deming to be the father of quality. A statistics professor and physicist by trade, Deming combined the concepts he learned from Shewhart and taught that by adopting appropriate principles of data-based management, organizations could increase quality and customer loyalty and simultaneously decrease costs by reducing waste, rework, and staff attrition. One of several statisticians and advisers who provided guidance at the request of Japanese industry leaders in the 1950s, he taught top management how to improve design (and thus service), product quality, testing, and sales (the latter through global markets). Deming (2000b) stressed the importance of practicing continuous improvement and thinking of manufacturing as a system. In the 1970s, Deming developed his "14 Points for Western Management" in response to requests from US managers for the secret to the radical improvement that Japanese companies were achieving in a number of industries. Deming's 14 points were a unified body of knowledge that ran counter to the conventional wisdom of most US managers (Neave 1990).

As part of his "system of profound knowledge," Deming (2000a) promoted that "around 15% of poor quality was because of workers, and the rest of 85% was due to bad management, improper systems and processes." His system is based on four components:

1. Appreciation for a system
2. Knowledge about variation
3. Theory of knowledge
4. Psychology

Deming described the Plan-Do-Study-Act (PDSA) cycle, which can be traced to Shewhart. He referred to PDSA as a cycle for learning and improvement. Some have changed the "S" to "C" (Plan-Do-Check-Act [PDCA] cycle), but Deming preferred to use *study* instead of *check* (Neave 1990).

Joseph M. Juran (1904–2008)

After receiving a bachelor of science in electrical engineering from the University of Minnesota, Joseph M. Juran joined Western Electric's inspection department and ultimately became the head of the company's industrial engineering department. As an internal consultant to Deming on the subject of industrial engineering, Juran formulated ideas that prompted the creation of the concept now known as the Pareto principle (80/20 rule).

Juran was the coauthor of *Juran's Quality Control Handbook* (Juran and Gryna 1951) and consulted with Japanese companies in the 1950s. He defined quality as consisting of two different but related concepts. The first form of quality is income oriented. It includes features of the product that meet customer needs and thereby produces income (i.e., customers are willing to pay for items and services they need). The second form of quality is cost oriented and emphasizes freedom from failures and deficiencies (i.e., higher-quality production ultimately costs less and lasts longer) (ASQ 2014).

Another of Juran's (1989) notable contributions to the quality movement is the "Juran Trilogy." The trilogy describes three interrelated processes: quality planning, quality improvement, and quality control. See Exhibit 4.1.

Taiichi Ohno (1912–1990)

Taiichi Ohno is generally credited with developing the Toyota Production System (TPS). Ohno's development of TPS and continuous (one-piece) flow began in 1948 after he was promoted to manage Toyota's engine manufacturing department. Known for saying "common sense is always wrong," Ohno expressed concern about poor productivity and perceived waste—activities

Quality Planning	• Identify who the customers are. • Determine the needs of those customers. • Translate those needs into our language. • Develop a product that can respond to those needs. • Optimize the product features to meet our needs and customer needs.
Quality Improvement	• Develop a process that is able to produce the product. • Optimize the process.
Quality Control	• Prove that the process can produce the product under operating conditions with minimal inspection. • Transfer the process to operations.

EXHIBIT 4.1
Juran's Quality Trilogy

that do not add value—in operations' "batch and queue" (grouping of individual component development) process and categorized the types of waste (*muda* in Japanese) (Womack and Jones 2003):

- Overproduction
- Inventory
- Repairs/rejects
- Motion
- Processing
- Waiting
- Transport

In contrast to the batch-and-queue process, Ohno created a standardized process in which products are produced through one continuous system one at a time, ultimately producing less waste, greater efficiency, and higher output.

Kaoru Ishikawa (1915–1989)

Kaoru Ishikawa, known for his study of scientific analysis of causes of industrial process problems, was a student of Deming and a member of the Union of Japanese Scientists and Engineers. One of his most noted contributions to the quality movement was the creation of the Ishikawa diagram (fishbone diagram) (Tague 2004). Ishikawa's discussions of total quality control (TQC) focused on the importance of participation by all levels of an organization in quality improvement initiatives and the use of statistical and precise measurement in the decision-making process.

Professor Ishikawa obtained his doctorate in engineering from Tokyo University. In 1968, building on a series of articles on quality control, he authored a textbook that ultimately became the *Guide to Quality Control*. Although the concept of quality circles can be traced to the United States, Professor Ishikawa is noted for introducing the concept to Japan as part of his TQC efforts to ensure participation in and an understanding of quality control at all levels of an organization.

Armand V. Feigenbaum (1922–)

The concept of TQC originated in a 1951 book by Armand V. Feigenbaum. He approached quality as a strategic business tool that everyone in a company should be aware of, in the same manner that most companies view cost and revenue. He stated that quality reaches beyond managing defects in production and should be a philosophy and a commitment to excellence. Feigenbaum defined TQC as excellence driven rather than defect driven—a system that integrates quality development, quality improvement, and quality maintenance (ASQ Quality Management Division 1999). The book *Total Quality Control* (Feigenbaum 1951), originally published as *Quality Control: Principles, Practice, and Administration*, outlines his approach to quality (ASQ 2014). Feigenbaum is known for introducing the concept of the "hidden plant"—that up to 40 percent of plant capacity waste can result when production is not performed correctly the first time (QualityGurus.com 2014).

Philip B. Crosby (1926–2001)

Philip B. Crosby introduced the idea of zero defects in 1961. He defined quality as "conformance to requirements" and measured quality as the "price of nonconformance" (Crosby 1996). Crosby equated quality management with prevention, believing that inspecting, checking, and other nonpreventive techniques have no place in quality management. He taught that quality improvement is a process and not a temporary program or project. His quality improvement process is based on the "four absolutes of quality management" (Crosby 1996):

- Quality is defined as conformance to requirements, not as goodness or elegance.
- The system for causing quality is prevention, not appraisal.
- The performance standard must be zero defects, not "that's close enough."
- The measurement of quality is the price of nonconformance, not indexes.

Crosby also believed that statistical levels of compliance tend to program people for failure and that there is absolutely no reason for having errors or defects in a product or service. He felt that to prevent nonconformance, companies should adopt a quality "vaccine" made of three ingredients: determination, education, and implementation (ASQ 2014).

Quality Improvement Processes and Approaches

"Form follows function," a concept founded in the field of architecture, describes the importance of understanding what you are trying to accomplish before you determine how you are going to do it. Understanding the purpose behind the effort—the goal—is important at the individual, departmental, and organizational level when deciding what quality improvement process or approach to adopt. The following discussion describes some of the many systems and processes that guide quality improvement efforts today.

The following approaches are derivatives and models of the ideas and theories developed by thought leaders in quality improvement:

- Shewhart cycle or PDCA/PDSA cycle
- Associates in Process Improvement's (API) improvement model
- FOCUS PDCA model
- Baldrige Criteria and related systems
- Lean/Toyota Production System
- Six Sigma

Shewhart Cycle or PDCA/PDSA Cycle

As discussed earlier, in the 1920s Shewhart developed the PDCA cycle used today as the basis for planning and directing performance improvement efforts. Since the creation of the PDCA/PDSA cycle, most formally recognized performance improvement models have some basis in or relation to this original quality improvement model. The stages of the cycle are broken down into the following activities:

Plan
- Establish an objective. What are you trying to accomplish? What is the goal?
- Ask questions and make predictions. What do you think will happen?
- Plan to carry out the cycle. Who will perform the functions? What steps will be performed? When will the plan be implemented and completed? Where will the plan/work take place?

Do
- Educate and train staff.
- Carry out the plan (e.g., try out the change on a small scale).
- Document problems and unexpected observations.
- Begin analysis of the data.

Check/Study
- Assess the effect of the change, and determine the level of success achieved as compared to the goal/objective.
- Compare the results with your predictions.
- Summarize the lessons learned.
- Determine what changes need to be made and what actions will be taken next.

Act

- Act on what you have learned.
- Determine whether the plan should be repeated with modification or a new plan should be created.
- Make necessary changes.
- Identify remaining gaps in the process or performance.
- Carry out additional PDCA/PDSA cycles until the goal/objective is met.

API Improvement Model

Tom Nolan and Lloyd Provost, cofounders of API, developed a simple model for improvement based on Deming's PDSA cycle. Three fundamental questions form the model's basis for improvement (see Exhibit 4.2): (1) What are we trying to accomplish? (2) How will we know that a change is an improvement? (3) What change can we make that will result in improvement? The focus on the three questions and the PDSA cycle allows the model's application to be as simple or sophisticated as necessary. The effort required to bring about improvement may vary on the basis of the problem's complexity, whether the focus is on a new or an old design, or the number of people involved in the process (Langley et al. 1996).

EXHIBIT 4.2
API Model for
Improvement

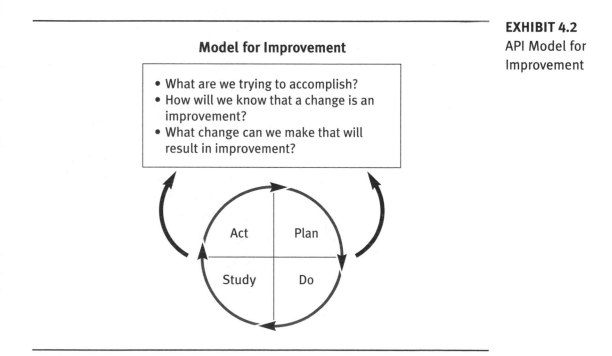

Model for Improvement

- What are we trying to accomplish?
- How will we know that a change is an improvement?
- What change can we make that will result in improvement?

Act | Plan

Study | Do

Source: Langley et al. (1996). Used with permisson.

FOCUS PDCA Model

Building on the PDSA cycle, Hospital Corporation of America designed the FOCUS PDCA model to create a more specific and more defined approach to process improvement. The key feature of FOCUS PDCA is the preexistence of a process that needs improvement. The intent of this model is to maximize the performance of a preexisting process, although the inclusion of PDCA provides the option of using this model for new or redesign projects (Brown 2003). The acronym FOCUS is broken down as follows:

F = FIND a process to improve.
O = ORGANIZE a team that knows the process.
C = CLARIFY current knowledge of the existing or redesigned process.
U = UNDERSTAND the variables and causes of process variation in the chosen process.
S = SELECT the process improvement and identify potential actions to achieve it.

Baldrige Criteria and Related Systems

The Malcolm Baldrige National Quality Award (www.nist.gov/baldrige)—named for Malcolm Baldrige, who served as Secretary of Commerce from 1981 until his death in 1987—was created by Public Law 100-107, which was signed in 1987 (Hertz 2010). This law led to the creation of a public–private partnership to improve the United States' competitiveness in the global marketplace.

The Baldrige Criteria were originally developed for and applied to businesses; however, in 1997, healthcare-specific criteria were created to help healthcare organizations address such challenges as developing core competencies, introducing new technologies, reducing costs, communicating and sharing information electronically, establishing new alliances with healthcare providers, and maintaining market advantage. The Baldrige Health Care Criteria focus on outcomes in five key areas, are built on a set of interrelated values and concepts, and are organized into seven interdependent categories. The key areas include (Baldrige Performance Excellence Program 2013)

- healthcare and processes,
- customers,
- workforce,
- leadership and governance, and
- finance and markets.

The set of interrelated values and concepts includes (Baldrige Performance Excellence Program 2013)

- visionary leadership,
- patient-focused excellence,
- organizational and personal learning,
- valuing of staff and partners,
- agility,
- focus on the future,
- managing for innovation,
- management by fact,
- social responsibility and community health,
- creating value and results, and
- systems perspective.

The seven interdependent categories include (Baldrige Performance Excellence Program 2013)

1. leadership;
2. strategic planning;
3. customer focus;
4. measurement, analysis, and knowledge management;
5. workforce focus;
6. operations focus; and
7. outcomes.

Evaluation and scoring on the seven criteria are based on two dimensions: process and results. For the process criteria, applicants are evaluated on the basis of their description of their organizational approach, deployment, learning, and integration. For the results criteria, applicants are evaluated on the basis of their description and display of organizational performance levels, trends, comparisons, and integration. The Baldrige scoring system is based on a 1,000-point scale. The most heavily weighted criterion is the outcomes category (450 possible points). The weight of this category is based on the emphasis Baldrige places on results and an organization's ability to demonstrate performance and improvement in the following areas:

- Product and service outcomes
- Customer-focused outcomes
- Financial and market outcomes
- Workforce-focused outcomes
- Process effectiveness outcomes
- Leadership outcomes

All Baldrige applicants receive a feedback report evaluating the strengths and weaknesses of their responses to each of the seven categories. The purpose of the feedback report is to document the analysis of the applicant's response so that it can be used to evaluate the organization's responses to future applications and identify potential gaps in the organization's strategic planning and improvement activities.

The national Baldrige criteria serve as the framework for many state and local quality awards. In 2012, eligibility requirements for the Baldrige Award were changed; applicants now must have received a "top-tier award" from a state or local Baldrige-based award program or meet one of five conditions related to past national or state-based award performance.

Lean/Toyota Production System

The Massachusetts Institute of Technology developed the term *Lean* in 1987 to describe product development and production methods that, when compared with traditional mass production processes, produce more products with fewer defects in a shorter time. The goal was to develop a way to specify value, align steps/processes in the best sequence, conduct these activities without interruption whenever someone requests them, and perform them more effectively (Womack and Jones 2003). Lean thinking, sometimes called *Lean manufacturing* or the *Toyota Production System* (*TPS*), focuses on the removal of waste (*muda*), which is defined as anything that is not needed to produce a product or service. Taiichi Ohno (cofounder of TPS) identified seven types of waste: (1) overproduction, (2) waiting, (3) unnecessary transport, (4) overprocessing, (5) excess inventory, (6) unnecessary movement, and (7) defects.

The focus of Lean methodology is a "back to basics" approach that places the needs of the customer first through the following five steps:

1. Define *value* as determined by the customer, identified by the provider's ability to deliver the right product or service at an appropriate price.
2. Identify the *value stream*, the set of specific actions required to bring a specific product or service from concept to completion.
3. Make value-added steps *flow* from beginning to end.
4. Let the customer *pull* the product from the supplier; do not push products.
5. Pursue *perfection* of the process.

Although Lean focuses on removing waste and improving flow, it also has some secondary effects. Quality is improved. The product spends less time in process, reducing the chances of damage or obsolescence. The simplification of processes reduces variation and inventory and increases the uniformity of outputs (Heim 1999).

Six Sigma

Six Sigma (3.4 defects per million) is a system for improvement developed by Hewlett-Packard, Motorola, General Electric, and others over the course of the 1980s and 1990s (Pande, Neuman, and Cavanagh 2000). The tools used in Six Sigma are not new. The thinking behind this system builds on the foundations of quality improvement established in the 1930s through the 1950s. What makes Six Sigma appear new is the rigor of tying improvement projects to key business processes and clear roles and responsibilities for executives, champions, master black belts, black belts, and green belts.

The aim of Six Sigma is to reduce variation (eliminate defects) in key business processes. By using a set of statistical tools to understand the fluctuation of a process, managers can predict the expected outcome of that process. If the outcome is not satisfactory, management can use associated tools to learn more about the elements influencing the process. Six Sigma includes five steps—define, measure, analyze, improve, and control—commonly known as DMAIC:

1. *Define*: Identify the customers and their problems. Determine the key characteristics important to the customer along with the processes that support those key characteristics. Identify existing output conditions along with process elements.
2. *Measure*: Categorize key characteristics, verify measurement systems, and collect data.
3. *Analyze*: Convert raw data into information that provides insights into the process. These insights include identifying the fundamental and most important causes of the defects or problems.
4. *Improve*: Develop solutions to the problem, and make changes to the process. Measure process changes, and judge whether the changes are beneficial or another set of changes is necessary.
5. *Control*: If the process is performing at a desired and predictable level, monitor the process to ensure that no unexpected changes occur.

The primary theory of Six Sigma is that a focus on reducing variation leads to more uniform process output. Secondary effects include less waste, less throughput time, and less inventory (Heim 1999).

Quality Tools

One of the difficult things about quality is explaining how a **tool** is different from a **process** or a **system**. We can observe people using tools and methods for improvement. We can see them making a flowchart, plotting a control chart, or using a checklist. These tools and procedures are the logical outcomes of process and system changes that people have put in place or implemented to make improvements or identify a problem. People may use several tools and procedures to make improvements, and these tools may form one part of an improvement system. Although we can observe people using the tools of the system, the system (e.g., Six Sigma, Lean) itself is invisible and cannot be observed. Many of the more than 50 quality tools available today were developed to "see" the quality system they are designed to support. The American Society for Quality (Tague 2004) has classified quality tools into six categories:

1. Cause analysis
2. Evaluation and decision making
3. Process analysis
4. Data collection and analysis
5. Idea creation
6. Project planning and implementation

This section of the chapter is not intended to be a comprehensive reference on quality tools and techniques but rather highlights some of the more widely used tools. The following discussion organizes the tools into three categories:

1. Basic quality tools
2. Management and planning tools
3. Other quality tools

Basic Quality Tools

Basic quality tools are used to define and analyze discrete processes that usually produce quantitative data. These tools primarily are used to explain a process, identify potential causes for process performance problems, and collect and display data indicating which causes are most prevalent.

5 Whys

Simple to understand and perform, the *5 Whys* exercise was developed as a basic method for drilling down through the symptoms of a process or design failure to identify the root cause. By asking why or what caused the problem, users of this technique can quickly identify possible root causes and make improvements that will correct the real problem, not just address the symptoms. Key to successful use of this technique is not to stop the analysis too early so as to misidentify the root cause.

Control Chart

Also referred to as *statistical process control, control charts* are graphs used to display data for the purpose of identifying how processes or outcomes change over time. Control charts contain three lines: a central/control line (average), an upper control limit, and a lower control limit. These boundaries are used to measure and monitor performance to identify performance tendencies and variation. Control charts also can be used to assess the impact of a process change on performance, enabling the user to correct or identify any problems that arise (Tague 2004).

Histogram

A *histogram* is a graphical display of the frequency distribution of a quality characteristic of interest. A histogram makes variation in a group of data apparent and aids analysis of the distribution of data around an average or median value.

Cause-and-Effect/Fishbone Diagram

Cause-and-effect diagrams are sometimes referred to as *Ishikawa*, or *fishbone*, *diagrams.* In a cause-and-effect diagram, the problem (effect) is stated in a box on the right side of the chart, and likely causes are listed around major headings (bones) that lead to the effect. Cause-and-effect diagrams can help organize the causes contributing to a complex problem (ASQ 2014).

Pareto Chart

Vilfredo Pareto, an Italian economist in the 1880s, observed that 80 percent of the wealth in Italy was held by 20 percent of the population. Juran later applied this principle to other applications and found that 80 percent of the variation of any characteristic is caused by only 20 percent of the possible variables. A *Pareto chart* is a display of occurrence frequency that shows this small number of significant contributors to a problem, enabling management to concentrate resources and identify the frequency with which specific errors are occurring (Tague 2004).

Checksheet

Checksheets are a generic tool designed for multiple data-collection purposes. They are used to capture data measured repeatedly over time for purposes of identifying patterns, trends, defects, or causes of defects. Data collected using a checksheet can be easily converted into data performance tools such as histograms or Pareto charts (Tague 2004).

Management and Planning Tools

Managers use management and planning tools to organize the decision-making process and create a hierarchy when faced with competing priorities. These tools also are useful for dealing with issues involving multiple departments in an organization and for creating an organization-wide quality culture.

Balanced Scorecard

Renowned management consultant Peter Drucker is often quoted as having said "you can't manage what you don't measure." Developed by Dr. Robert Kaplan and Dr. David Norton, the *balanced scorecard* is used to collect, measure, and analyze the strategic planning and management of an organization. This tool transfers high-level organizational performance expectations to the individual department level to measure the impact of day-to-day operations and deliverables. Through visual display of performance measures in the areas of finance, customers, internal (business) processes, and employee learning and growth, an organization can reinforce its priorities and design specific systems and processes around its vision and strategy (Balanced Scorecard Institute 2014).

Affinity Diagram

Affinity diagrams can encourage people to develop creative solutions to problems. For example, the use of an affinity diagram is a way to create order out of a brainstorming session. An issue or problem is identified, and then individuals record their own ideas about the issue/problem on small note cards. As a group, team members study the cards and then group the recorded ideas into common categories.

Matrix Relations Diagram

The *matrix relations diagram* helps us answer two important questions when sets of data are compared: (1) Are the data related? and (2) How strong is the relationship? The House of Quality, a quality function deployment tool, is an example of a matrix relations diagram. It lists customers' needs on one axis and an organization's/product's capabilities on the second axis. The diagram compares what the customer wants with how the vendor will meet those expectations. The matrix relations diagram can identify not only relationships between sets of data but also patterns in the relationships and serves as a useful checklist for ensuring that tasks are being completed (Tague 2004).

Stratification

When gathering data from multiple sources or conditions, researchers may use the technique of *stratification* to analyze and determine whether data variation exists among the sources. Stratification can help researchers identify patterns in the data and prevent misrepresentation of study findings when data from multiple sources are presented together.

Scatter Diagram

Scatter diagrams enable users to identify whether a correlation exists between pairs of numerical data. Also known as a *scatter plot* or *X-Y graph*, the scatter diagram can be used in a root cause analysis to determine the cause-and-effect relationship that two elements may have. The greater the correlation between the two elements, the more the data will display as a tight line or curve, whereas two disparate elements will display as a more scattered or "shotgun" distribution.

Priorities Matrix

Use of a *priorities matrix* involves the application of a series of planning tools built around the matrix chart. When tasks outnumber available resources, managers can use this matrix to prioritize work on the basis of data rather than emotion. Priorities matrixes enable managers to systematically discuss, identify, and prioritize the criteria that most influence their decisions about which tasks to complete and to study different possibilities for prioritizing tasks (ASQ 2014).

Other Quality Tools
Benchmarking

Organizations use *benchmarking* to compare the processes and successes of their competitors or of similar top-performing organizations to their own processes to identify process variation and organizational opportunities for improvement.

Failure Mode and Effects Analysis

Failure mode and effects analysis (FMEA) examines potential problems and their causes and predicts undesired results. FMEA normally is used to predict product failure from past part failure, but it also can be used to analyze future system failures. This method of failure analysis generally is performed on product design and work processes. By basing their activities on FMEA, organizations can focus their efforts on steps in a process that have the greatest potential for failure before failure actually occurs. Prioritization of failure modes to address and mitigate is based on the detectability of the potential failure, its severity, and its likelihood of occurrence.

Flowchart

Flowcharts are used to visually display the steps of a process in sequential order. Each step in a flowchart is displayed as a symbol that represents a particular action (e.g., process step, direction, decision, delay). For quality improvement purposes, flowcharts are useful tools for identifying unnecessary steps in a process, developing procedures, and facilitating communication between staff involved in the same process (Tague 2004).

Spaghetti Diagram

First developed in the manufacturing industry to display the path of an item through a factory, *spaghetti diagrams* are used to identify unnecessary repetition in a process and opportunities for improved efficiency (i.e., removal of unnecessary steps). By visually displaying multiple simultaneous processes, spaghetti diagrams can reveal potential causes of delay or unnecessary motion.

5S

The Japanese tool *5S* (each step starts with the letter "S") is a systematic program that helps workers take control of their workspace so that it helps them complete their jobs instead of being a neutral or, as is commonly the case, a competing factor:

1. *Seiri* (sort) means to keep only items necessary for completing one's work.
2. *Seiton* (straighten) means to arrange and identify items so that they can be easily retrieved when needed.
3. *Seiso* (shine) means to keep items and workspaces clean and in working order.
4. *Seiketsu* (standardize) means to use best practices consistently.
5. *Shitsuke* (sustain) means to maintain gains and make a commitment to continue to apply the first four Ss.

Mistake Proofing (Poka Yoke)

A concept developed in the 1960s by Japanese industrial engineer and TPS cofounder Shigeo Shingo, *mistake proofing* is the creation of techniques and devices to ensure that processes work right from the first time they are implemented. Mistake proofing techniques can be used to address potential failures identified during FMEA. The goal of mistake proofing is to make an error impossible to occur or easily detectable before significant consequences result.

Knowledge Transfer and Spread Techniques

A key aspect of any quality improvement effort is the ability to replicate successes in other areas of the organization. Barriers to spread and adoption (e.g., organizational culture, communication, leadership support) exist in any unit, organization, or system. However, failure to transfer knowledge effectively may cause an organization to produce waste, perform inconsistently, and miss opportunities to achieve benchmark levels of operational performance.

The concept of *transfer of learning*, developed in 1901, explores how individuals can apply lessons learned in one context to another context. The theory relies on the notion that the characteristics of the new setting are similar enough to those of the previous setting that processes can be replicated and similar efficiencies can be gained in the new setting (Thorndike and Woodworth 1901).

In 1999, the Institute for Healthcare Improvement (IHI) chartered a team to create a "framework for spread." In 2006, IHI published "A Framework for Spread: From Local Improvements to System-Wide Change," a white paper that identified "the ability of healthcare providers and their organizations to rapidly spread innovations and new ideas" as a "key factor in closing the gap between *best* practice and *common* practice" (Massoud et al. 2006, 1). The report noted the following questions as important for organizations to address when attempting to spread ideas to their target populations (Massoud et al. 2006, 6):

- Can the organization or community structure be used to facilitate spread?
- How are decisions about the adoption of improvements made?
- What infrastructure enhancements will assist in achieving the spread aim?
- What transition issues need to be addressed?
- How will the spread efforts be transitioned to operational responsibilities?

The following discussion presents techniques that can be used to facilitate spread within a department, across an organization, or throughout a system. The decision to use any of these techniques depends on the goals and complexity of the changes to be disseminated. Like the group of quality improvement systems and tools presented earlier in the chapter, this selection of knowledge transfer techniques is only a representative sample of the many methods available for this purpose.

Kaizen Blitz/Event

Kaizen, translated as "continuous improvement," was developed in Japan shortly after World War II. Kaizen in any organization involves ongoing improvement that is supported and implemented at all levels of an organization. The key aspect of Kaizen is the continual focus on improving a system or process regardless of how well the system or process is currently functioning. A Kaizen "blitz" or event is a highly focused improvement effort aimed at addressing a specific problem. Kaizen events are short in duration—typically three to five days. As such, Kaizen blitzes/events are intended to produce rapid changes that produce quick results. The approach to improvement taken during a Kaizen blitz/event typically involves common improvement methodologies (e.g., DMAIC, PDCA, value stream mapping) and the participation of teams with decision-making authority from multiple departments and levels of leadership.

Rapid-Cycle Testing/Improvement

Two important characteristics of an effective spread model are staff buy-in and proof that the change will improve performance. Developed by IHI, *rapid-cycle testing* (or *rapid-cycle improvement*) was designed to create various small tests involving small sample sizes and multiple PDSA cycles that build on the lessons learned in a short period while gaining buy-in from staff involved in the change (see Exhibit 4.3). Successful tests are applied to other units in the organization, whereas unsuccessful tests continue to be revised for potential spread and further implementation. Rapid-cycle testing is designed to reduce the cycle time of new process implementation from months to days. To prevent unnecessary delays in testing or implementation, teams or units using rapid-cycle testing must remain focused on testing solutions and avoid overanalysis. Rapid-cycle testing can be resource intensive (i.e., involves high resource consumption in a short period) and therefore may require top-level leadership support.

Case Study: Reengineering Discharge in a Community-Wide Collaborative Project to Reduce Hospital Readmissions

In August 2008, TMF Health Quality Institute initiated Care Transitions, an 18-month project to reduce 30-day all-cause readmissions in the Harlingen referral region of the Lower Rio Grande Valley in South Texas. The goal of the project was to engage inpatient hospitals and their "downstream" or discharge providers (e.g., home health agencies, long-term care facilities,

EXHIBIT 4.3
Example of
Rapid-Cycle
Testing

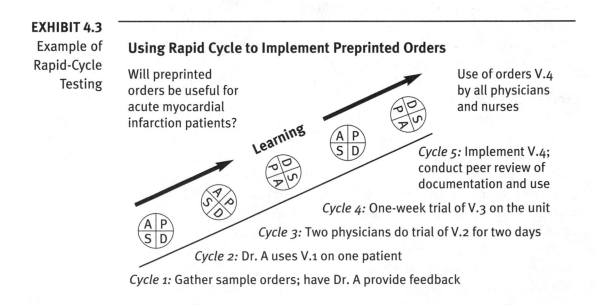

Using Rapid Cycle to Implement Preprinted Orders

Will preprinted orders be useful for acute myocardial infarction patients?

Learning

Use of orders V.4 by all physicians and nurses

Cycle 5: Implement V.4; conduct peer review of documentation and use

Cycle 4: One-week trial of V.3 on the unit

Cycle 3: Two physicians do trial of V.2 for two days

Cycle 2: Dr. A uses V.1 on one patient

Cycle 1: Gather sample orders; have Dr. A provide feedback

Note: V.1, V.2, V.3, and *V.4* refer to the consecutive versions of the preprinted order sets being tested. Each time the orders are modified during a test, a new version of the orders is created.

inpatient rehabilitation facilities) in identifying gaps in care coordination and implementing evidence-based interventions to reduce unnecessary hospital readmissions. As part of the Centers for Medicare & Medicaid Services' Quality Improvement Organization Program's 9th Scope of Work, TMF proposed that home health agencies, hospices, skilled nursing facilities (SNFs), inpatient rehabilitation facilities (IRFs), and hospitals working in collaboration with each other and with physicians could achieve the goals of the Care Transitions project through

- improved communication during the transition of patients from one setting to another,
- use of community and provider-specific data reports to increase accountability and feedback on progress toward goals, and
- implementation of provider-specific evidence-based interventions focused on improving the quality of care during transitions.

During the recruitment phase of the project, TMF engaged 5 inpatient hospitals, 28 home health agencies, 11 SNFs, and 2 IRFs. Initial planning at the participating hospitals involved conducting a process-of-care investigation to determine the root causes of their readmission rates. The investigation included the following activities:

- Conducting staff interviews and interdisciplinary meetings to discuss the current discharge process in comparison to Project RED (Re-Engineered Discharge) and to identify barriers and areas for improvement
- Analyzing project data provided by TMF (calendar year 2007 Medicare claims), which included the facility's 30-day readmission rate and discharge disposition (i.e., home, SNF, IRF, and long-term acute care hospital) in relation to the 30-day readmission rate
- Evaluating current Hospital Consumer Assessment of Healthcare Providers and Systems scores related to the hospital discharge process

The hospitals identified the following root causes (TMF 2010):

- A weak or fragmented discharge plan
- Miscommunication or failure to communicate key information at the time of transition
- Discharged patients' unpreparedness for discharge or self-management
- Inadequate medical follow-up with discharged patients after discharge
- Inadequate or poor communication with patients and/or caregivers when relating information about medicines, tests, and red flags

Following the process-of-care and root cause investigations, the participating providers reviewed multiple hospital-based interventions designed to reduce unnecessary readmissions, such as (TMF 2010)

- Project RED,
- Project BOOST (Better Outcomes for Older adults through Safe Transitions),
- Care Transitions program's Care Transitions Intervention, and
- IHI's guide to creating an ideal transition home.

Following review of the interventions, all hospitals participating in the Texas Care Transitions project chose to implement components of Project RED. Developed from a study conducted by Boston Medical Center, Project RED includes 11 components targeting patient education, discharge planning, and postdischarge reinforcement:

1. Educate the patient about his or her diagnosis throughout the hospital stay.
2. Make appointments for clinical follow-up visits and testing prior to hospital discharge.
3. Discuss any tests or studies with the patient that have been completed in the hospital, and identify who will be responsible for following up on the results.
4. Organize postdischarge services.
5. Confirm the patient's medication plan.
6. Reconcile the discharge plan with national guidelines and critical pathways.
7. Review with the patient the steps he or she should follow if a problem arises after discharge.
8. Expedite dissemination of the discharge summary to the patient's physician and other clinicians involved in the patient's follow-up care after discharge.
9. Give the patient a written discharge plan at the time of discharge.
10. Implement "teach back" of the patient's discharge plan by asking the patient to explain the details of the plan in his or her own words.
11. Follow up on the discharge plan with the patient via telephone two to three days after discharge.

Throughout the Care Transitions project, TMF provided the following support to participating providers:

- On-site technical support for team leaders, facility leaders, and Care Transitions committees
- Regional meetings in which community providers could work together across the care continuum to develop region- or community-specific solutions
- Reports identifying the percentage of patients readmitted within 30 days who received a visit from a physician between hospital discharge and readmission
- Quarterly data reports and run charts (based on Medicare claims data) displaying readmission rate performance
- Medical staff education and provider education sessions (e.g., medication reconciliation and health literacy)
- Data collection tools for monitoring the effectiveness of the implemented project components
- A patient discharge survey tool for monitoring the effectiveness of the implemented project components and ensuring that discharge plans met hospital core measurement requirements and national guidelines for patients with acute myocardial infarction, congestive heart failure, or pneumonia

    Project results from one of the participating hospitals (see Exhibits 4.4 and 4.5) suggest that the implementation of a community-based project in which providers across the patient care continuum work together can reduce unnecessary hospital readmissions. Support from leadership, accountability for implementation of evidence-based interventions, and concurrent monitoring are critical to sustaining process redesign efforts. Collaboration among providers across the community on behalf of the patient fosters an awareness of other individual and organizational efforts and successes in overcoming

EXHIBIT 4.4

Percentage of 30-Day Readmissions at One Participating Hospital (semiannual rate ending in the listed quarter)

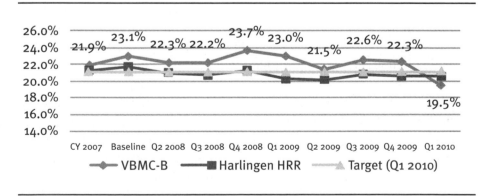

Source: TMF Health Quality Institute. Used with permission.

EXHIBIT 4.5
Percentage of
Discharges with
a 30-Day
Readmission
to One
Participating
Hospital

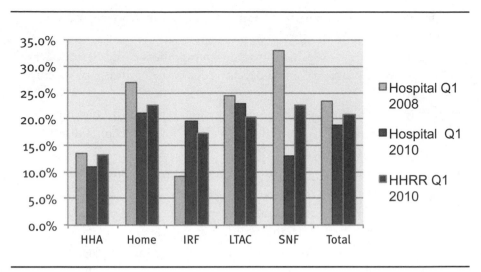

Source: TMF Health Quality Institute. Used with permission.

mutual impediments to improvement. Collective problem solving can expedite the application of evidence-based care practices and the use of process redesign methods.

Conclusion

An organization's success depends on the foundation on which it was built and the strength of the systems, processes, tools, and methods it uses to sustain benchmark levels of performance and to identify and improve performance when expectations are not being met. Although quality improvement theory and methodology have been available since the early 1900s, their widespread acceptance and application by the healthcare industry have not occurred as rapidly and effectively as in other industries (e.g., manufacturing). The release of two Institute of Medicine publications (*Crossing the Quality Chasm* [IOM 2001] and *To Err Is Human* [Kohn, Corrigan, and Donaldson 2000]) describing significant concerns about the US healthcare system incited a movement toward improvement that greatly increased healthcare institutions' focus on better care and patient safety (Berwick and Leape 2005). However, because of a combination of technical complexity, system fragmentation, a tradition of autonomy, and hierarchical authority structures, overcoming the "daunting barrier to creating the habits and beliefs of common purpose, teamwork and individual accountability" necessary for spread and sustainability will require a continual focus and commitment (Berwick and Leape 2005). Sustainable improvement is further defined through will, ideas, and execution. "You have to have the *will* to improve, you have to have *ideas* about alternatives to the status quo, and then you have to make it real—*execution*" (Nolan 2007). The principles described in this chapter have demonstrated success in many healthcare organizations. As healthcare technology advances and access to care improves, healthcare must continue to build on these principles as it strives to reach and maintain benchmark levels of performance. Successful coordination of care across the healthcare continuum will provide the right care for every patient at the right time, every time.

Study Questions

1. How would you select and implement one or more of the approaches described in this chapter in your own institution?
2. What are some of the challenges to spreading change? Identify two key questions/issues that need to be considered when applying change concepts in an organization or system.
3. How would a healthcare organization choose elements to measure and measurement tools when seeking to improve the quality of care?
4. How would you encourage your organization to work with other healthcare organizations across the healthcare continuum? Name two factors that are key to ensuring collaboration/coordination among healthcare providers.
5. What are some of the key elements common to the different tools discussed in this chapter?
6. What is the difference between a quality improvement system and a quality improvement tool? Provide examples of each.

References

American Society for Quality (ASQ). 2014. "A. V. Feigenbaum: Laying the Foundations of Modern Quality Control." Accessed January 30. http://asq.org/about-asq/who-we-are/bio_feigen.html.

American Society for Quality (ASQ) Quality Management Division. 1999. *The Certified Quality Manager Handbook*. Milwaukee, WI: ASQ Quality Press.

Balanced Scorecard Institute. 2014. "Balanced Scorecard Basics." Accessed January 30. http://balancedscorecard.org/Resources/AbouttheBalancedScorecard/tabid/55/Default.aspx.

Baldrige Performance Excellence Program. 2013. *2013–2014 Health Care Criteria for Performance Excellence*. Gaithersburg, MD: US Department of Commerce, National Institute of Standards and Technology.

Berwick, D. A., and L. L. Leape. 2005. "Five Years After *To Err Is Human*: What Have We Learned?" *Journal of the American Medical Association* 293 (19): 2384–90.

Brown, J. A. 2003. *The Healthcare Quality Handbook: A Professional Resource and Study Guide.* Pasadena, CA: JB Enterprises.

Crosby, P. B. 1996. *Quality Is Still Free: Making Quality Certain in Uncertain Times.* New York: McGraw-Hill.

Cutler, A. N. 2001. "Biography of Walter A. Shewhart." www.sigma-engineering. co.uk/ light/shewhartbiog.htm.

Deming, W. E. 2000a. *The New Economics for Industry, Government, Education,* second edition. Cambridge, MA: MIT Press.

———. 2000b. *Out of the Crisis.* Cambridge, MA: MIT Press.

Feigenbaum, A. V. 1951. *Total Quality Control.* New York: McGraw-Hill.

Heim, K. 1999. "Creating Continuous Improvement Synergy with Lean and TOC." Paper presented at the American Society for Quality Annual Quality Congress, Anaheim, California, May.

Hertz, H. S. (ed.). 2010. *Education Criteria for Performance Excellence (2009– 2010): Baldrige National Quality Program.* Darby, PA: DIANE Publishing.

Institute of Medicine (IOM). 2001. *Crossing the Quality Chasm: A New Health System for the 21st Century.* Washington, DC: National Academies Press.

Juran, J. M. 1989. *Juran on Leadership for Quality.* New York: Free Press.

Juran, J. M., and F. M. Gryna (eds.). 1951. *Juran's Quality Control Handbook.* New York: McGraw-Hill.

Kilian, C. 1988. *The World of W. Edwards Deming.* Knoxville, TN: SPC Press.

Kohn, L.T., J.M. Corrigan, and M.S. Donaldson (eds.). 2000. *To Err Is Human: Building a Safer Health System.* Washington, DC: National Academies Press.

Langley, G., K. Nolan, T. Nolan, C. Norman, and L. Provost. 1996. *The Improvement Guide: A Practical Approach to Enhancing Organizational Performance.* San Francisco: Jossey-Bass.

Massoud, M. R., G. A. Nielson, K. Nolan, T. Nolan, M. W. Schall, and C. Sevin. 2006. "A Framework for Spread: From Local Improvements to System-Wide Change." IHI Innovation Series white paper. Cambridge, MA: Institute for Healthcare Improvement.

Neave, H. R. 1990. *The Deming Dimension.* Knoxville, TN: SPC Press.

Nolan, T. W. 2007. "Execution of Strategic Improvement Initiatives to Produce System-Level Results." IHI Innovation Series white paper. Cambridge, MA: Institute for Healthcare Improvement.

Pande, P. S., R. P. Neuman, and R. R. Cavanagh. 2000. *The Six Sigma Way: How GE, Motorola, and Other Top Companies Are Honing Their Performance.* New York: McGraw-Hill.

QualityGurus.com. 2014. "Armand V. Feigenbaum." Accessed January 30. www. qualitygurus.com/gurus/list-of-gurus/armand-v-feigenbaum.

Tague, N. R. 2004. *The Quality Toolbox*, second edition. Milwaukee, WI: ASQ Quality Press.

Thorndike, E. L., and R. S. Woodworth. 1901. "The Influence of Improvement in One Mental Function upon the Efficiency of Other Functions." *Psychological Review* 8: 247–61.

TMF Health Quality Institute (TMF). 2010. *Re-Engineering Discharges in a Community-wide Project Reduces 30-Day Hospital Readmission Rate SQUIRE.* Austin, TX: TMF Health Quality Institute.

Womack, J. P., and D. T. Jones. 2003. *Lean Thinking: Banish Waste and Create Wealth in Your Corporation.* New York: Free Press.

HEALTHCARE QUALITY AT THE ORGANIZATION AND MICROSYSTEM LEVELS

DATA COLLECTION

John J. Byrnes

Everywhere you turn, everyone wants data. What do they really mean? Where do you get data? Is chart review the gold standard, the best source? Are administrative databases reliable; can they be the gold standard? What about health plan claims databases—are they accurate? What is the best source for inpatient data that reflects the quality of patient care from both a process and an outcome perspective? When working in the outpatient environment, where and how would you obtain data that reflect the level of quality delivered in physician office practices? These questions challenge many healthcare leaders as they struggle to develop quality improvement and measurement programs. This chapter clarifies these issues and common industry myths and provides a practical framework for obtaining valid, accurate, and useful data for quality improvement work.

Categories of Data: Case Example

Quality measurements can be grouped into four categories or domains: (1) clinical quality (including both process and outcome measures); (2) financial performance; (3) patient, physician, and staff satisfaction; and (4) functional status. To report on each of these categories, one may need to collect data from several separate sources. The challenge is to collect as many data elements from as few data sources as possible with the objectives of consistency and continuity in mind. For most large and mature quality improvement projects, teams will want to report their organization's performance in all four domains.

Spectrum Health's clinical reporting (CR) system illustrates this point. The CR system contains more than 50 disease-specific dashboards that report performance at the system, hospital, and physician levels (see Exhibit 5.1). In Exhibit 5.2, a dashboard for total hip replacement provides examples of clinical quality and financial performance measures. To produce the CR system, Spectrum Health used a variety of data sources, including extracts from its finance and electronic health record (EHR) systems. The decision support department processed the data, applying a series of rigorous data cleanup

EXHIBIT 5.1

Spectrum Health's Clinical Reporting System— Available Disease and Project Reports

1. Chest pain	29. Pediatric asthma
2. Heart attack	30. Very low birth weight neonates
3. PCI	31. Pediatric appendectomy
4. Heart failure	32. RSV/bronchiolitis
5. Pneumonia	33. Pediatric chemotherapy
6. Normal delivery	34. Pediatric VP shunts
7. C-section	35. Pediatric hospitalist conditions
8. Bypass surgery	a. Bronchitis and asthma
9. Valve surgery	b. Esophagitis and gastroenteritis
10. Stroke—ischemic	c. Kidney and UTI
11. Total hip replacement	d. Nutritional and miscellaneous metabolic disorders
12. Total knee replacement	e. Otitis media and URI
13. Hip fracture	f. Pediatric pneumonia
14. Abd. hysterectomy—non-CA	g. Seizure and headache
15. Abd. hysterectomy—CA	h. Fever of unknown origin
16. Lap hysterectomy	36. NICU, PICU, and adult ICU (medical, surgical, and burn)
17. Cholecystectomy—lap	37. AHRQ patient safety indicators
18. Cholecystectomy—open	38. Pain management
19. Lumbar fusion	39. Sickle cell
20. Lumbar laminectomy	40. Sepsis
21. Bariatric surgery	41. 100,000 Lives Campaign
22. Colon resection	42. 5 Million Lives Campaign
23. Diabetes and glycemic control	43. National Patient Safety Goals
24. DVT	44. Rapid response team
25. COPD	
26. Upper GI bleed	
27. SCIP	
28. Peripheral vascular procedures	

algorithms, adjusting for severity, and adding industry benchmarks. The resulting report contains measures of clinical processes (antibiotic utilization, deep vein thrombosis [DVT] prophylaxis, beta-blocker administration, autologous blood collection, and blood product administration), financial performance (lengths of stay, total patient charges, pharmacy charges, lab charges, X-ray charges, and intravenous therapy charges), and clinical outcomes (DVT, acute myocardial infarction [AMI], and readmission within 31 days). From more than 200 indicators available in the database, the total joint quality improvement team selected these measures as the most important for assessing the quality and cost of care delivered. The measures also include some Joint Commission core measures.[1]

To obtain patient satisfaction information, the team uses industry-standard patient satisfaction surveys. The outbound call center administers these surveys by telephone within one week of a patient's discharge. The results can be reported by nursing unit or physician, are updated monthly, and can be charted over the past eight quarters.

EXHIBIT 5.2
Clinical Dash-
board — Hip
Replacement

✪ Spectrum Health   Clinical Outcomes Report (COR)–**Hip Replacement**

March 1, 2006 to February 28, 2007

Administrative Data   Process

Name	No. of patients	1st gen. Ceph	Vancomycin	Coumadin	Heparin	Low mol. wt. heparin	Coumadin or LMW heparin	Beta blocker	Autologous blood coll.	Blood prod. given	DVT prophylaxis*	Hip revision
BL	617	95.5%	9.9%	14.6%	23.0%	91.2%	96.6%	39.9%	1.8%	33.2%	99.7%	20.4%
BW	136	90.4%	11.8%	5.9%	5.1%	100.0%	100.0%	41.9%	4.4%	30.9%	100.0%	13.2%
SH-GR	753	94.6%	10.2%	13.0%	19.8%	92.8%	97.2%	40.2%	2.3%	32.8%	99.7%	19.1%

Administrative Data   Outcome | Education

Name	No. of patients	DVT	AccPuncLac	Any 30 days	readmit 2nd DX	AMI Los
BL	617	0.6%	0.0%	4.2%	0.0%	3.67
BW	136	0.0%	0.0%	4.4%	0.7%	3.78
SH-GR	753	0.5%	0.0%	4.2%	0.1%	3.69

Education participation rate*

59.3%

** The education rate reflects all total joint replacement patients who had their surgery within the time period stated on this dashboard.

JCAHO SCIP   JCAHO Surgical Care Improvement Project

Name	No. of patients	Preop dose (SCIP-INF-1)*		Antibiotic Selection (SCIP-INF-2)		Postop duration (SCIP-INF-3)*	
SH-GR	Varies	96.0%	n = 75	100.0%	n = 76	97.2%	n = 72

Administrative Data   Direct Costs

Name	No. of patients	ICU cost	Laboratory cost	OR cost	Pharmacy cost	Radiology cost	R&B cost	Supplies cost	Therapy cost	Other cost	Total cost
BL	617	$71	$180	$2,219	$384	$79	$1,460	$1,944	$394	$217	$6,948
BW	136	$101	$127	$1,140	$405	$101	$1,801	$5,062	$389	$285	$9,410
SH-GR	753	$76	$170	$2,024	$388	$83	$1,521	$2,507	$393	$230	$7,393

Administrative Data   Fully Allocated Costs

Name	No. of patients	ICU cost	Laboratory cost	OR cost	Pharmacy cost	Radiology cost	R&B cost	Supplies cost	Therapy cost	Other cost	Total cost
BL	617	$117	$251	$3,711	$492	$162	$3,020	$2,078	$559	$326	$10,715
BW	136	$189	$176	$2,279	$515	$171	$3,215	$5,263	$578	$416	$12,802
SH-GR	753	$130	$237	$3,452	$496	$163	$3,055	$2,653	$562	$342	$11,092

Administrative Data   Potential Direct Cost Savings

Name	No. of patients	DVT		AccPuncLac		AMI 2nd DX		Total cost (Patients above average)	
BL	Varies	$51,618	n = 4	$0	n = 0	$0	n = 0	$679,916	n = 189
BW	Varies	$0	n = 0	$0	n = 0	$9,653	n = 1	$165,825	n = 61
SH-GR	Varies	$49,770	n = 4	$0	n = 0	$11,614	n = 1	$920,655	n = 270

* Denotes indicators selected for "The Joint Commission"

Prepared June 10, 2007 by the Spectrum Health Quality Department.

Source: Spectrum Health, Grand Rapids, MI. Copyright 2008 Spectrum Health. Used with permission.

To complete the measurement set, the team includes the results of patients' functional status (following their treatments). This information can be obtained from patients' EHRs (if it has been included in them) or by using survey tools during follow-up visits. Many hospital procedures are performed to improve patients' functional status. A patient who undergoes a total knee replacement, for example, should experience less knee pain when he or she walks, have a good range of joint motion, and be able to perform the activities of daily living that most of us take for granted. For this report, the team examines patients' functional status before and after hospitalization to demonstrate that their treatments were effective.

In summary, when designing data collection efforts, quality improvement teams need to maintain a balanced perspective of the process of care by collecting data in all four categories: clinical quality, financial performance, patient satisfaction, and functional status. Teams that fail to maintain this balance may overlook critical information. For instance, a health system in the Southwest initially reported that it had completed a series of successful quality improvement projects—clinical care had improved, patient satisfaction was at an all-time high, and patient outcomes were at national benchmark levels. However, subsequent review of the projects identified that some of the interventions had negatively affected the system's financial outcomes. Revenue had significantly decreased as a result of several interventions, and other interventions had increased the cost of care. If financial measures had been included in the reporting process, the negative financial effect could have been minimized and the same outstanding quality improvements would have resulted. In the end, the projects were considered only marginally successful because they lacked a balanced approach to process improvement and measurement.

Considerations in Data Collection

Time and Cost Involved in Data Collection

All data collection efforts take time and money. The key is to balance the cost of data collection and the value of the data to your improvement efforts. In other words, are the cost and time spent collecting data worth the effort? Will the data have the power to drive change and improvement? Although this cost–benefit analysis may not be as tangible as it is in the world of business and finance, the value equation must be considered. Generally, medical record review and prospective data collection are considered the most time-intensive and expensive ways to collect information. Many reserve these methods for highly specialized improvement projects or use them to answer questions that have surfaced following review of administrative data sets. Use of administrative data[2] is often considered cost-effective, especially because the credibility of administrative databases has improved and continues to improve through the efforts of coding and billing regulations, initiatives,[3] and rule-based software development. Additionally, third-party vendors can provide data cleanup and severity adjustment. Successful data collection strategies often combine both code- and chart-based sources into a data collection plan that capitalizes on the strengths and cost-effectiveness of each.

The following situation illustrates how the cost-effectiveness of an administrative system can be combined with the detailed information available in a medical record review. A data analyst using a clinical decision support system (administrative database) discovered a higher-than-expected incidence of renal failure (a serious complication) following coronary artery bypass surgery. The rate was well above 10 percent for the most recent 12 months (more than 800 patients were included in the data set) and had slowly increased over the past six quarters. However, the clinical decision support system did not contain enough detail to explain why such a large number of patients were experiencing this complication—whether this complication resulted from the coronary artery bypass graft procedure or was a chronic condition present on admission. To find the answer, the data analyst used chart review to (1) verify that the rate of renal failure as reported in the administrative data system was correct, (2) isolate cases of postoperative incidence, (3) identify the root cause(s) of the renal failure, and (4) answer additional questions about the patient population that were of interest to the physicians involved in the patients' care. In this example, the analyst used the administrative system to identify unwanted complications in a large patient population (a screening or surveillance function) and reserved chart review for a much smaller focused study (80 charts) to validate the incidence and determine why the patients were experiencing the complication. This excellent example shows effective use of two common data sources and demonstrates how the analyst is able to capitalize on the strengths of both while using each most efficiently.

Collecting the Critical Few Rather than Collecting for a Rainy Day

Many quality improvement efforts collect every possible data element in case it might be needed. Ironically, justification for this approach is often based on saving time—the chart has already been pulled, so one might as well be thorough. This syndrome of stockpiling "just in case" versus fulfilling requirements "just in time" has been studied in supply chain management and proven to be ineffective and inefficient. It also creates quality issues (Denison 2002). This approach provides little value to the data collection effort and is one of the biggest mistakes quality improvement teams make. Rather than provide a rich source of information, this approach unnecessarily drives up the cost of data collection, slows the data collection process, creates data management issues, and overwhelms the quality improvement team with too much information.

For all quality improvement projects, it is critical to collect only the data required to identify and correct quality issues. As a rule in ongoing data collection efforts, quality improvement teams should be able to link every data element collected to a report, thereby ensuring that teams do not collect data that will not be used (James 2003). In the reporting project discussed earlier, the hospital team was limited to selecting no more than 15 measures for each clinical condition. It also selected indicators that (1) have been shown by evidence-based literature to have the greatest effect on patient outcomes (e.g., in congestive heart failure, the use of angiotensin converting enzyme [ACE] inhibitors and beta blockers and evaluation of left ventricular ejection fraction); (2) reflect areas in which significant improvements are needed; (3) will be reported in the public domain (Joint Commission core measures); and (4) together provide a balanced view of the clinical process of care, financial performance, and patient outcomes.

Inpatient Versus Outpatient Data

The distinction between inpatient and outpatient data is an important consideration in planning the data collection process because the data sources and approaches to data collection can be different.

The case of a team working on a diabetes disease management project illustrates this point. First, disease management projects tend to focus on the entire continuum of care, so the team needs data from both inpatient and outpatient settings. Second, the team needs to identify whether patients receive the majority of care in one setting or the other and decide whether data collection priorities should be established with this setting in mind. For diabetes, the outpatient setting has the most influence on patient outcomes, so collection of outpatient data is a priority. Third, the team must select the measures that reflect the aspects of care that have the most influence on patient outcomes. Remembering to collect the critical few (as discussed in the previous section), the team would consult the American Diabetes Association (ADA) guidelines for expert direction. Fourth, the team must recognize that the sources of outpatient data are much different from the sources of inpatient data, and outpatient data tend to be more fragmented and harder to obtain. However, with the advent of outpatient EHRs and patient registries, the ease of collecting outpatient data is improving.

To identify outpatient data sources, the team should consider the following questions:

- Are the physicians in organized medical groups that have outpatient EHRs? Can their financial or billing systems identify all patients with diabetes in their practices? If not, can the health plans in the area supply the data by practice site or individual physician?
- Some of the most important diabetes measures are based on laboratory testing. Do the physicians have their own labs? If so, do they archive the lab data for a 12- to 24-month snapshot? If they do not do their own lab testing, do they use a common reference lab that would be able to supply the data?

Once the team answers these questions, it will be ready to proceed with data collection in the outpatient setting.

Sources of Data

As just discussed, the sources of data for quality improvement projects are extensive. Some sources are simple to access, while accessing others is complex; some data sources are inexpensive to use, while others are expensive. In the average hospital or health system, data sources include medical records, prospective data collection, surveys of various types, telephone interviews, focus groups, administrative databases, health plan claims databases, cost accounting systems, patient registries, stand-alone clinical databases, EHRs, and lab and pharmacy databases.

The following objectives are essential to a successful quality improvement project and data collection initiative:

- Identify the purpose of the data measurement activity (i.e., for monitoring at regular intervals, investigation over a limited period, or a onetime study).
- Identify data sources that are most appropriate for the activity.
- Identify the most important measures to collect (the critical few).
- Design a common-sense strategy that will ensure collection of complete, accurate, and timely information.

By following these steps, project teams will gather actionable data and the information required to drive quality improvements.

Medical Record Review (Retrospective)

Retrospective data collection involves identification and selection of a patient's medical record or group of records after the patient has been discharged from the hospital or clinic. Records generally cannot be reviewed until all medical and financial coding is complete because codes are used as a starting point for identifying the study cohort.

For several reasons, many quality improvement projects depend on medical record review for data collection. First, many proponents of medical record review believe it to be the most accurate method of data collection. They believe that because administrative databases have been designed for financial and administrative purposes rather than for quality improvement, the databases contain inadequate detail, many errors, and "dirty data"—that is, data that make no sense or appear to have come from other sources.

Second, some improvement projects rely on medical record review because many of the data elements are not available from administrative databases. For example, most administrative databases do not contain measures that require a time stamp, such as administration of antibiotics within one hour before surgical incision.

Third, several national quality improvement database projects— including the Healthcare Effectiveness Data and Information Set (HEDIS), Joint Commission core measures, Leapfrog Hospital Survey,[4] and National Quality Forum's (NQF) National Voluntary Consensus Standards for Hospital Care—depend on retrospective medical record review for collecting a significant portion of the data elements required to be reported. The records not only contain measures requiring a time stamp but, for some measures, also require the data collector to include or exclude patients on the basis of criteria that administrative databases do not capture consistently. The percentage of patients with congestive heart failure who are receiving an ACE inhibitor is an example of this type of measure. The use of ACE inhibitors in this population is indicated for all patients with an ejection fraction of less than 40 percent. The ejection fraction is not part of the typical administrative database. Sometimes this information is contained in a generally inaccessible, stand-alone database in the cardiology department, or it may be contained only in a transcribed report in the patient's medical record. Hence, accurate reporting of this measure, one of the most critical interventions that a patient with congestive heart failure will receive, depends completely on retrospective chart review. A consensus document presented to NQF[5] suggested that clinical importance should rate foremost among criteria for effectiveness and that measures that score poorly on feasibility[6] because of the burden of medical record review should not be excluded solely on that basis if their clinical importance is high (NQF Consumer, Purchaser, and Research Council Members 2002).

Fourth, focused medical record review is the primary tool for answering the "why" of given situations (e.g., why patients were experiencing a particular complication, why a certain intervention negatively affected patient outcomes). Medical record review continues to be a key component of many data collection projects, but it needs to be used judiciously because of the time and cost involved.

The approach to medical record review involves a series of well-conceived steps, beginning with the development of a data collection tool and ending with the compilation of collected data elements into a registry or electronic database for review and analysis.

Prospective Data Collection, Data Collection Forms, and Scanners

Prospective data collection also relies on medical record review, but it is completed during a patient's hospitalization or visit rather than retrospectively. Nursing staff, dedicated research assistants, or full-time data analysts commonly collect the data. The downside to asking nursing staff to collect data is the effort involved; it is a time-consuming task that can distract nurses from their direct patient care responsibilities. A better approach would be to hire research assistants or full-time data analysts who can collect the data and be responsible for data entry and analysis. Because this job is their sole responsibility, the accuracy of data collection is greater. If they also are responsible for presenting their analyses to various quality committees, they are likely to review the data more rigorously.

Obviously, this method of data collection is expensive, but if staff can minimize the time required for data entry, it can focus on accuracy and analysis/reporting. Converting the data collection forms into a format that can be scanned is one way to save time. With this approach, data entry can be as simple as feeding the forms into a scanner and viewing the results on a computer screen. Successful execution hinges on careful design of the forms and careful completion to ensure that the scanner captures all data elements. Alternatively, data collection forms can be developed for tablet technology that automatically downloads the collected data to project databases.

The most efficient data collection tools follow the actual flow of patient care and medical record documentation, whether the data are collected retrospectively or prospectively. There are numerous advantages to prospective data collection. First, detailed information not routinely available from administrative databases can be gathered. Physiologic parameters can be captured, such as the range of blood pressures for a patient on vasoactive infusions or 24-hour intake and output for patients with heart failure. As discussed earlier, data requiring a time stamp also can be captured. Timely administration of certain therapies (e.g., administration of antibiotics within one hour before surgical incision or within eight hours of hospital arrival for patients with pneumonia) has shown to improve patient outcomes. The timing of "clot buster" administration to certain stroke patients can mean the difference between full recovery and no recovery, and the window of opportunity for these patients is small; they usually must receive thrombolytic therapy within three hours of symptom onset. For patients with AMI, the administration of aspirin and beta blockers within the first 24 hours is critical to survival.

Through prospective chart review, the data collection staff can spot patient trends as they develop rather than receive the information after patients have been discharged. For instance, they may detect an increasing incidence of ventilator-associated pneumonia sooner, or they may spot an increase in the rate of aspiration in stroke patients as it occurs.

Unfortunately, the downside to this data collection approach is cost. Prospective data collection is costly and time consuming and often requires healthcare organizations to hire several full-time data analysts.

Administrative Databases

Administrative databases are a common source of data for quality improvement projects. *Administrative data* are information collected, processed, and stored in automated information systems. These data include enrollment or eligibility information, claims information, and information on managed care encounters. They may relate to hospital and other facility services, professional services, prescription drug services, or laboratory services.

Examples of administrative data sources are hospital and physician office billing systems, health plan claims databases, health information management or medical record systems, and registration systems (admission/discharge/transfer). Ideally, hospitals also maintain a cost accounting system that integrates the previously mentioned systems into one database and provides the important elements of patient cost. Although each of these sources has unique characteristics, for the purposes of this discussion they will be considered collectively as administrative databases (with the exception of health plan claims databases, which are covered later in this chapter).

Administrative databases are an excellent source of data for reporting on clinical quality, financial performance, and certain patient outcomes. They are the backbone of many quality improvement programs, including the CR system described at the beginning of this chapter.

The use of administrative databases is advantageous for the following reasons:

- Their use is less expensive than the use of alternative methods, such as chart review or prospective data collection.
- They incorporate transaction systems already used in a healthcare organization's daily business operations (frequently referred to as *legacy systems*).
- Most of the code sets embedded in administrative databases are standardized,[7] simplifying internal comparison between multi-facility organizations and external benchmarking with purchased or government data sets.
- Most administrative databases are maintained by individuals who are skilled at sophisticated database queries.
- Expert database administrators in information technology departments provide database architecture and support.
- The volume of available indicators is 100 times greater than that available through other data collection techniques.
- Data reporting tools are available as part of the purchased system or through third-party add-ons or services.
- Many administrative databases—especially well-managed financial and cost accounting systems—are subject to regular reconciliation, audit, and data cleanup procedures that enhance the integrity of their data.

Because of these advantages, many healthcare organizations make extensive use of administrative data systems as the primary source of data for quality improvement projects. For example, SCL Health System's CR system uses two administrative data sources: the billing system and the medical record system. Information from these sources is extracted and subjected to extensive cleanup. Severity adjustment, statistical analysis, and benchmarks also are applied.

The system contains more than 50 of the most common clinical conditions (medical and surgical procedures) and at least 100 measures of clinical quality, financial performance, and patient outcomes for each condition. The decision support system contains a total of more than 5,000 standardized performance measures, with functionality to report performance at the system level, by individual hospital, by individual physician, by resident, and by nursing unit. SCL Health System updates the database monthly and archives historical data in its data warehouse for future quality improvement projects and clinical studies.

The yearly cost to maintain this system is approximately $300,000, or the equivalent of four to five data analysts' combined salaries, yet the system's reporting power surpasses anything that five analysts performing chart review could accomplish. This system is a good value proposition because successful implementation of one or two quality improvement projects carefully selected from the many opportunities identified by the system can reimburse its full cost. One of the first projects identified by the system was the need to improve blood product utilization. The savings realized as a result of this project will more than cover the cost of the system for the first year.

Some argue that administrative data are less reliable than data gathered by chart review. However, when administrative data are properly cleaned and validated, the indicator definitions are clear and concise, and the limitations of the data are understood, administrative data can be just as reliable as data from chart review. These characteristics form a primary basis for the commercial outcome reporting systems available today. For example, the most common measures from the system described earlier were validated using four approaches: (1) chart review using an appropriate sampling methodology, (2) chart review performed for the core measures, (3) comparison to similar measures in stand-alone databases that rely on chart abstraction or prospective data collection strategies (e.g., National Registry of Myocardial Infarction), and (4) face validation performed by physicians with expertise in the clinical condition being studied. Results proved the administrative data sources to be just as reliable. In fact, if systems are not in place to ensure inter-rater reliability, such as third-party audits, chart review data can be very inaccurate.

Patient Surveys: Satisfaction and Functional Status
Patient Satisfaction Surveys

Patient satisfaction surveys have long been a favorite tool of quality improvement professionals, especially teams interested in the perceptions of patients, either in terms of the quality of care or the quality of service provided.

However, underestimation of the scientific complexity underlying survey research often leads to undesirable results. There is an art (and science) to constructing surveys that produce valid, reliable, relevant information. Likewise, survey validation itself is a time-consuming and complex undertaking. For an in-depth review of survey development and validation, many excellent textbooks on the concepts of reliability, validity, sampling methodology, and bias are available.

When an organization or a quality improvement team is considering the use of surveys, it has several choices on how to proceed. The team can design the survey tool itself, hire an outside expert to design the survey, or purchase an existing, well-validated survey or survey service. Usually, the fastest and least expensive approach is to purchase existing, well-validated survey instruments or to hire a survey organization to provide a solution. Press Ganey is one such organization.[8]

The frequency with which surveys are conducted and reported to the organization is also important. When patient satisfaction surveys are conducted on a continual basis using a proper sampling methodology, the organization is able to respond rapidly to changes in patients' wants and needs. It also can respond rapidly to poor service.

The ability to report survey results at an actionable level is critical; in most cases, *actionable level* means the nursing unit or location of service. Furthermore, full engagement at the management and support staff levels is important to ensuring that results are regularly reviewed and action plans are developed.

One of the most successful patient satisfaction survey projects was the point-of-service patient satisfaction surveys at Lovelace Health Systems in the late 1990s. Any patient who received care within the system could comment immediately following the encounter on the quality of the care and service. The survey forms were short (one page), concise, and easy to read, and patients could complete them in a few minutes. The questions assessed the most important determinants of satisfaction (as selected by the survey research staff), and patients could provide comments at the end of the survey. Unit managers collected and reviewed the surveys on a daily or weekly basis to identify emerging trends and quickly correct negative outcomes. Survey results were tabulated monthly and posted in the units for all to see, including patients who visited the clinics and inpatient areas. Senior management also reviewed the results on a unit-by-unit basis each month.

Functional Status Surveys

The measurement of functional status following medical treatment is the fourth category of data collection for clinical quality improvement projects. As a general rule, the purpose of medical treatments and hospital procedures is to improve patients' functional status or quality of life. For example, patients hospitalized for congestive heart failure should be able to walk farther, have more energy, and experience less shortness of breath following hospital treatment. Patients who undergo total knee replacements should have less knee pain when they walk, have a good range of joint motion, and be able to perform activities of daily living such as walking several miles, dancing, doing yard work, and performing normal household chores.

Functional status is usually measured before and at several points following the treatment or procedure. For some surgical procedures, such as total joint replacement, a baseline assessment commonly is made before the procedure, and then assessments are made at regular intervals following surgery, often at 1, 3, 6, and 12 months postoperatively. The survey can be collected by several means, including mail, telephone, and Internet.

The most widely recognized pioneer of functional status surveys is John Ware, PhD, the principal developer of the SF-36, SF-12, SF-8, and disease-specific health outcome surveys.[9]

Health Plan Databases

Health plan databases can be an excellent source of data for quality improvement projects, particularly projects that have a population health management focus. For many years, health plans have used a variety of means to collect data on their performance, track the management of the care received by their members, and direct programs on disease management and care management. Because of this experience, health plan data have become more and more reliable. Most health plans now have sophisticated data warehouses and a staff of expert data analysts.

Health plan databases are valuable because they contain detailed information on all care received by health plan members. They track care through bills (claims). Bills are generated for all services provided to a patient. When the bill is submitted to the health plan for payment, it is captured in a claims-processing system. As a result of this process, all care received by a population of patients—including hospitalizations, outpatient procedures, physician office visits, lab testing, and prescriptions—is documented in the health plan claims database.

Why is this process so important? From a population management perspective, the health plan claims database is often the only source of information on the care received by a patient and, for that matter, an entire population of patients. It is therefore an excellent source of data for disease management teams whose goal is to improve the health of a specific population. It provides a comprehensive record of patient activity and can be used to identify and select patients for enrollment in disease management programs. Claims databases are excellent tracking tools for examining the continuum of care and, until the advent of outpatient EHRs, were the only available external source of information on physician office practice. In essence, a claims database is the single best source of information on the total care received by a patient. Several illustrative examples follow.

Health plan databases commonly are used to identify patients who have not received preventive services, such as mammograms, colon cancer screening, and immunizations. They can identify patients who are not receiving the appropriate medications for many chronic medical conditions, such as heart failure and asthma. They also can be used to support physicians in their office practices. Exhibit 5.3 is an example of a report[10] for a diabetes disease management program. It provides participating physicians with a quarterly snapshot of (1) the percentage of their patients who are receiving all treatments and tests recommended by ADA guidelines, (2) how the physician's performance compares to the performance of his or her peers, and (3) all patients whose treatment has not met ADA standards in the previous quarter and who need recommended tests or treatments.

What are the limitations of health plan databases? Many of the considerations covered in the discussion of hospital administrative databases apply to health plan databases, including questions associated with accuracy, detail, and timeliness. Users of health plan claims databases also must keep in mind that changes to reimbursement rules (and the provider's response to those changes) may affect the integrity of the data over time. Recoding may make some historical data inaccurate, especially as they relate to the tracking and trending of complication rates and the categorization of certain types of complications. Furthermore, health plan databases track events, the type of procedure performed, or completion of a lab test. They do not contain detailed information on the outcomes of care or the results of tests (e.g., lab tests, radiology examinations, biopsies). Nevertheless, health plan claims data are inexpensive to acquire, are available electronically, and encompass large populations across the continuum of care. Used properly, they are a rich source of data for population management, disease management, and quality improvement projects.

Patient Registries

Many organizations establish condition-specific patient registries for their more sophisticated quality improvement projects because they do not have a reliable source of clinical information, available data are not timely, or they wish to collect patient outcome information over several months following a hospitalization or procedure. Often, the desire to develop a patient registry involves all of these considerations, and the registry includes data collected through all of the aforementioned approaches. Because of their detail and straightforward design, patient registries can be a powerful source of quality improvement data. Registries usually are specialty or procedure specific.

Rolling Calendar Year July 1, 2001–June 30, 2002

PCP:
Provider Group:

EXHIBIT 5.3
Diabetes
Provider
Support Report

I. Provider-Specific Data

Criteria	ADA Standards	Points	Tested	In Standard	Percentage
Education	1/2 year	48	42	42	88
Eye exams	Annual	48	30	30	63
Hemoglobin A1C ordered	Annual	48	45	45	94
Hemoglobin A1C level	≤7.0	48	45	37	82
Microalbumin ordered	Annual	48	31	31	65
Microalbumin >30	Rx filled	10	10	5	50
LDL ordered	Annual	48	42	42	88
LDL level	<100	48	42	31	73

*Patients in this report have had at least two diagnoses of diabetes.

II. Percentage of Patients Within Standard

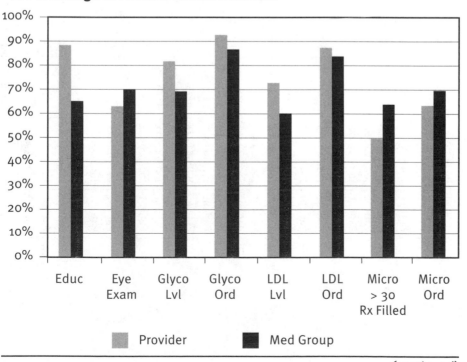

(continued)

EXHIBIT 5.3
Diabetes Provider Support Report *(continued)*

III. High-Risk Patient Detail—Patients Outside ADA Standards in Current Quarter

Criteria for inclusion—one or more of the following: (1) no education in last two years; (2) no eye exam in last one year; (3) Hemoglobin A1C > 7.0 or no Hemoglobin A1C ordered in last year; (4) no microalbumin in last one year; (5) microalbumin > 30 and no ACE/ARB filled; or (6) LDL ≥ 100 or no LDL ordered in last year.

Name	MR No.	Education	Eye Exam	Hemoglobin Ordered	Hemoglobin Level	Microalbumin Ordered	Microalbumin > 30, Rx Filled	Lipids Ordered	Lipids Results
Patient	100-319-xxx		7/21/99	7/15/99	6.7	5/28/99	N	2/29/00	120
Patient	100-427-xxx					2/22/00		2/22/00	118
Patient	100-587-xxx								
Patient	100-595-xxx	8/12/99		8/21/99	7.0				
Patient	100-623-xxx			2/2/00	10.8			1/21/00	142
Patient	100-666-xxx	7/14/99		12/15/99	10.7				
Patient	100-782-xxx	2/12/00		11/27/99	11.0				
Patient	100-847-xxx	2/12/00		3/12/99	7.0				
Patient	100-849-xxx	12/27/99		8/1/99	6.1			5/24/99	118
Patient	100-882-xxx	10/15/98		8/31/99	6.8			3/21/00	132
Patient	100-882-xxx	4/25/99		4/23/00	6.3				
Patient	100-893-xxx	7/31/98		9/19/99	12.4			8/25/99	123
Patient	100-901-xxx	6/15/99		6/2/00	6.3				
Patient	100-901-xxx	1/15/00		1/23/00	12.0			9/19/99	98
Patient	100-902-xxx	1/18/00		5/15/99	12.4			7/31/99	92
Patient	100-909-xxx							2/15/00	145
Patient	100-914-xxx	12/27/99		10/10/99	11.9			10/6/99	150
Patient	100-914-xxx			2/4/00	10.8			4/14/00	92
Patient	100-919-xxx			4/29/00	6.2			6/1/00	89
Patient	100-809-xxx	6/13/00	6/15/00	6/2/00	6.9	4/2/00	N	2/11/00	126
Patient	100-914-xxx	1/15/00	12/20/99	12/12/99	11.2	12/12/99	N	1/16/00	132
Patient	100-917-xxx	1/18/00	2/13/00	1/18/00	6.9	1/15/00	N	11/21/99	160
Patient	100-929-xxx	7/22/99	8/1/99	7/21/99	10.0	7/21/99	N	12/5/99	98

Note: ADA = American Diabetes Association; LDL = low-density lipoprotein (bad cholesterol).
Source: Spectrum Health, Grand Rapids, MI. Copyright 2008 Spectrum Health. Used with permission.

AMI, total joint replacement, coronary artery bypass graft, and congestive heart failure are common examples of conditions/procedures for which specific registries are created.

Use of patient registries is advantageous for the following reasons:

- They are a rich source of information because they are customized.
- They can collect all the data that the physician or health system determines are most important.
- They can be used for quality improvement and research purposes.
- They are not subject to the shortcomings of administrative or health plan databases.
- A multitude of data sources and collection techniques can be combined to provide a complete picture of the patient experience, including the quality of care provided and long-term patient outcomes (often up to a year following the procedure).

Patient registries are versatile and flexible because just about any reliable data source or collection methodology can be used to populate the registry, including administrative data, outbound call centers, prospective data collection, retrospective chart review, and a variety of survey instruments, particularly those used to assess patient satisfaction and functional status. However, with all customized database projects, the volume of data collected and the insight they will provide or the change they will drive must be weighed against the cost of collecting the data. A team overseeing a registry project must collect only the data necessary to the success of its project.

Use of an orthopedic patient registry illustrates how the considerations mentioned earlier were addressed. First, a team including a service line director, medical director, and physicians was established to oversee the project. The inclusion of physicians from the beginning created a tremendous level of physician involvement, to the point that the physicians felt great pride of ownership in the project. Second, the scope of data collection was narrowed to focus on only total knee and hip replacements. Third, the purpose and use of the registry were clearly outlined; its function was limited to identifying clinical issues and improving the quality of patient care. Fourth, the number of data elements was restricted to the critical few—elements most important to assessing patient outcomes and the integrity of the patient care processes— which meant the team would report and review them regularly.

Data collection was accomplished through several means, as illustrated in Exhibits 5.4 and 5.5. Patients were identified through the administrative database. Data collection was completed prospectively during hospitalization, and missing elements were captured from charts retrospectively. The team eased the data-entry burden by having all data collected on forms that could

Orthopedic Database Characteristics	
Total data elements	329
Manual data elements	216
Electronic data elements	113
No. of patients (monthly)	106
Data sources	
• Patient	
• Case managers	
• OR system	
• Billing/cost accounting system	
• Call center	
Number of Data Elements by Category	
Patient history	32
Demographic	56
Functional status	42
Procedures/OR	26
Complications	3
Devices/equipment	13
Postoperative	45
Follow-up	28 (× 4) = 112
Number of Data Elements by Source	
Patient	35
Case managers	69
OR system	48
Billing/cost accounting system	65
Call center	112

Source: Spectrum Health, Grand Rapids, MI. Copyright 2008 Spectrum Health. Used with permission.

be scanned. The outbound call center tracked outcomes over time through a variety of patient interview tools and survey instruments, making calls 1, 3, 6, and 12 months after the primary procedure. Ultimately, the data were combined in a database product available to all and audited for completeness and accuracy.

Case Study in Clinical Reporting

So far, this chapter has covered the different categories of data, considerations for data collection, and six data sources. Let's pull all this information together in a current hospital setting.

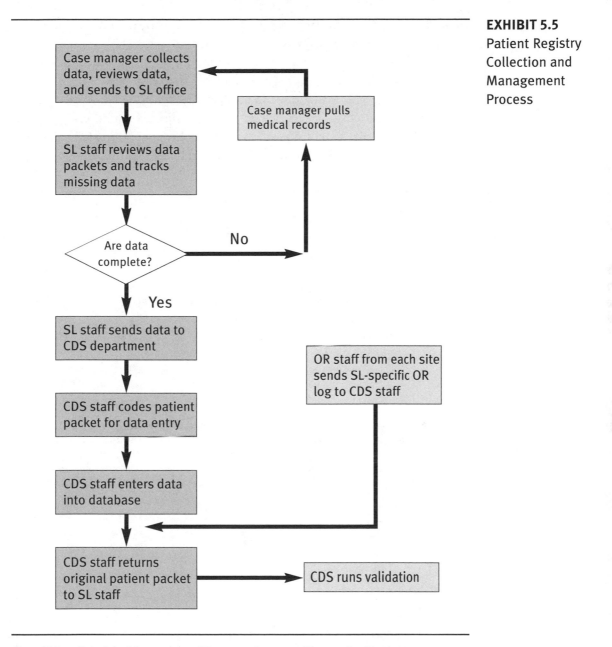

EXHIBIT 5.5
Patient Registry
Collection and
Management
Process

Note: CDS = clinical decision support; OR = operating room; SL = service line.

Earlier, this chapter introduced a CR system. The CR system consists of a data mart assembled from a variety of data sources and more than 50 disease-specific dashboards. The most commonly used reports include a clinical dashboard with health system–level and hospital-level data and physician-level reports. The clinical dashboard shown in Exhibit 5.2 contains measures of clinical quality for hip replacement. Ideally, the executive leadership team and medical directors review the executive dashboard monthly. It also is shared with the hospital quality committee and the board quality committee.

In addition to the dashboard's spreadsheet-like display, the CR system shows trends for each measure over the past 24 months (see Exhibit 5.6).

The physician-level reports can contain any of the indicators in the database, including indicators generated for the hospital-level dashboard. The physician-level information can be shared at medical staff or peer review committees. The physician-level data also are adjusted for severity, so they clearly identify patients considered "sicker" at hospital admission. The presentation format is similar to that of the hospital dashboard.

EXHIBIT 5.6
Clinical Report:
Example of
Trended Data
Over 24 Months

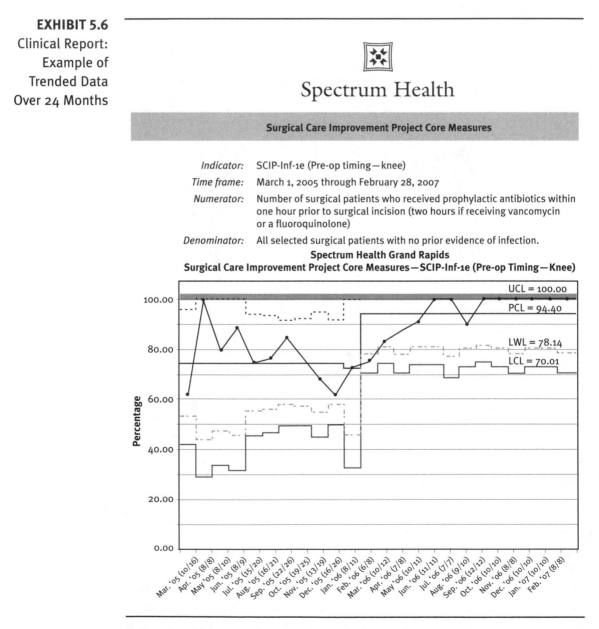

Spectrum Health

Surgical Care Improvement Project Core Measures

Indicator: SCIP-Inf-1e (Pre-op timing—knee)

Time frame: March 1, 2005 through February 28, 2007

Numerator: Number of surgical patients who received prophylactic antibiotics within one hour prior to surgical incision (two hours if receiving vancomycin or a fluoroquinolone)

Denominator: All selected surgical patients with no prior evidence of infection.

Spectrum Health Grand Rapids
Surgical Care Improvement Project Core Measures—SCIP-Inf-1e (Pre-op Timing—Knee)

Source: Copyright 2008 Spectrum Health. Used with permission.

Conclusion

There are many data sources and data collection approaches from which to choose. Rarely does one method serve all purposes, so it is important to understand the advantages and disadvantages of all methods. For this reason, the Spectrum Health case, like all successful quality improvement initiatives, uses a combination of data and data collection techniques, capitalizing on strengths and minimizing weaknesses. Knowledge of the different sources and techniques will help you use data more effectively and efficiently in your clinical quality improvement efforts.

Study Questions

1. What are notable advantages and disadvantages of using medical records versus administrative sources for collecting quality data?
2. Give two examples of areas in which you can identify a balanced set of measures.
3. Will EHRs improve data collection? Why or why not?

Acknowledgments

Special thanks go to Lori Anderson for her diligent review, suggestions, and contributions, as well as to Monica Carpenter for her editorial assistance.

Notes

1. Creation of the Joint Commission core measures was an initial attempt to integrate outcomes and other performance measurement into the accreditation process by requiring hospitals to collect and submit 25 measures distributed across five core measurement areas.
2. Administrative data generally reflect the content of discharge abstracts (e.g., demographic information on patients such as age, sex, and zip code; information about the episode of care such as admission source, length of stay, charges, and discharge status; diagnostic and procedural codes). The Uniform Hospital Discharge Data Set and the Uniform Bill (UB-92) of the Centers for Medicare & Medicaid Services provide specifications for the abstraction of administrative/billing data.
3. Examples include the Health Insurance Portability and Accountability Act (HIPAA) of 1996 (Public Law 104-191); the International

Classification of Diseases developed by the World Health Organization (WHO), which is scheduled to transition to ICD-10 on October 1, 2014 (Centers for Medicare & Medicaid Services 2013); the Systematized Nomenclature of Medicine (SNOMED) project; and the Unified Medical Language System (UMLS).

4. The Leapfrog Group is a coalition of more than 140 public and private organizations that provide healthcare benefits. It was created to help save lives and reduce preventable medical mistakes by mobilizing employer purchasing power to initiate breakthrough improvements in the safety of healthcare and by giving consumers information so that they may make more informed hospital choices.

5. NQF is a private, not-for-profit membership organization created to develop and implement a national strategy for healthcare quality measurement and reporting. Its mission is to improve US healthcare through endorsement of consensus-based national standards for measurement and public reporting of healthcare performance data that provide meaningful information about whether care is safe, timely, effective, patient centered, equitable, and efficient.

6. Feasibility infers that the cost of data collection and reporting is justified by the potential improvements in care and outcomes that result from the act of measurement.

7. The Uniform Hospital Discharge Data Set and UB-92 standardize the abstraction of administrative/billing data, including admission source, charges (national revenue codes), discharge status, and diagnostic and procedural codes (ICD-9, CPT-4, NCD, and HCPCS).

8. For more information, see www.pressganey.com.

9. For more information on Ware's work and a description of available surveys, visit www.qualitymetric.com.

10. This report was developed as part of a diabetes collaborative. Lovelace Health System developed the original design in Albuquerque, New Mexico, as part of the Episode of Care Disease Management Program.

References

Centers for Medicare & Medicaid Services. 2013. "About ICD-10." Updated September 9. www.cms.gov/Medicare/Coding/ICD10/index.html?redirect=/ICD10/.

Denison, D. C. 2002. "On the Supply Chain, Just-in-Time Enters New Era." *Boston Globe* May 5.

James, B. 2003. "Designing Data Systems. Advanced Training Program in Health Care Delivery Research." Salt Lake City, UT: Intermountain Healthcare.

National Quality Forum (NQF) Consumer, Purchaser and Research Council Members. 2002. "Hospital Performance Measurement Project. Proposal to NQF." Washington, DC: National Quality Forum.

Suggested Reading

Carey, R. G., and R. C. Lloyd. 2001. *Measuring Quality Improvement in Healthcare: A Guide to Statistical Process Control Applications.* Milwaukee, WI: ASQ Quality Press.

Eddy, D. M. 1998. "Performance Measurement: Problems and Solutions." *Health Affairs (Millwood)* 17 (4): 7–25.

Fuller, S. 1998. "Practice Brief: Designing a Data Collection Process." *Journal of the American Health Information Management Association* 70 (May): 12–16.

Gunter, M., J. Byrnes, M. Shainline, and J. Lucas. 1996. "Improving Outcomes Through Disease-Specific Clinical Practice Improvement Teams: The Lovelace Episodes of Care Disease Management Program." *Journal of Outcomes Management* 3 (3): 10–17.

Iz, P. H., J. Warren, and L. Sokol. 2001. "Data Mining for Healthcare Quality, Efficiency, and Practice Support." 34th Annual Hawaii International Conference on System Sciences (HICSS-34), January 3–6.

Joint Commission. 2012. *2013 Hospital Accreditation Standards.* Oakbrook Terrace, IL: The Joint Commission.

Lucas, J., M. J. Gunter, J. Byrnes, M. Coyle, and N. Friedman. 1995. "Integrating Outcomes Measurement into Clinical Practice Improvement Across the Continuum of Care: A Disease-Specific Episode of Care Model." *Managed Care Quarterly* 3 (2): 14–22.

Micheletti, J. A., T. J. Shlala, and C. R. Goodall. 1998. "Evaluating Performance Outcomes Measurement Systems: Concerns and Considerations." *Journal of Healthcare Quality* 20 (2): 6–12.

Mulder, C., M. Mycyk, and A. Roberts. 2003. "Data Warehousing and More." *Healthcare Informatics* 1 (March): 6–8.

STATISTICAL TOOLS FOR QUALITY IMPROVEMENT[1]

Stephen Schmaltz, Linda S. Hanold, Richard G. Koss, and Jerod M. Loeb

Fundamentals of Performance Measurement

Purpose of Measurement

Organizations measure performance to meet multiple internal and external needs and demands. Internal quality improvement literature identifies three fundamental purposes for conducting performance measurement: (1) assessment of current performance, (2) demonstration and verification of performance improvement, and (3) control of performance.

These purposes complement and support internal performance improvement activities. The first step in a structured performance improvement project is to assess current performance. This assessment identifies the strengths and weaknesses of the current process, thus targeting areas for intervention. It also provides the baseline data against which the organization will compare future measurement data after it has implemented interventions. The comparison of postintervention measurement data to baseline data will demonstrate and verify whether the intervention brought about an improvement. Measurement of performance control provides an early warning and correction system that highlights undesirable changes in process operations. This measurement is critical to sustaining improvements realized through process improvement activities.

Organizations also measure performance to meet external needs and demands—including healthcare provider accountability (e.g., pay for performance), decision making, public reporting, and organizational evaluation—and to support national performance improvement goals and activities. Healthcare purchasers and payers are demanding that providers demonstrate their ability to provide high-quality patient care at fair prices. Specifically, they are seeking objective evidence that hospitals and other healthcare organizations manage their costs well, satisfy their customers, and have desirable outcomes. Consumers are interested in care-related information for selection purposes. In other words, they use information to identify where they believe they will have the greatest probability of a good outcome for treatment of their condition. Evaluators such as The Joint Commission and the National Committee on Quality Assurance factor this information into their evaluation and accreditation activities. Performance measurement data can fulfill these needs if the measure construct is sound, the data analyses and interpretations are scientifically credible, and the data are reported in a useable format that is easy to understand.

Generally, effective performance measurement benefits organizations in the following ways (Joint Commission 2000):

- Provides factual evidence of performance
- Promotes ongoing organizational self-evaluation and improvement
- Demonstrates improvement
- Facilitates cost–benefit analysis
- Helps to meet external requirements and demands for performance evaluation
- May facilitate the establishment of long-term relationships with various external stakeholders
- May differentiate the organization from competitors
- May contribute to the awarding of business contracts
- Fosters organizational survival

Framework for Measurement

Performance improvement can be considered a philosophy. The organization-wide application of this philosophy composes the organizational framework for measurement. Healthcare organizations committed to ongoing performance improvement have incorporated this philosophy or framework into their overall strategic planning process. Performance improvement projects are not isolated but rather are a part of a cohesive performance improvement program. A cohesive performance improvement program comprises a performance improvement process, a plan, and projects (Joint Commission 2000).

The *performance improvement process* is a carefully chosen, strategically driven, values-based, systemic, organization-wide approach to the achievement of specific, meaningful, high-priority organizational improvements. The performance improvement plan is derived from this overall context.

The *performance improvement plan* consists of a detailed strategy for undertaking specific projects to address improvement opportunities. This plan should include the (1) identified and prioritized opportunities for improvement, (2) staff needed to coordinate and conduct the improvement project,

(3) expected time frames, and (4) needed financial and material resources. An organization should integrate its performance improvement plan with the organization-wide strategic plan so that the performance improvement priorities are viewed as being as important as other organizational priorities and so that they are given equal consideration in the allocation of resources and in the short- and long-term planning processes.

Performance improvement projects evolve from the establishment and articulation of the performance improvement plan. Projects are the diverse, individual, focused initiatives in which hospitals invest to achieve clearly defined, important, measurable improvements.

The following components support successful implementation of performance improvement programs and attainment of project goals and objectives:

- *Leadership commitment*: Leaders must create the setting that demands and supports continuous improvement. Leaders affect how staff work, which in turn affects how patients experience the care and services delivered. Literature identifies senior management leadership as the most critical factor in organizational performance improvement success.

- *Staff understanding and participation*: Another critical component to successful performance improvement is staff involvement. Each employee is responsible for an organization's performance and, therefore, for the improvement of that performance. Employees must understand the healthcare organization's mission, vision, and values and their work's contribution to achieving those objectives. They need to understand the value of continuous organizational improvement and their role in this context. They must become familiar with improvement principles, tools, and techniques and become adept at using them to measure, assess, and improve.

- *Establishment of partnerships with key stakeholders*: Establishment of such partnerships will provide an understanding of each stakeholder's specific and unique performance data and information needs and allow the organization to produce customized, meaningful performance reports that present the information in the most easily understood and informative format for various external audiences.

- *Establishment of a performance improvement oversight entity*: This group oversees all aspects of the healthcare organization's performance improvement process, including determination of improvement priorities, integration of performance improvement efforts with daily work activities, initiation and facilitation of performance improvement projects, performance improvement education, development of performance improvement protocols, monitoring the progress of improvement efforts, quantification of resource consumption for each project, communication of improvement internally and externally, and assurance that process improvements are sustained.

- *Selection and use of a performance improvement methodology*: Use of a single improvement methodology across all improvement initiatives is critical to facilitating a cohesive and consistent approach to improvement within the organization. An organization can develop improvement methodologies internally or can adapt or adopt those of external sources, such as The Joint Commission's FOCUS PDCA method, the robust process improvement method (Chassin and Loeb 2011), or other approaches.

- *Development of performance improvement protocols*: Performance improvement protocols describe how the organization implements its performance improvement process. They typically describe the purpose and responsibilities of the oversight entity, the process for proposing improvement projects, the process for reviewing and selecting projects, methods for convening project teams, the roles and responsibilities of team members, the selected performance improvement method and how to implement it, and reporting and communication requirements.

- *Identification of and response to performance improvement resource needs*: Performance improvement requires investment and support, including an expert resource person, employees who are allocated dedicated time to work on the project, education, information and knowledge, equipment, and financial resources.

- *Recognition and acknowledgment of performance improvement successes and efforts*: Acknowledgment of improvement successes builds organizational momentum for future successes, engenders a sense of meaningful contribution in individual employees, and bonds the organization in celebration. In-house or public recognition of improvement successes rewards teams by showing respect and appreciation for their unique talents, skills, and perspectives. In turn, this recognition fosters employee dedication and loyalty.

- *Continuous assessment of improvement efforts' effectiveness*: Healthcare organizations are not static, and neither are the functions performed in them. Improvement efforts must be reviewed routinely to determine that successes are sustained in the rapidly changing environment of today's healthcare organization (Joint Commission 2000).

Selecting Performance Measures

Numerous opportunities for improvement exist in every healthcare organization. However, not all improvements are of the same magnitude. Improvements that are powerful and worthy of organizational resources include those that will positively affect a large number of patients, eliminate or reduce instability in critical clinical or business processes, decrease risk, and ameliorate serious problems. In short, a focus on high-risk, high-volume, problem-prone areas is most appropriate to maximize the return on performance improvement investment.

Because performance measurement lies at the heart of any performance improvement process, performance measures must be selected in a thoughtful and deliberate manner. An organization may develop performance measures internally or adopt them from a multitude of external resources. However, regardless of the source of performance measures, each measure should be evaluated against certain characteristics to ensure a credible and beneficial measurement effort. The following characteristics are critical to performance measures (Joint Commission 2010):

- *Relevant*: Selected measures should relate directly to the organization's improvement goals and should be linked to the organization's mission, vision, values, and strategic goals and objectives.
- *Reliable*: Reliability refers to data constancy and consistency. Reliable measures accurately and consistently identify the events they were designed to identify across multiple healthcare settings.
- *Valid*: Valid measures identify opportunities for improvement (i.e., events that merit further review) relative to the services provided and the quality of the healthcare results achieved. Valid measures raise good questions about current processes and, therefore, underlie the identification of improvement opportunities.
- *Cost-effective*: Performance measurement requires resource investment and, therefore, implies that the ultimate value of the measurement activity should justify the related resource expenditure. Some measurement activities are not worth the investment necessary to collect and analyze the data. The cost versus the benefit (i.e., the value) of all measurement activities must be considered.
- *Under the provider's control*: There is little value in collecting data on processes or outcomes over which the organization has little or no control. A provider must be able to influence (i.e., implement interventions on) the processes and outcomes tracked by any performance measure it uses.
- *Precisely defined and specified*: Performance measures and their data elements must be specified precisely through predefined and standardized requirements for data collection and must measure calculation to ensure uniform application from measurement period to measurement period and to ensure comparability across organizations. Precisely defined and specified measures ensure that the organization

will collect and calculate the measures the same way each time and that other organizations will do the same.

- *Interpretable*: Interpretability refers to the extent to which users of the data and information understand the measures' rationale and results.
- *Risk adjusted or stratified*: Adjustment/stratification refers to the extent to which the influences of factors that differ among comparison groups can be controlled or taken into account (Iezzoni 2013).

The presence or absence of some of these characteristics may not be obvious before implementation. Pilot testing may help with this determination. Pilot testing may disclose that a particular measure is not appropriate before significant resources have been invested in the activity.

Finally, an organization should consider various types of performance measures in its performance measure selection process. Avedis Donabedian (1980) first described three components of quality: structure, process, and outcome. An organization can develop meaningful measures for each of these components. *Structure* describes hospital characteristics such as organization structure, specialty services provided, and patient census. *Process* includes components of clinical care (i.e., how care and services are provided) such as assessments and evaluations, diagnoses, and therapeutic and palliative interventions. Clinical *outcome* is multidimensional and describes how delivered care affects the patient's health status, functionality, and well-being. Structure, process, and outcome measures can be defined further as either *continuous-variable measures* or *rate-based measures*.

- *Continuous-variable measures*: Each value of a continuous-variable measure is a precise measurement that can fall anywhere along a continuous scale. An example is the number of days from surgery to discharge of patients undergoing coronary artery bypass graft procedures.
- *Rate-based measures*: The value of a rate-based measure reflects the frequency of an event or condition and is expressed as a proportion or ratio. A *proportion* shows the number of occurrences over the entire group within which the occurrence could take place (for example, surgical patients receiving prophylactic antibiotics within one hour of surgery over all surgical patients). A *ratio* shows occurrences compared with a different but related phenomenon (for example, patients who fall over patient days).

Statistical Process Control

Statistical process control (SPC) is the use of numbers and data to study the things we do to make them behave the way we want (McNeese and Klein

1991). In other words, SPC is a method of using data to track processes (the things we do) so that we can improve the quality of products and services (make them behave the way we want). SPC uses simple statistical tools to help us understand any process that generates products or services.

SPC evolved from work done by Walter Shewhart in the 1920s at Bell Labs in New York. Developed as a quality control tool in manufacturing, SPC was introduced into healthcare in the early 1990s. During World War I, Shewhart was directed to design a radio headset for the military. One of the key pieces of information he needed to design a headset was the width of people's heads. Shewhart measured them and discovered not only that head width varied but also that it varied according to a pattern. The size of most people's heads fell within a relatively narrow range, but some people had heads that were larger or smaller than the norm, a few considerably so. Shewhart found that this pattern of variation, now known as the normal distribution (or bell-shaped curve), also was present in many manufacturing processes (McNeese and Klein 1991).

Later, Shewhart developed a control chart based on this pattern of variation. Control charts, one of the SPC tools discussed later in this chapter, are used to track and analyze variation in processes over time. Control charts were not widely used until World War II, when they assisted in the production of wartime goods.

After World War II, the Japanese began to use SPC extensively to improve the quality of their products as they were rebuilding their economy. Japanese industry underwent massive statistical training as a result of the influence and efforts of Shewhart, W. Edwards Deming, and Joseph M. Juran. SPC did not catch on in the West until the 1980s, by which time the United States and Europe were scrambling to catch up with the quality standards set by Japanese manufacturers.

The theory behind SPC is straightforward. It requires a change in thinking from error detection to error prevention. In manufacturing, once a product is made, correcting errors is wasteful, time consuming, and expensive. The same is true in healthcare. Making the product or providing the service correctly the first time is better and more cost-effective.

SPC changes the approach toward producing a product or service. The approach moves from inspecting the product or evaluating the service after it is produced to understanding the process itself so that the process can be improved. Problems should be identified and resolved before the product is produced or the service is provided, which requires monitoring how the process is performing through routine, selective measurements.

All processes, whether in manufacturing or healthcare, produce data. SPC uses data generated by the process to improve the process. Process improvement, in turn, leads to improved products and services. Exhibit 6.1

EXHIBIT 6.1
Continuous
Process
Improvement
Cycle

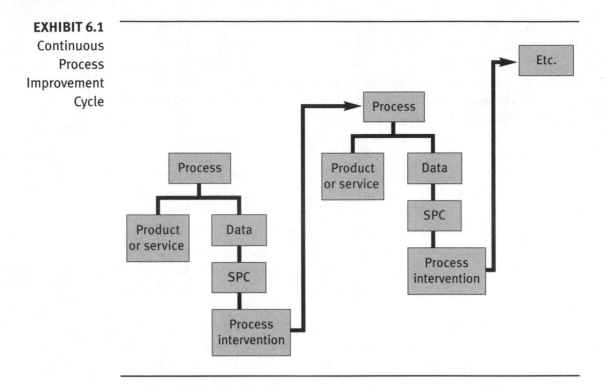

illustrates how a process that generates a product or service simultaneously generates data that can be analyzed using SPC tools and used to improve that process continuously.

In summary, the use of SPC in healthcare has a number of benefits, including (1) increased quality awareness on the part of healthcare organizations and practitioners, (2) increased focus on patients, (3) the ability to base decisions on data, (4) the implementation of predictable healthcare processes, (5) cost reduction, (6) fewer errors and increased patient safety, and (7) improved processes that result in improved healthcare outcomes and better quality care.

Control Chart Analysis

Every process varies. For example, a healthcare organization is unlikely to have the same number of patient falls every month. However, not every process will vary in the same way. For example, suppose that in a given year, the number of patient falls averaged 20 per month and ranged between 17 and 23 per month. These data suggest a stable process because the variation is predictable within given limits. In SPC terminology, this type of variation is called *common cause variation*. Common cause variation does not imply that the process is functioning at either a desirable or an undesirable level; it describes only the nature of variation—that it is stable and predictable within given limits.

Next, suppose that during the following year, the average number of falls stayed the same, but in one month, there were 35 falls. This type of variation is called *special cause variation*. The process has changed and is no longer predictable within limits. In this case, the special cause is a negative finding. The healthcare organization should not make changes to its fall prevention protocols until it identifies and eliminates the special cause.

On the other hand, if the observed variation were only common cause variation (as in the first case), introduction of a new fall prevention program to improve the process would be appropriate. After introducing a fall prevention program, if the number of falls in the second year decreased to an average of 17 per month with a range of 14 to 19, this change would be a positive special cause. This special cause would signal the success of the intervention.

In summary, the control chart will tell a healthcare organization whether the observed variation results from a common or special cause so that it knows how to approach a process improvement. If there is a special cause, the healthcare organization should investigate and eliminate it, not change the process. If there is common cause variation, implementation of a process change to improve it is appropriate. A control chart will reveal whether the change was effective.

Elements of a Control Chart

A control chart is a line graph with a centerline that represents the overall process average (or mean). It shows the flow of a process over time, as distinguished from a distribution, which is a collection of data not necessarily organized in the order they were collected. A control chart is a dynamic presentation of data; a distribution is a static presentation. The measure of the process being monitored or evaluated appears on the vertical axis.

A control chart also has an upper control limit (UCL) and a lower control limit (LCL). The control limits are not the same as the confidence limits of a distribution. The *control limits* describe the variability of a process over time and usually are set at three standard deviations (or sigmas), whereas the *confidence limits* of a distribution describe the degree of certainty that a given point is different from the average score—in other words, an outlier. Data falling outside the three-sigma limits are a signal that the process has changed significantly. This data point is properly referred to as a special cause, not an outlier. However, the three-sigma rule is only one test to detect special cause variation. See Exhibit 6.2 for an example of a control chart.

Tests for a Special Cause

There are two errors (or mistakes) that we can make in trying to detect a special cause. First, we can conclude that there is a special cause when one is not present (Type I error). Second, we can conclude that there is no special cause when in fact one is present (Type II error). Shewhart, who developed

EXHIBIT 6.2
Pneumococcal
Vaccination
Rate Control
Chart

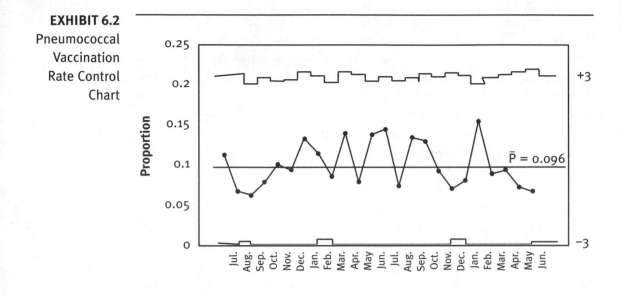

Source: Data from Lee and McGreevey (2000).

the control chart, recommended that using three-sigma control limits offered the best balance between making either the first or the second mistake.

Shewhart's disciples at Western Electric developed other tests, such as observation of eight consecutive points either above or below the mean, four of five consecutive points beyond one sigma, or two of three consecutive points beyond two sigmas.

A *trend* is defined as six consecutive data points incrementally increasing or decreasing. Those unfamiliar with control charts tend to see "trends" of fewer than six points, which often results in the incorrect identification of common cause patterns as special causes. See Exhibit 6.3.

Number of Data Points

Shewhart recommended that 20 to 25 data points be used to evaluate the stability of a given process. If a process with 25 points has only common cause variation, one can be reasonably certain that a process is "in control." One then can estimate the capability of the process—that is, how it is likely to perform in the near future. Even with fewer than 25 points, examination of a process for the presence of special causes is useful. However, with fewer than 25 points, the upper and lower control limits should be referred to as *trial limits*. If one observes a special cause with, for example, only 12 points, one should take the time to investigate it. However, with only 12 data points, there is a higher probability of missing a special cause when it is present (Type II error), and one cannot estimate process capability confidently.

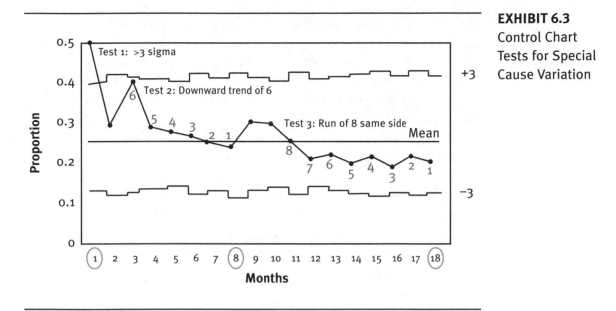

EXHIBIT 6.3
Control Chart
Tests for Special
Cause Variation

Source: Data from Lee and McGreevey (2000).

Choosing the Correct Control Chart

Many different control charts are available. However, in its initial efforts, the average facility can manage well with only four:

1. p-chart
2. u-chart
3. Individual values and moving range chart (XmR chart)
4. X-bar and S chart

The first two charts analyze attributes data. The second two charts analyze variables data. The details behind the calculation of the p-, u-, X-bar, and S charts are given in Appendix 1, and worked examples are given in Appendix 3.

Attributes Data

Attributes data are discrete whole numbers, not continuous measurements. They are counts of an event of interest that can be considered as either desirable or undesirable. One can keep score of these counts in two ways:

1. *The number of times a unique event of interest occurs*—for example, the surgical patient was given an antibiotic within one hour of surgery (For any given patient, the event either did or did not occur and can be counted only one time per patient.)
2. *The total number of nonunique events*—for example, the total number of patient falls (This event may occur multiple times for a patient.)

When counting unique events, one uses a p-chart. The number plotted on a chart would be either a proportion or a percentage. When counting total events (e.g., the number of falls per patient day each month), one plots a ratio on a u-chart.

Examples of attributes data plotted as percentages on p-charts include figures such as

- percentage of pneumonia patients who died;
- percentage of surgical patients who received an antibiotic within one hour of surgery;
- percentage of scripts that had one or more medication errors; and
- percentage of patients readmitted to the hospital within 30 days.

Examples of attributes data plotted as ratio data on u-charts include figures such as

- total number of patient falls per patient day;
- total number of medication errors per total number of scripts; and
- total number of surgical complications divided by the total number of surgeries.

Variables Data

Variables data are measurements that can be plotted on a continuous scale. They can be either whole numbers or decimals. Variables data are plotted on either an X-bar and S chart or an XmR chart.

Examples of variables data include measurements such as

- length of stay,
- emergency department wait time,
- length of intubation time, and
- average door-to-thrombolytic time for acute myocardial infarction patients.

An XmR chart is used when there is only one measurement for each period.

The X-bar and S charts are complementary and always used together. In other words, the X-bar chart reveals whether there is a special cause across months, whereas the S chart reveals whether there are special causes within each month.

To interpret the X-bar chart successfully, the S chart must be free of data points beyond the upper control limit (the only test used on the S chart). If the S chart has a data point beyond three standard deviations from the mean, that data point or points should be investigated for a special cause. A special cause on the S chart must be identified and eliminated before the X-bar chart can be interpreted accurately (Lee and McGreevey 2000).

Comparison Chart Analysis

The objective of comparison analysis is to evaluate whether a healthcare organization's performance is different from the expected level derived from other organizations' data. This analysis is interorganizational because analysis is performed on the basis of data from multiple organizations. This analysis also is cross-sectional because comparisons are made at a specific point in time (e.g., month). When an organization's performance level is significantly different from the expected level, it is called an *outlier performance*. An outlier performance may be either favorable or unfavorable depending on the measure's direction of improvement.

The use of comparison analysis in addition to the control chart can be a powerful approach. The two analyses are alike in that an organization's actual (or observed) performance level is evaluated against a comparative norm, but they are fundamentally different in how such a norm is established. In control chart analysis, the norm is determined from an organization's own historic data (i.e., process mean) to assess the organization's internal process stability. On the other hand, in comparison analysis, the norm is determined on the basis of several organizations' performance data to evaluate an organization's relative performance level. Therefore, the two analyses evaluate organizational performance from two distinct perspectives and, as a result, provide a more comprehensive framework to assess overall performance level.

Because of the analyses' different focuses, the control and comparison analyses may portray different pictures about an organization's performance. For example, an organization's control chart may show a favorable pattern (i.e., in control) at the same time the comparison chart shows unfavorable performance (i.e., a bad outlier). This seeming discrepancy may appear when an organization's performance is consistently lower than that of other organizations and suggests that a new process may need to be implemented to achieve a performance improvement. On the other hand, an organization without an outlier performance in the comparison analysis may show an out-of-control pattern in the control chart. In this case, the organization needs to investigate any presence of special cause variation in the process before making conclusions about its performance level. In general, the control chart analysis should be done before the comparison analysis to ensure process stability so that the observed performance data truly represent the organization's performance capability.

Statistical Assumptions About Data

Statistical analyses differ depending on assumptions made about data. For instance, if a normal distribution is assumed for a data set, comparison analysis is performed using a Z-test. Different assumptions are made depending on the type of measure—proportion, ratio, or continuous variable:

- *Proportion measures*: Proportion measures are assumed to follow a binomial distribution, which is the probability distribution of the number of "successes" (i.e., numerator) in a series of independent trials (i.e., denominator), each of which can result in either a "success" or a "failure" with a constant probability. For example, for a pneumococcal vaccination rate proportion measure, each individual is assumed to have an equal probability of receiving a vaccination under the binomial assumption. Under certain circumstances (e.g., large sample size), a binomial distribution can be approximated using a normal distribution to simplify statistical analysis.

- *Ratio measures*: Ratio measures are similar to proportion measures in that both are based on count (or attributes) data, but they differ in that the numerator and the denominator address different attributes. An example is the number of adverse drug reactions (ADRs) per 1,000 patient days. For this type of measure, the probability of a "failure" (e.g., an ADR) is very small, whereas the area of opportunity (e.g., patient days) is usually large. Ratio measures are assumed to follow a Poisson distribution. Like the binomial distribution, the Poisson distribution can be approximated by a normal distribution.

- *Continuous variable measures*: Continuous variable measures deal with interval scale data and generally are not restricted to particular values. Examples include emergency department wait time and the number of minutes before administration of antibiotics. An appropriate distribution assumption for this type of measure is a normal distribution (or *t* distribution for a small sample size).

What Data Are Compared?

The comparative norm (e.g., expected rate) in the comparison analysis is the *predicted rate* if the measure is risk adjusted and the *comparison group mean* if the measure is not risk adjusted. Because performance measurement systems develop the comparative data and The Joint Commission receives only summary-level data, the accuracy of comparison analysis depends on the quality of data submitted by individual measurement systems. Whenever appropriate, as a comparative norm, risk-adjusted data are preferable to the summary data from comparison groups because a valid and reliable risk-adjustment procedure can reduce organization- or patient-level variability (e.g., different levels of severity of illness). In this case, the comparison data are customized for individual organizations, and thus more accurate, fairer performance comparisons can be made.

How Are Statistical Outliers Determined?

In comparison analysis, the underlying hypothesis (i.e., null hypothesis) about an organization's performance is that the observed performance is not different (statistically) from the expected level. By applying a set of statistical procedures (i.e., hypothesis testing) to actual performance data, one determines whether the null hypothesis is likely to be true for individual organizations. If it is not true, the performance is called an *outlier*. In general, statistical outliers can be determined using two approaches. One approach is based on the p-value, and the other is based on the expected range. These two approaches always result in the same conclusion about the outlier status.

1. *Outlier decision based on p-value*: A p-value is the probability of obtaining data that are the same or more extreme than the observed data when the null hypothesis is true (i.e., when the organization's actual performance is not different from the expected performance). Therefore, a p-value that is very small (e.g., less than 0.01) indicates that the actual performance is likely to be different from the expected level. In this case, the null hypothesis is rejected and an outlier is determined. A p-value is calculated on the basis of an assumption about the probability distribution of data. If a normal distribution is assumed, a p-value less than 0.01 is equivalent to a Z-score greater than 2.576 or less than –2.576 (for a two-sided test). See Exhibit 6.4.

2. *Outlier decision based on expected range*: An expected range (also called *acceptance interval*) is an interval with upper and lower limits that represents the set of values for which the null hypothesis is accepted. Usually, the midpoint of the interval is the expected rate (or value) for the organization. When the observed data are outside the expected range, an outlier is determined. The expected range can be useful for displaying an organization's outlier status in a chart. See Exhibit 6.5.

Comparison Chart Construction

A comparison chart is a graphical summary of comparison analysis. It displays tabular information from the comparison analysis in a standardized graphical format so that a visually intuitive assessment may be made about an organization's performance.

A comparison chart consists of actual (or observed) rates, expected rates, and expected ranges (i.e., upper and lower limits) for a given time frame. Unlike control charts, which require at least 12 data points (i.e.,

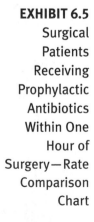

EXHIBIT 6.4
Use of p-Values
to Determine
Statistical
Outliers

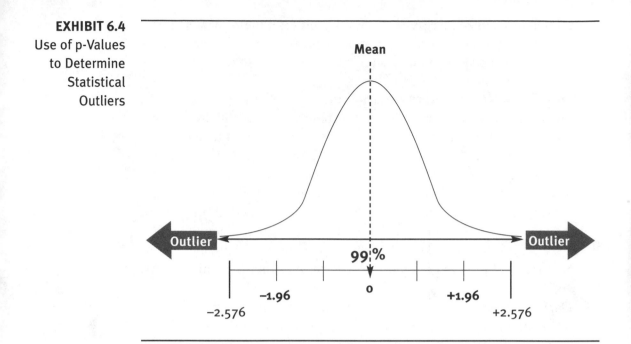

months) for a meaningful interpretation, comparison charts can be created with just a single valid data point because of its cross-sectional nature.

To create a comparison chart, one must calculate the expected range. An expected range is determined using the following two-step process:

- *Step one*: Calculate confidence limits for the observed rate (or value) using the formulas provided in Appendix 2. (Here, the observed rate is considered as a random variable, whereas the expected rate is assumed to be a constant value.) If the confidence interval includes

EXHIBIT 6.5
Surgical
Patients
Receiving
Prophylactic
Antibiotics
Within One
Hour of
Surgery—Rate
Comparison
Chart

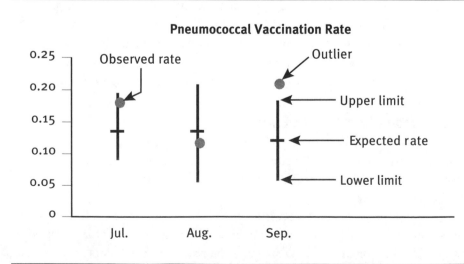

values outside the allowable range, the interval must be truncated. For proportion measures, the values must be between 0 and 1. For ratio measures, the values must be 0 or any positive numbers. Continuous variable measures may include any positive or negative numbers.

- *Step two*: Convert the confidence interval into the expected range. The mathematical formulas for the calculation of a comparison chart are given in Appendix 2, and worked examples are given in Appendix 3.

Comparison Chart Interpretation

Depending on the direction of a measure's improvement, outlier interpretations can be positive, negative, or neutral.

- *Positive measures*: A rate increase signals improvement. In other words, a larger rate is better than a smaller rate. The measure of surgical patients receiving prophylactic antibiotics within one hour of surgery is an example. For this measure, an observed rate above the expected range indicates a favorable outlier, whereas a rate below the range indicates an unfavorable outlier.

- *Negative measures*: A rate decrease signals improvement. In other words, a smaller rate is better than a larger rate. Mortality rate measures are an example. For these measures, an observed rate above the expected range indicates an unfavorable outlier, whereas a rate below the range indicates a favorable outlier.

- *Neutral measures*: Either an increase or a decrease in rate could be a signal of improvement. In other words, there is no clear direction of improvement for these measures. For example, whether a vaginal birth after cesarean section (VBAC) rate of 5 percent is better (or worse) than a VBAC rate of 95 percent is difficult to determine. In this case, an observed rate either above or below the expected range is an unfavorable outlier. For these measures, no favorable outliers can be identified.

The comparison analysis will result in one of the following scenarios, regardless of the type of measure:

- *No outlier*: Actual performance is within the expected range.
- *Favorable outlier*: Actual performance is better than the expected performance.
- *Unfavorable outlier*: Actual performance is worse than the expected performance.
- *Incomplete data*: Data cannot be analyzed because of a data error.
- *Small sample size*: Data cannot be analyzed because of a small sample size.

Data are "incomplete" if data elements used in the comparison analysis are missing or invalid. Small sample sizes are defined as fewer than 25 denominator cases for proportion measures, fewer than 4 numerator cases for ratio measures, and fewer than 10 cases for continuous variable measures. In addition, representation of fewer than 10 organizations in the comparison group data for non-risk-adjusted measures is considered a small sample size (Lee and McGreevey 2000).

Using Data for Performance Improvement

Once collected, performance measurement data require interpretation and analysis if they are to be used to improve the processes and outcomes of healthcare. There are a number of ways to use data for improvement purposes, all of which involve comparison. Data can be used to compare (1) an organization's performance against itself over time, (2) the performance of one organization against the performance of a group of organizations collecting data on the same measures in the same way, and (3) an organization's performance against established benchmarks or guidelines.

As a first step, an organization must determine whether the process it is measuring is in control. To improve a process, it first must be understood. Processes characterized by special cause variation are unstable, unpredictable, and therefore difficult to understand. Control charts should be used to determine whether processes are stable and in statistical control or whether special cause variation exists. If special cause variation does exist, it must be investigated and eliminated. Once special cause variation has been eliminated, organizations can be confident that the data accurately reflect performance.

Consider a hypothetical situation in which a hospital uses a control chart to track the rates of a performance measure. The control chart in Exhibit 6.6 indicates existence of special cause variation at time 9 as the observed rate deviates from the upper control limit. Suppose that the hospital conducted a root cause analysis after time 8 to identify the source of the special cause and found that there was a serious problem in the hospital's coding practice. The hospital then implemented an intervention plan at time 10, and the hospital's rates shifted to within the control limits (times 11 to 20). In addition, the process mean (i.e., centerline) shifted from 0.42 to 0.75 after the intervention. The hospital should continue to monitor its pneumococcal vaccination rates using the new process mean as part of a continuous quality improvement plan.

Control charts, however, tell us only about the stability of the process; they tell us nothing about quality of care. After determining that the process of interest is stable and in control, organizations need to use other SPC

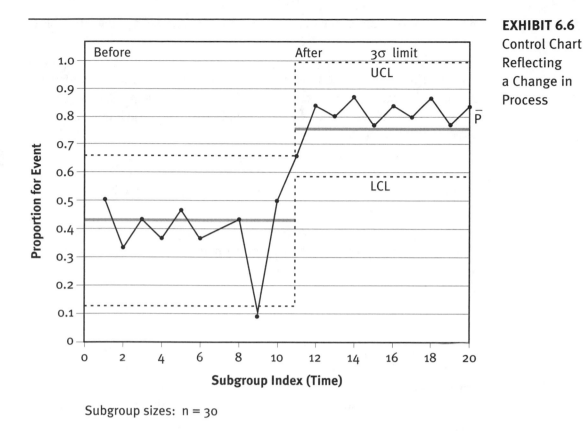

EXHIBIT 6.6
Control Chart
Reflecting
a Change in
Process

Subgroup sizes: n = 30

tools and data analysis techniques to determine whether they are performing as they want to perform. One way a healthcare organization can measure whether it is meeting its goals and targets is to compare its performance against itself over time. By consistently tracking the same measures on an ongoing basis, an organization can spot trends, cycles, and patterns, all of which will help determine whether it is meeting its preset targets and whether its performance is improving or declining. It also can monitor the impact of quality improvement interventions it has implemented and track the sustainability of those improvements.

Another way to use data for improvement purposes is to compare the performance of one organization to the performance of a group of organizations collecting data on the same measures in the same way. In this way, the healthcare organization can track how it is performing as compared with other organizations providing the same services. These comparisons can be local, regional, national, or based on any number of other strata. Statistical analyses can pinpoint whether a healthcare entity is performing in a way that is comparable to other organizations or whether it is at a level that is, statistically speaking, significantly above or below others in the comparison group.

An organization's discovery that it is performing at a level significantly below that of its peers is often a powerful incentive to improve.

A third method of comparing performance is through benchmarking. Definitions of benchmarking vary, but, generally speaking, benchmarking compares an organization's performance in relation to a specified service or function to that of industry leaders or exemplary organizations. Benchmarking is goal directed and promotes performance improvement by (Czarnecki 1994)

- providing an environment amenable to organizational change through continuous improvement and striving to match industry-leading practices and results,
- creating objective measures of performance that are driven by industry-leading targets instead of by past performance,
- providing a customer/external focus,
- substantiating the need for improvement, and
- establishing data-driven decision-making processes.

In healthcare, professional societies and expert panels routinely develop scientifically based guidelines of patient care practices for given treatments or procedures. The goal of these guideline-setting efforts is to provide healthcare organizations with tools that, if appropriately applied, can help raise their performance to the level of industry leaders. Organizations can use performance measure data to track how often, and how well, they comply with the guidelines.

Conclusion

This chapter provided a framework for performance measurement in the context of performance improvement and advice on the selection of performance measures. It described two statistical tools—the control chart and the comparison chart—and their use in tracking performance measures data.

Study Questions

1. What are common data-quality problems in healthcare performance measurement? How should the sufficiency of data quality be evaluated? What consequences are associated with the use of poor-quality data?
2. When an organization uses sample data in performance measurement, how can it determine appropriate sample sizes and how can it ensure

that the sample data represent the entire population? How should it handle small sample sizes in the analysis and use of control and comparison charts?

3. How does the rigorous use of control and comparison charts for performance management and improvement contradict, if at all, the art-of-medicine philosophy that each patient is unique?

Appendix 1: Control Chart Formulas[2]

Attributes Data: Proportion Measures (p-Chart)

Proportion measures are analyzed using a p-chart. The following data elements (organization level) are used to construct a p-chart:

Data Element	Notation*
Number of denominator cases for a month	n_i
Number of numerator cases for a month	x_i
Observed rate for a month	p_i

*The subscript i represents individual months.

Statistical formulas for calculating the centerline and control limits are given below. Note that the control limits are calculated for individual months and that the limits vary by month unless the number of denominator cases for each month is the same for all months.

Centerline of the Chart

$$\bar{p} = \frac{\sum x_i}{\sum n_i} = \frac{x_1 + x_2 + \ldots + x_m}{n_1 + n_2 + \ldots + n_m},$$

where m is the number of months (or data points).

Upper and Lower Control Limits for Each Month

$$\bar{p} \pm 3 \times \sqrt{\frac{\bar{p} \times (1 - \bar{p})}{n_i}}$$

Small Sample Size Adjustments

When the sample sizes are very small, a standard p-chart cannot be used because the statistical assumption needed to create a p-chart (i.e., normal approximation to the binomial distribution) is not valid. Specifically, the small sample sizes are defined as follows:

$$\bar{n} \times \bar{p} < 4 \text{ or } \bar{n} \times (1 - \bar{p}) < 4,$$

where n-bar is the average number of denominator cases and p-bar is the centerline (i.e., weighted average of individual months' observed rates).

In this situation, an adjusted p-chart using an exact binomial probability (i.e., probability limit method) is used. To calculate the upper and the lower control limits using the probability limit method, the smallest x_U and the largest x_L satisfying the following two binomial probability distribution functions should be calculated first:

$$\sum_{x=x_u}^{n} \left[\frac{n}{x} \right] p^x (1-p)^{n-x} \leq 0.00135 \text{ and } \sum_{x=0}^{x_L} \left[\frac{n}{x} \right] p^x (1-p)^{n-x} \leq 0.00135.$$

Next, the upper and lower control limits for the observed rate are obtained by dividing x_U and x_L by the number of denominator cases n for the month. Alternatively, instead of the binomial probability distribution, an incomplete beta distribution may be used to calculate the probability limits (SAS Institute 2013).

Attributes Data: Ratio Measures (u-Chart)

Ratio measures are analyzed using the u-chart. A u-chart is created using the following data elements (organization level):

Data Element	Notation*
Number of denominator cases for a month	n_i
Number of numerator cases for a month	x_i
Observed rate for a month	u_i

*The subscript i represents individual months.

Centerline of a u-Chart

$$\bar{u} = \frac{\sum x_i}{\sum n_i} = \frac{x_1 + x_2 + \ldots + x_m}{n_1 + n_2 + \ldots + n_m},$$

where m is the number of months (or data points).

Control Limits for Each Month

$$\bar{u} \pm 3 \times \sqrt{\frac{\bar{\bar{u}}}{n_i}}$$

If the ratio is to be calculated on a prespecified denominator basis (or on a scaling factor basis), the control chart must be scaled appropriately using that information. For example, the denominator basis for the ratio measure "number of falls per 100 resident days" is 100. In this case, all values in the control chart—including the centerline and control limits—and the observed ratio must be multiplied by 100.

Small Sample Size Adjustments
Like p-charts, a standard u-chart should not be used when the sample size is very small because the statistical assumption for a u-chart (normal approximation to the Poisson distribution) fails if the sample size is very small. Small sample size for ratio measures is defined as

$$\bar{n} \times \bar{u} < 4,$$

where n-bar is the average number of denominator cases and u-bar is the centerline of the u-chart.

In this situation, an adjusted u-chart based on Poisson probability is used. The upper and lower control limits are obtained by first calculating x_U and x_L and then dividing each value by the number of denominator cases n for the month. To obtain x_U and x_L, the following two Poisson probability distribution functions should be solved in such a way that the smallest x_U and the largest x_L satisfying these conditions are obtained:

$$\sum_{x=x_u}^{\infty} \frac{e^{-u} u^x}{x!} \leq 0.00135 \text{ and } \sum_{x=0}^{x_L} \frac{e^{-u} u^x}{x!} \leq 0.00135.$$

Alternatively, a chi-square distribution may be used instead of the Poisson probability distribution to calculate the probability limits (SAS Institute 2013).

Variables Data (X-Bar and S Chart)
Variables data, or *continuous variable measures*, are analyzed using the X-bar and S chart. To construct an X-bar and S chart, the following data elements (organization level) are needed:

Data Element	Notation*
Number of cases for a month	n_i
Mean of observed values for a month	x_i
Standard deviation of observed values for a month	s_i

*The subscript *i* represents individual months.

The centerline and control limits for an X-bar and S chart are calculated using the following formulas. Note that the control limits vary by months, depending on the denominator cases for individual months.

Centerline

1. X-bar chart

$$\bar{x} = \frac{\sum n_i \times x_i}{\sum n_i}.$$

2. S chart

   a. Minimum variance linear unbiased estimate (SAS Institute 2013)

$$\bar{s}_i = c_4 \times \frac{\sum h_i \times \dfrac{S_i}{c_4}}{\sum h_i}, \text{ where } h_i = \frac{c_4^2}{1 - c_4^2}.$$

   b. Pooled standard deviation (Montgomery 2012)

$$\bar{s} = \sqrt{\frac{\sum (n_i - 1) \times s_i^2}{\sum n_i - m}}.$$

These two methods result in slightly different values, but the differences generally are negligible.

c_4 is a constant that depends on the sample size. As the sample size increases, c_4 approaches 1. The exact formula for c_4 is

$$c_4 = \sqrt{\frac{2}{n_i - 1}} \times \frac{\Gamma\left(\dfrac{n_i}{2}\right)}{\Gamma\left(\dfrac{n_i - 1}{2}\right)}.$$

Control Limits

1. X-bar chart

$$\bar{x} \pm 3 \times \frac{\bar{s}}{c_4 \sqrt{n_i}}$$

2. S chart

$$\bar{s} \times (1 \pm \frac{3}{c_4} \times \sqrt{1 - c_4^2})$$

Small Sample Size Adjustments

If the sample size is 1 for all data points (i.e., the observed value is a single observation for each month), an XmR chart is used instead of an X-bar and S chart (Lee and McGreevey 2000).

Appendix 2: Comparison Chart Formulas[2]

Comparison Analysis: Proportion Measures

Three data elements are used in the comparison chart analysis for proportion measures. The expected rate is either the risk-adjusted rate (if risk adjusted) or the overall observed rate for the comparison group (if not risk adjusted or if risk-adjusted data are not available).

Data Element	Notation
Number of denominator cases for a month	n
Observed rate for a month	p_o
Expected rate for a month A) risk-adjusted rate, or B) overall observed rate for a comparative group (e.g., national average)	p_e p_e

Analysis is based on the score test (Agresti and Coull 1998). This test is based on the difference between the observed and the expected rates, divided by the standard error of the expected rate as shown here:

$$Z = \frac{p_o - p_e}{\sqrt{\frac{p_e \times (1 - p_e)}{n}}}$$

This value (or Z-statistic) follows a normal distribution when the sample size is not very small. A value less than -2.576 or greater than 2.576 signals a statistically significant difference between the two rates at a 1 percent significance level.

The confidence interval for the observed rate is determined by expanding the above formula with respect to the expected rate (Agresti and Coull 1998; Bickel and Doksum 2000). Its upper limit (U_o) and lower limit (L_o) for a month are calculated as follows:

$$U_o = \frac{\left(p_o + \dfrac{Z^2_{1-\frac{\alpha}{2}}}{2 \times n}\right) + Z_{1-\frac{\alpha}{2}} \times \sqrt{\dfrac{Z^2_{1-\frac{\alpha}{2}}}{4 \times n^2} + \dfrac{p_o \times (1 - p_o)}{n}}}{1 + \dfrac{Z^2_{1-\frac{\alpha}{2}}}{n}}, \text{ where } Z_{1-\frac{\alpha}{2}} = 2.576.$$

$$L_o = \frac{\left(p_o + \dfrac{Z^2_{1-\frac{\alpha}{2}}}{2 \times n}\right) - Z_{1-\frac{\alpha}{2}} \times \sqrt{\dfrac{Z^2_{1-\frac{\alpha}{2}}}{4 \times n^2} + \dfrac{p_o \times (1 - p_o)}{n}}}{1 + \dfrac{Z^2_{1-\frac{\alpha}{2}}}{n}}, \text{ where } Z_{1-\frac{\alpha}{2}} = 2.576.$$

Statistical significance also can be determined by comparing the expected rate (p_e) with the confidence interval (L_o, U_o). If p_e is within the interval, the observed rate is not different from the expected rates; therefore, it is not an outlier. If p_e is outside the interval, it is an outlier.

This information is depicted on the comparison chart by converting the confidence interval around the observed rate into the expected range (or acceptance interval) around the expected rate (Holubkov et al. 1998). The upper limit (U_e) and lower limit (L_e) of the expected range are calculated as follows:

$U_e = p_e + (p_o - L_o)$. [If $U_e > 1$, then $U_e = 1$.]

$L_e = p_e + (p_o - U_o)$. [If $L_e < 0$, then $L_e = 0$.]

The interpretation of the comparison chart now involves the relative location of the observed rate with respect to the expected range. If the observed rate (p_o) is within the expected range (L_e, U_e), it is not a statistical outlier (i.e., not a statistically significant difference) at a 1 percent significance level. If the observed rate is outside the expected range, the observed rate is a statistical outlier.

Comparison Analysis: Ratio Measures

Three data elements are used in the comparison chart analysis for ratio measures. The expected rate is either the risk-adjusted rate (if risk adjusted) or the overall observed rate for the comparison group (if not risk adjusted or if risk-adjusted data are not available).

Data Element	Notation
Number of denominator cases for a month	n
Observed rate (ratio) for a month	u_o
Expected rate (ratio) for a month A) risk-adjusted rate, or B) overall observed rate for a comparative group (e.g., national average)	u_e u_e

As with proportion measures, analysis for ratio measures is based on the score test (Joint Commission 2000). This test is based on the difference between the observed and expected number of numerator cases divided by the standard error of the expected number of events.

This value (or Z-statistic) is assumed to follow a normal distribution when the sample size is not very small. A value less than –2.576 or greater than 2.576 signals a statistically significant difference between the two rates at a 1 percent significance level.

$$Z = \frac{n \times u_o - n \times u_e}{\sqrt{n \times u_e}}.$$

The confidence interval is derived from the above test statistic (Agresti and Coull 1998; Bickel and Doksum 2000). The upper and lower limits of the confidence interval are calculated as follows:

$$U_o = \frac{(n \times u_o + \frac{Z^2_{1-\frac{\alpha}{2}}}{2}) + \frac{Z_{1-\frac{\alpha}{2}}}{2} \times \sqrt{Z^2_{1-\frac{\alpha}{2}} + 4 \times n \times u_o}}{n}, \text{ where } Z_{1-\frac{\alpha}{2}} = 2.576.$$

$$L_o = \frac{(n \times u_o + \frac{Z^2_{1-\frac{\alpha}{2}}}{2}) - \frac{Z_{1-\frac{\alpha}{2}}}{2} \times \sqrt{Z^2_{1-\frac{\alpha}{2}} + 4 \times n \times u_o}}{n}, \text{ where } Z_{1-\frac{\alpha}{2}} = 2.576.$$

The upper limit (U_e) and lower limit (L_e) of the expected range are calculated as follows (Holubkov et al. 1998):

$$U_e = u_e + (u_o - L_o).$$

$$L_e = u_e + (u_o - U_o). \text{ [If } L_e < 0, \text{ then } L_e = 0.]$$

Using the comparison chart, one can determine statistical significance by comparing the observed rate (u_o) to the expected range (L_e, U_e). If the observed ratio (u_o) is within the expected range (L_e, U_e), it is not a statistical outlier at a 1 percent significance level. If the observed ratio is outside the expected range, the observed rate is a statistical outlier.

Continuous Variable Measures

Four data elements are used in the comparison chart analysis for continuous variable measures. The expected value is either the risk-adjusted value (if risk adjusted) or the overall mean observed value for the comparison group (if not risk adjusted or if risk-adjusted data are not available).

Data Element	Notation
Number of cases for a month	n
Mean of observed values for a month	X_o
Standard deviation of observed values	S_o
Mean of expected values for a month A) mean risk-adjusted value, or B) overall mean observed value for a comparative group (e.g., national average)	X_e X_e

1. The statistical test is based on normal distribution. Specifically, the following formulas are used depending on the sample size:
   a. $n \geq 25$.

$$Z = \frac{X_o - X_e}{S_o / \sqrt{n}}.$$

This value (or Z-statistic) is assumed to follow a normal distribution when the sample size is not very small. A value less than −2.576 or greater than 2.576 signals a statistically significant difference between the two rates at a 1 percent significance level.

b. $n < 25$.

$$t = \frac{X_o - X_e}{S_o / \sqrt{n}}.$$

This value (or t-statistic) is assumed to follow a t distribution. Unlike a normal distribution, the t distribution depends on the sample size. For example, if the sample size is 15, a value less than –2.977 or greater than 2.977 signals a statistically significant difference between the two rates at a 1 percent significance level.

2. Based on the test statistic, the expected range is calculated using the following formula:

Expected upper limit: $U_e = x_e + (x_o - L_o)$, and
expected lower limit: $L_e = x_e + (x_o - U_o)$, where

$$U_o = x_o + Z_{1-\frac{\alpha}{2}} \times \frac{S_o}{\sqrt{n}} \text{ and } L_o = x_o - Z_{1-\frac{\alpha}{2}} \times \frac{S_o}{\sqrt{n}} \text{ if } n \geq 25$$

or

$$U_o = x_o + t_{1-\frac{\alpha}{2},\, n-1} \times \frac{S_o}{\sqrt{n}} \text{ and } L_o = x_o - t_{1-\frac{\alpha}{2},\, n-1} \times \frac{S_o}{\sqrt{n}} \text{ if } n < 25.$$

If the observed value (x_o) is within the expected range (L_e, U_e), it is not a statistical outlier (i.e., not a statistically significant difference) at a 1 percent significance level. If the observed value is outside the expected range, the observed rate is a statistical outlier (Lee and McGreevey 2000).

Appendix 3: Case Studies[2]

Case 1: Prophylactic Antibiotic Received Within One Hour Prior to Surgical Incision Rate—Proportion Measure

A healthcare organization started to collect data for the proportion measure "prophylactic antibiotic received within one hour prior to surgical incision" on July 1, 2011. As of June 1, 2012, this organization collected 12 months of observed measure rates (p_o). The organization's calculated observed rates (p_o) for individual months as well as the overall monthly national averages (p_e) are as follows:

	7/11	8/11	9/11	10/11	11/11	12/11
n	93	82	82	91	78	84
x	70	52	65	66	54	62
p_o	0.7527	0.6341	0.7927	0.7253	0.6923	0.7381
p_e	0.8205	0.8073	0.8878	0.8406	0.8065	0.8750

	1/12	2/12	3/12	4/12	5/12	6/12
n	75	73	85	82	71	80
x	61	60	65	61	56	62
p_o	0.8133	0.8219	0.7647	0.7439	0.7887	0.7750
p_e	0.8454	0.8670	0.8355	0.8521	0.8969	0.8572

Control Chart (p-Chart)

A standard p-chart can be created for this organization because (1) at least 12 months passed since the data-collection begin date, (2) more than two nonmissing data points are available, and (3) the sample sizes are not small.

Centerline

$$\bar{p} = \frac{70+52+65+66+54+62+61+60+65+61+56+62}{93+82+82+91+78+84+75+73+85+82+71+80} = 0.7520$$

Control Limits

1. UCL for July 2011

$$UCL = 0.7520 + 3 \times \sqrt{\frac{0.7520 \times (1 - 0.7520)}{93}} = 0.8864.$$

2. LCL for July 2011

$$LCL = 0.7520 - 3 \times \sqrt{\frac{0.7520 \times (1 - 0.7520)}{93}} = 0.6177.$$

3. UCL for June 2012

$$UCL = 0.7250 + 3 \times \sqrt{\frac{0.7520 \times (1 - 0.7520)}{80}} = 0.8969.$$

4. LCL for June 2012

$$LCL = 0.7520 - 3 \times \sqrt{\frac{0.7520 \times (1 - 0.7520)}{80}} = 0.6072.$$

These calculations were rounded to four decimal points for illustration. A p-chart using the above data is shown here. (The centerline is rounded to two decimal points.)

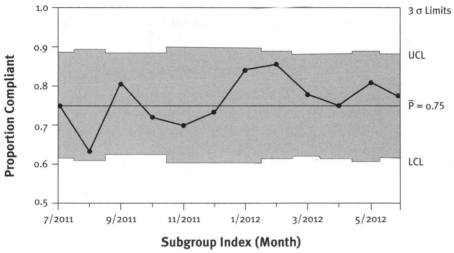

Subgroup Sizes: Min n = 71   Max n = 89

Comparison Chart

For July 2011:

$$U_o = \frac{0.7527 + \dfrac{2.576^2}{2 \times 93} + 2.576 \times \sqrt{\dfrac{2.576^2}{4 \times 93^2} + \dfrac{0.7527 \times (1 - 0.7527)}{93}}}{1 + \dfrac{2.576^2}{93}} = 0.8485.$$

$$L_o = \frac{0.7527 + \dfrac{2.576^2}{2 \times 93} - 2.576 \times \sqrt{\dfrac{2.576^2}{4 \times 93^2} + \dfrac{0.7527 \times (1 - 0.7527)}{93}}}{1 + \dfrac{2.576^2}{93}} = 0.6233.$$

The expected range is

$$U_e = 0.8205 + 0.7527 - 0.6233 = 0.9499,$$

and

$L_e = 0.8205 + 0.7527 - 0.8485 = 0.7247.$

Because $|Z| = 1.515 < 2.576$, the measure rate for July 2011 is not a statistical outlier at a 1 percent significance level. The same conclusion can be drawn about the July 2011 performance using the expected range approach because the observed rate 0.7527 is within the expected range (0.7247, 0.9499). Note that the UCL calculations for September 2011, December 2011, February 2012, and May 2012 were reduced to 100 percent, the highest possible value. The comparison chart using these data is shown here:

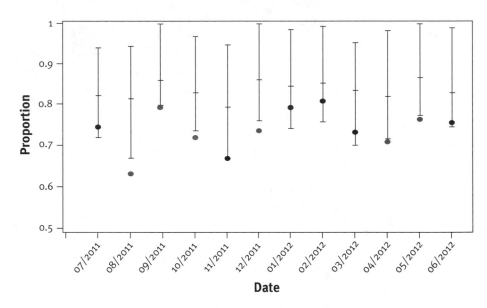

Case 2: Patient Falls per 100 Patient Days—Ratio Measure

Suppose a healthcare organization collected data for the ratio measure "patient falls per 100 patient days" for the period from July 1, 2011, to June 30, 2012. U_o and U_e represent the actual rate and comparison group rate, respectively.

	7/11	8/11	9/11	10/11	11/11	12/11
n	286	297	236	217	249	195
x	9	13	13	9	16	6
U_o	0.0315	0.0438	0.0551	0.0415	0.643	0.0308
U_e	0.0484	0.0579	0.0539	0.0422	0.0589	0.0511

	1/12	2/12	3/12	4/12	5/12	6/12
n	269	206	183	245	226	185
x	19	17	7	17	15	4
U_o	0.0706	0.0825	0.0383	0.0694	0.0664	0.0216
U_e	0.0545	0.0592	0.0591	0.0416	0.0535	0.0457

Control Chart (u-Chart)

A standard u-chart can be created for this organization because (1) at least 12 months passed since the data-collection begin date, (2) more than two nonmissing data points are available, and (3) the sample sizes are not small.

Centerline

$$\bar{u} = \frac{9 + 13 + \ldots + 4}{286 + 297 + \ldots + 185} = 0.0519 \text{ (5.19 falls per 100 patient days)}.$$

Control Limits for Each Month

1. UCL for July 2011

$$UCL = 0.0519 + 3 \times \sqrt{\frac{0.0519}{286}} = 0.0923 \text{ (9.23 falls per 100 patient days)}.$$

2. LCL for July 2011

$$LCL = 0.0519 - 3 \times \sqrt{\frac{0.0519}{286}} = 0.0115 \text{ (1.15 falls per 100 patient days)}.$$

3. UCL for June 2012

$$UCL = 0.0519 + 3 \times \sqrt{\frac{0.0519}{185}} = 0.1021 \text{ (10.21 falls per 100 patient days)}.$$

4. LCL for June 2012

$$LCL = 0.0519 - 3 \times \sqrt{\frac{0.0519}{185}} = 0.0017 \text{ (0.17 falls per 100 patient days)}.$$

Following is a u-chart created using these data:

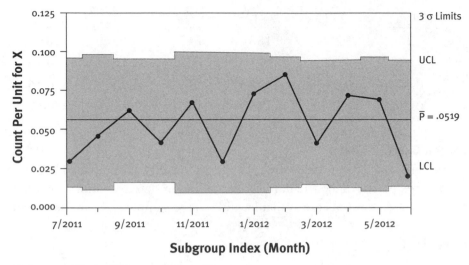

Subgroup Sizes: Min n = 183   Max n = 297

Comparison Analysis

For July 2011:

$$Z = \frac{286 \times 0.0315 - 286 \times 0.0484}{\sqrt{286 \times 0.0484}} = -1.301,$$

$$U_o = \frac{\left(286 \times 0.0315 + \dfrac{2.576^2}{2}\right) + \dfrac{2.576}{2} \times \sqrt{2.576^2 + 4 \times 286 \times 0.0315}}{286} = 0.0725, \text{ and}$$

$$L_o = \frac{\left(286 \times 0.0315 + \dfrac{2.576^2}{2}\right) - \dfrac{2.576}{2} \times \sqrt{2.576^2 + 4 \times 286 \times 0.0315}}{286} = 0.0137.$$

The expected range is

$U_e = 0.0315 + 0.0484 - 0.0137 = 0.0662$ (6.62 falls per 100 patient days),

and

$L_e = 0.0315 + 0.0484 - 0.0725 = 0.0074$ (0.74 falls per 100 patient days).

Because $|Z| = 1.301 < 2.576$, the observed ratio for July 2011 is not a statistical outlier at a 1 percent significance level. The same conclusion for July 2011 performance can be drawn using the expected range approach because the observed ratio 0.0315 (3.15 falls per 100 patient days) is within the expected range (0.0074, 0.0662). The comparison chart using these data is shown below with the ratio expressed in falls per 100 patient days. Note that the LCL calculations for some months resulted in a negative value and were replaced by zero because a u-chart must include only non-negative values.

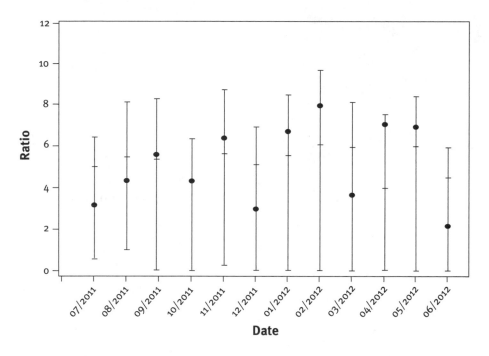

Case 3: Emergency Department Wait Time—Continuous Variable Measure

Suppose a healthcare organization has collected data for the continuous variable measure "emergency department wait time in minutes" during the 12-month period from July 1, 2011, to June 30, 2012 (see below):

	7/11	8/11	9/11	10/11	11/11	12/11
n	35	36	45	32	36	45
x_o	249.0	143.1	154.5	107.4	99.2	179.5
s_o	206.6	270.6	201.5	191.7	199.9	205.2
x_e	174.0	180.1	170.4	172.5	164.4	165.9

	1/12	2/12	3/12	4/12	5/12	6/12
n	32	36	45	32	36	45
x_o	124.1	230.5	130.9	118.0	138.7	202.8
s_o	229.2	238.5	178.2	212.7	240.7	194.9
x_e	190.0	177.5	180.9	187.3	169.0	183.1

Control Chart (X-Bar and S Chart)

An X-bar and S chart can be created for this organization because (1) at least 12 months passed since the data-collection begin date, (2) more than two nonmissing data points are available, and (3) the sample sizes are not small.

Centerline

X-bar chart

$$\bar{x} = \frac{35 \times 249.0 + 36 \times 143.1 + \ldots + 45 \times 202.8}{35 + 36 + \ldots + 45} = 158.2$$

S chart (June 2012)

$$\bar{s}_{12} = 0.9943 \times \left[\frac{\dfrac{0.9927^2}{1 - 0.9927^2} \times \dfrac{206.6}{0.9927} + \ldots + \dfrac{0.9943^2}{1 - 0.9943^2} \times \dfrac{194.9}{0.9943}}{\dfrac{0.9927^2}{1 - 0.9927^2} + \ldots + \dfrac{0.9943^2}{1 - 0.9943^2}} \right] = 213.0$$

c_4 is 0.9927 for $n = 35$ and 0.9943 for $n = 45$.

Control Limits

X-bar chart

$$UCL(\bar{x}) = 158.2 + 3 \times \frac{213.0}{0.9943 \sqrt{45}} = 254.0$$

$$LCL(\bar{x}) = 158.2 - 3 \times \frac{213.0}{0.9943 \sqrt{45}} = 62.4$$

S chart

$$UCL(\bar{s}) = 213.0 \times \left(1 + \frac{3}{0.9943} \sqrt{1 - 0.9943^2} \right) = 281.5$$

$$LCL(\bar{s}) = 213.0 \times \left(1 - \frac{3}{0.9943} \sqrt{1 - 0.9943^2} \right) = 144.5$$

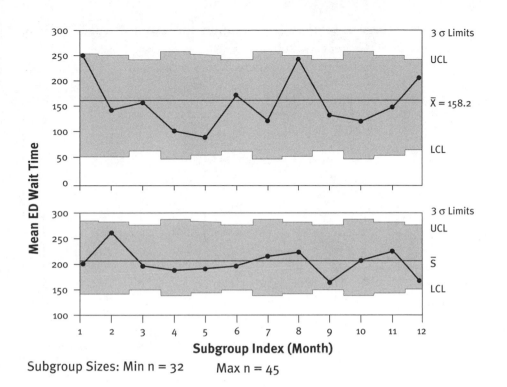

Subgroup Sizes: Min n = 32   Max n = 45

Comparison Analysis

For June 2012:

$$Z = \frac{202.8 - 194.9}{194.9 / \sqrt{45}} = 0.679$$

$$U_o = 202.8 + 2.576 \times \frac{194.9}{\sqrt{45}} = 277.7$$

$$L_o = 202.8 - 2.576 \times \frac{194.9}{\sqrt{45}} = 128.0$$

Then, the expected range is

$$U_e = 183.1 + 202.8 - 128.0 = 257.9$$

$$L_e = 183.1 + 202.8 - 257.5 = 108.3$$

Because $|Z| = 0.678 < 2.576$, the observed value for June 2012 is not a statistical outlier at a 1 percent significance level. The same conclusion for June 2012 performance can be drawn using the expected range approach because the observed value 202.8 is within the expected range (108.3, 257.9) (Lee and McGreevey 2000).

The comparison chart using these data is shown here:

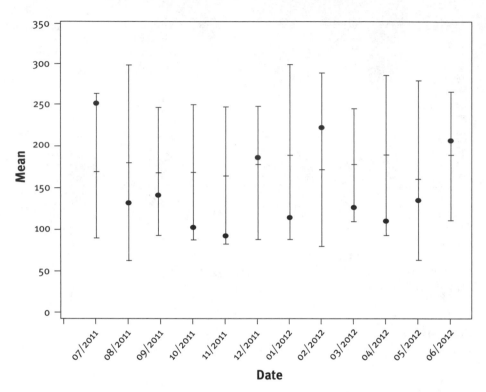

Notes

1. Kwan Y. Lee, formerly of The Joint Commission, contributed as the first author in the first edition of this chapter.
2. The content of Appendixes 1, 2, and 3 is largely based on a Joint Commission specification manual titled *Mining ORYX Data 2000—A Guide for Performance Measurement Systems* (The Joint Commission, Oakbrook Terrace, IL, 2000).

References

Agresti, A., and B. A. Coull. 1998. "Approximate Is Better Than 'Exact' for Interval Estimation of Binomial Proportions." *The American Statistician* 52 (2): 119–25.

Bickel, P. J., and K. A. Doksum. 2000. *Mathematical Statistics*, second edition. San Francisco: Holden-Day.

Chassin, M. R., and J. M. Loeb. 2011. "The Ongoing Quality Improvement Journey: Next Stop, High Reliability." *Health Affairs* 30 (4): 559–68.

Czarnecki, M. T. 1994. *Benchmarking Strategies for Health Care Management*. Gaithersburg, MD: Aspen.

Donabedian, A. 1980. *The Definition of Quality and Approaches to Its Assessment. Explorations in Quality Assessment and Monitoring 1*. Chicago: Health Administration Press.

Holubkov, R., V. L. Holt, F. A. Connell, and J. P. LoGerfo. 1998. "Analysis, Assessment, and Presentation of Risk-Adjusted Statewide Obstetrical Care Data: The StORQS II Study in Washington State." *Health Services Research* 33 (3, Pt. I): 531–48.

Iezzoni, L. I. 2013. *Risk Adjustment for Measuring Healthcare Outcomes*, fourth edition. Chicago: Health Administration Press.

Joint Commission. 2010. "Attributes of Core Performance Measures and Associated Evaluation Criteria." Updated November 3. www.jointcommission.org/Attributes_of_Core_Performance_Measures_and_Associated_Evaluation_Criteria/.

———. 2000. *A Guide to Performance Measurement for Hospitals*. Oakbrook Terrace, IL: The Joint Commission.

Lee, K. Y., and C. McGreevey. 2000. *Mining ORYX Data 2000—A Guide for Performance Measurement Systems*. Oakbrook Terrace, IL: The Joint Commission.

McNeese, W. C., and R. A. Klein. 1991. *Statistical Methods for the Process Industries*. Boca Raton, FL: CRC Press.

Montgomery, D. C. 2012. *Introduction to Statistical Quality Control*, seventh edition, New York: Wiley & Sons.

SAS Institute. 2013. *SAS/QC 12.3 User's Guide*. Cary, NC: SAS Institute Inc.

PHYSICIAN AND PROVIDER PROFILING

David B. Nash, Richard Jacoby, and Bettina Berman

Physician profiles can improve physician performance, especially in the context of continuous quality management and value-based purchasing of healthcare. Profile development is not without problems, however, and profiles are not always fully implemented in healthcare organizations.

Background and Terminology

National healthcare spending reached 17.9 percent of the gross domestic product (GDP) in 2011 (Fuchs 2013) and is projected to reach 19.8 percent of the GDP by 2020 (Keehan et al. 2011). With this increased spending on healthcare, many Americans are beginning to question whether they are receiving appropriate quality and value for their healthcare dollars. The Institute of Medicine (IOM) detailed that anywhere from 44,000 to 98,000 people die each year from preventable medical errors (Kohn, Corrigan, and Donaldson 2000). Because of the significance of reports like the IOM report, which details problems with medical errors and adverse events, the government, employers, and the public are concerned about the effects of suboptimal care and demanding more affordable healthcare of the highest quality.

The Physician's Role in Improving Quality

Despite advances in medical technology and science, healthcare in the United States is characterized by uneven and often poor quality. Although clinical guidelines and best practices exist, major barriers are preventing these practices from being implemented across the nation (RWJF 2009). Healthcare quality and cost vary widely across the country. Physicians' practice patterns have been shown to be a major contributor to unexplained clinical variation in healthcare. Unexplained clinical variation exists among providers by specialty, geographic region, and practice setting and is not associated with better quality of care and health outcomes (Skinner and Fisher 2010). Unexplained clinical variation exists for patients with many different conditions. Although variation can lead to similar outcomes, it often can lead to problems with care.

The increase in data being collected on cost and quality measures has begun to expose widespread variations in practice. Performance measurement is a critical component of national and local efforts to improve care at the institutional level and at the individual provider level. Provider profiles generated by these measurement efforts are currently used for public report cards, credentialing, and board certification as well as in pay-for-performance programs that link quality rankings to financial incentives (Fung et al. 2010).

In response to the public's demand for greater physician accountability, initial attempts to change physician behavior resulted in the development of physician report cards (Ransom 1999). However, the medical community has found fault with these report cards, and considerable debate surrounds the use of performance profiles, especially at the individual physician level (Fung et al. 2010; Ofri 2010). Proponents of performance assessment feel that physician profiling, despite its limitations, is a useful tool to change provider behavior and improve quality of care. Opponents of profiling claim that providers are unfairly penalized and have raised concerns that the ultimate goal of performance measurement is to control the cost of care. Their complaints center largely on the gauges of quality used to measure physician performance, such as measure attribution, sample size, and the inconsistency in risk-adjustment methods used to compare outcomes among physicians (Berman and Friedman 2010).

Physician Profiling

Physician profiling is the collection of provider-specific and practice-level data used to analyze physician practice patterns, utilization of services, and outcomes of care. The goals of physician profiling are to improve physician performance through accountability and feedback and to decrease practice variation through adherence to evidence-based standards of care.

The purpose of establishing consistent treatment guidelines for physicians is to achieve high-quality, high-value healthcare. Through profiling, physicians' performance can be measured against their colleagues' performance on local, state, and national levels. The idea is that physicians, who are often highly driven, goal-oriented individuals, will be motivated to improve their performance in areas in which they do not currently rank the highest. Examples of categories in which physicians would be evaluated include patient satisfaction and amount of resources used (Gevirtz and Nash 2000).

Numerous studies have highlighted differences between what physicians think they do and what they actually do (Gevirtz and Nash 2000). Many physicians overrate their performance. Profile development enables a physician's treatment pattern to be assessed and evaluated. Profiling compares providers' adherence to the current evidence-based best practices in medicine and helps to reduce practice variation. Such feedback gives physicians the opportunity to make changes to their practice patterns and to improve patient satisfaction. Profile development also provides a framework for physician evaluation through credentialing, board certification, and organizational quality improvement.

The establishment of measures to assess physician performance could lead to greater accountability and improved physician performance. Since the dissemination of the IOM's 2001 publication *Crossing the Quality Chasm*, which detailed the problems with processes of care and unexplained clinical variation in the US healthcare system, more employers, consumers, and patients have been seeking information on which to base healthcare and provider choices. Published information about provider performance assessments will help healthcare stakeholders make informed decisions based on quality.

Scope and Use of Profiling in Healthcare

Value-Based Purchasing

The government, large employers, and the public are concerned about whether healthcare providers offer high-quality, affordable care. Included in the new healthcare reform law is a requirement for increased measurement and public reporting of doctors' and hospitals' performance (RWJF 2011). Because many employees receive health insurance through their employers, employers have a stake in purchasing high-quality care.

Evidence is growing that healthcare buyers are beginning to use value-based purchasing to make healthcare decisions. In addition to cost, employers are interested in incorporating outcomes and value into their decisions when selecting provider contracts.

Efforts to determine quality measures for hospitals and healthcare plans are now being expanded to include physicians through the Centers for Medicare & Medicaid Services (CMS) Physician Quality Reporting System (PQRS) program (CMS 2013). The PQRS, initiated in 2007 as a voluntary pay-for-reporting program, is a key program under CMS's value-based purchasing strategy. Common strategies that large employers use to compare quality among physicians and hospitals include asking health plans to identify low-cost physicians and hospitals and encouraging their employees to seek care from those providers (Miller, Brennan, and Milstein 2009).

These strategies have a significant effect on physician practice patterns and decision making. Information regarding higher-quality providers enables employers to make objective decisions regarding higher-quality care in the best interest of their employees. In addition, collection of reliable and accurate data on physician performance gives purchasers an advantage in contract negotiations with physicians.

In some situations, such data could facilitate a working relationship between healthcare purchasers and providers to improve the quality of care individuals are receiving. Physician performance measurement could lead to the development of continuous quality improvement (CQI) programs that could improve various aspects of patient care and clinical outcomes. Financial rewards for physicians who meet the highest standards of performance also would encourage greater physician participation.

Profiling as Part of Continuous Quality Improvement

Physicians realize that a problem with quality exists in the United States, but the medical profession lacks a culture of quality improvement. Many physicians are suspicious of quality improvement efforts and public reporting focused on their practice patterns. Most physicians question whether quality measures are, in fact, accurate reflections of the quality of care they provide and are skeptical that data sources lack methodological rigor (Barr et al. 2008). Several physicians also question the clinical relevance of some of the measures (RWJF 2009). Often providers feel that they are being held accountable for factors that are beyond their control, such as patient compliance with physician recommendations (Ofri 2010). Other concerns relate to data validity, risk adjustment, credibility of the data source, and sampling issues (Barr et al. 2008). As a result, many physicians have dismissed conclusions about their performance as interpretations of inaccurate data, which adds to their concern about public release of quality information.

In response to increased public reporting on quality measures and patient satisfaction indicators by CMS (2011), many healthcare organizations have developed a CQI strategy that encourages a systems solution to improving healthcare. Many hospitals are concerned about unexplained variation of care and are developing strategies to address the issue (Gauld et al. 2011). CQI integrates structure, process, and outcomes of care into a management system that allows processes to be analyzed and outcomes to be improved. *Structure* relates to the array of organizational resources, such as facilities, equipment, human resources, and organizational structure, in the setting where care is provided. *Process* refers to the patient's and provider's activities in the process of receiving and providing care. *Outcomes* indicate the effects of care on the patient's health status (Berman and Friedman 2010). This approach involves everyone in an organization and focuses on process failures, not individual failures. An understanding of process problems can help identify and improve factors that contribute to poor quality.

As part of their CQI strategies, healthcare organizations use many mechanisms to maintain the most competent physician staff. Some of the tools and strategies, described briefly here, include credentialing, physician report cards, benchmarking, and clinical pathways.

Credentialing

Credentialing refers to the process of hiring a well-qualified medical staff that is able to deliver the highest-quality care. Physicians are offered positions based on criteria such as peer review, board certification, and hours spent in continuing medical education. By developing standards for competency, the hospital or the provider organization is able to maintain the highest level of quality among the physicians in its system.

Physician Report Cards

Physician report cards (which may be a component of a physician profile) compare physicians on outcomes related to measures such as quality, patient satisfaction, and cost-utilization patterns. This information can encourage changes in physician behavior because physicians who do not perform well in rankings against their peers likely will take steps to improve their performance. However, providers have disapproved of report cards because of concerns about the validity and reliability of physician performance profiles. Multiple factors, such as evidence-based quality measures, accurate data sources, and standardized data collection, are required to accurately compare physician-level performance (Scholle et al. 2008).

Benchmarking

Benchmarking uses quantitative measures of best practices to evaluate physician performance. When physicians' performance is compared to the best practices of their peers, underperforming physicians may be more willing to change their practice patterns. For example, in ambulatory care, achieving and maintaining an optimal blood level of HbA1c has been identified as an important measurement in controlling the incidence of complications in patients with diabetes. If a physician's rate of achieving this level for his or her diabetic population lags that of his or her peer group, the physician can theoretically identify and rectify the causes so that subsequent measurements more closely resemble the best practices of the peer group.

Clinical Pathways

Clinical pathways are treatment plans designed to reduce variations in clinical care. By combining physician input with evidence-based medicine, organizations create new treatment pathways to increase quality, improve outcomes, and decrease costs. Increasingly, the use of information technology in the form of electronic health records (EHRs) that incorporate clinical pathways will facilitate the deployment of this tool.

Use in Healthcare Organizations

Physician profiling is one of the many tools used in CQI. It is valuable to healthcare purchasers and in educating physicians. Because unexplained clinical variation can lead to poorer outcomes for patients and to a payment differential for hospitals, measuring what providers actually do in practice is an essential part of improving physicians' performance and an organization's overall processes of care. Although physicians typically do not like to examine their own performance, numerous studies have documented that, when presented with information about their performance relative to that of their colleagues, peer pressure can stimulate physician behavior changes to meet a specified outcome (Miller, Brennan, and Milstein 2009).

The most effective profiles document variations in provider performance on individual, local, and national levels. If shown how they perform compared with a group of peers, physicians might be more likely to improve in areas in which they rank low. Profiles should be easy to understand and provide specific suggestions. If profiles outline physicians' strengths and weaknesses in a way that is easy to understand and that is supported by evidence-based medicine, physicians might be more likely to change their practice patterns.

Healthcare organizations can use physician profiles as a valuable educational tool. Doing things correctly the first time will yield the lowest costs. Profiles provide physicians with the information to determine which conditions they are treating appropriately and how they compare against set benchmarks or with their peers.

Profile comparison displays current trends among providers and can encourage physicians to follow evidence-based guidelines. Based on those trends, an organization can develop quality improvement strategies to educate physicians on how to improve their performance and the health of the population they care for.

The creation of an information technology infrastructure to analyze the performance of all physicians in a healthcare system can be useful in identifying the conditions the hospital, physician, or physician group treats most. EHRs can be valuable in creating disease registries and in giving physicians an overview of patient outcomes at the population level.

Clinical and Operational Issues

Best-practice standards in healthcare continue to evolve in response to new research and treatment options. Organizations can use physician profiles to compare various processes and determine the most efficient, cost-effective ways to practice medicine. In addition, the development of ongoing measurements to evaluate physicians will encourage physicians to stay current on the most recent evidence in medicine.

Before beginning to use profiles, an organization and its physicians must adopt a commitment to CQI. This commitment entails improving patient satisfaction, working with the physicians on staff at the hospital or the physician group, and determining quality indicators.

The following list identifies a number of concerns related to the creation of physician profiles (Gevirtz and Nash 2000):

- What do you want to measure, and why is this important?
- Are these the most appropriate measures of quality improvement?
- How will you measure performance? (What is the gold standard?)
- How and when will you collect the measures?
- How reliable are the profiles you are creating?
- What are the most appropriate measures of physician performance?
- Can you measure these variables? (How will you collect the data?)
- What is the appropriate design (e.g., measuring percentages, means)?
- How will you interpret the results (e.g., risk adjustment, acceptable results)?
- How will these findings influence change?

The implementation and use of profiles should be part of a CQI process. A step-by-step approach is the most effective approach to profiling. An approach that moves slowly and involves a diverse group of members of the healthcare organization will be more likely to gain support and produce change within the system.

Choosing Which Measures to Profile

Within a healthcare organization, many areas lend themselves to quality improvement. These areas include clinical processes of care and patient outcomes. Examples are appropriate prescribing of antibiotics, surgical outcomes, patient safety, and patient satisfaction. The organization's quality improvement committee should identify the areas most appropriate for profiling and the areas in which to improve performance. Committee members must understand that not all medical conditions are appropriate for profiling and that they should profile only conditions for which evidence-based guidelines exist. The criteria for the profiles could come from nationally recognized practice guidelines or other practice parameters.

Guidelines serve as a checklist of objectives against which the committee can compare its actions. Without guidelines, committee members cannot be sure that they are including all components of the care process. This emphasis on rational decision making will foster greater support from physicians and is more likely to bring about performance improvement.

Collecting the Data

The quality improvement committee should identify the techniques to be used in gathering and disseminating data. The gathering of information should not interfere with the daily operations of patient care. Traditional methods of data collection have relied on medical records and claims data. Newer methods involve collating data in EHRs and reporting quality measures through specialized software programs. Data collection by any method can be difficult, and the committee must assess which data are most applicable for measuring performance. The committee also should identify how much data must be gathered to produce statistically valid results.

Interpreting the Results

Once the data are gathered, the quality improvement committee must develop an objective and appropriate way to interpret the results. Physician performance should be assessed in relation to the accepted national benchmarks for the condition or the target determined by the committee. Profiles should be developed only for physicians who have a large volume of patients with the disease or other target. A physician who sees 200 patients with a condition is more likely to value the data on his or her performance than will a physician who sees 20 patients with the same condition. Physicians themselves can help the committee construct profiles by including diseases for which there is potential for improved treatment processes and outcomes, agreeing on benchmarks and gauges of quality, and encouraging other physicians to participate in the quality improvement process. From this information, the committee can determine statistically and clinically significant outcomes. The data also must be risk adjusted to compensate for the diverse populations of patients that physicians encounter. Risk adjusting will validate the physicians' results and improve the likelihood that physicians will accept the data.

Communicating the Results

After developing the profile, the quality improvement committee must decide which format will be most valuable to the physician. Graphical presentations of data in dashboard format are easy to understand and allow physicians to view trends over a specific period. The information conveyed to the physician must be kept simple. Exhibit 7.1 is an example of a physician-group profile that illustrates prescribing behaviors.

In addition, the committee must decide whether the information distributed in the profiles will be blinded or nonblinded. Some physicians may resent having their performance publicly available for other physicians to see, especially if they rank lower in certain areas. Ideally, physicians will use nonblinded information to find physicians who have better outcomes and to learn ways to improve. Also, physicians who rank lower will want to improve because they do not want to be seen as performing at a lower level than that of their peers. For this part of the process, physician buy-in is crucial.

Meetings should be scheduled on a monthly or quarterly basis so that physicians have the opportunity to comment on how the profiling system is

EXHIBIT 7.1

Example of a Physician-Group Profile for Generic Drug Prescribing

Practice X
Generic Drug Prescribing Report
Group Summary and Peer Comparison
Based on Paid Claims Incurred Between 01/01/2013 and 06/30/2013

Provider	Provider Count	Unique Member Count	Generic Prescription Count	Brand Prescription Count	Generic Drug %	Brand Drug %
Practice X	13	348	688	210	76.61%	23.39%
Peer Comparison	154	11,931	29,314	11,097	72.54%	27.46%

Peer Percentiles

50th Percentile	70th Percentile	75th Percentile	80th Percentile	85th Percentile	90th Percentile	95th Percentile
75.94%	81.54%	82.51%	85.10%	87.68%	91.30%	93.59%

Top-Level Summary (calculation based on Q1 2013 data)

Practice X would have needed to increase generic prescribing about 2 percentage points to achieve an incentive (70th percentile) during this time frame.

Practice X would need to have written an additional 44 generic prescriptions during this time frame.

93% of the brands prescribed most in Practice X, accounting for 13 scripts, have generic equivalents that should be considered.

Practice X Generic Drug Prescribing

2013	Generic Drug %	Min. Target
Q2	76.61%	81.54%
Q1	75.99%	80.99%
2012		
Q4	67.66%	79.09%
Q3	69.98%	78.10%
Q2	67.34%	77.00%
Q1	67.49%	76.32%
2011		
Q4	69.43%	76.52%
Q3	68.83%	76.19%
Q2	69.80%	75.26%
Q1	72.31%	74.07%

working. These meetings also will provide time for physicians to obtain feedback on their performance and discuss ways to improve.

Implementation

Keys to Success

Administrators or quality improvement committees who wish to develop profiles should work closely with physicians. At the start of the project, teams should approach physician leaders who express interest in quality improvement. Involvement of physicians who are open to change, respected by their peers, and knowledgeable about quality will increase the chance that other physicians in the organization will participate.

Specialty providers require different levels of information and different methodologies to analyze outcomes. Involvement of many different specialists in the quality process will result in greater data validity and increased physician participation.

After developing a profile, the quality improvement committee should determine a time frame for all physicians to review the information before the profile becomes an official tool of the organization. If the committee allows physicians to participate in profile development, they may be more likely to approve of profiling. Once the physicians have submitted their reviews, the committee should meet to finalize the profiles and set a date to begin using them.

Once the profile has been in use for a defined period, the committee should present a series of educational sessions. Organized follow-up activities communicate to physicians that the profiling program is designed for quality improvement. Modification of physician behavior is a process that will happen over time, and the organization needs to reassure physicians on a regular basis that they are following the best treatment protocols for their patients. Providing physicians with incentives to improve their performance, such as award recognition, also will boost quality improvement.

The profiling system should not be threatening to physicians. If profiles are to be successful in improving healthcare processes and outcomes, physicians must see them as nonpunitive and primarily for educational purposes. Physicians have to believe that profiling is designed to help them improve their performance and target conditions that offer opportunity for improvement.

Challenges

The use of profiling has many critics. No consensus exists on what constitutes a profile, what it should measure, and the groups to which the information should be targeted. Employers and consumers want different levels of information with which to make healthcare decisions. Employers are interested in differences in quality and outcomes across providers and favor public reporting and transparency, although only 20 percent of employers offer information to employees on quality and cost (Miller, Brennan, and Milstein 2009).

Consumers' interest in performance measurement has been limited. The average consumer is interested in provider recommendations from other patients, rather than ones based on publicly available quality metrics (Miller, Brennan, and Milstein 2009).

Many physicians are skeptical of profiling. They feel that they know what is best for their patients because they see them on a regular basis. Adherence to generally accepted guidelines may not be appropriate for the population of patients they serve.

Individuals with chronic conditions who see several doctors pose another problem. Examination of the practice pattern of a physician and related outcomes in such cases may lead to inaccurate conclusions. In addition, because many patients frequently switch providers, it may be difficult to develop profiles over a period long enough to be meaningful (Gevirtz and Nash 2000).

Physicians also may be skeptical of the calculation of their results. Physicians who treat a low volume of patients with a specific condition may resent being compared to physicians who treat a larger volume of patients with the same condition.

Reaching agreement on the best treatment for a particular medical condition is a difficult task. New technologies, drugs, and payment schemes significantly affect a physician's practice and make reaching consensus on a specific treatment challenging. Consequently, some physicians may be reluctant to accept national treatment guidelines.

Finally, successful patient outcomes rely partly on patient compliance. A well-designed profile has to recognize the point at which a physician's efforts to improve quality reach their maximum because beyond that point the patients' actions largely determine the outcomes.

Provider Profiling in the Era of Healthcare Reform

Over the last decade, many advances have been made to improve the quality and value of healthcare; however, the passage of the Affordable Care Act (ACA) may become the greatest change agent. The ACA reforms many aspects of both the private health insurance industry and public health insurance programs. While the law has far-reaching ramifications, its ultimate goal is to increase the value of healthcare by improving quality and controlling costs (US Congress 2010). Notable aspects of the legislation that affect physician and provider profiling are outlined here.

Development of New Patient Care Models
A major provision of the ACA is the establishment of the new Center for Medicare & Medicaid Innovation. This center will begin testing new ways of delivering care to patients. The new methods will be evaluated to see if they improve the quality of care and reduce the rate of growth in healthcare costs. The center aims to test models that deal broadly with both delivery of care, such as patient-centered medical homes (PCMHs) and accountable care organizations (ACOs), and alternative models for provider payment.

Linking Payments to Quality
The ACA also requires the establishment of a Hospital Value-Based Purchasing Program, which creates incentives for hospitals to meet certain performance measures for quality of care, efficiency, and patient satisfaction. Hospitals that do not meet the required standards will be penalized financially. In addition, CMS will publish the performance of all hospitals, including those with substandard performance. Although this aspect of the legislation does not affect individual providers financially, it will be a major focus of hospital administrators and quality improvement committees.

Individual providers, however, will be affected by other strategies that tie provider payment to performance. Thus, providers who did not participate in the CMS PQRS in 2013 will be subject to payment adjustments in 2015. Providers will also be held accountable for measures of both quality of care and cost under the so-called Value-Based Payment Modifier (VBPM). As established by the ACA, the VBPM provides differential payments to physicians based on quality of care compared to cost. By 2015, providers in group practices of 100 or more eligible providers will be subject to the VBPM based on their 2013 performance on quality and cost metrics. In 2017, the VBPM will be applied to all providers based on performance in 2015. CMS will provide feedback reports called Quality and Resource Use Reports (QRURs). The QRURs present data about the care provided to Medicare fee-for-service patients and show how a provider's Medicare spending compares to average Medicare spending.

Continued growth in healthcare spending combined with uneven quality of care has led to an increased focus on improving the value of care. Measuring performance through the use of quality indicators has become a key part of efforts to reform healthcare delivery and payment models. Provider profiles generated by these efforts are increasingly being tied to financial incentives, and penalties for noncompliance with quality reporting will be imposed in the near future. To remain successful and competitive in a value-conscious era, providers and healthcare organizations must collaborate to create a culture of accountability that will lead to improved value of care.

Case Study

This section highlights a theoretical scenario involving physician profiles in an ambulatory care setting. As part of pay-for-performance programs, two different payers developed physician profiles for two different groups of primary care physicians. One set of physicians participated in a large academic group practice, and the other set consisted of physicians in private practice who worked both individually and in small groups.

The first payer was a large commercial health plan that dominated the local market. It developed its profiles using administrative claims data. The second payer was Medicare, which developed profiles from data submitted by physicians on billing forms as part of the CMS PQRS.

The commercial health plan's profiles involved a variety of measures from the Healthcare Effectiveness Data and Information Set (HEDIS). The measures and goals were chosen in conjunction with representatives from the academic group and applied to all the academic and private practice physicians. The health plan calculated performance on each measure for each physician. It displayed the information in graphical, nonblinded formats that compared the performance of individual physicians to those of their colleagues. A sample of the type of data physicians received is shown in Exhibit 7.2. The physicians received such reports quarterly.

A second report, also sent quarterly, not only provided physicians' numerical scores for each measure but also benchmarked their performance (scores) against the scores of local physicians in their specialty as well as against national benchmarks. These reports also contained information about their pay-for-performance bonuses. For purposes of determining the bonus amounts, the score for each measure was given a weight. A weighted average of a physician's scores was then developed, displayed in a profile, and compared against the appropriate aggregated benchmarks (Exhibit 7.3). Bonuses were based on a sliding scale that related performance to the benchmarks at the conclusion of the measurement cycle. The maximum achievable bonus was 5 percent of the total fees the commercial plan paid a physician for that cycle. A small percentage of each bonus was based on cost management. Physicians whose performance did not qualify them for a bonus were not penalized.

In graphics like those shown in Exhibit 7.2, physicians could see whether they were performing up to the best standards and how they compared to their peers. Some physicians did not like being compared to their peers and having their results shown publicly, but the commercial health plan emphasized that such reports were meant to be nonpunitive and aimed at CQI.

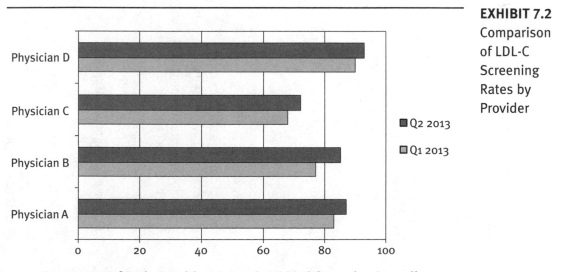

EXHIBIT 7.2
Comparison of LDL-C Screening Rates by Provider

Percentage of Patients with at Least One LDL-C Screening Annually

Note: LDL-C = low-density lipoprotein cholesterol.

EXHIBIT 7.3
Physician C
Profile: Pay-for-
Performance
Results
Through Third
Quarter—2013

Measures	Weights	Target Local Peer-Group Performance	Target HEDIS 90th Percentile Benchmark Performance	Dr. C Results
Quality Measures				
Persistence of beta-blocker treatment after a heart attack	11.2%	51.5%	81.0%	57.1%
Comprehensive diabetes care: LDL-C screening performed	11.2%	95.4%	96.0%	83.3%
Colorectal cancer screening	11.2%	56.8%	63.5%	57.9%
Use of appropriate medications for people with asthma	11.2%	91.8%	94.1%	89.5%
Breast cancer screening	11.2%	70.6%	80.1%	73.0%
Comprehensive diabetes care: HbA1c control (<9.0%)	6.0%	70.0%	86.1%	82.0%
Comprehensive diabetes care: eye exam (retinal) performed	6.0%	62.7%	69.3%	43.6%
Osteoporosis management in women who had a fracture	6.0%	29.0%	30.4%	30.0%
Cholesterol management for patients with cardiovascular conditions	6.0%	54.4%	56.5%	46.5%
Resource Management Measures				
Pharmacy management	10.0%	53.2%	55.2%	52.8%
Relative cost-of-care index (ETGs)	10.0%			Calculated at year end

Note: HEDIS = Healthcare Effectiveness Data and Information Set; LDL-C = low-density lipoprotein cholesterol; ETG = episode treatment group.

A quality improvement team trained in CQI supported the physicians in the academic group practice. When the initial results were received, the team instituted a CQI education and implementation program. As a result, over the next several years, the practice incrementally improved its performance on the quality measures and all members eventually received the maximum bonus from the pay-for-performance program. The physicians took pride in their accomplishments.

The physicians in the private practice settings had a slightly different experience. Although their performance on quality measures in the first year paralleled that of their colleagues practicing in the academic setting, they did not perform as well in subsequent years. Lack of an infrastructure supporting CQI caused their performance on the measures to stagnate. They did not qualify for bonus payments, and their profiles reflected subpar performance when compared to national and local benchmarks.

Both the academic and the private practice groups had difficulty implementing the CMS PQRS program (more accurately described as a pay-for-reporting program than a pay-for-performance program when initiated) because the program required more active engagement on the part of physicians and their staff. Both groups' engagement in the PQRS program fell short because the physicians' offices had to gather and submit the required data on billing forms, whereas the commercial health plan simply aggregated administrative data. Neither the academic nor the private practice physicians used EHRs, which made data collection labor intensive.

Initially, participation in the PQRS program was voluntary and required physicians and staff to be educated in quality and its measurement. Physicians primarily used the CMS website to acquire this education. CMS reported the results once per year.

In the academic practice group, the quality improvement team provided supplemental educational materials to physicians as well as chart tools that facilitated identification and capture of the data required for reporting. At first, the physicians used the tools inconsistently. As a result, relatively few physicians reported on enough measures to earn bonuses, and the physician profiles developed by CMS were incomplete.

In an attempt to monitor ongoing performance, the quality improvement team developed a database by using reports from the billing system. It programmed a sophisticated analytic tool to capture the data and report them in a format that could be monitored quarterly so that CQI could be implemented. With this feedback and support, physicians in the academic group practice began to consistently report on measures. Through monitoring, feedback, and interaction with the quality improvement team, the physicians were able to improve their performance where indicated and receive bonus payments. In addition, their CMS profiles identified them as physicians practicing high-quality medicine.

The primary care physicians practicing both individually and in small groups in private practice participated minimally in the PQRS program. Many were unaware of the program, and many who were aware of it found it difficult to comprehend. Of the few who took the time to understand it, most concluded that the 0.5 percent bonus being offered did not cover the costs of gathering the required data. Some physicians and physician groups reported on the required measures, figuring that this type of reporting and profiling would be mandatory at some time in the near future. They appreciated that the quality performance measures would benefit their patients and decided that learning the program would be worth the effort sooner rather than later. In general, the lack of a supporting educational infrastructure impeded the adoption of PQRS in the private practice group.

The success of the academic group practice in both the commercial health plan and the PQRS profiling programs is a good example of how having a quality infrastructure and fostering and supporting a culture of quality in an organization can enhance the delivery of healthcare. Development of incentives to improve physician performance and investment in information systems are valuable initiatives that will help to improve outcomes and make processes of care more efficient.

Study Questions

1. What challenges may a quality improvement committee encounter when attempting to measure physician performance?
2. Describe the relationship between continuous quality improvement and physician profiling.
3. Describe the strengths and weaknesses of the profiles discussed in this chapter.

References

Barr, J. K., S. L. Bernard, S. Sofaer, T. E. Giannotti, N. F. Lenfestey, and D. J. Miranda. 2008. "Physicians' Views on Public Reporting of Hospital Quality Data." *Medical Care Research and Review* 65 (6): 655–73.

Berman, B., and C. D. Friedman. 2010. "Value-Based Purchasing Paradigms for Facial Plastic Surgery." *Facial Plastic Surgery* 26 (4): 283–88.

Centers for Medicare & Medicaid Services (CMS). 2013. "Physician Quality Reporting System." Page modified November 18. www.cms.gov/Medicare/Quality-Initiatives-Patient-Assessment-Instruments/PQRS/index.html.

———. 2011. "Medicare Program; Hospital Inpatient Value-Based Purchasing Program; Final Rule." *Federal Register* 76 (88): 26490–547. Published May 6. www.gpo.gov/fdsys/pkg/FR-2011-05-06/pdf/2011-10568.pdf.

Fuchs, V. R. 2013. "The Gross Domestic Product and Health Care Spending." *New England Journal of Medicine* 369 (2): 107–9.

Fung, V., J. A. Schmittdiel, B. Fireman, A. Meer, S. Thomas, J. Hsu, and J. V. Selby. 2010. "Meaningful Variation in Performance: A Systematic Literature Review." *Medical Care* 48 (2): 140–48.

Gauld, R., J. Horwitt, S. Williams, and A. B. Cohen. 2011. "What Strategies Do U.S. Hospitals Employ to Reduce Unwarranted Clinical Practice Variations?" *American Journal of Medical Quality* 26 (2): 120–26.

Gevirtz, F., and D. B. Nash. 2000. "Enhancing Physician Performance Through Practice Profiling." In *Enhancing Physician Performance: Advanced Principles of Medical Management*, edited by S. Ransom, W. Pinsky, and J. Tropman, 91–116. Tampa, FL: American College of Physician Executives.

Institute of Medicine (IOM). 2001. *Crossing the Quality Chasm: A New Health System for the 21st Century*. Washington, DC: National Academies Press.

Keehan, S. P., A. M. Sisko, C. J. Truffer, J. A. Poisal, G. A. Cuckler, A. J. Madison, J. M. Lizonitz, and S. D. Smith. 2011. "National Health Spending Projections Through 2020: Economic Recovery and Reform Drive Faster Spending Growth." *Health Affairs* 30 (8): 1594–605.

Kohn, L. T., J. M. Corrigan, and M. S. Donaldson (eds.). 2000. *To Err Is Human: Building a Safer Health System*. Washington, DC: National Academies Press.

Miller, T. P., T. A. Brennan, and A. Milstein. 2009. "How Can We Make More Progress in Measuring Physicians' Performance to Improve the Value of Care?" *Health Affairs* 28 (5): 1429–37.

Ofri, D. 2010. "Quality Measures and the Individual Physician." *New England Journal of Medicine* 363 (7): 606–7.

Ransom, S. 1999. "Enhancing Physician Performance." In *Clinical Resource and Quality Management*, edited by S. Ransom and W. Pinsky, 139–69. Tampa, FL: American College of Physician Executives.

Robert Wood Johnson Foundation (RWJF). 2011. "Report on Americans' Views on the Quality of Health Care." Published March 22. www.rwjf.org/en/research-publications/find-rwjf-research/2011/03/report-on-americans--views-on-the-quality-of-health-care.html.

———. 2009. "Communicating with Physicians About Performance Measurement." Posted Winter. www.rwjf.org/en/research-publications/find-rwjf-research/2009/12/communicating-with-physicians-about-performance-measurement.html.

Scholle, S. H., J. Roski, J. L. Adams, D. L. Dunn, E. A. Kerr, D. P. Dugan, and R. E. Jensen. 2008. "Benchmarking Physician Performance: Reliability of

Individual and Composite Measures." *American Journal of Managed Care* 14 (12): 829–38.

Skinner, J., and E. S. Fisher. 2010. "Reflections on Geographic Variations in U.S. Health Care." Dartmouth Institute for Health Policy and Clinical Practice. www.dartmouthatlas.org/downloads/press/Skinner_Fisher_DA_05_10.pdf.

US Congress. 2010. "Compilation of Patient Protection and Affordable Care Act." Prepared by the Office of the Legislative Counsel for the US House of Representatives, as amended through May 1. http://docs.house.gov/energycommerce/ppacacon.pdf.

THE CULTURE CONNECTION: HARDWIRING CONSISTENT QUALITY DELIVERY

Quint Studer

Providing top-notch clinical quality has always been the main goal of healthcare organizations. In our industry, it has to be. Patient care is not just another product or service. Making sure we do the best possible quality work matters on a different level. It is about saving lives—and there can be no higher calling.

As healthcare leaders, we have always had a moral imperative to constantly improve quality. But with all the changes shaking up our industry, how do we stay focused on our overall goal of providing the best care to the patient? How do we strive to hardwire excellence into our organizations without feeling pressured to jump from one quality initiative to the next, especially as we are being held accountable for quality in a way that is more rigorous and quantifiable than ever before?

How Is Quality Defined Today?

Now that we have moved into a pay-for-performance reimbursement era— one in which the requirements become ever more stringent—we must ask ourselves: What does high quality mean now? And how best can we achieve it consistently?

Quality can be defined as "the cumulative impact of all that happens to a patient while in an organization's care" (Porter 2012). This definition includes the care provided as well as the outcomes achieved. Patient experience-of-care results, safety metrics, the presence of hospital-acquired conditions (HACs), and preventable readmissions are measures that help define quality of care.

When the Centers for Medicare & Medicaid Services (CMS) released the Hospital Value-Based Purchasing Program, the quality metrics for 2013 included the Hospital Consumer Assessment of Healthcare Providers and Systems (HCAHPS)—a survey that measures the patient experience or perception of quality care—and 12 process-of-care measures. Three mortality outcome measures were scheduled to be added to these indicators representing quality care in 2014, and the addition of HACs (specifically, central-line-associated bloodstream infections) was scheduled for 2015.

There is, in fact, a proven link between patient perception of care and clinical quality care—these outcomes go hand in hand. Exhibits 8.1 and 8.2 show that as patients' HCAHPS percentile rankings of providers' responsiveness increase, both vascular-catheter-associated infections and manifestations of poor glycemic control decrease.

We can infer another important point from Exhibits 8.1 and 8.2: Responsiveness itself seems to drive improved quality results. When **all** staff members are trained to respond to call lights—keeping in mind that patients do not make distinctions between clinical care providers and nonclinical employees—outcomes will improve in all quality areas.

For example, a Studer Group® study on reducing the incidence of call lights and the impact that the Hourly Rounding® model (see sidebar "What Is Hourly Rounding?") has on patient satisfaction and quality of care (Meade, Bursell, and Ketelsen 2006) found that providers who implemented Hourly Rounding were able to decrease call lights by 37.8 percent, decrease falls by 50 percent, decrease hospital-acquired decubiti by 14 percent, and improve patient satisfaction by an average of 12 points.

Over the years, results have shown that Hourly Rounding, coupled with a no-pass zone tactic that involves all staff in responding to a patient's

EXHIBIT 8.1
Relation Between Vascular Catheter-Associated Infections and HCAHPS Percentiles

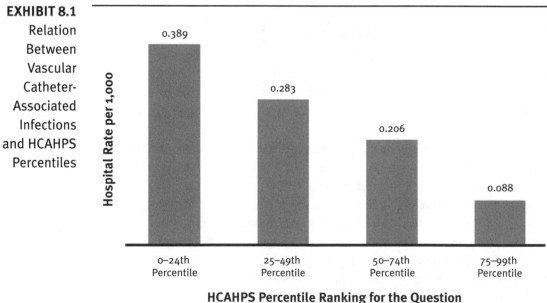

Source: Data from CMS (2013) for discharges between October 1, 2008, and June 30, 2010.

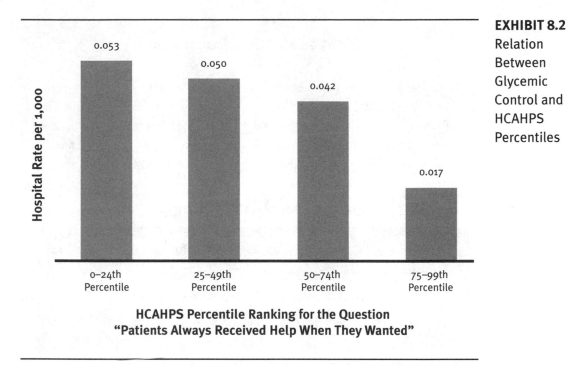

EXHIBIT 8.2
Relation
Between
Glycemic
Control and
HCAHPS
Percentiles

Source: Data from CMS (2013) for discharges between October 1, 2008, and June 30, 2010.

needs, yields tremendous results. Patients feel they are always being assisted and cared for as soon as they need help (and sometimes before they even have to ask). Of course, this is just one example of a set of tactics that improve both patient perception of care and clinical quality results.

We can conclude that quality is the culmination of everything that affects patients during their stay. So, with this linkage in mind, how does a hospital get to the point that it consistently provides high-quality care in all areas? How does it ensure that its care is consistently responsive and that evidence-based care and processes are hardwired throughout the entire organization? The answer requires a laser focus on creating an accountable culture.

Why Accountability Matters

Leaders often know which tactics will improve quality in specific areas. Sometimes they even see quick results when those tactics are implemented. Consistency, reliability, and sustainability—the hallmarks of an organization that has hardwired excellence—are the real challenges. Achieving isolated surges of improved quality is one thing. Making sure the behaviors that create quality are hardwired across the organization and the improvements will last over time is quite another.

WHAT IS HOURLY ROUNDING?

Hourly Rounding involves staff (nurses, nurse assistants, other appropriate team members) rounding on patients every hour during the day and every two hours at night using eight key behaviors. This tactic is a way to provide consistent, proactive care by bundling a patient's needs into one visit and setting expectations about frequency of visits.

Eight Behaviors for Hourly Rounding

Hourly Rounding Behavior	Expected Results
Use opening key words	Improved efficiency
Accomplish scheduled tasks	Improved efficiency
Address three Ps (pain, potty, position)	Improved quality indicators—falls, decubitis, pain management
Address additional comfort needs	Improved patient experience with pain, concern, and caring
Conduct environmental assessment	Improved efficiency and teamwork
Ask, "Is there anything else I can do for you before I go? I have time."	Improved efficiency; improved patient experience with teamwork and communication
Tell patient when you will be back	Improved efficiency
Document the round	Improved quality and accountability

Hourly Rounding is a trademark of Studer Group.

Some organizations really "get" the value of hardwiring behaviors and holding people accountable for performing them. For example, organizations that have implemented comprehensive hand-hygiene compliance programs—complete with unit-based initiatives, intensive marketing campaigns, and accountability measures on their leader evaluations—have achieved dramatic decreases in various hospital-acquired infection rates.

To create and sustain such improvements, leaders have to make sure everyone is practicing the right behaviors with every patient, every time. This approach requires everyone in the organization—from senior leaders to middle managers, from physicians to frontline care givers to ancillary service providers—to be passionate about working together to accomplish great things for the patient. But passion is not enough: All staff also need to be aligned in goals and accountability.

In short, everyone must execute the behaviors proven to achieve great quality outcomes. Critical to the execution of these behaviors is ensuring that all involved fully understand why they are important. And everyone must be held accountable for the results. Leaders must define the behaviors desired, engage staff by thoroughly explaining why, and then ensure compliance through accountability.

The bottom line is that culture drives quality. If an organization does not have a culture in which people hold themselves accountable, it will not have the foundation necessary to achieve and sustain high-level quality outcomes.

What Does an Accountable Culture Look Like?

In a hospital where everything seems to be focused on providing the absolute best care for the patient, processes and procedures happen in a smooth and organized fashion. Employees come across as competent, caring, and positive. Even patients, despite the (obvious) fact that they are not feeling their best, seem less anxious and more confident than patients in other hospitals—as if they trust they are in good hands.

That kind of hospital is the result of a culture in which accountability reigns—and it does not just happen. It is deliberately created from the top down. The following are some of its characteristics:

- *The organization is aligned from top to bottom.* Everyone knows the mission, and actionable goals are set to support it organization-wide. Those goals are cascaded from level to level through the organization so that everyone works together to achieve the same outcomes.

- *People know the why behind everything they do.* If they are asked to make a change, they are told exactly how it will benefit the patient. Knowing the why forces them to make the behavior a must-do. Once people understand their personal role in the patient's outcome, their values will not allow them **not** to perform as expected.

- *Leaders are well trained and able to cascade that training to their staff.* Even the best clinicians do not automatically have the skills to lead. Organizations that consistently provide high-quality care also provide leadership training.

- *Everyone practices specific behaviors proven to get results.* Whether it is rounding for outcomes or postvisit calls, leaders make an effort to standardize behaviors so that all employees and patients have a consistent experience. These behaviors are validated and rewarded to ensure they are repeated until they are hardwired throughout the organization (see sidebar "Five Evidence-Based Tactics That Improve Quality").

- *The majority of employees are deeply engaged.* They feel like a team that is committed and working together to achieve the same outcomes. They practice proven behaviors even when no one is looking. In short, they act like owners.

- *People are held accountable for their performance.* High-quality, high-reliability organizations use evaluation systems that are based on objective, weighted performance metrics that are aligned with the overall goals of the organization. Furthermore, low performers are not tolerated—high-quality organizations have effective systems in place for moving performance up and moving low performers out.

- *Processes are standardized across the organization.* Whether it is hand-hygiene practices or responding to call lights, everyone in every department is trained to perform tasks the same way. Doctors, nurses, or cleaning staff—all employees follow the same procedures.

- *The organization is geared to innovate.* People at all levels understand the need to constantly improve and strive for ever-greater efficiency and cost savings. The willingness, and even the thirst, to change is built into the culture. This has always been an important characteristic of great healthcare organizations, but it is even more critical in an environment of pay for performance, where the bar will continue to be raised.

As an organization seeks to create this kind of culture, nothing is more critical than being able to help every staff member connect to the purpose—the why. It is this ability that makes continuous transformation possible.

Connecting staff to purpose requires more than just making vague, overarching statements such as "Do this, it's better for the patient." It means saying, "As a member of the housekeeping staff, you reduce infections and help patients heal when you follow the protocols for sanitizing patient rooms" or "As a lab technician, you can prevent unnecessary delays in diagnosis when you always return the samples you collect to the lab within an hour." The key in connecting staff to purpose is to express the why at the individual level so that staff can see how they personally affect patient care.

People who work in healthcare feel a strong sense not only of professional responsibility but also of human responsibility. Our mission is to provide the best possible care for patients, and when we understand that the changes we are being asked to make result in better outcomes for patients, our values will not allow us **not** to make them.

FIVE EVIDENCE-BASED TACTICS THAT IMPROVE QUALITY

The following tactics have been developed, refined, and proven effective based on evidence gained from observing and working with the more than 850 hospitals that make up Studer Group's National Learning Lab. While many organizations practice a form of these tactics, implementing them in very specific ways is necessary to maximize effectiveness.

1. **Hourly Rounding:** The organization makes a commitment to have a staff member visit every patient every one to two hours. This commitment does not mean just checking in—it means practicing a series of eight very specific behaviors (see sidebar "What Is Hourly Rounding?").

2. **Nurse leader rounding on patients:** Nurse leader rounding is a proactive plan to engage, listen to, communicate with, build relationships with, and support patients and their families. It is a structured mechanism to ensure that quality, safe, and compassionate care is delivered to every patient, every time.

3. **AIDET®:** This acronym stands for **A**cknowledge, **I**ntroduce, **D**uration, **E**xplanation, and **T**hank You. It is a communication framework that improves the patient experience, helps reduce anxiety (thus improving outcomes), builds patient loyalty, and ensures that staff members are delivering consistent messages of concern and appreciation.

4. **Bedside Shift Report℠:** When one nurse transfers care delivery to another nurse during shift change, all necessary information is exchanged at the patient's bedside—patient identifiers, safety checks, medications, tests, and so forth. The patient is an active participant in the conversation. This real-time exchange of information increases patient safety, improves quality of care, increases accountability, and strengthens teamwork.

5. **Postvisit patient phone calls:** Staff members connect with patients following discharge to confirm compliance with and understanding of discharge instructions, demonstrate empathy, and afford an opportunity for service recovery, if appropriate. Results include fewer readmissions, better compliance with discharge instructions, improved clinical outcomes, fewer complaints and claims, and improved perceptions of care.

Evidence-Based Leadership

So how does an organization go about systematically building an accountability-centered, quality-focused culture? One proven way is to use Studer Group's Evidence-Based Leadership[SM] (EBL) framework, an approach to leadership that developed out of work with hospitals across the United States and in Canada, Australia, New Zealand, and beyond. EBL and culture go hand in hand. As an organization begins to implement this or a similar framework, the desired culture naturally evolves, strengthens, and grows. It happens simultaneously, and it happens organically.

EBL is an approach to leadership that is modeled after the concept of evidence-based medicine. Evidence-based medicine aims to apply the best available evidence to clinical decision making. It examines external scientific research for evidence of the risks and benefits of a specific test or treatment, and assesses the findings to determine whether the test or treatment is likely to do more good than harm. Individual clinical expertise factors into decisions as well, as do the patient's values and expectations.

David M. Eddy, MD, PhD, widely considered the father of evidence-based medicine, was interviewed for the PBS feature *Healthcare Crisis: Who's at Risk?* He said (Eddy 2013):

> Evidence-based medicine is in fact a very simple, common sense concept. It says when we have a treatment where we know its effects and it has benefit, we should do it. We should give patients those treatments. When we have evidence that something is not beneficial or is harmful, we should not do it. And when we don't know what the effects of a treatment are, when we don't know whether giving a treatment to a patient will make them come out ahead or come out behind, we should be conservative.

A comparison of evidence-based medicine and EBL is presented in Exhibit 8.3.

Similarly, EBL is based on hardwiring the behaviors that evidence has shown to have the greatest impact on patient outcomes. Organizations that embrace EBL are seeking the same results as high-reliability organizations in, for instance, the airline and nuclear power industries. Consider how similar their definitions are:

- EBL organizations hardwire practices that are proven to result in the best possible outcomes.
- High-reliability organizations reduce variance to create greater predictability in outcomes.

Organizations that use the EBL framework are also building a high-reliability culture. Whether the aim is to regularly get people safely to their

EXHIBIT 8.3
Evidence-Based
Leadership
Echoes
Evidence-Based
Medicine

Evidence-Based Medicine

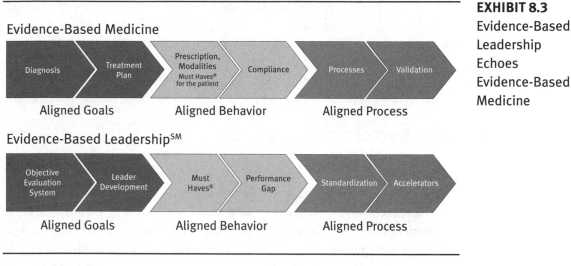

Source: Studer Group.

destinations hundreds of miles away or to bring them through life-saving medical procedures, the endgame is consistency in behaviors and processes. In both cases, accountability takes on great importance.

The EBL framework serves two purposes: It provides the structure for hardwiring behaviors, and it aligns the culture with the accountability mind-set.

To achieve and sustain the quality outcomes necessary to survive and thrive in the pay-for-performance environment, every individual in the organization needs to execute properly every time. Getting people to consistently perform the right behavior in the right way is key. The EBL framework drives consistency in any behavior—in experience of care as well as in processes of care, flow, and safety.

While new behaviors can be forced on others, at least for a short time, people cannot be forced to choose those behaviors of their own free will. Only they can decide to practice the desired behaviors when they are not being watched. Only they can hold others accountable for performing the desired behaviors because it is the right thing to do for the patient. As EBL is practiced—as the tools and tactics are taught, reinforced, and measured—the engagement and passion that fuel accountability begin to manifest.

For example, Team Member A may see Team Member B leave a patient's room without washing his hands. Team Member A will immediately smile and kindly say, "Don't forget to wash your hands! Hand washing is a big part of our patient-safety policy. It really does help us provide excellent patient care." When an accountable culture is in place, the recipient is open to this feedback. There is no blame or defensiveness—just friendly reminders and self-corrections.

When such engagement takes place, when people will not tolerate the nonperformance of desired behavior, we know that a cultural shift has taken place. We know that the necessary mind-set and the behavior are both hardwired. The culture makes it unacceptable for desired behavior not to happen—it is the glue of the quality-focused, high-reliability organization.

Of course, building this culture takes time—but if the EBL framework is followed with a very strong focus on the why, it happens organically. Every action needed is taken because it is the right thing to do for the patient.

EBL in Practice

As an organization seeks to improve quality, it may implement a new process without addressing leadership issues or explaining the why behind the changes it's asking people to make. Leaders may set a goal for reducing medication errors and ask people to practice a new tactic that is proven to accomplish that goal. However, if they have not thoughtfully explained why it matters that people execute the new behavior, trained them how to do it, or put in place a system for validating it, the changes will not happen—or they will not last for long.

Following the EBL framework changes that reality, for these reasons:

- It ensures that everyone is aligned with the goals that drive the organization's mission.
- It requires that the right leaders are paired with the right goals and are held accountable for meeting them.
- It ensures that everyone is well trained in the processes and behaviors they are being asked to implement.
- It ensures that the why is communicated over and over, at many levels and in many different forms—during team meetings, during rounding, at employee forums, and in newsletters and e-mails.
- It ensures that everyone knows how success is measured, that behavior is validated, and that gaps in performance are addressed.

As an example, suppose an organization's chief nursing officer (CNO) and chief quality officer (CQO) want to address performance gaps resulting in patient falls. The organization has implemented the eight behaviors of Hourly Rounding (see "What Is Hourly Rounding?" sidebar). In addition, it has a falls prevention program. The program includes posting fall-risk signage on patients' doors as well as using colored, nonslip booties and colored armbands to identify and protect patients identified as at risk for falls.

The CNO and the CQO round on the unit's staff and patients to see how consistently the staff practice the expected behaviors. What they discover is that none of the patients know the purpose of their colored armband. Staff members are not always placing armbands on the patients who should get them, and when they do, they are failing to use the proper keywords to explain why. In other words, this leader rounding has revealed two areas in the process that need to be fixed.

The CNO and CQO must now go back and close the loop. They address the staff and share that the behaviors are not being practiced consistently. They also reinforce the why behind the tactics. They may solidify their point by reminding staff members of the evidence that shows these tactics get results (evidence that was first discussed when the tactics were introduced).

This validation process usually needs to be repeated only a couple of times before the staff understand it. They do not need to be retrained so much as they need to be reminded and held accountable.

Organizations that validate whether new practices are being implemented usually find that the vast majority of people will practice the new behavior right away. A small percentage will need one coaching conversation to reach hardwired status. Of this small percentage, the majority will respond positively and begin practicing the desired behavior.

Once an organization has addressed performance gaps and reached the point where inconsistencies in behavior are not tolerated, behavior becomes truly standardized. The organization can then innovate to move outcomes faster. (This is the "Accelerators" part of EBL [see Exhibit 8.3]. For example, staff might start using tablets or mobile devices to make rounding more efficient.)

How EBL Hardwires Improved Quality Outcomes

Once the EBL framework has been established and the organization is focused on the mission and knows the why, any improvement can be achieved. Regardless of the initiative, the process is the same.

Suppose an organization wants to decrease infections. One behavior that helps achieve this goal is hand washing, as previously mentioned. The organization sets a very specific target metric and monitors it monthly. It holds the staff accountable for performance on this goal by including the hand-washing metric in their evaluations and giving it enough weight to make hand washing a priority.

The organization then trains leaders in the proper hand-washing technique as well as in how to cascade this technique to those they lead. A big part of this training involves conveying the why. People need to understand how hand washing affects patients and feel strongly enough to address those not practicing the behavior. If an organization is willing to take all of these steps and to validate that people are doing what it has asked them to do, its infection rates will decrease.

So how does one validate? As an example, if an organization wishes to reduce ventilator-associated pneumonia (VAP) infections, it would again include VAP rates in the evaluations of ancillary leaders, the CEO, the CNO, and possibly even the emergency department (ED) leaders, if they have ventilators in their department. The organization would start by talking with leaders about validating ventilator protocol. As leaders round on patients, they need to look for conditions and behaviors that reduce VAP infection: The head of the patient's bed should be up 30 degrees, the patient should be practicing good oral hygiene, and all staff members should be washing their hands.

Leaders can see easily enough whether those practices and behaviors are in place. Is the head of the bed elevated? Is oral-hygiene equipment by the bedside? For less obvious practices and behaviors, they can ask patients and family members if all staff wash their hands every time they come into the room.

Rounding on patients allows leaders to reinforce desirable behaviors and to close the loop with feedback when they discover that a staff member is not practicing them. It allows them to say, "Abby, the patient told me (or I noticed) that when you went into the room you didn't wash your hands. This is an important part of decreasing infections on the unit. I really need you to wash your hands in and out, because this is our policy."

The other type of rounding leaders do—rounding on staff—provides a built-in opportunity to connect with employees about how their efforts are going. It gives them a chance to ask, "What is going well with the VAP infection initiative? Is there anything I can do to help?" Rounding is also a good opportunity for leaders to pass along any words of recognition or praise for a person's good performance in infection-reducing practices.

Rounding on employees engages staff. Rounding on patients is designed to validate, verify, and give them a voice.

How Lean and Continuous Improvement Tools Fit In

Many hospitals use Lean, Six Sigma, and other tools or initiatives to improve their process-of-care measures. These strategies can be tremendously valuable quality accelerators—but only if people actually choose to implement the new behaviors that the strategies require.

This is where EBL comes in. It creates the culture that drives people to consistently and faithfully execute the new Lean or Six Sigma behavior.

For example, Six Sigma created a process aimed at reducing medication errors. It involves putting a mark on the floor by the medication-dispensing system that indicates a no-talk zone. The goal is to eliminate distractions for the person loading the machine while they do their delicate work.

Now, how does the hospital make sure that every single person who loads the machine does not talk while inside the zone? And how does it ensure that no one else tries to talk to that person? The only way is to make sure the culture will not allow it.

An accountability-centered culture means nurse leaders are held accountable for medication errors through the inclusion of a related metric in their evaluations. It means everyone is made to understand **why** talking is not allowed—because it could harm or even end the life of a patient. It means that during rounding leaders ask, "When you are loading the medication-dispensing machine, do you stand in the circle 100 percent of the time? When you're in the circle, do people talk to you?" It means that the leader rounds on other staff members and asks them if they have seen anyone talking to the person standing inside the circle. And it means that, if the answer is yes, they have conversations with the talkers to close the loop and correct the behaviors.

Culture is critical. And when the right kind of culture is in place, people will want to make any initiative succeed as long as they can see that it fits with their values.

Staying Focused

Of course, medication errors are just one small part of the picture. Organizations now have a number of process-of-care measures that require heightened focus in the environment of pay for performance. HACs and safety issues must also be considered, as well as HCAHPS results. How can an organization focus on all of these issues? And given that new measures and processes will be added and removed as changes in value-based purchasing are phased in, people may well feel they are jumping from one goal to another.

Leaders would do best to identify the two or three process-of-care measures and perception-of-care measures that they are struggling with the most. Those are the ones to focus on and improve. Although leaders must continue to monitor other measures, the main focus should remain on moving up those that are lagging.

For an organization struggling to bring up one of the process-of-care measures for pneumonia, it is required that blood cultures be obtained prior to the initiation of antibiotics for pneumonia patients in the ED. It sounds simple, yet if the nursing, pharmacy, and lab staff are not working together, the antibiotics may be started before the blood culture is drawn. This happens in EDs across the nation. Effective identification of patients with pneumonia, workflow processes that support multidepartment care collaboration, and accountability are key to ensuring that this process-of-care measure is carried out 100 percent of the time.

Any department that affects this process-of-care measure at all will have goals that are heavily focused on improving it. Departments that do not affect this metric (such as labor and delivery), and those that do affect it but are excelling in that area, will focus on their own lowest measures. (Of course, everyone should be aware of where the organization as a whole is not doing well and of the plan for improvement so that they can support the effort.)

In other words, all units pick the measures for which they are not hitting goals and focus on them. Renewed focus and emphasis are placed on the crucial behaviors proven to reach those goals and the why behind them. Of course, validation occurs, and those not practicing the behaviors are given feedback. Measures, focus, and validation all take place in a cyclical way until the outcomes improve.

The good news is that when a new behavior is hardwired, people will keep doing it automatically—even after the organization moves on to its next focus. The behavior has become second nature.

One of the great things about taking a cultural approach to quality is that people actually want to get better and better. In fact, they are passionate about it. An organization may have to coach heavily at first as it validates, but that part of the process is small and short lived. It is similar to the way a personal trainer works. In the beginning, clients need a lot of guidance, but eventually the trainer only has to check in for refreshers and course corrections. By using EBL principles to get people engaged and keep them engaged, an organization can set them up for success with minimal coaching long-term (except, perhaps, in a few very rare instances).

The knowledge that they are creating better conditions for the patient is what keeps people pushing forward. It is always there in front of them, motivating and inspiring them to do their best work. Leaders' most important job is to keep everyone's eyes focused on that sense of purpose. If leaders have trained employees to maintain this focus, excellent quality will be the natural outcome.

Study Questions

1. Describe the relationship between clinical quality and patient experience of care.
2. What role does accountability play in ensuring the consistent delivery of quality care? What are some of the hallmarks of a culture built on this concept? List a few tactics that create such a culture.
3. Considering the ever-increasing demand created by healthcare reform, how do organizations stay focused on one area long enough to see results? What prevents them from feeling that they are jumping from one goal to another?

References

Centers for Medicare & Medicaid Services (CMS). 2013. "Official Hospital Compare Data." Accessed August 5. https://data.medicare.gov/data/hospital-compare.

Eddy, D. M. 2013. *Healthcare Crisis: Who's at Risk?* PBS. Accessed November 19. www.pbs.org/healthcarecrisis/Exprts_intrvw/d_eddy.htm.

Meade, C. M., A. L. Bursell, and L. Ketelsen. 2006. "Effects of Nursing Rounds on Patients' Call Light Use, Satisfaction, and Safety." *American Journal of Nursing* 106 (9): 58–70.

Porter, B. G. 2012. "Building a Quality Framework: The Structure and Focus That Create a High-Performing Organization." Studer Group. Released August 1. December 4. www.studergroup.com/resources/news-media/articles/building-a-quality-framework-the-structure-and-foc.

MEASURING AND IMPROVING PATIENT EXPERIENCES OF CARE

Susan Edgman-Levitan

A ccording to Gerteis and colleagues (1993),

> Quality in health care has two dimensions. Technical excellence: the skill and
> competence of health professionals and the ability of diagnostic or therapeutic
> equipment, procedures, and systems to accomplish what they are meant to accom-
> plish, reliably and effectively. The other dimension relates to the subjective expe-
> rience, and in health care, it is quality in this subjective dimension that patients
> experience most directly—in their perception of illness or well-being and in their
> encounters with health care professionals and institutions, i.e., the experience of
> illness and healthcare *through the patient's eyes*. Health care professionals and
> managers are often uneasy about addressing this "soft" subject, given the hard,
> intractable, and unyielding problems of financing, access, and clinical effective-
> ness in health care. But the experiential dimension of quality is not trivial. It is
> the heart of what patients want from health care—enhancement of their sense of
> well-being, relief from their suffering. *Any* health care system, however it may be
> financed or structured, must address both aspects of quality to achieve legitimacy
> in the eyes of those it serves.

Patient satisfaction or patient experience-of-care surveys are the most
common method used to evaluate quality from the patient's perspective. Since
the 1980s, there has been a strong push to develop surveys that measure the
processes of care that matter most to patients and their families in place of
older instruments that tended to focus on processes of care or departments
that healthcare managers had some control over or that they decided on their
own were important (e.g., food services, housekeeping, admitting). These
departments and services all contribute to a positive experience, but they may
or may not be what matters most to patients and their families.

In 1987, the Picker Commonwealth Program for Patient-Centered
Care—which later became the Picker Institute—set out to explore patients'
needs and concerns, as patients themselves define them, to inform the

development of new surveys that could be linked to quality improvement efforts to enhance the patient's experience of care. Through extensive interviews and focus groups with diverse patients and their families, the research program defined eight dimensions of measurable patient-centered care:

1. Access to care
2. Respect for patients' values, preferences, and expressed needs
3. Coordination of care and integration of services
4. Information, communication, and education
5. Physical comfort
6. Emotional support and alleviation of fear and anxiety
7. Involvement of family and friends
8. Transition and continuity

The Picker Institute further explored and enhanced these dimensions of care, and the Institute of Medicine used them as the basis of its definition of patient centeredness in its 2001 publication *Crossing the Quality Chasm*.

An important design feature of these survey instruments is the use of a combination of *reports* and *ratings* to assess patients' experiences within important dimensions of care, their overall satisfaction with services, and the relative importance of each dimension in relation to satisfaction. In focus groups of healthcare managers, physicians, and nurses that were organized to facilitate the design of "actionable" responses, complaints about the difficulty of interpreting patients' *satisfaction ratings* came up repeatedly. Clinicians and managers expressed well-founded concern about the inherent bias in ratings of satisfaction and asked for more objective measures describing what did and did not happen from the patient's perspective. The end result has been the development of questions that enable patients to *report* their care experiences. For example, a report-style question asks, "Did your doctor explain your diagnosis to you in a way you could understand?" instead of "Rate your satisfaction with the quality of information you received from your doctor."

Regulatory and Federal Patient Survey Initiatives

Most healthcare organizations and settings in the United States routinely measure patient experiences of care in some fashion. Nationally, much of the standardization of survey instruments and processes has occurred as a result of the Consumer Assessment of Healthcare Providers and Systems (CAHPS) initiative, funded by the Agency for Healthcare Research and Quality. The CAHPS program is a multiyear, public–private initiative to develop standardized surveys of patients' experiences with ambulatory and facility-level care.

Healthcare organizations, public and private purchasers, consumers, and researchers use CAHPS results to

- assess the patient centeredness of care,
- compare and report on performance, and
- improve quality of care.

Additional information can be found at www.cahps.ahrq.gov.

By providing consumers with standardized data and presenting them in a way that is easy to understand and use, CAHPS can help people make decisions that support better healthcare and better health. This emphasis on the consumer's point of view differentiates CAHPS reports from other sources of information about clinical measures of quality. The CAHPS program is also working to integrate CAHPS results into the quality improvement programs of sponsors and healthcare providers. The Centers for Medicare & Medicaid Services (CMS) and the CAHPS team also published *The CAHPS Improvement Guide* (Edgman-Levitan et al. 2003) to help health plans and group practices improve their performance on the surveys. All CAHPS products are in the public domain, free, and available for use by anyone.[1]

CAHPS has been tested more completely than any previously used consumer survey (Hays et al. 1999). Surveys and consumer reports are now completed to measure and report customers' care experiences with commercial health plans, Medicare and Medicaid, and behavioral health services. Over a dozen CAHPS surveys have been developed or are in development for different healthcare settings. Common CAHPS surveys currently used include a hospital survey, a nursing home survey, a health plan survey, and a clinician and group survey. These instruments were developed as part of a national plan to publicly report results to consumers to foster quality improvement and help consumers improve their decision making about choice of plan, hospital, or provider.

The value of national efforts such as CAHPS lies in the development of standardized surveys and data collection protocols that enable rigorous comparisons among organizations and the creation of trustworthy, accurate benchmark data. Standardized surveys allow healthcare organizations to share strategies that are known to improve scores, and publicly reported quality measures enable consumers to make better plan and clinician choices. They also have proven to be a powerful stimulant to internal quality improvement efforts and frequently result in increased budgets for quality improvement work.

The National Committee for Quality Assurance requires that all health plans report CAHPS data as part of their Healthcare Effectiveness Data and Information Set (HEDIS) submission for accreditation. CMS uses CAHPS to collect data from all Medicare beneficiaries in both managed care plans and fee-for-service settings, and approximately half of state Medicaid programs collect CAHPS data from Medicaid recipients. The CAHPS Hospital Survey, also known as HCAHPS, is a standardized survey instrument and data collection methodology for measuring and publicly reporting patients' perspectives of hospital care. Although many hospitals collect information on patient satisfaction, until the HCAHPS initiative there had been no national standard for collecting or publicly reporting information that would allow valid comparisons to be made among hospitals.

The HCAHPS survey is composed of 27 questions: 18 substantive items that encompass critical aspects of the hospital experience (communication with doctors, communication with nurses, responsiveness of hospital staff, cleanliness and quietness of hospital environment, pain management, communication about medicines, discharge information, overall rating of hospital, and recommendation of hospital), 4 items that skip patients to appropriate questions, 3 items that adjust for the mix of patients across hospitals, and 2 items that support congressionally mandated reports. There are four approved modes of HCAHPS administration: (1) mail only, (2) telephone only, (3) mixed (mail followed by telephone), and (4) active interactive voice response. Hospitals began reporting HCAHPS data publicly in 2008 to allow consumers to make "apples to apples" comparisons on patients' perspectives of hospital care. Additional information can be found at www.hcahpsonline.org.

Collecting patient experience-of-care data also is becoming a standard evaluation measure in the education and certification of medical, nursing, and allied health students. The American College of Graduate Medical Education has incorporated extensive standards into its requirements for residency training that focus on the doctor–patient relationship, and the American Board of Internal Medicine is piloting patient experience-of-care surveys for incorporation into the recertification process for Board-certified physicians.

Using Patient Feedback for Quality Improvement

Although nationally standardized instruments and comparative databases are essential for public accountability and benchmarking, measurement for the purposes of monitoring quality improvement interventions does not necessarily require the same sort of standardized data collection and sampling. Many institutions prefer more frequent feedback of results (e.g., quarterly, monthly, weekly), with more precise, in-depth sampling (e.g., at the unit or clinic level) to target areas that need improvement. Staff usually are eager to obtain data frequently, but the cost of administration and the burden of response on patients must be weighed against the knowledge that substantial changes in scores usually take at least a quarter, if not longer, to appear in the data.

Survey Terminology

Familiarity with terms describing the psychometric properties of survey instruments and methods for data collection can help an organization choose a survey that will provide it with credible information for quality improvement. There are two different and complementary approaches to assessing the reliability and validity of a questionnaire: (1) cognitive testing, which bases assessments on feedback from interviews with people who are asked to react to the survey questions; and (2) psychometric testing, which bases assessments on the analysis of data collected by the questionnaire. Although many existing consumer questionnaires about healthcare have been tested primarily or exclusively using a psychometric approach, many survey researchers view the combination of cognitive and psychometric approaches as essential to producing the best possible survey instruments. Consequently, both methods have been included in the development of CAHPS and other instruments (Fowler 1995, 2001).

The cognitive testing method provides useful information on respondents' perceptions of the response task, how respondents recall and report events, and how they interpret specified reference periods. It also helps identify words that can be used to describe healthcare providers accurately and consistently across a range of consumers (e.g., commercially insured, Medicaid, fee for service, managed care; lower socioeconomic status, middle socioeconomic status; low literacy, high literacy) and helps determine whether key words and concepts included in the core questions work equally well in English and Spanish. For example, in the cognitive interviews to test CAHPS, researchers learned that parents did not think pediatricians were primary care providers. They evaluated the care they were receiving from pediatricians in the questions about specialists, not primary care doctors. Survey language was amended to ask about "your personal doctor," not "your primary care provider," as a result of this discovery (Fowler 1992).

Validity

In conventional use, the term *validity* refers to the extent to which an empirical measure accurately reflects the meaning of the concept under consideration (Babbie 1995). In other words, validity refers to the degree to which the measurement made by a survey corresponds to some true or real value. For example, a bathroom scale that always reads 185 pounds is reliable, but it is not valid if the person does not weigh 185 pounds.

The different types of validity are described here.

- *Face validity* is the agreement between empirical measurers and mental images associated with a particular concept. Does the measure look valid to the people who will be using it? A survey has face validity if it appears on the surface to measure what it has been designed to measure.
- *Construct validity* is based on the logical relationships among variables (or questions) and refers to the extent to which a scale measures the construct, or theoretical framework, it is designed to measure (e.g., satisfaction). Valid questions should have answers that correspond to what they are intended to measure. Researchers measure construct validity by testing the correlations between different items and other established constructs. Because there is no objective way of validating answers to the majority of survey questions, researchers can assess *answer validity* only through their correlations with other answers a person gives. We would expect high *convergent validity*, or strong correlation, between survey items such as waiting times and overall ratings of access. We would expect *discriminant validity*, or little correlation, between patient reports about coordination of care in the emergency department (ED) and the adequacy of pain control on an inpatient unit.
- *Content validity* refers to the degree to which a measure covers the range of meanings included within the concept. A survey with high content validity would represent topics related to satisfaction in appropriate proportions. For example, we would expect an inpatient survey to have a number of questions about nursing care, but we would not expect a majority of the questions to ask about telephone service in the patient's room.
- *Criterion validity* refers to whether a newly developed scale is strongly correlated with another measure that already has been demonstrated to be highly reliable and valid. Criterion validity can be viewed as how well a question measures up to a gold standard. For example, if you wanted to ask patients about the interns and residents who cared for them, you would want to be sure that patients could distinguish between staff and trainee physicians. You could measure the criterion validity of questions that ask about the identity of physicians by comparing patients' answers to hospital records.
- *Discriminant validity* is the degree of difference between survey results when the scales are applied in different settings. Survey scores should reflect differences among different institutions, where care is presumably different. Discriminant validity is the extent to which groups of respondents who are expected to differ on a certain measure do in fact differ in their answers (Fowler 1995).

Reliability

Reliability is a matter of whether a particular technique applied repeatedly to the same object yields the same results each time. The reliability of a survey instrument is initially addressed during the questionnaire development phase. Use of ambiguous questions, words with many different meanings, or words that are not universally understood will yield unreliable results. Use of simple, short words that are widely understood is a sound approach to question-naire design, even with well-educated sample populations (Fowler 1992). An instrument is reliable if consistency across respondents exists (i.e., the questions mean the same thing to every respondent). This consistency will ensure that differences in answers can be attributed to differences in respondents or their experiences.

Instrument reliability, or the reliability of a measure, refers to the stability and equivalence of repeated measures of the same concept. In other words, instrument reliability is the consistency of the answers people give to the same question when they are asked it at different points in time, assuming no real changes have occurred that should cause them to answer the questions differently. Reliable survey questions always produce the same answers from the same respondents when answered under similar circumstances. Thus, reliability is also the degree to which respondents answer survey questions consistently in similar situations. Inadequate wording of questions and poorly defined terms can compromise reliability. The goal is to ensure (through pilot testing) that questions mean the same thing to all respondents.

The *test–retest reliability coefficient* is a method to measure instrument reliability. This method measures the degree of correspondence between answers to the same questions asked of the same respondents at different points in time. If there is no reason to expect the information to change (and the methodology for obtaining the information is correct), the same responses should result at all points in time. If answers vary, the measurement is unstable and thus unreliable.

Internal consistency is the intercorrelation among a number of differ-ent questions intended to measure (or reflect) the same concept. The internal consistency of a measurement tool may be assessed using *Cronbach's alpha reliability coefficient*. Cronbach's alpha tests the internal consistency of a model or survey. Sometimes called a *scale reliability coefficient*, Cronbach's alpha assesses the reliability of a rating summarizing a group of test or survey answers that measure some underlying factor (e.g., some attribute of the test taker) (Cortina 1993; Cronbach 1951).

Readability of Survey Instruments

The readability of survey questions has a direct effect on the reliability of the instrument. Unreliable survey questions use words that are ambiguous and not universally understood. No simple measure of literacy exists. The

Microsoft Word program comes with a spelling and grammar checker that will produce a statistical analysis of a document. The spelling and grammar checker can calculate the Flesch-Kincaid index for any document, including questionnaires. The Flesch-Kincaid index (Flesch 1948) is a formula that uses sentence length (words per sentence) and complexity, along with the number of syllables per word, to derive a number corresponding to grade level. Documents containing shorter sentences with shorter words have lower Flesch-Kincaid scores.

Weighting Survey Results

Weighting of scores is frequently recommended if members of a (patient) population have unequal probabilities of being selected for the sample. If necessary, weights are assigned to the different observations to provide a representative picture of the total population. The weight assigned to a particular sample member should be the inverse of its probability of selection.

Weighting should be considered when an unequal distribution of patients exists by discharge service, nursing unit, or clinic. When computing an overall score for a hospital or a group of clinics with an unequal distribution of patients, weighting by probability of selection is appropriate. The probability of selection is estimated by dividing the number of patients sampled by the total number of patients. When the probability of selection of patients from different services or units is equal, patients from different services or units will be represented in the sample in the same proportion they occur in the population. If the probability of selection of patients from different hospitals or medical groups is different, the sample size for different hospitals or medical groups will vary according to the number of total discharges from each.

Similarity—presenting results stratified by service, unit, or clinic—provides an accurate and representative picture of the total population. For example, the most straightforward method for comparing units to an overall score is to compare medical units to all medical patients, surgical units to all surgical patients, and childbirth units to all childbirth patients.

The weighting issue also arises when comparing hospitals or clinics within a system. If the service case mix is similar, we can compare by hospital without accounting for case-mix difference. If service case mix is not similar across institutions, scores should be weighted before comparisons are made among hospitals. Alternatively, comparisons could be made at the service level.

Response Rates

The response rate for mailed surveys is calculated by dividing the number of useable returned questionnaires by the number of patients who were mailed questionnaires. Adjustments are made to the denominator to exclude ineligible cases—questionnaires that were not delivered and patients who should not have been sent a questionnaire, such as deceased patients.

The calculation is different for telephone surveys. The following cases are often removed before calculating rates: nonworking numbers, numbers that were never answered or were answered by a machine, patients who were too ill or confused to be interviewed, and patients the interviewer determined were ineligible for some other reason.

Low response rates compromise the internal validity of the sample. Survey results based on response rates of 30 percent or less may not be representative of patient satisfaction (at that institution). Although a representative sample is chosen, certain population groups are more likely to self-select out of the survey process. An expected (and typical) response bias is seen in all mailed surveys. For example, young people and Medicaid patients are less likely to respond to mailed surveys.

An optimal response rate is necessary to have a representative sample; therefore, boosting response rates should be a priority. Methods to improve response rates include

- making telephone reminder calls for certain types of surveys;
- using the Dillman (1978) method, a three-wave mailing protocol designed to boost response rates;
- ensuring that telephone numbers or addresses are drawn from as accurate a source as possible; and
- offering incentives appropriate for the survey population (e.g., drugstore coupons, free parking coupons).

Survey Bias

Bias refers to the extent to which survey results do not accurately represent a population. Conducting a perfectly unbiased survey is impossible. Considering potential sources of bias during the survey design phase can minimize its effect. The potential biases in survey results should be considered as well.

Sampling Bias

All patients who have been selected to provide feedback should have an equal opportunity to respond. Any situation that makes certain patients less likely to be included in a sample leads to bias. For example, patients whose addresses are outdated or whose phone numbers are obsolete or incomplete in the database are less likely to be reached. Up-to-date patient lists are essential. Survey vendors also can minimize sampling bias through probability sampling—that is, giving all patients who meet the study criteria an opportunity to be included in the sample.

Nonresponse Bias

In every survey, some people agree to be respondents but do not answer every question. Although nonresponse to individual questions is usually low, occasionally it can be high and can affect estimates. Three categories of patients selected to be in the sample do not actually provide data:

1. Patients whom the data collection procedures do not reach, thereby not giving them a chance to answer questions
2. Patients asked to provide data who refuse to do so (who do not respond to the survey)
3. Patients asked to provide data who are unable to perform the task required of them (e.g., people who are too ill to respond to a survey or whose reading and writing skills preclude them from filling out self-administered questionnaires)

Regardless of how representative the sampling frame is, bias usually is introduced by selected patients' choice not to respond to the survey. Demographic information on all patients in the sample pool can help estimate the size and type of nonresponse bias. The profile of respondents and nonrespondents should be considered in relation to demographic variables that are important (e.g., age, gender, payer, discharge service).

Administration Method Bias or Mode Effects

The way a survey is administered inevitably introduces bias. Comparison of data that have been collected using different modes of administration (e.g., mail and telephone) will reveal differences that are either real or the result of different modes of administration. An instrument that produces comparable data regardless of mode effect introduces no bias. For example, patients who are not literate or do not have a mailing address are excluded from mail surveys. People who do not have phones introduce bias in telephone surveys. In face-to-face interviews, interviewers can influence respondents by their body language and facial expressions. In surveys conducted at the clinic or hospital, respondents may be reluctant to answer questions candidly. A combination of methods, such as phone follow-up to mailed surveys or phone interviews for low-literacy patients, can reduce some of these biases.

A major concern about comparability is that telephone interviews often collect more favorable responses (or answers that reflect more positively on respondents) than do mail surveys. CAHPS testing showed that the majority of the differences could be linked to the way question skips were handled. The telephone interview used explicit screening questions, whereas the mail version asked respondents to check a box labeled "inapplicable" when the question did not apply. The explicit screening question identified many more people to whom questions did not apply than were reflected in the mail data.

Proxy-Response Bias

Studies comparing self-reports with proxy reports do not consistently support the hypothesis that self-reports are more accurate than proxy reports. However, conclusions drawn from studies in which responses were verified using hospital and physician records show that, on average, (1) self-reports tend to be more accurate than proxy reports and (2) health events are underreported in both populations. In terms of reporting problems with care, most studies comparing proxy responses to patients' responses show that proxies tend to report more problems with care than patients do (Vom Eigen et al. 1999). Therefore, the percentage of response by proxy needs to be taken into consideration in the interpretation of survey results.

Recall Bias

Typically, patients receive questionnaires from two weeks to four months after discharge from the hospital. This delay raises concern about the reliability of the patient's memory. Memory studies have shown that the greater the effect of the hospitalization and the nature of the condition are, the greater the patient's ability is to recall health events. Studies also suggest that most people find it difficult to remember precise details, such as minor symptoms or the number of times a specific event occurred. For ambulatory surveys, patients should be surveyed as soon after the visit or event as possible.

Case-Mix Adjustment

Case-mix adjustment accounts for the different types of patients in institutions. Adjustments should be considered when hospital survey results are being released to the public. The characteristics commonly associated with patient reports on quality of care are (1) patient age (i.e., older patients tend to report fewer problems with care) and (2) discharge service (e.g., childbirth patients evaluate their experience more favorably than do medical or surgical patients; medical patients report the most problems with care) (Hargraves et al. 2001).

Scope and Use of Patient Experiences in Healthcare

Customer Service and Patient Satisfaction

Healthcare organizations' ability to deliver high-quality, patient-centered care to their members and patients depends in part on their understanding of basic customer service principles and their ability to integrate these principles into clinical settings.

Healthcare organizations should pay attention to customer service for several reasons. First, better service translates into higher satisfaction for the patient and, subsequently, for the employer who pays most of the bills. Second, as in any other service industry, a satisfied (and loyal) member or patient creates value over the course of a lifetime. In the context of healthcare, this value may manifest itself in the form of repeat visits, trusting relationships, and positive word of mouth. A dissatisfied member or patient, on the other hand, generates potential new costs. Many health plans, for example, have found that the cost of replacing members lost to disenrollment can be high. Patients who are not involved in decision making the way they want to be; who cannot get an appointment with their clinician when they are sick; or who are not treated with respect and dignity by their hospital, plan, or clinician may not follow clinical advice, can develop worse outcomes, and frequently share their negative stories with friends and family members. Third, existing patients and members are an invaluable source of information healthcare organizations can use to learn how to improve what they do and reduce waste by eliminating services that are unnecessary or not valued (Heskett et al. 1994).

Exhibit 9.1 depicts the relationship between satisfaction and loyalty. Individuals who are the most satisfied have the highest correlation to loyalty to a product, service, or provider (the zone of affection). Accordingly, individuals who are the most dissatisfied have the highest correlation to abandonment of their current service, product, or provider (the zone of defection).

EXHIBIT 9.1
Relationship Between Patient/ Member Satisfaction and Retention

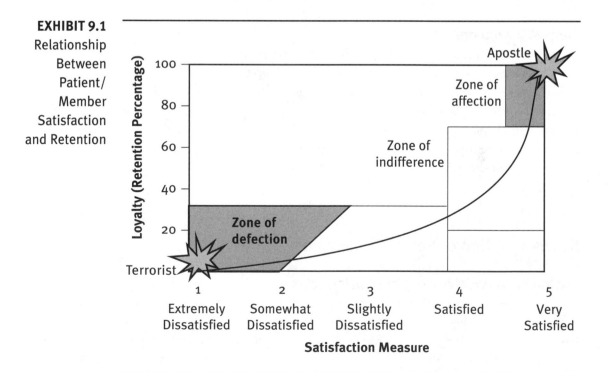

Source: Heskett et al. (1994, 167). Used with permission.

The zone of indifference reflects the greatest percentage of people who are neither highly satisfied (loyal) nor highly dissatisfied (disloyal).

Finally, poor customer service raises the risk of a negative "grapevine effect." More than 50 percent of people who have bad experiences will not complain openly to the plan or the medical group. However, research shows that nearly all (96 percent) are likely to tell at least ten other people about them. Several years of experience in collecting CAHPS data have revealed that even patient surveys do not adequately capture the full story about problems because, contrary to what many staff and clinicians think, the angriest patients are often the least likely to respond to patient surveys.

Word-of-mouth reputation is important because studies continue to find that the most trusted sources of information for people choosing a health plan, medical group, doctor, or hospital are close family, friends, and work colleagues. When a survey asked people whom they would go to for this kind of information, more than two-thirds of respondents said they would rely on the opinions of family members and friends (Kaiser Family Foundation and Agency for Healthcare Research and Quality 2000). General Electric concluded from one of its studies that "the impact of word-of-mouth on a customer's purchase decision was twice as important as corporate advertising" (Goodman, Malech, and Marra 1987).

Healthcare organizations also need to pay attention to customer service because service quality and employee satisfaction go hand in hand. When employee satisfaction is low, satisfied patients are almost impossible to find. Employees often are frustrated and angry about the same issues that bother patients and members: chaotic work environments, poor systems, and ineffective training. No amount of money, signing bonuses, or other tools currently used to recruit hard-to-find staff will offset the negative effect of these problems on employees. The real cost of high turnover may not be the replacement costs of finding new staff but the expenses associated with lost organizational knowledge, lower productivity, and decreased customer satisfaction.

Achieving Better Customer Service

The most successful service organizations pay attention to the factors that ensure their success: investing in people with an aptitude for service, technology that supports frontline staff, training practices that incorporate well-designed experiences for the patient or member, and compensation linked to performance. In particular, they recognize that their staff value achievement of good results, and they equip them to meet the needs of members and patients. For health plans, better customer service could mean developing information systems that allow staff to answer members' questions and settle claims quickly and easily; for provider organizations, better customer service could mean providing the resources and materials that clinicians need to provide high-quality care in a compassionate, safe environment.

Experts on delivering superior customer service suggest that healthcare organizations adopt the following set of principles (Leebov, Scott, and Olson 1998):

1. Hire service-savvy people. Aptitude is everything; people can be taught technical skills.
2. Establish high standards of customer service.
3. Help staff hear the voice of the customer.
4. Remove barriers so that staff can serve customers.
5. Design processes of care to reduce patient and family anxiety and thus increase satisfaction.
6. Help staff cope better in a stressful atmosphere.
7. Maintain a focus on service.

Many customer service programs have been developed for companies outside healthcare. Although the strategies are similar, Leebov, Scott, and Olson (1998) have adapted this work for healthcare settings in ways that increase its credibility and buy-in, especially from clinical staff. Their books and articles include practical, step-by-step instructions about how to identify and solve customer service problems in the healthcare delivery system (Leebov 1998).

"Listening Posts" Used to Incorporate Patient and Family Perspective into Quality Improvement Work

Patient satisfaction and patient experience-of-care surveys are the most common *quantitative* measures healthcare organizations use, but they can use other important *qualitative* methods, or *listening posts*, to obtain important information from patients and their families to guide improvement work. Although patient satisfaction surveys provide useful data, they are not the best source of information for innovative ideas about improving the delivery of care. Also, even healthcare organizations with high satisfaction scores have opportunities to improve services, which survey data may not reveal.

Quality improvement activities that focus on the needs and experiences of customers (i.e., members and patients) are effective only in environments that emphasize the concepts and responsibilities of customer service. One critical element of effective customer service is the capacity to elicit detailed, constructive feedback in a way that assures people that someone is listening to them. Members and patients are more likely to report a positive experience to customer service teams that have this skill.

However, this hands-on approach can be a major challenge for healthcare organizations that are not accustomed to communicating with their members or patients in this way. Many assume they understand how to fix the problem and do not probe beneath the surface of complaints and survey responses. Organizations should not be surprised by negative reports. Complaints about unhelpful office staff could stem from many sources:

- Employees did not provide clear directions to patients on how to get to the practice.
- Patients were not able to get an appointment when they needed one.
- Employees put patients on hold in the middle of medical emergencies.
- Employees were rude or disrespectful during a visit or on the phone.

The solutions to these problems vary. Without consulting with patients or members further to understand the true problem, healthcare organizations or quality improvement teams could waste a lot of money on the wrong fixes.

The term *listening posts* refers to a variety of ways to learn about the experiences of patients and staff and involve them in the improvement process. Listening posts already exist in some form in most health plans or clinical practices. The most difficult issue with listening posts is building a system to routinely synthesize the feedback received from them into a coherent picture of what they reveal about the delivery of care. Once this system is in place, root-cause analyses can be performed to identify particular problems, such as a staff member or medical group that contributes to problems, or problems that are systemic to the delivery of care, such as an antiquated manual appointment system. Listening post strategies include

- surveys,
- focus groups,
- walk-throughs,
- complaint/compliment letters, and
- patient and family advisory councils.

Surveys

Analyzing data from the CAHPS and other patient satisfaction or patient experience-of-care surveys can be beneficial, as can more frequent, small-scale use of individual questions to monitor a specific intervention.

Focus Groups

Staff or patients can be brought together in a moderator-led discussion group to collect more precise information about a specific problem and new ideas for improvement strategies. A focus group allows for more in-depth exploration of the causes of dissatisfaction and can provide excellent ideas for reengineering services. In addition, videotapes of focus groups can be effective at changing the attitudes and beliefs of staff members because the stories participants tell animate the emotional effect of excellent service as well as service failures (Bader and Rossi 2001; Krueger and Casey 2000).

Walk-Throughs

A walk-through may be the fastest way to identify system, flow, and attitude problems, many of which can be fixed almost overnight. Performing a walk-through is an effective way for staff to re-create the emotional and physical experiences of being a patient or family member. Walk-throughs provide a different perspective and uncover rules and procedures that may have outlived their usefulness. This method of observation was developed by David Gustafson, PhD, at the University of Wisconsin in Madison (Ford et al. 2007) and adapted here to incorporate the staff perspective.

During a walk-through, one staff member plays the role of the patient and another accompanies him or her as the family member. They go through a clinic, service, or procedure exactly as a patient and family do, and they follow the same rules. They do this openly, not as a mystery patient and family, and ask staff questions throughout the process to encourage reflection on the systems of care and identify improvement opportunities.

The staff members conducting the walk-through take notes to document what they see and how they feel during the process. They then share these notes with the leadership of the organization and quality improvement teams to help develop improvement plans. For many conducting walk-throughs, they will enter their clinics, procedure rooms, or labs for the first time as a patient and family member. Clinicians are routinely surprised at how clearly they can hear staff comments about patients from public areas and waiting rooms. Walk-throughs usually reveal problems with flow and signage as well as wasteful procedures and policies that can be fixed promptly.

An alternative to a walk-through is a similar technique called *patient shadowing*. A staff member asks permission to accompany a patient through the visit and take notes on the patient's experience. Because this approach does not take a slot away from a real patient, it can be useful in settings where visits are at a premium.

Complaint/Compliment Letters

Systematic review of letters can provide a better picture of where more background research is needed with staff and patient focus groups or a walk-through versus when a manager should be involved to address a personnel problem.

Patient and Family Advisory Councils

Some patients and health plan members are not concerned about being heard. Rather, their dissatisfaction with their healthcare experience reflects frustration with a system that does not involve them in decisions that will affect the design and delivery of care. From their perspective, the system is superficially responsive; it acknowledges that a problem with service or care exists but does not bother to investigate whether a proposed solution will really address the problem from the patient's or member's point of view.

A patient and family advisory council is one of the most effective strategies for involving families and patients in the design of care (Webster and Johnson 2000). An increased emphasis on patient and family engagement has resulted in the implementation of numerous successful patient and family advisory councils across the country (Haycock and Wahl 2013; Moore et al. 2003). First designed and advanced by the Institute for Family-Centered Care, these councils are composed of patients and families who represent the constituencies served by the plan or medical group. Families and patients both should be involved because they see different things, and each has an important perspective to consider.

The goal of the councils is to integrate patients and families into the healthcare organization's evaluation and redesign processes to improve the experience of care and customer service. In addition to meeting regularly with senior leadership, council members serve as listening posts for the staff and provide a structure and process for ongoing dialogue and creative problem solving between the organization and its patients and families. The councils can play many roles, but they do not function as boards, nor do they have fiduciary responsibility for the organization.

Council responsibilities may include input on or involvement in

- program development, implementation, and evaluation;
- planning for a major renovation or the design of a new building or service;
- staff selection and training;
- marketing plan or practice services;
- participation in staff orientation and in-service training programs; and
- design of new materials or tools that support the doctor–patient relationship.[2]

These councils help organizations overcome a common problem that they face when they begin to develop patient- and family-centered processes—they do not have direct experience of illness or the healthcare system. Consequently, healthcare professionals often approach the design process from their own perspective, not those of patients or families. Improvement committees with the best of intentions may disagree about who understands the needs of the family and patient best. Family members and patients rarely understand professional boundaries. Their suggestions are usually inexpensive, straightforward, and easy to implement because they are not bound by the usual rules and sensitivities.

Usually, employees recommend potential members of the family advisory council, and then those family members form the group. Depending on the size of the organization, most councils have between 12 and 30 patient or family members and 3 or 4 members from the staff of the organization. The council members are usually asked to commit to one two- to three-hour meeting per month, usually over dinner, and participation on one committee. Most councils start with one-year terms for all members to allow for departures in case a member is not well suited for the council.

People who can listen and respect different opinions should be sought. They should offer constructive input and be supportive of the institution's mission. Staff members frequently describe good council members as people who know how to provide constructive critiques. Council members also need to be comfortable speaking to groups and in front of professionals.

Keys to Successful Implementation

Avoid Failure by Establishing Clear Goals

Feedback from patients and their families will provide rich information for quality improvement work. For these efforts to be successful, you should consider the following questions:

- What is your aim for improvement?
- What types of information from patients, families, and staff will help you achieve your aim?
- How frequently do you need to measure your performance to achieve your aim?
- Who will review the data?
- What is your budget?

Once you know the answers to these questions, you can plan your data collection strategy.

What Is Your Aim for Improvement?

If you are trying to improve overall satisfaction with care, or your patients' willingness to recommend your organization to their family members and friends, or both, you must focus your measurement efforts on all dimensions of care that matter to patients and choose a survey that accurately measures these dimensions. If you are trying to improve a specific dimension of the patient's experience of care or the performance of a specific unit (e.g., ED, surgical unit, outpatient clinic), you must think carefully about what type of survey you need.

Be sure to determine the strongest drivers of overall satisfaction from the results of the survey you are using and focus on them. In general, many studies document the importance of access to care, doctor–patient communication, and respect for patient preferences; however, you may decide that preparing patients for discharge from the hospital is so important to clinical outcomes that it will take precedence over the other dimensions.

What Type of Information Will Help You Achieve Your Aim?

Match the type of feedback you are collecting to your aim. If you are trying to improve overall satisfaction with care, you may need a combination of survey data, focus group information, and information from compliment/complaint letters. If you are trying to improve a specific unit, you may need a combination of survey data, focus group information, walk-through results, and information from a targeted patient and family advisory council.

Choose a survey instrument that measures the processes of care that matter most to your patients. Make sure that it is a validated instrument and that the comparative data are truly comparable. Determine how many organizations like yours are in the database and whether the data can be broken down to give you customized benchmarks. For example, a community hospital near a ski resort measuring patient experiences of ED care is probably more interested in benchmarks from other EDs that see lots of orthopedic problems than benchmarks from large urban EDs with many trauma victims.

Pick a survey that has a mode of administration that suits your patient population, and make sure you have tested the questions for administration in that mode. For example, if you have a patient population with low literacy, you may want to choose a telephone survey or a survey that is administered through interactive voice response.

How Frequently Do You Need to Measure Your Performance?

Plan your data collection carefully. Avoid asking patients to answer too many surveys or appearing uncoordinated in your efforts to improve care. If you are trying to improve overall satisfaction with care, quarterly surveys are appropriate; you are unlikely to see changes in the data with more frequent data collection. On the other hand, you may determine that continuous sampling is more appropriate than a onetime snapshot in a quarter or that you need to survey or interview five patients every Monday, ten patients a week, or all of the patients seen in a specific clinic. If you are testing a specific intervention, try various small tests. Develop a sampling strategy by service, unit, or condition, depending on your aim.

Never underestimate the potential for response bias when surveying patients about their experiences. Many people are concerned that negative responses will jeopardize the quality of care they receive in the future. Make sure that the surveys are administered in a way that provides anonymity and confidentiality. Also, ensure that the measures are taken at a time when the person can evaluate his or her experiences clearly. For example, many vendors try to send surveys to recently discharged patients as quickly as possible. However, patients may not have recovered enough to know whether they have received all the information they need to manage their condition or to know when they may resume activities of daily living or return to work.

Who Will Review the Data?

Make sure you understand the needs and perspectives of the audience who will receive the data. Include open-ended comments, stories, and anecdotes wherever possible in reports; they are powerful motivators for behavior change, and most staff members enjoy reading them. In his studies, Richard Nisbett at the University of Michigan found that data alone were the least persuasive motivator of cultural or behavioral change; stories combined with data were moderately persuasive; and stories alone were the most persuasive (Nisbett and Borgida 1975). More recent literature has identified eight key elements for change, which include developing a vision for change and creating a culture of continuous commitment to change (Weber and Joshi 2000). Both data and patient stories are tools for leading and motivating change. Accordingly, consider how you can combine stories from your walk-throughs, focus groups, and patient and family advisory councils to enrich your staff's understanding of the experiences of care, both positive and negative. If you are trying to attract the attention of senior leaders or clinicians, the scientific rigor of the data collection is important, and comparative data are usually essential to clarify whether the myths about the organization's performance measure up to reality.

You also should consider how the reports are formatted and presented to different audiences. Web-based reports support widespread and rapid dissemination of data. Some audiences need sophisticated graphical presentations; others are most interested in open-ended comments.

What Is Your Budget?

Do everything you can to create a budget that supports the type of data collection necessary to achieve your goals. If you are reporting patient experience-of-care data to the public, you need to maximize the rigor of the data collection to ensure excellent response rates and sampling, and you may need to spend more money to accomplish that goal. If you are collecting the data primarily for quality improvement purposes, you need to consider vendors that can supply the data via the Internet using reporting formats that facilitate quality improvement, such as putting the results into control charts. All these features have different budget implications that need to be considered before putting together a request for proposals.

Be careful not to include any in-house data collection activities (postage, printing the surveys, mailing them) or analyses as "free." Sometimes organizations actually spend more money by choosing a lower-cost vendor that requires a lot of in-house support and in-kind contributions that are not factored into the overall cost of the data collection. Most healthcare organizations are not sophisticated about these issues, and their internal staff often take far longer to accomplish the same tasks a good survey vendor could complete much more economically. For example, vendors sometimes drop the cost of postage and mailing the surveys out of their overall budget for a project, expecting the healthcare organization to pick up these costs. These tactics can lower a project bid falsely and need to be screened carefully.

Lessons Learned, or "The Roads Not to Take"

Honest criticism is hard to take, particularly from a relative, a friend, an acquaintance, or a stranger.

—Franklin P. Jones

Resistance to lower-than-expected results is common and reasonable. It is not necessarily a sign of complacency or lack of commitment to high-quality, patient-centered care. Most healthcare clinicians and staff are working harder than they ever have, and the systems they are using to deliver care are not necessarily designed to give patients or staff a positive experience. The expectations of patients and families also have increased over the last decade in response to greater access to clinical information and excellent service experiences in other industries such as banking, financial services, retail stores, and Internet retailers.

Feedback from patients stating that their clinical care falls short of expectations is frustrating and demoralizing for healthcare clinicians and employees to receive. With this in mind, both positive and negative results from patient surveys or listening posts should be presented and, whenever possible, strategies and systematic supports that make it easier for staff to perform at the desired levels should be included. Executives, senior clinicians, and managers need to be prepared to respond effectively to the common arguments clinical and administrative staff use to deny the validity of patients' feedback. Most of this resistance comes in two forms: (1) *people resistance*, or arguments about patients' ability to accurately judge their interactions with healthcare clinicians and staff or the importance of such perceptions, and (2) *data resistance*, or arguments that attempt to undermine the scientific credibility of the data.

How to Address People Resistance

- "No one comes here for a good time." One certainly does not, and patients and family members will be the first to agree. Most people want to have as little contact with the healthcare system as possible, but when they need care, they want patient- and family-centered care designed to meet their needs, and they want it delivered in a compassionate, considerate manner.

- "But I was very nice." *Nice* is not the only aspect of quality care. Patients and their families have clearly articulated needs with respect to the care they receive. If the staff members they encounter are nice but do not meet their needs, these staff members have delivered care ineffectively. Usually, staff members emphasize this point when "being nice" was their only recourse to redress other important service failures (e.g., delays, absence of equipment the patient needed, missing lab work or X-rays). To solve this problem, staff must have the resources, systems, and training required to meet the needs of patients.

- "This patient/family is very difficult or dysfunctional." Asking staff members to describe patients or families they like and do not like can be helpful. They usually like patients and families who are grateful, patients from the same culture, or patients who speak the same language, but beyond those characteristics, the attributes of popular patients and families become pretty grim. The most popular patients never ring their call lights, never ask for help, never ask questions or challenge their nurses and doctors, never read medical books, and never use the Internet for help. Their families are not present, and they do not have friends. In fact, they are as close to dead as possible.

- Many people who work in healthcare forget how anxiety-provoking an encounter with the healthcare system is, from finding a parking spot to receiving bad news. For most patients and families, a visit to the doctor or hospital is more like visiting a foreign country or going to jail than a positive, healing experience. They do not speak the same language, and few helpful guidebooks exist to show patients the way.

- We also do everything we can to force people to comply with our rules and regulations, no matter how outdated or meaningless they are, and then we are surprised when they react in anger or dismay. Why should a heart patient have to use a wheelchair to enter the hospital, when he or she has been walking around the community for months, and then be required to walk out the door only a few days after surgery? Why are we surprised when families fight over chairs or sofas in an ICU waiting room when we provide only a fraction of the chairs or couches necessary for at least two family members per patient? Why do we characterize patients as difficult when they express anger at being forced to go to the ED for a simple acute problem after office hours?

- Pointing out the effect of these unspoken beliefs and rules is helpful, as is reminding everyone that the patients who are least likely to get better are the ones we like. Passive patients rarely do as well in the long run as active, assertive patients who want to learn as much as possible about how to improve their health or be more autonomous.

- "How can patients rate the skill of their doctors/nurses?" Patient and family surveys and the other listening posts described in this chapter are not designed to evaluate the technical skills of clinicians, and patients are the first to acknowledge that they do not know how to do so. Surveys ask patients to evaluate the processes of care and their communication with doctors and nurses (as well as the communication between doctors and nurses)—aspects of care that only they can evaluate. Chart documentation about patient education is worthless if the patient did not understand what was being taught.

How to Address Data Resistance

- "The sample size is too small—you can't learn anything from it." Interestingly, doctors and other clinical staff trained in statistical methods are often the first to say they will not believe survey data until every patient has been interviewed. Sampling methodology in the social sciences and for survey research is no different from the sampling used in the diagnostic and laboratory tests clinicians trust every day. No one draws all of someone's blood to check hematocrit; a teaspoon or two is plenty.

- "Only angry people respond to surveys." Actually, the opposite is often true. Patients sometimes are afraid that negative responses to surveys will affect the quality of care they receive—a sad indicator of the trust they have in their healthcare providers—and we never hear from patients who likely had problems, such as patients who were discharged to nursing homes, people who speak foreign languages, and patients who died. In fact, the data most people see represent the happiest patients. This inherent bias is another important reason to draw samples that are as representative as possible of the patient population.

- "You really can't determine where something went wrong." Well-designed survey tools that measure things patients care about can provide a good picture of where to start looking. Also, remember to use the other listening posts to determine the sources of the problems, as well as ways to fix them, from the perspective of staff and patients.

- "It's not statistically significant." Again, if you pay attention to the reliability and validity of your survey tools, the sampling strategy, and the quality of your vendor's comparative database, and do everything you can to increase response rates, you will have an excellent idea about the statistical significance of trends and comparative benchmarks.

- "These patients aren't mine; my patients are different." Most people think their patients are different and that all survey data come from someone else's service or patient panel. Stratified results and comparative data can quiet some of these protests. A synthesis of data sources also can be helpful. Staff are more likely to believe that the problems are real if survey data reveal problems in the same areas addressed by complaint letters.

Other Reasons for Failure

- "We survey only because we have to." Organizations that survey only because an outside entity requires them to do so will never be successful in their efforts to become truly patient centered. Surveying is a waste of time and money until leadership takes the importance of patient- and family-centered care seriously.
- "Our bonuses are based on the results. We have to look good whether we are or not." When the incentives are aligned to reward people for appearing to be excellent instead of for collecting honest feedback and working to improve it, improvement efforts will never be successful. As with efforts to improve patient safety, rewarding people for continuing the status quo or hiding problems will never work.
- "The report sits on the shelf." Reports must be user friendly and easily accessible. Fortunately, most survey results are now available on the Internet, facilitating dissemination across an organization and customization of results to meet the needs of different audiences. The chief of primary care probably does not care about the results of the orthopedic clinic; doctors want to see results about the dimensions of care important to them, not dimensions that evaluate other disciplines or things over which they have no control (e.g., the claims processing service in a health plan).
- "Patient experience-of-care data do not appear credible to clinicians and senior leaders." If data and stories collected from patients and their families meet rigorous scientific standards and focus on issues that have relevance to clinicians, clinicians and senior leaders are more likely to take them seriously. The more they perceive the information to have relevance to clinical outcomes (help to reduce pain and suffering and improve patients' ability to manage their ongoing health problems), the more the organization will value it. If feedback is only collected about "safe" issues (e.g., food and parking), staff will be less willing to use it for improvement. Involve all end users of the data in the process of

selecting survey instruments and vendors. Have them participate in other listening post activities. Videotape focus groups, and have clinical staff do walk-throughs or attend patient and family advisory council meetings.

- "Patient satisfaction is valued more than employee and clinical satisfaction." Again, patient satisfaction will never be high unless staff and clinicians also feel nurtured and supported by the organization. Patient and staff satisfaction go hand in hand, and acknowledgment of this relationship will reinforce and motivate improvement efforts in both areas.

Case Study

A walk-through is an excellent method to use at the start of a quality improvement project because it is a simple and inexpensive but powerful way to provide clinicians and other staff with insights about the experience of care. Walk-throughs always yield ideas for improvement, many of which can be implemented quickly. Walk-throughs also build support and enthusiasm for redesigning care through the eyes of the patient much more rapidly than do data or directives from managers to "be nice to patients."

As you do the walk-through, ask questions of staff you encounter. The following questions incorporate the staff's perspective about their own work improvement opportunities into the process:

- What made you mad today?
- What took too long?
- What caused complaints today?
- What was misunderstood today?
- What cost too much?
- What was wasted?
- What was too complicated?
- What was just plain silly?
- What job involved too many people?
- What job involved too many actions?

Keep careful notes, and you will have a long list of things you can fix the next day.

Several years ago, the medical director and head nurse of a public community hospital ED joined an Institute for Healthcare Improvement Service Excellence Collaborative to improve the care in their ED. At the start of the collaborative, they did a walk-through in which the doctor played a patient with asthma and the nurse played his family member. They encountered several surprises along the way, and their experience ultimately guided a redesign of the ED's physical environment and processes of care. They came to one realization right at the beginning of the walk-through: The "patient" and the "family member," both clinical leaders of the ED, had never entered the ED through the patient entrance.

When the patient called the hospital number (from his office) and told the operator he was having an acute asthma attack, the operator put him on hold without explanation for several minutes. Although the operator did transfer his call to the ED, his anxiety increased because he did not understand what was happening.

When he was finally connected to the ED, his family member took the phone to get directions to the entrance from an address in the neighborhood. The ED staff member was incapable of helping her and finally found someone else to give her directions. After this delay, as they followed the directions, they discovered they were incorrect. Also, as they drove up to the hospital, they realized that all of the signage to the ED entrance was covered with shrubs and plants. They had no idea where to park or what to do.

The ED entrance and waiting area were filthy and chaotic. The signage was menacing and told them what not to do rather than where they could find help. They felt like they had arrived at the county jail.

As the patient was gasping for air, they were told to wait and not to ask for how long. At this point in the walk-through, the doctor described his anxiety as so intense he thought he actually might need care.

The family member went to the restroom, but it was so dirty she had to leave; she realized that this simple but important condition made her lose all confidence in the clinical care at the ED. If staff could not keep the bathroom clean, how could it do a good job with more complicated clinical problems?

The most painful part of the walk-through occurred when the nurse told the patient to take his clothes off. He realized there was no hook, hanger, or place for them; he had to put them on the floor. For years he had judged his patients negatively because of the way they threw their clothes on the floor, only to discover that this behavior was, in essence, his fault.

The story could continue indefinitely. Many of the problems the medical director and head nurse experienced were relatively easy to fix quickly: standardized, written directions to the emergency department in different languages for staff to read; different signage in the waiting areas and outside the hospital; and better housekeeping and other comfort issues such as clothes hooks in the exam areas. Other problems took longer to redress, but one simple walk-through helped refocus the hospital's improvement aims and its perspective on the importance of the patient's experience of care.

Conclusion

Apart from the obvious humane desire to be compassionate toward people who are sick, improving the patient experience of care results in better clinical outcomes, reduced medical errors, and increased market share. The leadership, focus, and human resource strategies required to build a patient-centered culture also result in improved employee satisfaction because we cannot begin to meet the needs of our patients until we provide excellent training and support for our clinical staff and all employees. Improving the patient's experience of care could be the key to transforming our current healthcare systems into the healthcare systems we all seek.

Study Questions

1. What is the difference between patient reports about experiences with care and patient ratings of satisfaction?
2. What criteria should you use when selecting a patient survey?
3. List four methods other than surveys to acquire feedback from patients and families to help improve care.
4. What are four arguments for the importance of collecting feedback from patients and families about their experiences with care?

Notes

1. The CAHPS Survey and Reporting Kit 2002 contains everything necessary to conduct a CAHPS survey, including the CAHPS 3.0 questionnaires in English and Spanish. To learn more about CAHPS, access a bibliography of publications about the CAHPS products, or download or order a free copy of the kit, go to www.cahps.ahrq.gov.
2. The Peace Health Shared Care Plan is an example of such material and is available at www.peoplepowered.org.

References

Babbie, E. R. 1995. *Survey Research Methods*, second edition. Belmont, CA: Wadsworth.

Bader, G. E., and C. A. Rossi. 2001. *Focus Groups: A Step-by-Step Guide*, third edition. San Diego: Bader Group.

Cortina, J. M. 1993. "What Is Co-Efficient Alpha? An Examination of Theory and Applications." *Journal of Applied Psychology* 78 (1): 98–104.

Cronbach, L. J. 1951. "Coefficient Alpha and the Internal Structure of Tests." *Psychometrika* 16 (3): 297–334.

Dillman, D. A. 1978. *Mail and Telephone Surveys: The Total Design Method.* New York: John Wiley & Sons.

Edgman-Levitan, S., D. Shaller, K. McInnes, R. Joyce, K. Coltin, and P. D. Cleary. 2003. *The CAHPS Improvement Guide: Practical Strategies for Improving the Patient Care Experience.* Baltimore, MD: Centers for Medicare & Medicaid Services.

Flesch, R. F. 1948. "A New Readability Yardstick." *Journal of Applied Psychology* 32 (3): 221–33.

Ford, J. H., C. Green, K. Hoffman, J. Wisdom, K. Riley, L. Bergmann, and T. Molfenter. 2007. "Process Improvement Needs in Substance Abuse Treatment: Admissions Walk-Through Results." *Journal of Substance Abuse Treatment* 33 (4): 379–89.

Fowler, F. J., Jr. 2001. *Survey Research Methods.* Thousand Oaks, CA: Sage.

———. 1995. *Improving Survey Questions: Design and Evaluation.* Thousand Oaks, CA: Sage.

———. 1992. "How Unclear Terms Affect Survey Data." *Public Opinion Quarterly* 56 (2): 218–31.

Gerteis, M., S. Edgman-Levitan, J. Daley, and T. Delbanco. 1993. *Through the Patient's Eyes: Understanding and Promoting Patient-Centered Care.* San Francisco: Jossey-Bass.

Goodman, J., A. Malech, and T. Marra. 1987. "Setting Priorities for Satisfaction Improvement." *Quality Review* (Winter).

Hargraves, J. L., I. B. Wilson, A. Zaslavsky, C. James, J. D. Walker, G. Rogers, and P. D. Cleary. 2001. "Adjusting for Patient Characteristics When Analyzing Reports from Patients About Hospital Care." *Medical Care* 39 (6): 635–41.

Haycock, C., and C. Wahl. 2013. "Achieving Patient and Family Engagement Through the Implementation and Evolution of Advisory Councils Across a Large Health Care System." *Nursing Administration Quarterly* 37 (3): 242–46.

Hays, R. D., J. A. Shaul, V. S. Williams, J. S. Lubalin, L. D. Harris-Kojetin, S. F. Sweeny, and P. D. Cleary. 1999. "Psychometric Properties of the CAHPS 1.0 Survey Measures. Consumer Assessment of Health Plans Study." *Medical Care* 37 (3, Suppl.): MS22–MS31.

Heskett, J. L., T. O. Jones, G. Loveman, E. Sasser, Jr., and J. A. Schlesinger. 1994. "Putting the Service-Profit Chain to Work." *Harvard Business Review* 72 (2): 164–74.

Institute of Medicine. 2001. *Crossing the Quality Chasm: A New Health System for the 21st Century.* Washington, DC: National Academies Press.

Kaiser Family Foundation and Agency for Healthcare Research and Quality. 2000. *Americans as Health Care Consumers: An Update on the Role of Quality Information, 2000.* Rockville, MD: Agency for Healthcare Research and Quality.

Krueger, R. A., and M. A. Casey. 2000. *Focus Groups: A Practical Guide for Applied Research.* Thousand Oaks, CA: Sage.

Leebov, W. 1998. *Service Savvy Health Care: One Goal at a Time.* San Francisco: Jossey-Bass/AHA Press.

Leebov, W., G. Scott, and L. Olson. 1998. *Achieving Impressive Customer Service: 7 Strategies for the Health Care Manager.* San Francisco: Jossey-Bass.

Moore, K. A., K. Coker, A. B. DuBuisson, B. Swett, and W. H. Edwards. 2003. "Implementing Potentially Better Practices for Improving Family-Centered Care in Neonatal Intensive Care Units: Successes and Challenges." *Pediatrics* 111 (4 Part 2): e450–e460.

Nisbett, R., and E. Borgida. 1975. "Attribution and the Psychology of Prediction." *Journal of Personality and Social Psychology* 32 (5): 932–43.

Vom Eigen, K. A., J. D. Walker, S. Edgman-Levitan, P. D. Cleary, and T. L. Delbanco. 1999. "Carepartner Experiences with Hospital Care." *Medical Care* 37 (1): 33–38.

Weber, V., and M. S. Joshi. 2000. "Effecting and Leading Change in Health Care Organizations." *Joint Commission Journal on Quality Improvement* 26 (7): 388–99.

Webster, P. D., and B. Johnson. 2000. *Developing and Sustaining a Patient and Family Advisory Council.* Bethesda, MD: Institute for Family-Centered Care.

Suggested Reading

Barry, M. J., and S. Edgman-Levitan. 2012. "Shared Decision Making—the Pinnacle of Patient-Centered Care." *New England Journal of Medicine* 366 (9): 780–81.

Charles, C., M. Gauld, L. Chambers, B. O'Brien, R. B. Haynes, and R. Labelle. 1994. "How Was Your Hospital Stay? Patients' Reports About Their Care in Canadian Hospitals." *Canadian Medical Association Journal* 150 (11): 1813–22.

Cleary, P. D. 2003. "A Hospitalization from Hell: A Patient's Perspective on Quality." *Annals of Internal Medicine* 138 (1): 33–39.

Cleary, P. D., and S. Edgman-Levitan. 1997. "Health Care Quality. Incorporating Consumer Perspectives." *Journal of the American Medical Association* 278 (19): 1608–12.

Cleary, P. D., S. Edgman-Levitan, J. D. Walker, M. Gerteis, and T. L. Delbanco. 1993. "Using Patient Reports to Improve Medical Care: A Preliminary

Report from 10 Hospitals." *Quality Management in Health Care* 2 (1): 31–38.

Coulter, A., and P. D. Cleary. 2001. "Patients' Experiences with Hospital Care in Five Countries." *Health Affairs (Millwood)* 20 (3): 244–52.

Delbanco, T. L., D. M. Stokes, P. D. Cleary, S. Edgman-Levitan, J. D. Walker, M. Gerteis, and J. Daley. 1995. "Medical Patients' Assessments of Their Care During Hospitalization: Insights for Internists." *Journal of General Internal Medicine* 10 (12): 679–85.

Edgman-Levitan, S. 1996. "What Information Do Consumers Want and Need?" *Health Affairs (Millwood)* 15 (4): 42–56.

Elliott, M. N., W. G. Lehrman, E. H. Goldstein, L. A. Giordano, M. K. Beckett, C. W. Cohea, and P. D. Cleary. 2010. "Hospital Survey Shows Improvements in Patient Experience." *Health Affairs* 29 (11): 2061–67.

Frampton, S., L. Gilpin, and P. Charmel. 2003. *Putting Patients First: Designing and Practicing Patient-Centered Care.* San Francisco: Jossey-Bass.

Fremont, A. M., P. D. Cleary, J. L. Hargraves, R. M. Rowe, N. B. Jacobson, and J. Z. Ayanian. 2001. "Patient-Centered Processes of Care and Long-Term Outcomes of Myocardial Infarction." *Journal of General Internal Medicine* 16 (12): 800–8.

Fremont, A. M., P. D. Cleary, J. L. Hargraves, R. M. Rowe, N. B. Jacobson, J. Z. Ayanian, J. H. Gilmore, and B. J. Pine II. 1997. "The Four Faces of Mass Customization." *Harvard Business Review* 75 (1): 91–101.

Goodman, J. 1999. "Basic Facts on Customer Complaint Behavior and the Impact of Service on the Bottom Line." *Competitive Advantage: ASQ Newsletter* 8 (June): 1.

Health Research & Educational Trust. 2013. *Leadership Resource for Patient and Family Engagement Strategies.* Published July. Chicago: Health Research & Educational Trust. www.hpoe.org/Reports-HPOE/Patient_Family_Engagement_2013.pdf.

Homer, C. J., B. Marino, P. D. Cleary, H. R. Alpert, B. Smith, C. M. Crowley-Ganser, R. M. Brustowicz, and D. A. Goldmann. 1999. "Quality of Care at a Children's Hospital: The Parent's Perspective." *Archives of Pediatric and Adolescent Medicine* 153 (11): 1123–29.

Johnson, B., M. Abraham, J. Conway, L. Simmons, S. Edgman-Levitan, P. Sodomka, J. Schlucter, and D. Ford. 2008. "Partnering with Patients and Families to Design a Patient- and Family-Centered Health Care System: Recommendations and Promising Practices." Institute for Patient- and Family-Centered Care. Published April. www.ipfcc.org/pdf/PartneringwithPatientsandFamilies.pdf.

Kenagy, J. W., D. M. Berwick, and M. R. Shore. 1999. "Service Quality in Health Care." *Journal of the American Medical Association* 281 (7): 661–65.

Larson, C. O., E. C. Nelson, D. Gustafson, and P. B. Batalden. 1996. "The Relationship Between Meeting Patients' Information Needs and Their Satisfaction with Hospital Care and General Health Status Outcomes." *International Journal of Quality in Health Care* 8 (5): 447–56.

Leebov, W., and G. Scott. 1993. *Service Quality Improvement: The Customer Satisfaction Strategy for Health Care*. San Francisco: Jossey-Bass/AHA Press.

Nash, D. B. 2010. "Increasing Patient and Family Engagement in Health Care." *Pharmacy and Therapeutics* 35 (4): 185.

Roth, M. S., and W. P. Amoroso. 1993. "Linking Core Competencies to Customer Needs: Strategic Marketing of Health Care Services." *Journal of Health Care Marketing* 13 (2): 49–54.

Seelos, L., and C. Adamson. 1994. "Redefining NHS Complaint Handling—The Real Challenge." *International Journal of Health Care Quality Assurance* 7 (6): 26–31.

Seybold, P. B. 2001. "Get Inside the Lives of Your Customers." *Harvard Business Review* 79 (5): 80–89, 164.

Veroff, D. R., P. M. Gallagher, V. Wilson, M. Uyeda, J. Merselis, E. Guadagnoli, S. Edgman-Levitan, A. Zaslavsky, S. Kleimann, and P. D. Cleary. 1998. "Effective Reports for Health Care Quality Data: Lessons from a CAHPS Demonstration in Washington State." *International Journal of Quality in Health Care* 10 (6): 555–60.

Wasson, J. H., M. M. Godfrey, E. C. Nelson, J. J. Mohr, and P. B. Batalden. 2003. "Microsystems in Health Care: Part 4. Planning Patient-Centered Care." *Joint Commission Journal of Quality and Safety* 29 (5): 227–37.

DASHBOARDS AND SCORECARDS: TOOLS FOR CREATING ALIGNMENT

Michael D. Pugh

Measurement is a critical leadership function. Most healthcare organizations use measurement tools to track their performance in dimensions beyond mere financial results. Those dimensions commonly include clinical quality, patient satisfaction, patient safety, employee satisfaction, and organizational culture. As a means of organizing and using measurement to drive change, dashboards and scorecards are useful tools. When used properly, they can contribute to better alignment of effort, accelerated rates of improvement, and focused execution of organizational strategies.

Background and Terminology

Robert S. Kaplan and David P. Norton first used the term *balanced scorecard* in their January–February 1992 *Harvard Business Review* article, "The Balanced Scorecard—Measures That Drive Performance." Based on a multicompany study, the article examined approaches to organizational performance management beyond the use of standard financial and accounting measures. Kaplan and Norton's theory was that reliance on traditional financial measures alone to drive performance limits a company's ability to increase shareholder value. This investigational premise is consistent with quality guru Dr. W. Edwards Deming's idea that companies cannot be run by visible numbers alone (Aguayo 1991). To overcome this limitation, successful organizations use a broader index of performance metrics to create a balance between financial and other important dimensions of performance.

Kaplan and Norton's 1996 follow-up book, *The Balanced Scorecard—Translating Strategy into Action*, further examined the development of performance measures linked to organizational strategy. Kaplan and Norton observed that, to achieve results, the balanced scorecard should be central to the leadership system rather than merely a balanced set of outcome measures for the organization. Kaplan and Norton (1996) observed that most organizations collect performance measures of important nonfinancial dimensions, such as customers, service, and product quality. However, those measures are usually reviewed separately from financial results and with less emphasis on leadership. Kaplan and Norton also observe that leaders can increase organizational alignment by simultaneously reviewing and monitoring critical measures across multiple dimensions of performance, not just financial dimensions. According to Kaplan and Norton, the balanced scorecard is more than a way to monitor a broader set of outcome or process measures—it is central to deploying organizational strategy.

Dashboards

Although the terms *dashboard* and *scorecard*[1] are used interchangeably in practice, they actually refer to two different things. The term *dashboard* brings to mind the instrument panel on an automobile, which, when the car is moving, enables the driver to monitor key performance metrics such as speed, fuel level, and direction. The driver also could monitor many other metrics, such as tire pressure, RPM, engine temperature, oil pressure, and transmission efficiency. Those measures may be useful to a NASCAR driver in a high-performance race car, but they are generally not critical to the average driver's journey from point A to point B. Instead, everyday drivers rely on a core set of high-level measures to track the real-time process of driving the car.

The pilot of an airplane depends on a much more complex collection of instruments to track critical operating information. The driver of a car and the pilot of an airplane monitor multiple performance indicators simultaneously to arrive at their intended destination successfully. At any given point in the journey, the driver or the pilot may focus on one indicator, but their overall success depends on the collective performance of the systems represented by the indicators. Similarly, in the business world, dashboards are tools that report on the ongoing performance of the critical processes that lead to organizational success rather than on the success itself.

Scorecards

The term *scorecard* brings to mind a different image. Scorecards are used to record and report on prior periods or past performance rather than on real-time performance. Generally, scorecards reflect outcome measures rather than process measures. School report cards, for example, which use a specific grading standard to report how an individual student performed, are issued after all work is completed. Although there is a lag time between the performance and the reporting, the information in the report card can still be used to make changes that will influence future outcomes, such as improvements in study habits, class attendance, allocation of study time to specific subject matter, outside tutoring, and homework preparation. However, the possible changes result from investigation of the current process rather than review of information about past performance presented in the report card.

Golf scorecards are another example. They reflect the outcome of the previous holes played, compare the score for each hole to a target score (par), and compare performance against other players or an overall stroke target for the game. In a competitive match, a player can use this report of past performance to evaluate how aggressively to play on future holes. Also, a player can monitor the cumulative score during play to judge the likelihood of achieving a desired overall score for the round. However, because the scorecard focuses on past results, it generally does not tell a player much about the changes she needs to make to improve success on future holes. For many of us, golf might be more fun if we did not keep score. If we never keep score, though, we will never know how our play compares to the target (par) or other players' performance, or how our play varies from round to round.

The differences between scorecards as measures of outcomes or results and dashboards as measures of process may be logical, but in practical application in healthcare they are rarely distinct. Healthcare organizations are complex, and a metric often may be a process measure and the proxy for an outcome measure at the same time. As a result, many organizational scorecards contain a mix of outcome-, strategic-, and process-related measures. The key issue is how leadership uses individual measures and measurement sets to align priorities and achieve desired organizational results.

Scope and Use of Dashboards and Scorecards in Healthcare

Performance Scorecard: Central to Strategic Leadership System

A typical hospital routinely collects hundreds of quality and performance measures for external reporting to regulatory agencies and for internal quality monitoring. Most commonly, healthcare organizations use some form of quality scorecard or dashboard at the senior leadership level to support the governance function. These scorecards are often voluminous, populated with as many as a hundred narrow outcome- or process-based measures. They tend to be reports of past achievement or quality-control measures rather than drivers of future efforts, and they are not used routinely in the strategic manner contemplated by Kaplan and Norton. For example, a quality-control measure such as the hospital infection rate or the hospital inpatient mortality rate is commonly included on a leadership report, even absent an active improvement effort or link to organizational strategy. Healthcare organizations have monitored infection rates and mortality rates for years, but they tend to take action only when an infectious outbreak occurs or when an incident report or the medical staff peer-review process reveals known instances of avoidable patient death.

Simply tracking an indicator is not enough. Organizations often show a wide gap between the existence of a measurement set that they consider to be a scorecard or dashboard and their actual use of the tool to create alignment or drive improvement and change.

Exhibit 10.1 is one depiction of the leadership system in a healthcare organization. The leadership system drives both organizational culture and alignment in daily work to achieve a desired level of organizational performance. One of the key elements of the leadership system is the measurement process, which includes the tools of dashboards and scorecards.

The challenge for healthcare leaders is to make sense of the multitude of measures and metrics that are routinely available in most organizations. Scorecards and dashboards are useful tools for organizing important metrics. However, healthcare leaders struggle with the question: What should we measure? That answer is tied to the answer to another question: For what purpose? Form should follow function.

Scorecards and dashboards should drive leadership behavior and be used to create alignment in organizations. Financial and volume measures traditionally have driven management behavior in healthcare. Governing boards traditionally have spent considerably more time reviewing and discussing financial reports than quality or patient satisfaction reports. Even though financial review still tends to dominate, a shift has occurred over the last ten years. Increasing numbers of hospital boards and senior leadership teams are recognizing that performance in healthcare involves much more

EXHIBIT 10.1
Leadership
System in One
Healthcare
Organization

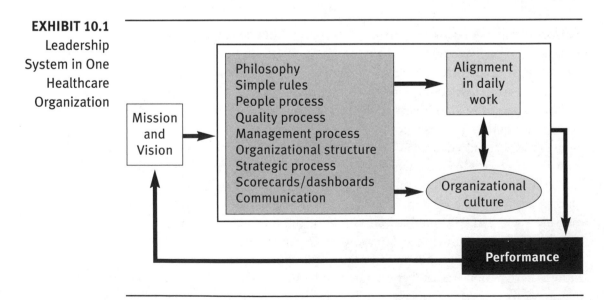

Source: Pugh Ettinger McCarthy Associates, LLC. Used with permission.

than the financial bottom line and are now devoting more time to reviewing quality, workplace culture, and patient satisfaction data. Despite the increased emphasis on patient safety and harm prevention, patient safety indicators are still underrepresented on most organizational performance scorecards.

Commonly Used Quality-Measurement Sets

Hospitals routinely collect and review patient satisfaction and financial indicators and monitor a large, diverse set of quality indicators. As a condition of accreditation, The Joint Commission requires organizations to collect and monitor specific sets of quality indicators and report them to the commission. Currently, the Centers for Medicare & Medicaid Services (CMS) requires both hospitals and long-term care facilities to collect a broad set of quality and clinical indicators that are then made publicly available through the CMS website Hospital Compare (www.medicare.gov/hospitalcompare). Multiple states—as well as state hospital associations, hospital trade groups, commercial sites such as HealthGrades.com, and business coalitions such as the Leapfrog Group—also publish sets of quality measures. Transparency about quality and performance is intended to spur healthcare organizations to pay attention to important quality indicators and provide consumers the information they need to make better healthcare-purchasing decisions. However, many in healthcare view public reporting of performance data as a questionable regulatory process rather than a meaningful reflection of an organization's performance. There is a significant difference between compliance with regulatory reporting and focusing an organization on a set of key performance indicators that leadership uses to guide improvement efforts.

On March 23, 2010, President Barack Obama signed the Affordable Care Act, which contains sweeping provisions for increased public reporting of quality measures by hospitals. The law also includes reforms that tie payment levels and methodologies to physician and hospital performance and the clinical results for specified populations of patients.

The National Committee for Quality Assurance (NCQA) sponsors the Healthcare Effectiveness Data and Information Set (HEDIS), which is used by more than 90 percent of US health plans and managed care organizations to measure performance in important dimensions of care and service. To demonstrate effectiveness of care for their members, health plans collect (along with many other measures) the percentage of eligible members who received screening for breast cancer and colorectal cancer, and they also measure whether members received appropriate treatment for diabetes, cholesterol management in heart disease, and upper respiratory infections in children. HEDIS measures extend to individual physician practices and organized medical groups, which also are measured on patient satisfaction as well as the HEDIS clinical data set. Medical groups and outpatient care systems may also collect and track workflow and process indicators, such as the average waiting time until the next open appointment, number of clinic visits per day, average waiting time before the patient is seen by the clinician, or other clinic flow measures.

Organizing Measures by Categories

Creating useful information out of the myriad measures and data routinely collected for internal improvement efforts and external reporting to CMS or others is a challenge for healthcare organizations. The availability of electronic health records and health information exchanges is making it easier for organizations to track and collect some quality and performance measures, but taking full advantage of technology to track and report quality measures is still a mirage in the distance. Healthcare organizations traditionally sort the measures they collect into five categories: financial, volume, satisfaction, patient safety, and clinical quality. Some healthcare organizations have developed summary dashboards of key indicators, organized by category, to sharpen focus and facilitate reporting and day-to-day management of various functions. Quality scorecards and safety dashboards have become popular ways of reporting on clinical quality to medical staff committees and to the board.

Dashboards and scorecards may be organized in formats ranging from simple tables to web-based graphical reports embedded in computerized decision-support systems. Data report formats include tables, radar charts, bar graphs, run or control charts, and color-coded indicators designed to highlight metrics that do not meet targets or expectations.[2] In some organizations, each operating unit has a scorecard of key indicators that mirrors the organizational scorecard.

Formatting available measures into a summary dashboard (departmental, category-specific, or cross-dimensional) is a start. However, senior leaders can harness the real power of measures by organizing their leadership systems to achieve results.

Applications of Scorecards and Dashboards

Governance and Leadership Measures

Healthcare organizations should consider the use of three basic sets of measures when designing a scorecard or dashboard. Exhibit 10.2 summarizes the three basic types of performance metrics and the relationships between them. At the governance level, a set of organizational performance measures should be defined and monitored. The organization should link those measures to how it defines performance within the context of its mission, vision, and values. A governance-level scorecard of performance measures should be a basic tool for all healthcare governing boards.

At the senior leadership level, a different set of measures should be used to align priorities, lead the organization, and embody the concept of a balanced scorecard. The organization should link these measures to its critical

EXHIBIT 10.2
Different Sets
of Measures
for Different
Purposes

Organizational Performance Measures	Strategic Measures	Process and Operational Measures
• Link to mission and vision • Cover key dimensions • Outcome measures • Used to judge overall organizational performance and results	• Link to vital few • Drive overall performance measures • Focal point of leadership system • Used to create alignment and focus	• Important to daily work • Quality control • Quality improvement • Traditional performance/ quality improvement • Key processes • Problem indicators
Governance	**Leadership**	**Management**

Source: Pugh Ettinger McCarthy Associates, LLC. Used with permission.

strategies, or "vital few" initiatives, and use them to drive desired results. As Kaplan and Norton (1992, 1996) suggest, strategic measures should be at the center of the organization's leadership system. Although leadership's main role is to deploy strategy, monitoring deployment is also its responsibility. A dashboard of strategic measures is a tool leaders can use to set priorities and drive change.

The board may use the same dashboard as a scorecard to monitor the deployment of strategy and assess leadership effectiveness. An important relationship exists between the overall organizational performance measures and the strategic measures. Strategy should focus on what drives desired results. The test of good strategy and strategic measures is whether successful deployment of the strategies results in improved performance as measured by the scorecard.

Process and Management Measures

Typical metrics found on dashboards of critical process measures include quality-control metrics, efficiency metrics, traditional quality improvement and performance improvement measures, labor statistics, customer satisfaction indexes, and other routine statistics used in day-to-day operations. The monitored operational and process measures should be linked to the strategic measures. Organizational alignment is enhanced when, at the day-to-day level, key processes that have a direct link to a specific organizational strategy are monitored and the successful deployment of strategy improves one or more organizational performance metrics.

Dimensions of Performance in Healthcare

What is good performance in healthcare? How do we know whether we are doing a good job? How should we organize our important measures to have the greatest effect? What should be on our organizational scorecard?

These questions are critical for healthcare leaders. Exhibit 10.1 indicates that performance is an outcome of the leadership process and ultimately should be measured by the organization's ability to achieve its mission and vision. Another way to think about performance is by important dimensions. Healthcare is about more than the bottom line. Use of the word *performance* in Exhibit 10.1 instead of *quality* emphasizes that performance is a broader term that encompasses quality, although some advocates of quality improvement theory may disagree. The point is that performance and quality in healthcare should be considered broadly; therefore, organizations should identify the multiple dimensions of performance.

One method of defining performance is in terms of traditional financial, satisfaction, human resource, and clinical dimensions. However, many organizations have benefited from a broader view of the important dimensions of performance in healthcare. Exhibit 10.3 lists some of the critical dimensions that healthcare organizations can use to define performance.

In *Crossing the Quality Chasm*, the Institute of Medicine (IOM 2001) suggested a second approach to thinking about performance in healthcare. It recommended that patient care be reorganized and redesigned to focus on six specific aims:

1. Safety
2. Effectiveness
3. Patient centeredness
4. Timeliness
5. Efficiency
6. Equity

Some organizations have found these six aims useful in defining organizational performance and the metrics that should be included on their scorecards.

A third approach to organizing performance results is the Baldrige Performance Excellence Program. The criteria for Category 7—Results— define specific classes of performance results that healthcare organization

• Patient and customer (satisfaction)	• Employee and staff satisfaction (culture)
• Effectiveness (clinical outcomes)	• Efficiency (cost)
• Appropriateness (evidence and process)	• Financial
• Safety (patient and staff)	• Flow (wait times, cycle times, and throughput)
• Equity	• Community/population health

EXHIBIT 10.3
Critical Dimensions of Performance in Healthcare Organizations

Source: Pugh Ettinger McCarthy Associates, LLC. Used with permission.

applicants are expected to track and report. Exhibit 10.4 shows the relationships between the various results required by the Baldrige Performance Excellence Program as a balanced-strategy diagram.

Organizations can use other methods besides the three discussed above to develop and define the important dimensions of performance. Traditional financial, human resource, satisfaction, and clinical dimensions are the foundations of most methods. In addition, religiously affiliated healthcare organizations often include dimensions of performance related to the mission of their sponsoring organization.

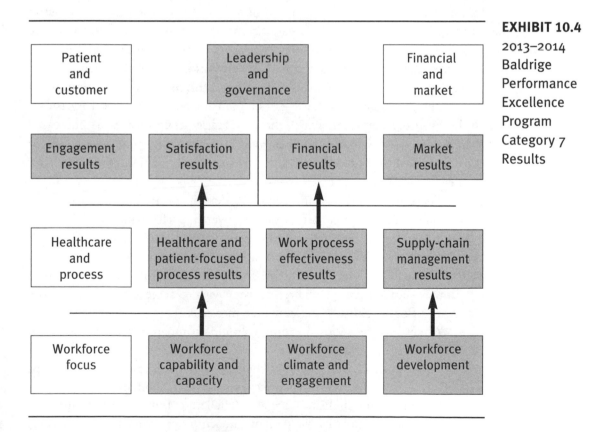

EXHIBIT 10.4
2013–2014 Baldrige Performance Excellence Program Category 7 Results

Clinical and Operational Issues

Creating an Organizational Scorecard

The development of an organizational scorecard should involve more than a simple transfer of existing measures into a new format or framework. The first step is to decide on an appropriate framework. Next, senior leadership and the governing body should define the dimensions of performance that are relevant to the organization's mission and the results they wish to achieve. Once they have agreed on these dimensions, they should select appropriate outcome measures for each of the chosen dimensions.

At the organizational level, the ideal cycle time for performance measurement is quarterly. However, some metrics may be too difficult or expensive to obtain every quarter, so the organization may be forced to make exceptions and settle for one or more annual measures. Sometimes the appropriate outcome measure for a dimension does not exist, in which case the organization must use a proxy measure or invest in the development of new metrics.

Healthcare leaders and trustees should include enough measures in an organizational scorecard to define the desired results for each of the important dimensions. Initially, in their enthusiasm for the new approach and desire to include great detail, most organizations identify more measures than are practical to track and tend to include process measures rather than outcome measures. Additional measures may be interesting, but the focus should remain on results. Organizations can maintain this focus by concentrating on the results they want to achieve rather than on potentially good measures. In the for-profit corporate world, the aim is fairly straightforward—increased shareholder value (which extends beyond ever-changing stock prices). In the not-for-profit healthcare world, the aims may be more numerous, but they are just as measurable.

The governing body and senior leadership of a healthcare organization should use a scorecard to monitor overall performance and balance. They also should use it to assess CEO and leadership performance. Although boards and senior leadership will continue to look at supporting reports of financial and clinical quality and other sources of additional performance detail, they should focus on the results they wish to achieve as defined by the scorecard of organizational performance measures.

When possible, organizations should compare their performance results to the best levels of performance, or benchmarks, reported by similar types of organizations. They should then deploy strategies to close the gaps between their current performance scores and the benchmarks.

Benchmarking in healthcare is a challenge but is becoming easier in some areas. Benchmarks for patient and employee satisfaction are available through the proprietary databases maintained by survey companies.

Comparative financial and workforce information is available through multiple sources, some free and some subscription based. And comparative clinical outcome metrics are becoming more widely available as well.

For some clinical and safety issues, the scorecard target should be 100 percent. For example, the administration of medication should be 100 percent error free, and the best evidence-based clinical care should be available to 100 percent of qualified patients. Setting best-in-class targets and high expectations on performance scorecards will help organizations achieve their desired results and thus increase healthcare reliability in key areas.

A healthcare organization could begin to create a scorecard by identifying potential measures for each of the six IOM aims. For example:

- *Safety*: adverse drug events per 1,000 doses
- *Effectiveness*: functional outcomes as defined by SF-12 health surveys, hospital mortality rates, compliance with best-practice guidelines, and disease-specific measures
- *Patient centeredness*: satisfaction levels reported on patient discharge survey
- *Timeliness*: number of days until the third next-available appointment
- *Efficiency*: hospital or clinic costs per discharge
- *Equity*: access to care and clinical outcomes compared by race/ ethnicity and gender

Exhibit 10.5 and Exhibit 10.6 present two examples of board-level scorecards used to drive organizational performance. In Exhibit 10.5, the key metrics are organized by culture, preventing harm (patient safety), clinical quality, and financial health, demonstrating a balance between the important dimensions of performance. The scorecard then shows the ultimate level of performance to be achieved in three years, the performance target for the current year, and the prior year's performance. The quarterly performance is coded to indicate whether it exceeded, met, or fell below target for that quarter.

Exhibit 10.6 is a simple but powerful one-page display of the key quality aims adopted by the board of a large, multihospital healthcare system. In this instance, the governing board set three-year aims for significant reduction of patient harm and improvement in patient outcomes throughout the system. Actual counts are being used to monitor improvement, and a simple line graphic provides instant feedback on directional performance.

Creating Alignment

Creating alignment in organizations is a critical leadership function. Leadership has been a focus of interest for many years, and innumerable works have been written about managing people and organizations and executing

EXHIBIT 10.5

Sample
Performance
Scorecard for a
Hospital Board

Main Street Hospital FY 2013 Board Performance Scorecard				FY 13 QTR 1	FY 13 QTR 2	FY 13 QTR 3	FY 13 QTR 4
CULTURE	**3-Year Goal**	**FY Target Range**	**Prior Year**				
Employee turnover rate (unplanned)	3% per quarter	5.5-6% per quarter	7.50%	2.41%	2.84%	NA	NA
Employee satisfaction (% recommend as place to work)	90%	60-70%	47%	75%	78%	NA	NA
PREVENTING HARM (Safety)	**3-Year Goal**	**FY Target Range**				NA	NA
Number of falls with injury	0	11	22 (FY)	5	5	NA	NA
Number of patients harmed from ADE	0	51	102(FY)	12	13	NA	NA
Number of central-line infections	0	0	9 (FY)	0	0	NA	NA
Number of ventilator-associated pneumonia	0	0	6 (FY)	1	1	NA	NA
Number of pressure ulcers	0	36	72 (FY)	20	26	NA	NA
CLINICAL QUALITY	**3-Year Goal**	**FY Target Range**				NA	NA
EVIDENCE-BASED CARE—% OF PATIENTS RECEIVING ALL REQUIRED ELEMENTS						NA	NA
Acute MI	100%	90-95%	88%	98%	98%	NA	NA
Pneumonia	100%	80-90%	75%	78%	74%	NA	NA
Congestive heart failure	100%	90-95%	85%	90%	98%	NA	NA
Hospital infection rate (per state reporting criteria)	5%	9-11%	14%	13.0%	14.5%	NA	NA
Unplanned readmission rate	0%	4-6.5%	8%	9.0%	5.0%	NA	NA
Number of inpatient deaths (unplanned, non-comfort care mortality)	0	2-4 quarter	28 (FY)	6	8	NA	NA
FINANCIAL HEALTH	**3-Year Goal**	**FY Target Range**				NA	NA
Contribution margin (%)	8%	2.5-4%	1.50%	2.50%	-2%	NA	NA
Days cash on hand	180 days	80-90	65	89	80	NA	NA

■ = Exceeds Target   ■ = Meets Target   ■ = Below Target

change. However, less literature exists about how leaders can create alignment between a compelling vision and an organization's day-to-day work.

Exhibit 10.7 identifies three categories of leadership functions: creating direction, creating alignment, and managing. Exhibit 10.8 shows the kinds of measurements that can be used to evaluate each category of functions in a scorecard or dashboard.

One approach to creating alignment is to use organizational performance dimensions as a framework for measurement throughout the

EXHIBIT 10.6

Sample
Dashboard of
Quality Aims for
the Board of a
Large Health-
care System

	FY 2013 Actual	20%	FY 2014 Target	Trend
Inpatient mortalities	1,254	251	1,003	
Inpatient all-cause readmissions	10,392	2,078	8,314	
Harm				
Related to medical management	679	136	543	
Hospital-acquired infections	1,549	310	1,239	
Related to patient care	905	181	724	
Other	14	3	11	
Total	3,147	629	2,518	
Sentinel events	162	32	130	
With harm	75	15	60	
Perfect care	81%	16	97%	

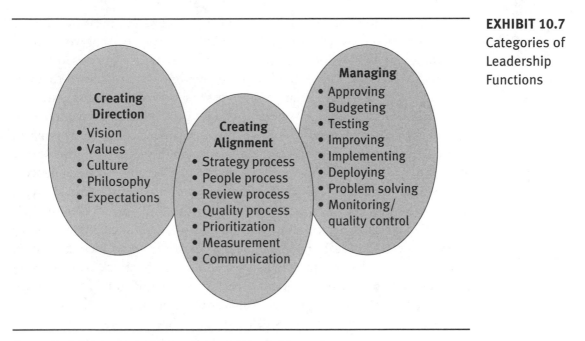

Source: Pugh Ettinger McCarthy Associates, LLC. Used with permission.

EXHIBIT 10.7
Categories of Leadership Functions

organization. Metrics may be different for every department or division, but they are linked by consistent focus at every level of the organization.

For example, many healthcare organizations have identified patient satisfaction as a key dimension of performance. In a competitive marketplace, an organization may determine that one of its critical strategies will be to improve patient satisfaction in order to build market share. Its strategic

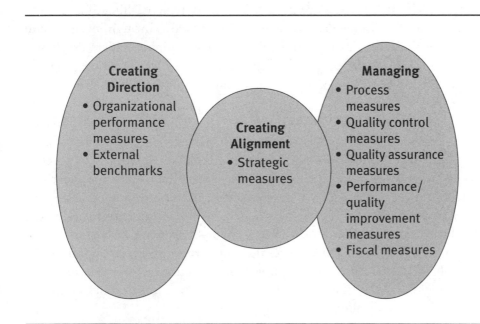

EXHIBIT 10.8
Different Measurement Sets Support Different Leadership Functions

Source: Pugh Ettinger McCarthy Associates, LLC. Used with permission.

dashboard would then include a set of metrics designed to measure whether patient satisfaction is improving. To link this strategy to daily work, every operating unit would monitor some metric that relates to patient satisfaction with its services and would monitor and improve processes known to affect satisfaction positively. For example, the dashboard for an emergency department (ED) would include a metric pertaining to patient satisfaction with emergency services. At the same time, the department could be working to improve flow, which in turn would reduce waiting time—a key process that affects the satisfaction of emergency patients. In this example, clear links exist between the organizational performance dimension of satisfaction, strategic measures, and the day-to-day improvement efforts and operation of the ED.

Exhibit 10.9 depicts a second method of aligning an organization's operations with a critical strategy or project. In this example, an organization has determined that reducing mortality among heart attack patients is an important aim for the population it serves. It has identified two key leverage points, or critical strategies, for reducing cardiac mortality in its organization: (1) ensure that all cardiac care is delivered according to evidence-based care plans and (2) reduce the time between a patient's presentation in the ED and the initiation of interventional therapy.

The first critical strategy, ensuring that all cardiac care is delivered according to evidence-based care plans, is measured by the percentage of patients who receive 100 percent of the required care elements. The second critical strategy, reducing the time between a patient's presentation in the ED and the initiation of interventional therapy, is measured by the percentage of patients who move from the door to the catheterization lab in less than 90 minutes. The two metrics are included on a strategic dashboard and regularly reviewed by senior management and the board. Through inclusion and review of these metrics on a strategic dashboard, senior leaders emphasize the importance of the project, establish a method of monitoring progress, and create a way to link desired results (lower mortality) to specific actions (strategies and tactics).

The targets associated with the two strategies are important because they alert managers to the significance of the change and the desired results. Department managers and clinical leaders can then identify the key processes needed to implement the strategies and the levels of reliability at which those processes must operate. Once leadership determines how key processes will be measured, those metrics can be added to the appropriate management dashboards and used on a real-time basis for further improvement or process control. In Exhibit 10.9, the critical supporting processes appear on the far right. The theory is that improvement and control of those processes will bring about the desired results in the strategic measures and ultimately reduce cardiac mortality.

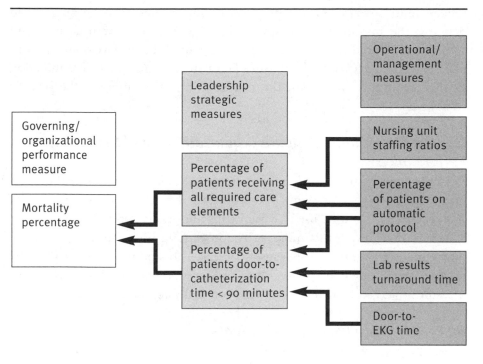

EXHIBIT 10.9
Creating
Organizational
Alignment
Around a
Critical Project:
Cardiac
Mortality

Source: Pugh Ettinger McCarthy Associates, LLC. Used with permission.

Keys to Successful Implementation and Lessons Learned

Successful development of performance scorecards and dashboards is dependent on many factors. This section describes some of the critical steps that organizations must take during the development and use of performance measures.

Develop a Clear Understanding of the Intended Use
The CEO, senior leadership team, and board must have a clear understanding of why a scorecard or dashboard is being created and how the measures will be used to drive execution and improvement. Many scorecards developed by organizations are sitting on shelves next to strategic plans, gathering dust.

Engage the Governing Board Early in the Development of Performance Measures
Organizations repeatedly make the mistake of having senior leadership present a performance scorecard to the board as an item of new business without adequate predevelopment discussion or involvement by the board. Ultimately, the governing body is responsible for the performance of the organization. This responsibility extends beyond simple fiduciary duties and includes clinical and service performance. Because scorecards should

reflect desired performance results, governing bodies must be involved in defining the important dimensions, choosing the relevant measures, and setting the desired levels of performance. Much of the development work may be assigned to leadership and clinical teams, but final determination of the important dimensions, the measures, and the targets is the board's responsibility.

Use the Scorecard to Evaluate Organizational and Leadership Performance

Once developed, the performance scorecard should be central to the organization's governance system. The scorecard should reflect the mission of the organization and be used by the board and leadership to evaluate progress toward achieving that mission. The governing board should review the scorecard at least quarterly. Because scorecards are about results, they can be useful in evaluating CEO performance and serve as a balanced set of objective measures that can be tied to compensation plans and performance criteria.

Be Prepared to Change the Measures

Developing a good organizational performance scorecard may sound like a simple idea, but it is difficult to do. An organization is unlikely to achieve a perfect set of measures the first time. Often, measures of desired results for a performance dimension do not exist and have to be developed. Other times, organizations realize after a couple of review cycles that they want better measures than those they currently use. Scorecard development is usually an iterative process rather than a single-shot job. Organizations should continue to improve their scorecards as they gain understanding of the desired results linked to each dimension and as better metrics are developed. Nevertheless, to quote the philosopher Voltaire, "Perfect is the enemy of good." Organizations should work toward creating a good scorecard, not a perfect one.

Make the Data Useful, Not Pretty

Scorecard formats should be useful and understandable. Many organizations struggle with fancy formats and attempts to create online versions. A good starting point is to construct simple run charts that display the measures over time and the desired target for each measure. Simple spreadsheet graphs can be dropped into a text document, four or six per page. The information conveyed, not the format, is important. Organizations have had mixed success with more sophisticated formats, such as radar charts. Some boards find radar charts invaluable because they display all the metrics and targets on a single page. Other boards have difficulty interpreting this type of graph. The admonition to start simple does not imply that other approaches will not work. One innovative computer-based display (see the Case Study section) uses a radar chart backed by hot-linked run and control charts for each performance metric.

Integrate the Measures to Achieve a Balanced View

Although some organizations like to use scorecard and dashboard formats for financial and quality reports, the routine display of metrics in separate, category-driven reports may reflect a lack of integration. Organizations that compile separate, detailed scorecards of financial, quality, and service metrics and review each independently, as tradition dictates, will probably place more emphasis on financial results and pay less attention to clinical, satisfaction, and other dimensions, except when a crisis erupts in a given area. However, if an organization has developed a broader set of high-level measures and the category-based reports support those measures, the use of detailed, separate scorecards can be useful.

Develop Clear and Measurable Strategies

Kaplan and Norton (1992, 1996) contend that strategic measures should be central to the leadership system. Strategic dashboards and balanced scorecards are key tools that leaders can use to align strategies and actions. Unfortunately, in healthcare, strategy and strategic planning are generally underdeveloped. Many organizations engage in a superficial annual process that results in a set of vague objectives that are task oriented rather than strategic. Often, the strategic plan is then set aside until it is time to prepare for the next board retreat. Organizations will have difficulty developing a balanced scorecard as envisioned by Kaplan and Norton if their strategies are not clear, measurable, and truly strategic. Most organizations do, in fact, have a simple set of critical strategies that, if successfully deployed, would accelerate progress toward their mission and vision. Organizations should clearly identify those critical strategies and develop a set of specific measures for each strategy.

Tracking progress on a specifically designed strategic dashboard can be very effective. The choice of measures is important because they reflect what the strategy is intended to accomplish. Most critical strategies inspire innumerable ideas and potential approaches. All proposed tactics, initiatives, and projects should directly affect one or more strategic measures. If not, leadership should look elsewhere to invest resources.

Use Organizational Performance Dimensions to Align Efforts

One approach to using scorecards and dashboards to create alignment is to build cascading sets of metrics that correspond to the key dimensions of performance on the scorecard. Each operating unit or department is required to develop a set of metrics for each of the key dimensions. For example, if patient safety is a key dimension, each nursing unit could track and seek to improve its fall rate or rate of adverse drug events. If employee well-being is a key performance dimension, each department could track voluntary turnover rates. Executive review of departmental performance should include the entire set of clinical, process, financial service, and safety measures rather than focus on a financial dimension one month and on a service or clinical quality dimension the next month.

Avoid Using Indicators Based on Averages

Because averages mask variation and are misleading, they should be avoided when developing scorecards and dashboards. For example, the average time from door to drug in the ED may be lower than the preset operating standard. However, examination of the individual data may reveal that a significant percentage of patients do not receive treatment within the prescribed amount of time. A better approach is to measure the percentage of patients who receive treatment within the time specified in the standard. Average waiting times, average length of stay, average satisfaction scores, and average cost are all suspect indicators.

Develop Composite Clinical Indicators for Processes and Outcome Indicators for Results

The approach to clinical indicators continues to evolve. Healthcare organizations are complex and generally provide care across a wide spectrum of conditions and treatment regimens. They often have difficulty determining which clinical indicators are truly important and representative of the processes of care provided. One approach is to develop composite indicators for high-volume, high-profile conditions. For example, the CMS review set for heart attack contains six cardiac indicators. Most hospital organizations track their performance against each of the indicators, which is appropriate at the operational level. However, at the senior leadership level, tracking the percentage of cardiac patients who received all six required elements may be more useful. This tracking accomplishes two things. First, it limits the number of metrics on a senior leadership or governing board scorecard. Second, it emphasizes that all patients should receive all required aspects of care, not just four out of six.

Organizations can use the same approach to track performance for chronic diseases such as diabetes. They can establish the critical aspects of care that should always be performed (e.g., timely hemoglobin testing, referral to the diabetes educator, eye and foot exams) and develop a composite measure that reflects the percentage of patients who receive complete care.

Another approach to developing clinical performance metrics is to consider the results rather than the process. Mortality and readmission rates are obvious results. Some organizations are beginning to look beyond such measures and are considering clinical results from the perspective of the patient. Development of experimental questionnaires and new approaches to assessing patient function are under way and may include the following types of patient-centered questions:

- Was pain controlled to my expectations?
- Am I better today as a result of the treatment I received?
- Am I able to function today at the level I expected?
- Is my function restored to the level it was at before I became ill or was injured?
- Did I receive the help I need to manage my ongoing condition?
- Am I aware of anything that went wrong in the course of my treatment that delayed my recovery or compromised my condition?

Use Comparative Data and External Benchmarks

When possible, use external benchmark data to establish standards and targets. Many organizations track mortality and readmission rates on their scorecards. Mortality is a much stronger performance measure when it is risk adjusted and compared to other organizations' performance to establish a frame of reference. Without that frame of reference, mortality tracking provides little useful information except for directional trends.

Beyond establishing a frame of reference, however, organizations should set targets based on best performance in class rather than peer-group averages. Comparison to a peer-group mean tends to reinforce mediocrity and deflects attention from the importance of the desired result monitored by the performance measure. One of the best examples is the peer averages and percentiles that most vendors of national patient satisfaction surveys provide. Being above average or in the top quartile does not necessarily equate to high patient satisfaction. A significant percentage of patients may be indifferent about or dissatisfied with the care they received. Instead of percentile-based targets (targets based on ranking), average raw score or the percentage of patients who express dissatisfaction may be better indicators.

Change Your Leadership System

There is a saying that goes something like, "If you always do what you have always done, you will always get what you always got." One mistake some organizations have made is to roll out an elaborate set of cascading dashboards and scorecards and then fail to change the way the leadership system functions. Scorecards and dashboards can quickly become another compliance effort or something done for The Joint Commission outside of the organization's "real work." Leadership must make the review of measurement sets an integral part of its function. When senior leaders review departments or operating units, the unit scorecard or dashboard should be their primary focus. If a strategic dashboard is developed, progress review should occur at least monthly or be coordinated with the measurement cycles of the indicators. Governing boards should review the organizational performance measures at least quarterly. Reviews should not be done solely for the sake of reviewing but for the purposes of driving change and setting priorities.

Focus on Results, Not on Activities

A well-developed system of dashboards and scorecards allows leadership to focus on results instead of activities. Many results-oriented, high-performing organizations work from a leadership philosophy of tight–loose–tight. Senior leaders are very clear and "tight" about the results they wish to achieve and measure them through the use of strategic and operational dashboards. At the same time, they are "loose" in their direct control of those doing the work, creating a sense of empowerment in those charged with achieving the results. In the absence of clear measures, leaders tend to control activities, micromanage, and disempower others in the organization. When desired results are clear, senior leaders can be "tight" about holding individuals and teams accountable for achieving them.

Cultivate Transparency

One characteristic of high-performing organizations, such as Baldrige Award recipients, is that every employee knows how his or her individual efforts fit into the bigger picture. Healthcare has a long tradition of secrecy about results, in part a reflection of the historical view that quality is about physician peer review and in part a reaction to the malpractice environment. Transparency is a big step for some organizations, but the results gathered on the organizational scorecard should be discussed openly and shared with employees and clinical staff. Ideally, the results should also be shared with the community served. Employees and clinical staff need to know what dimensions of performance are important to the organization, what process and management indicators are used for evaluation, what dashboards are related to their daily work, what the quarterly performance results are, and what those results mean. The same is true for strategic measures. Many organizations seek to keep their strategic measures confidential and do not routinely share them with employees. That approach is usually counterproductive. After all, successful deployment of strategy depends on what an organization itself does, not on what its competitors may do. Sometimes a specific tactic, such as building a new clinic in a competitive part of town, may need to be closely held because of market issues, but the critical strategy relating to growth of the enterprise should not be a secret. It is difficult to create awareness and improve key processes if the underlying strategy and strategic measures are kept secret.

Case Study: St. Joseph Hospital[3]

St. Joseph Hospital (SJH) in Orange, California, is the flagship hospital of the St. Joseph Health System (SJHS), sponsored by the sisters of St. Joseph of Orange. The system consists of 14 hospitals, all located in California with the exception of Covenant Health, which is located in Texas. SJH and the Covenant Health operation are the two largest organizations in the system.

SJHS was an early adopter and developer of a system-wide approach to collecting and reporting a set of common performance indicators. Using the four dimensions of the quality compass framework (financial, human resources, clinical, and satisfaction), the corporate office collects a monthly set of common performance indicators from each hospital in the system. Known internally as "the web," individual hospital radar charts are developed. On a periodic basis, the information is shared with the system's corporate board. The leadership and local governing boards of each hospital use the charts to track progress, and individual CEO performance reviews are based on the results. A run or control chart backs each indicator on the radar chart. The health system has been innovative in the development of its scorecard tool and posts monthly updates on its intranet. The indicators are fairly traditional, but SJHS continues to modify and change them as the system advances. Exhibit 10.10 shows a diagram of the monthly performance web for SJH.

Although both the corporate office and the governing boards of the hospitals considered the web useful for tracking performance across the system, they viewed it as a helpful but insufficient tool for driving change at SJH. Larry Ainsworth, the CEO, realized that a different set of measures tied to organizational strategy was required to continue to progress and remain competitive in the Orange County marketplace. Traditionally, SJH used an annual planning process that yielded a business plan of more than 20 pages of objectives and proposed actions. Management spent an enormous amount of time developing and tracking activities and objectives and reporting monthly to the board.

Instead of starting over, senior leadership examined the business plan and from it concluded that all of the proposed objectives could be sorted and grouped under six strategic themes: staff development and retention, information technology deployment, cardiac care improvement, cancer care improvement, physician recruitment and relations, and new business development (Exhibit 10.11).

EXHIBIT 10.10
The Web: St.
Joseph Health
System
Performance
Indicators

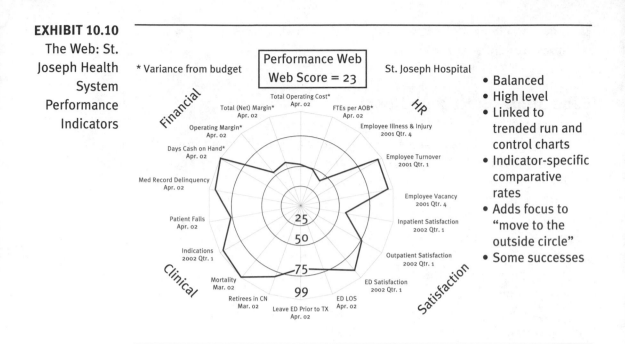

Source: St. Joseph Health System. Used with permission.

EXHIBIT 10.11
St. Joseph
Health System
Strategy Map:
The Vital Few

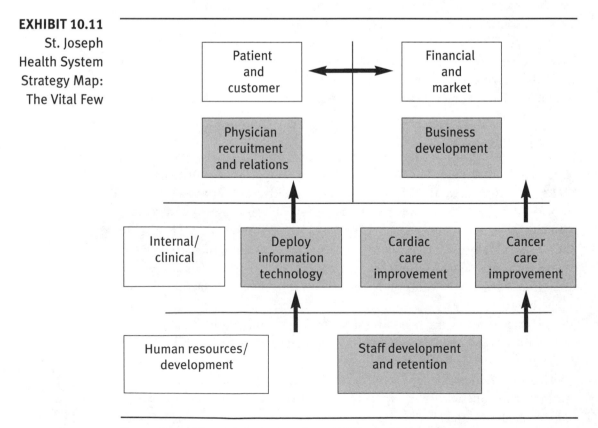

Source: Pugh Ettinger McCarthy Associates, LLC. Used with permission.

For each strategy, a team of senior leaders and clinicians was formed to develop specific proposed strategic measures and identify the required tactics for deployment. Many of the tactics were modifications of previously identified objectives and actions, but the team developed many new ones in consideration of how they would affect the strategic measures directly. Development of visual strategy maps and associated measures for each tactic helped the hospital accomplish its aim of integrating previously separate quality, business, and strategic plans into a single approach. Hospital leadership viewed the strategy maps as critical to creating alignment and focus.

For each strategy, a dashboard of key measures was developed. The senior leadership team reviews this dashboard monthly and shares results with the governing board on a quarterly basis. Exhibit 10.12 is a sample of the strategic dashboard used to drive progress on SJH's oncology strategy. The strategies must be measurable, and each proposed tactic is required to have a set of associated measures to guide deployment.

Ainsworth and his leadership team made changes in the leadership system and began a routine, scheduled, in-depth review of each strategy. The review started with the results of each of the strategic dashboard measures and continued with discussions of specific tactics and consideration of associated tactical measures. Identification of the five critical strategies and development of the strategy maps also changed the process by which the hospital board monitors progress.

Clarifying the key organizational strategies, developing key strategic measures for each, using the strategic measures to prioritize proposed tactics, and implementing changes in the leadership system to focus on strategy resulted in increased organization-wide alignment in SJH's improvement of important processes and increased organizational effectiveness. Those steps also had positive effects on the system-required web of performance indicators.

Conclusion

Healthcare organizations are complex service-delivery systems. Performance is measured across multiple dimensions, including financial, patient experience, clinical outcomes, employee engagement, and patient safety. Scorecards and dashboards are useful leadership and governance tools for creating focus and alignment within the organization on areas that need to be improved, and they are critical to tracking progress on strategic objectives. There should be a direct link between an organization's strategy and quality improvement efforts so that resources are committed to improvements that move the organizational and governance performance measures in the desired direction.

EXHIBIT 10.12
Strategic
Dashboard
Used to Drive
Progress on
Oncology
Strategy at St.
Joseph Health
System

What are we trying to accomplish:
To be recognized for clinical excellence with increased market share in the provision of coordinated cancer care (oncology) services for Orange County and surrounding communities

Promise:
You will receive timely, comprehensive, current knowledge-based, and compassionate care at St. Joseph Hospital

Volume, Profitability, and Market Share

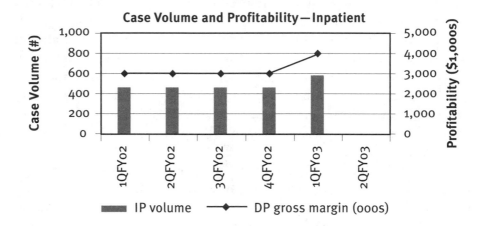

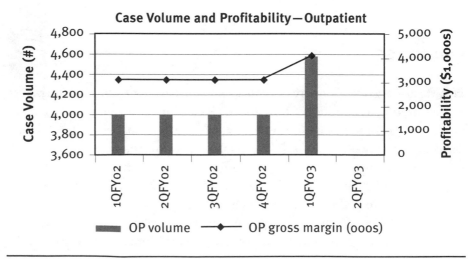

(Continued)

EXHIBIT 10.12
Strategic
Dashboard
Used to Drive
Progress on
Oncology
Strategy at St.
Joseph Health
System
(continued)

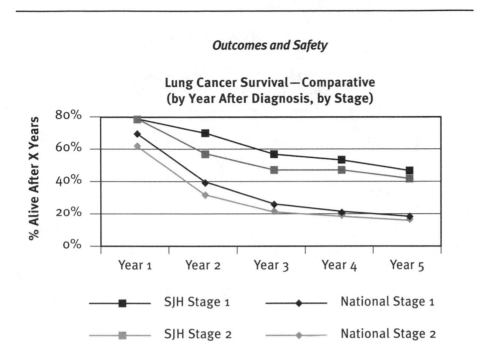

Outcomes and Safety

**Lung Cancer Survival—Comparative
(by Year After Diagnosis, by Stage)**

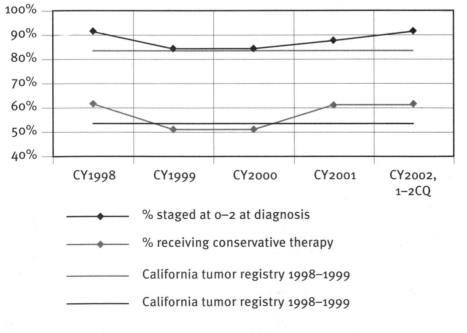

**Breast Care—Percentage Diagnosed at Stage 0–2 and Percentage
Receiving Conservative Therapy**

(Continued)

EXHIBIT 10.12
Strategic
Dashboard
Used to Drive
Progress on
Oncology
Strategy at St.
Joseph Health
System
(continued)

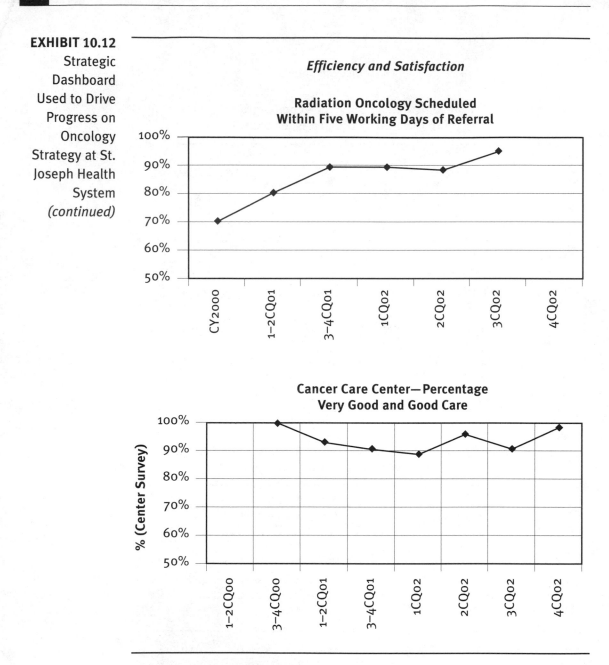

Efficiency and Satisfaction

**Radiation Oncology Scheduled
Within Five Working Days of Referral**

**Cancer Care Center—Percentage
Very Good and Good Care**

Source: St. Joseph Health System. Used with permission.

Study Questions

1. In your experience with healthcare, what are the important dimensions of performance? How would you know whether an organization is performing well? What indicators do you think are important for a hospital to track? For a physician practice? A home care agency? A long-term care facility? A managed care organization?

2. What could be good indicators of patient centeredness as recommended by IOM?

3. What are some of the pitfalls of overmeasurement? How do you determine what is important to measure in an organization?

4. Why is creating alignment an important leadership function? What are some methods of creating alignment, and how can the use of measurement support their deployment?

Notes

1. In deference to the work of Kaplan and Norton (1992, 1996) and the specific concept of leaders using a balanced scorecard of strategic measures, this chapter does not use the term *balanced scorecard* except in direct reference to Kaplan and Norton's concept. Instead, it discusses the use of dashboards and scorecards in broader, generic terms in its exploration of a variety of applications that create focus and alignment in healthcare organizations.

2. A popular approach has been to use the stoplight color scheme of red, yellow, and green to highlight indicators when performance is judged against a predetermined standard. Indicators that reflect negative performance are highlighted in red, whereas indicators judged to be satisfactory or above expectations are highlighted in green. Yellow can mean caution or need for further review. Although useful for identifying problems or failure to meet a target, this format does not provide trended information useful for assessing progress or decline and, depending on the standard chosen, may reinforce poor actual results.

3. This case study was developed from the author's consulting work with St. Joseph Health System. Used with permission.

References

Aguayo, R. 1991. *Dr. Deming: The American Who Taught the Japanese About Quality.* New York: Simon & Schuster.

Institute of Medicine (IOM). 2001. *Crossing the Quality Chasm: A New Health System for the 21st Century.* Washington, DC: National Academies Press.

Kaplan, R. S., and D. P. Norton. 1996. *The Balanced Scorecard—Translating Strategy into Action.* Boston: HBS Press.

———. 1992. "The Balanced Scorecard—Measures That Drive Performance." *Harvard Business Review* 70 (1): 71–79.

PATIENT SAFETY AND MEDICAL ERRORS

Frances A. Griffin

Background and Terminology

Harm is never the intention in healthcare delivery, but far too often it is the outcome. In addition to their fears of a terminal diagnosis and debilitating disease and pain, one of patients' greatest fears is that a mistake will occur and that the mistake will harm them. Horror stories of patients waking up in the middle of surgical procedures or having the wrong limb amputated, although rare, instill anxiety in individuals accessing the healthcare system. Media stories of patients who entered the hospital for elective surgery and then developed terrible or fatal infections have become more common. Fear of such events also plays on the minds of healthcare practitioners, who worry about malpractice claims, loss of licensure, and, worst of all, the guilt of having caused harm rather than having provided care and healing.

In 2000, the Institute of Medicine (IOM) published a landmark report on patient safety titled *To Err Is Human* (Kohn, Corrigan, and Donaldson 2000). Media attention to this report was swift and widespread, resulting in sudden public awareness that there was a problem. The public expressed shock at the estimate of up to 98,000 annual deaths in US hospitals resulting from medical errors. Reactions among healthcare providers ranged from those who argued (and continue to argue) that the numbers were grossly overestimated (Hayward and Hofer 2001) to those who were not surprised, and even relieved, that the information was now public and who hoped that action would be taken. The IOM followed this report with *Crossing the Quality Chasm* in 2001, which recommended strategies for improvement. In April 2011, *Health Affairs* devoted an entire issue to the progress made in the prior decade. Although examples of improvement were noted, a key study reported that adverse events in hospitals may be ten times higher than previously reported (Classen et al. 2011).

Published studies regarding medical errors, medication errors, and adverse events have been appearing in the literature for decades, providing the basis for the estimates in the IOM report and stimulating efforts to develop sensitive measurement strategies. In 1991, the Harvard Medical

Practice Study—of which Dr. Lucian Leape, a leading expert on medical errors and author of many studies and articles, was one of the principal authors—reviewed hospital records retrospectively for evidence of errors and adverse events (Brennan et al. 1991). The study's findings indicated that medical errors and adverse events were occurring far more often than reported and contributing to unnecessary deaths. Further studies demonstrated that errors and adverse events commonly occurred in other healthcare settings besides hospitals. In 2003, Gandhi and colleagues reported that 25 percent of patients in ambulatory care practices had experienced adverse drug events. Other studies, in both the United States and Australia, reported how adverse drug events resulted in additional visits to physicians' offices and emergency departments and increased hospital admissions (Kohn, Corrigan, and Donaldson 2000). The Commonwealth Fund found that 25 percent of patients across four countries reported that they had experienced some form of medical error in the past two years (Blendon et al. 2003). In addition to the 2011 *Health Affairs* study mentioned earlier, two studies published in 2010 found similar rates of nearly one-third of hospitalized patients being harmed by medical care and little improvement in one state over a five-year period (Landrigan et al. 2010; OIG 2010).

Patient Safety Defined

Patient safety is defined as "freedom from accidental injury" (Kohn, Corrigan, and Donaldson 2000). At the core is the experience of the patient and the goal that no patient will experience unnecessary harm, pain, or other suffering. A patient's experience of harm or injury from a medical intervention is an adverse event—that is, an occurrence not caused by an underlying medical condition (Kohn, Corrigan, and Donaldson 2000). Adverse events sometimes are the result of an error, in which case they would be considered preventable. Not all adverse events are clearly the result of error, though, and some medical interventions can cause harm even when planned and executed correctly (Shojania et al. 2002). Some argue that such events are not adverse and should not be regarded as harm but rather as known complications or associated risks of certain procedures and interventions. Still, those consequences are unintended, and patients who experience them receive little comfort from that argument.

Practitioners often link the determination that a harm was preventable with the assignment of culpability for the harm, though they are not related. If practitioners believe that most harm is unpreventable, they will stop searching for improved practices that create desired outcomes with no associated adverse events. For example, the early use of chemotherapy to treat cancer caused a good deal of harm in the form of excessive nausea and vomiting; patients became terribly ill and sometimes died from the treatment.

Hyperemesis was a known and associated risk of chemotherapy and, though often unpreventable, was judged acceptable. Years of research led to development of improved antiemetic agents and prophylactic protocols that prevent or significantly reduce such harm today.

Errors do not always reach the patient; for example, the wrong dose of a medication may be dispensed but detected before administration and corrected. Even when errors do reach the patient, they may not cause harm or injury; for example, if an incorrect dose of medication is administered, it may not differ enough from the intended dose to affect the patient adversely.

In the past few decades, much research has been conducted on human factors and the cognitive processes associated with errors. James Reason (1990), a renowned expert on human factors and error, defines *error* as "an occasion in which a planned sequence of events fails to achieve its intended outcome." According to Reason, errors originate from one of two basic types of failure: a planning failure or an execution failure. Let us consider examples in healthcare from a common process—use of antibiotics to treat an infection. When an antibiotic is prescribed, it should be one that is effective against the specific bacteria causing the patient's infection. However, sometimes an antibiotic is prescribed based on the physician's assessment of the most likely type of bacteria involved. Results of laboratory cultures identifying the specific organism and antibiotic susceptibility may not yet be available, and treatment needs to start because the patient is ill and experiencing symptoms. The prescribed antibiotic may be dispensed and administered in accordance with the physician's order, but test results may later reveal that the organism causing the infection is not susceptible to the antibiotic administered. A planning error has occurred because the physician initiated the wrong plan, and the plan may not achieve the aim (resolving the infection) even though it was carried out as intended.

An execution error occurs when a plan is correct but not carried out as intended. For example, if the physician selects the correct antibiotic, but the antibiotic is either not dispensed or not administered according to the order (e.g., wrong drug, wrong dose, wrong frequency), an error has occurred. Whether an error results from a planning failure or an execution failure, the patient may be placed at risk.

Etiology of Medical Errors

Addressing patient safety and medical error first requires an understanding of the underlying factors that contribute to errors and adverse events. Healthcare processes have become enormously complex over time, and the volume of information and knowledge currently available to practitioners is overwhelming. New and rapidly advancing technologies have led to new treatments that offer many benefits but require training and expertise to be used effectively and safely. Thousands of new medications are introduced each year, far more than anyone could recall accurately from memory. Working conditions play an important role as well; shortages of clinical personnel, high patient ratios, and long work hours all contribute to the risk that complex processes may not be executed as intended (i.e., that an error may occur).

When an error occurs, whether in planning or execution, it is most often a systems problem (Leape, Berwick, and Bates 2002). Healthcare has not recognized this important correlation sufficiently. The traditional response has been to blame an individual, usually the person at the end of a process that went wrong in many places, and often many times before. When an error leads to an adverse event or harm, emotions contribute to the situation: anger from patients and families, fear of lawsuits from risk managers and practitioners, and guilt from those involved. The common response has been to identify a person at fault and to take punitive action against that person, such as loss of licensure, fines, suspension, or employment termination. However, taking this sort of action prevents a deeper understanding of the real drivers of the event and mistakenly allows organizations and patients to feel safer until the same event occurs again but with different actors. Punishment for being involved in errors discourages people from reporting them (Findlay 2000).

Punitive action is appropriate if an individual has knowingly and intentionally taken action to cause harm, which would be criminal or negligent behavior, or has knowingly violated a procedure. Criminal behavior occurs, for example, when a practitioner injects a patient with a paralytic medication so that the practitioner can be the one to "save" the patient from the pulmonary arrest that occurs. Fortunately, such cases are exceptions and clearly warrant disciplinary and legal action. However, most adverse events do not fit into this category but rather result from a process breakdown. Blaming and punishing an individual and failing to change the process does not reverse the harm that has occurred and does nothing to decrease the likelihood that the same adverse event will occur again elsewhere in the organization.

Data on incidence of errors and adverse events are essential to identify the changes and improvements needed. Unfortunately, the systems of measurement commonly used in the United States grossly underestimate the numbers. In their 2011 study, Classen and colleagues found that voluntary reporting systems, which will be discussed in further detail in this chapter, detected only 1 percent of all adverse events. A common measurement tool is the Patient Safety Indicators software available from the Agency for Healthcare Research and Quality (AHRQ 2012). This popular tool is free and requires few resources for data collection because it uses data already collected for administrative billing purposes. However, the software may detect less than 10 percent of actual adverse events, and other methods have been developed that detect far more, such as the Institute for Healthcare Improvement (IHI) Global Trigger Tool (Griffin and Resar 2009).

Some state regulatory agencies, such as state departments of health, have mandated reporting for certain types of adverse events. As of January 2011, 30 states had mandated some type of reporting of hospital-associated infections, and most have a public reporting requirement. The Joint Commission has attempted to gain further information from accredited organizations through its Sentinel Event standards. Excessive jury awards, high settlements in malpractice cases, and sensational media coverage have contributed to the lack of reporting. When an error occurs that causes no harm, there may be little incentive to report it, if it is even recognized. The result is that the process remains unchanged such that the same error recurs and ultimately may cause harm. In addition, because only a minority of events are actually reported, those data cannot be used to track improvement robustly or to determine whether an institution is operating more safely today than it was at the same time last year.

In response to *To Err Is Human* and the ensuing patient-safety movement, several organizations led initiatives to promote and disseminate best practices for safety. For example, AHRQ released a report in 2001 on evidence-based safety practices. AHRQ defined a patient-safety practice as "a type of process or structure whose application reduces the probability of adverse events resulting from exposure to the health care system" (Shojania et al. 2002). This definition does not mention error because errors will continue to exist in healthcare. Processes will continue to have the potential to fail, and human factors always will contribute. However, adverse events and harm need not continue to occur. In a system designed for patient safety, errors are anticipated to occur, processes are designed and improved with human factors and safety in mind, and reporting is encouraged and rewarded. When safety is part of everyone's daily routine, errors exist but adverse events do not.

Scope and Use of Patient-Safety Systems

Healthcare is not the only industry to have struggled with a poor safety record and public image problem. At one time, aviation had nowhere near the safety record that it has today. During the mid-twentieth century, as commercial air travel increased in popularity, accidents and deaths occurred at significantly higher rates than they do today. To survive, the aviation industry had to make significant changes. It accomplished these changes by focusing on making systems safer and on developing a different culture. The results are obvious, considering the number of planes flown every day, the volume of passengers they transport, and the number of passengers who are injured or killed in airplane accidents. In the first half of the 1990s, the number of deaths was one-third what it had been in the mid-twentieth century (Kohn, Corrigan, and Donaldson 2000). We cannot say the same for healthcare and even wonder whether the opposite may be true.

Although the healthcare and aviation industries are different and the analogy is not perfect, many lessons from the aviation industry are applicable. In fact, anesthesiology already has applied many of them and is considered the benchmark for safe delivery of medical care, which was not always the case. In the mid-twentieth century, patients receiving general anesthesia were at a much greater risk of dying from the anesthesia than they are today. From the 1950s to the 1970s, changes were made that decreased the rate of anesthesia-related deaths from 1 in 3,500 to 1 in 10,000 (Findlay 2000), a significant improvement. The fact that anesthesiologists themselves led the change was a major factor in its success. They developed their own standards of practice and guidelines, which were more readily acceptable than those that might have been imposed on them by outside regulatory agencies. Protocols were adopted from the practices developed in aviation, such as use of standardized procedures and safety checklists. More recent data show that anesthesia-related deaths have decreased to 1 in 300,000, a staggering difference from the 1950s (Findlay 2000). No single breakthrough technology or newly discovered drug has been responsible for this improvement. Rather, the progress resulted from focusing on a system of care that recognizes human frailties and accounts for them in the design of care and from making many small changes over time that led to safer practices (Leape, Berwick, and Bates 2002).

Teamwork and Patient Safety

In any setting, the success of a team depends on the interactions of its members. When the members of a team do not function well together or do not perceive each other as having equally important roles, they do not handle unexpected situations well. The aviation industry learned this lesson the hard way. Reviews of the events in a cockpit before a plane accident or crash revealed that copilots and engineers often were unable to communicate warnings effectively to the pilot or the senior member of the team, or that the person responded negatively to their communication. Warnings that could have prevented the deaths of hundreds of passengers, including the crew itself, were frequently disregarded, poorly communicated, or not communicated. To change this environment, the industry initiated "cockpit resource management," later renamed "crew resource management" (CRM). In CRM, crews learn how to interact as a team, and all members have equally important roles and responsibilities to ensure the safety of all on board. Appropriate assertion of concerns is more than encouraged; it is expected.

Many hospitals have incorporated CRM and are using it in a variety of settings. Operating room teams are in some ways analogous to airline crews, and CRM training is improving how surgeons, anesthesiologists, nurses, and technicians work together to ensure the provision of safe care to the patient. Faculty at the University of Texas Center of Excellence in Patient Safety Research studied airline crews and operating room teams to evaluate how they interact with each other and respond to errors and unexpected events. Teams that reported high levels of teamwork still made errors but made fewer serious ones compared to teams that scored poorly on teamwork. In addition, operating room teams that scored high on teamwork were able to resolve conflict more often and prevent small errors from becoming adverse events. The correlation between teamwork scores and conflict resolution, however, appeared to be stronger in airplane crews than in operating room teams because the airline teams had been receiving CRM training for much longer (Sexton, Thomas, and Helmreich 2000).

In 2008, the World Health Organization (WHO) applied CRM concepts to improving patient safety in surgery worldwide. The WHO Surgical Safety Checklist has been adopted by many hospitals in the United States and around the globe to reinforce teamwork and communication among surgical team members and prevent surgery-related adverse events.

Communication styles between members of a team significantly affect how well the team functions, and in many adverse events (in both healthcare and other industries), communication failure is often identified as a leading contributing factor. Part of the reason for such failures in healthcare is that professional healthcare education does not include training in how to communicate effectively with others. Communication is even more difficult when there are perceived hierarchies or people are afraid to speak up.

An effective model for communication was developed by IHI (2013) faculty who adapted methods from CRM and strategies in other industries. This model is SBAR, which stands for Situation–Background–Assessment–Recommendation and provides a structured framework for healthcare professionals to communicate key patient information (IHI 2003). Many hospitals have trained staff in its use and found it valuable.

People derive their attitudes about teamwork from the overall culture of an organization and the unit in which they work. There can be enormous differences in culture from one unit or department to another, even within the same organization. Individuals are most affected by the culture of the department in which they spend most of their time. Culture in a unit may not be obvious. On the surface, it may appear that disputes between staff, physicians, and managers rarely occur. Absence of such overt problems, however, does not necessarily indicate a good underlying culture. Every department, unit, and organization should constantly work at developing and enhancing its culture, regardless of how effective it may appear or actually be, by improving how all members of the healthcare team interact and communicate with each other. Focusing on culture, and especially its interactional aspects, improves patient care and has many other benefits as well. When all team members feel valued and able to contribute, their work satisfaction improves, thereby decreasing turnover—a costly issue in any organization. Improved communication between practitioners results in better coordination of care, early recognition of errors, and more rapid interventions. At Johns Hopkins Hospital in Baltimore, Maryland, a comprehensive program to improve teamwork and culture in the intensive care unit resulted in a 50 percent decrease in patient length of stay, which allowed more than 650 additional admissions and provided $7 million in additional revenue (Pronovost et al. 2003).

Other hospitals have used similar approaches to improve teamwork and communication in operating room teams. One technique is to hold a safety briefing before every operation, during which the entire team meets to review the case and potential safety issues. Following implementation of this and other changes, staff members reported that they had less difficulty speaking up if they perceived a problem. Even more interesting, though, was the staff's perception that their workload had decreased, even though no changes to workload or staffing levels were made (Sexton 2002).

Leading Improved Patient Safety

Leadership is the driving force behind an organization's culture and the perceptions it creates. For staff in any healthcare organization to believe that patient safety is a priority, that message must come from the CEO, medical staff leaders, and the board. Furthermore, that message must be visible and consistent. A visible approach to patient safety does not mean memos sent out by the CEO emphasizing its importance or a periodic column in a staff newsletter. The only way frontline staff will know and believe that safety is important to the organization's senior leaders is if the senior leaders visit the departments and units where the work occurs and speak directly with the staff about safety. Through unit rounds and by soliciting input from staff, senior leaders can gain tremendous knowledge about what is happening in their organizations and take steps to make improvements (Frankel et al. 2003). To be convincing, these visits must be consistent and sustained. When leaders start to make rounds, staff may think the visits are just "the idea of the month" and expect them not to last, especially if previous initiatives have followed a similar path. Senior leaders can have a powerful effect on safety by setting aside just one hour per week to make rounds and talk with staff, as long as they do so routinely and provide feedback. Some senior leaders have found these visits so beneficial that they have increased the amount of time they spend on this activity.

Changing culture and perceptions can take a long time and requires tremendous effort and attention. Leaders' presence at the front line is essential, but it is only one piece of the package. Their response to anything that occurs—whether an error, an adverse event, or both—significantly affects staff beliefs. Acknowledging that errors and adverse events are systems problems and not people problems is a crucial first step, but follow-through on that acknowledgment—with appropriate response when something happens—is critical. Many organizations have created nonpunitive reporting policies to encourage staff to report errors and adverse events without fear of reprisal, even if the person reporting was involved in the event. Success of these policies has varied, especially at middle-management levels. Many managers, trained in the old paradigm of "blame the individual," struggle with the concept of nonpunitive policies because they mistakenly conclude that no employee will ever be disciplined, especially their "problem" employees. A true problem employee will usually violate enough other policies for the manager to take appropriate action. When it comes to errors and adverse events, however, other employees are just as likely as problem individuals to find themselves involved in a system failure. Such situations are not opportunities to get rid of a problem employee. In a just culture, every error or adverse event is analyzed as a system problem, and punitive action is not taken against anyone unless a policy was deliberately violated or there was intent to cause harm. Staff members will recall punitive action taken against anyone, even a problem employee, as an example of how someone was punished for being involved in an error or adverse event. They will remember that incident far longer than they will remember a senior leadership visit that occurred during the same week.

Punishment is important to consider from an employee's perspective. Managers sometimes think that formal disciplinary action, such as an official written warning, is the only type of punitive action. However, staff members often feel penalized in other ways, such as when they are criticized in front of others, when an error or adverse event in which they were involved is discussed at a staff meeting with emphasis on how "someone" made a mistake (even if no names are mentioned), or when details of reported errors or adverse events are attached to their performance appraisals. Anytime staff members walk away from an event feeling that they may have been at fault or that management views them that way, they perceive the environment as punitive and become less likely to voluntarily report a problem in the future.

Dealing with Adverse Events

Handling an adverse event in a healthcare organization can be enormously complicated. Emotions add further complexity when a patient has been harmed. External pressures can escalate the intensity of the situation when media and regulatory agencies become involved. All of these factors increase the natural tendency to blame someone. Leaders are pressured to identify the responsible parties and report on actions taken. At such times, leaders and managers must work with everyone involved to prevent a blame-focused or punitive response. Human factors expert James Reason (1997) provided resources on this subject in *Managing the Risks of Organizational Accidents*, including an algorithm to distinguish between systems issues and individual culpability when analyzing an error or event. With this tool, managers are prompted to consider key questions to determine whether a system failure occurred. Rather than assuming that an employee simply did not follow a policy, an investigator should evaluate aspects such as whether the policy was readily available, easily understandable, and workable. The investigator also should apply a substitution test to determine the likelihood that the same event would occur with three other employees with similar experience and training and in similar circumstances (e.g., hours on duty, fatigue, workload). If the same event is likely to occur, the problem is systems related.

Disclosure of harm to patients and families is another difficult task that hospital leaders and physicians must manage when an adverse event occurs. Disclosure often has been handled poorly, resulting in the perception that those in healthcare cover up for each other. Punitive responses from regulatory agencies, accreditation bodies, insurers, and licensing boards discourage healthcare organizations and practitioners from reporting events, unless mandated by law. Lawyers dissuade practitioners from apologizing to patients when an adverse event occurs, advising that doing so could be considered an admission of guilt and could place individuals and the organization at risk for lawsuits, punitive damage awards, and loss of public trust as well as market share.

Fearful of lawsuits, practitioners and representatives of healthcare organizations stay silent, say little, or speak vaguely about the event. Their reticence frustrates patients and families, who often know that something has gone wrong but are unable to obtain a straight answer, which leads to distrust and actually increases the likelihood that they will file a lawsuit. Many who have filed malpractice lawsuits have reported that they were not motivated by a desire for retribution or a large financial settlement but by the hope that filing suit would enable them to discover the truth about what happened, obtain an apology, and ensure that other patients and families would be spared the same experience. Public concern about disclosure of events led The Joint Commission to add standards that require accredited organizations to inform patients or their legal guardians of any unanticipated outcome, be it the result of an error or a known side effect of their treatment.

Involving patients and families in discussions about their care throughout the entire process is an essential element in cultural change. Patient centeredness is one of the changes recommended in the IOM's 2001 report *Crossing the Quality Chasm*. Every part of a patient's care should focus on the patient's needs first, not the needs of physicians, nurses, or other clinical personnel or those of hospitals or other healthcare agencies. Active participation by patients and families in rounds, goal setting, verification of identity before procedures, and verification of medications before administration are just a few examples of how patients' needs should be integrated into the process. A safety-focused culture must include patients, and open discussion in one area will encourage openness in other areas.

Reporting Errors and Adverse Events

Efforts to raise staff awareness of the need to report will increase reporting, but not substantially or for long. To improve their systems, organizations need to know as much as possible about the errors and adverse events that are occurring. Most rely on voluntary reporting systems to gather information, but as previously mentioned, those sources are not the most reliable and underreporting is a significant problem. To increase reporting, well-intentioned individuals in healthcare organizations typically try a variety of initiatives, including education fairs, posters, safety hotlines, shorter reporting forms, and raffles or prizes for departments that file the most reports. Strong emphasis is placed on the guaranteed anonymity of the reporting mechanisms and the nonpunitive nature of the system. For a short time, reporting increases, and the improved culture and new knowledge are celebrated. However, over time, reporting usually declines to where it was before, if not lower, leaving those who led the initiative feeling discouraged and disheartened. They may rally and try again, only to repeat the same cycle.

Why does a reporting initiative lead to this cycle instead of to sustained levels of increased reporting? The reason is the failure to address the core issue: the underlying culture. The emphasis on reporting causes a temporary increase but is not integrated into the daily routine, so unless follow-up initiatives keep the momentum going, reporting is eventually discussed less and less. Incentives may help, but their effectiveness is highest when they are new, and over time, people either forget about them or are no longer motivated by them. The reporting system itself may be complicated and burdensome, requiring too much time for practitioners to complete in a busy day. Also, the focus on guaranteed anonymity may cause the opposite of the desired effect. In a just culture, no one should need anonymity when reporting because there should be no fear of reprisal. Emphasizing guaranteed anonymity may be important in the early stages but may leave staff with the impression that the potential for punitive action still exists.

Hospitals that have seen significant and sustained increases in voluntary reporting rates have achieved these results not by concentrating efforts on reporting practices but rather by focusing on culture and creating a safety-conscious environment. Visible leadership commitment to safety and strategies to improve teamwork at all levels is a fundamental first step. Once the dialogue begins, feedback becomes critical. As frontline staff begin to call attention to safety issues and opportunities for improvement, belief in the new system will be established only if management provides feedback about suggestions. As these changes take root in the organization, the culture changes and voluntary reporting increases to levels not previously seen.

Even in a safety-conscious culture, errors will continue to occur; the difference is how they are handled. Reason (1990) describes two types of errors: active and latent. In an active error, the effects or consequences occur immediately. For example, an active error occurs when a driver steps on the gas pedal instead of the brake when shifting out of park and crashes through the garage wall. (This error is why automobiles now have a forcing function that locks the shift in park unless the driver's foot is on the brake.) In contrast, a latent error exists within a system for a long time without causing harm until a combination of other factors precipitate a chain of events that incorporates the latent error and results in disaster. The loss of the *Challenger* space shuttle was found to be the catastrophic result of latent errors, as have many other well-known disasters (Reason 1990). Retrospective reviews of adverse events in healthcare also usually reveal latent errors as contributing factors.

Each error or adverse event presents an opportunity for learning and sharing lessons both internally and externally. When creating a safety-oriented culture, an organization must ensure that information about errors and the actions taken to reduce them are shared openly. Frontline employees can learn a great deal from hearing about the experiences of others, and organizations should provide mechanisms that encourage such sharing. Incorporating patient-safety issues into change-of-shift reports and setting aside regular times for staff safety briefings are just a couple of the ways that communication and teamwork can be enhanced. Organizations should also find ways to disseminate information about errors and the actions taken to reduce them across departments, units, and divisions. Sharing a safety lesson from one area across the entire organization is an important step in reducing the risk that the same latent errors may exist in other departments.

Hospitals can learn more about patient-safety issues through deeper analysis of patient mortality. Overall mortality rates, especially those adjusted for severity by the hospital standardized mortality ratio (HSMR), can be useful to hospital leaders because they indicate whether one hospital's inpatient mortality is higher or lower than expected and how it compares to others. A hospital with a higher-than-expected HSMR should learn more about the inpatients who die to discover what opportunities for improvement may exist.

Of course, not all patients who die in the hospital die from adverse events or failures in care. In-hospital deaths occur from a variety of causes, including severe illness or injury and progression of disease. IHI's Hospital Mortality Review Tool helps to analyze patient deaths by looking at where an admitted patient was assigned (critical care or not) and whether the patient was admitted for comfort care associated with a terminal diagnosis. Those two questions place each case in one of four categories, or boxes, in a 2 × 2 matrix. For example, patients who were not admitted to critical care and who did not have a terminal diagnosis on admission were probably not expected to die in hospital. Such cases warrant analysis, and many hospitals have uncovered safety issues that can be addressed, such as earlier recognition of deterioration and improved communication between care team members. Analysis also can reveal opportunities for more effective use of hospital resources and the need for better support services outside the hospital for patients with terminal diagnoses.

Learning from the external environment is also important. Fortunately, the most serious adverse events, such as removal of the wrong limb, are rare. Even in hospitals where such an event has never occurred, however, avoiding complacency is essential. Anytime a serious adverse event occurs at any hospital anywhere, the lessons learned should be available to all hospitals so that all can analyze their own processes for areas that need improvement. Unfortunately, such information may not be easy to provide because legal concerns and privacy protections prevent or hinder many organizations from sharing details. To facilitate learning and improvement, organizations such as The Joint Commission and the Institute for Safe Medication Practices have published newsletter articles about serious adverse events without identifying the organizations or people involved. However, despite such worthwhile efforts, the same events continue to occur.

Looking to Other Industries

Healthcare should look to other industries for ideas about how to implement safer practices. A common argument against using approaches from other industries is that healthcare is different or that "we are not making widgets." Healthcare professionals do carry a special and unique responsibility because we are entrusted with the care of our fellow human beings. However, we still can learn from other industries.

Healthcare is not the only industry in which an error can result in the loss of life. For example, hundreds or even thousands of lives can be lost at once in fields such as aviation, in and around nuclear power plants, and on nuclear aircraft carriers. Yet despite their enormous risks and extremely complex processes, their safety records far exceed those in healthcare. In *Managing the Unexpected*, Weick and Sutcliffe (2001) describe organizations in these industries as *high-reliability organizations*. Daily work is centered around expectation and anticipation of failure rather than success, which results in regular, early identification of errors and error-producing processes and leads to continuous improvement of processes and routines. Healthcare leaders would be foolish not to learn more about how these organizations have achieved their safety records and which aspects are applicable to their own organizations.

One tool that was developed in industrial settings and has been applied in healthcare is failure modes and effects analysis (FMEA). FMEA is a systematic, prospective method of evaluating a process to predict where and how it might fail and of assessing the relative effects of those failures to identify which parts of the process need the most revision. FMEA includes review of

- steps in the process,
- failure modes (what could go wrong),
- failure causes (why the failure would happen), and
- failure effects (what the consequences of each failure would be).

An advantage of FMEA is that it alerts users to potential failures and enables users to prevent those failures by correcting the related processes, rather than merely react to adverse events after failures have occurred. FMEA thus contrasts with root cause analysis (RCA), which is conducted only after an event has occurred and which assumes that there was only one cause for an adverse event, which is rarely the case. Because FMEA looks at the entire process and every potential for failure, its perspective is broader. FMEA is particularly useful in evaluating a new process before its implementation and in assessing the outcome of a proposed change to an existing process. Using this approach, organizations can consider many options and assess potential consequences in a safe environment before making changes in the patient care process.

By emphasizing prevention, FMEA reduces the risk of harm to both patients and staff. Although prevention plays a key role in improving safety, not all errors can be prevented. When an error does occur, an important consideration is how visible it will be. When FMEA is used, each process is assigned a numeric value of risk called a risk priority number (RPN). The RPN is used to assess progress, and a drop in that number indicates improvement. An RPN is determined by answering three questions—one for each failure mode—and assigning each answer a value between 1 and 10, with 1 standing for very unlikely and 10 indicating very likely.

1. *Likelihood of occurrence*: What is the likelihood that this failure mode will occur?

2. *Likelihood of detection*: If this failure mode occurs, what is the likelihood that the failure will **not** be detected?

3. *Severity*: If this failure mode occurs, what is the likelihood that harm will occur?

The second question, about detection, relates directly to the issue of visibility. If an error is likely to occur and likely to go undetected, then in addition to devising prevention strategies, it is important to look for methods of alerting staff that an error has occurred. An example is the use of alert screens in computerized provider order entry (CPOE) systems. If a provider makes an error while ordering medications, an alert screen immediately announces the need to make a change.

Mitigation is a third and equally important factor in making practices safer. Despite well-designed prevention and detection strategies, some errors will slip through and reach the patient. The ultimate goal in patient safety is not to cause harm. When an error does reach a patient, quick recognition and appropriate intervention can prevent or significantly reduce harm to the patient. Training staff in response techniques through the use of drills and simulations and ensuring that the resources needed for interventions are readily available in patient-care areas can mitigate such events (Nolan 2000). A comprehensive approach to patient safety requires that changes be made to improve all three areas: prevention, detection, and mitigation.

Using Technology to Improve Patient Safety

Technology often is seen as a solution to safer care, and although advances have offered many ways to improve systems and processes, each new technology also introduces new occasions for error. A good basic rule before implementing a technological solution is never to automate a bad process. If frequent errors or process breakdowns reveal that a process is not working well, adding technology to it usually will not solve the underlying problems. Rather, the addition of technology may worsen the situation because more process failures may become more evident. Consequently, the technology is blamed for being worthless and is abandoned or not used. CPOE is an example of a technological addition. Almost every hospital in the United States has implemented this technology, which offers benefits such as decision support and elimination of illegible orders. Some hospitals have learned the hard way that implementation of CPOE should not coincide with the implementation of standardized processes that have not been used previously, such as order sets or protocols. Testing and implementing these approaches using existing systems (even paper ones) first is often best. This provides physicians and staff with an opportunity to learn and become accustomed to the new processes and integrate them into their routines. When CPOE is introduced later, the standard processes are in place and transferred to the new system so that users only need to learn the new prescribing method. Introducing standardized ordering processes and CPOE simultaneously has sometimes led to the failure of both.

Any new technology also introduces new chances for error and failure. Technological solutions often are used in systems and processes that are already complex, and a change to one part of the system can produce unexpected effects in another (Shojania et al. 2002). No technology will eliminate all errors; in fact, different ones will need to be addressed. In this situation, too, FMEA can aid staff in predicting potential failures of technology and developing processes to prevent, detect, and mitigate those failures.

The many features of technology must be used in a balanced manner. Overuse of any feature will diminish its effectiveness over time. For example, in a CPOE system, alerts and pop-up screens can provide critical prescribing information to users and even deal with high-risk situations by requiring the use of an override. However, if too many alerts appear, users will begin to ignore them and routinely proceed to the next screen without reading the alert information, which could allow a serious error to slip through the system. Audible alarms pose similar problems and should be programmed to sound only when attention is truly required. If equipment alarms go off too frequently or for reasons that do not require immediate attention, staff will become complacent about them. This behavior often can be observed in patient care units where many monitors, ventilators, and other equipment are used and alarms sound frequently and for long periods. Bypassing alert screens and not responding quickly to alarms cannot be blamed on the people involved; such reactions are the predictable by-products of improperly designed systems. We are overloaded with the visual and auditory stimulation of technology, and our natural defense mechanism is to shut some of it out. Alarm fatigue is of growing concern in healthcare and has been cited in a number of media stories about tragic events. Other industries already consider this behavior in their safety designs, and healthcare must too.

Designing Safe Processes

To prevent harm to patients, healthcare organizations must deliberately design patient care systems for safety. The foundation for success in this journey is the creation and development of a safety-conscious culture. Organizations must assess processes and systems for change according to the following principles:

1. Start with adoption of recommended, evidence-based practices and use resources to support implementation. Key practices for protecting patients from harm are well supported by evidence, have been recommended by multiple expert and clinical organizations, and

should be the starting point for any hospital striving to prevent harm. Organizations such as The Joint Commission, the National Quality Forum, and the Leapfrog Group have promoted and published these key practices, and the Centers for Medicare & Medicaid Services (CMS) and private insurers are using a number of them as the basis for reimbursement and reporting requirements. Other organizations, such as AHRQ, IHI, and the CMS Partnership for Patients, have made strategies for successful implementation of these practices widely available.

2. Incorporate human factors into training and procedures. Expect and plan for error, rather than react to it in surprise.

3. Design processes to be safely and reliably executed by staff with varying levels of experience, training, and environmental or personal stress. Every process should be designed so that a recently graduated nurse who is performing it for the second or third time will be able to do it as safely and reliably as a nurse with 20 years of experience who has done it hundreds of times. Safeguards to account for variations in human factors must be designed into the system.

4. Design technology and procedures for end users, planning for failures (Norman 1988). Until all medical-device manufacturers adopt this approach, healthcare organizations, as purchasers, are responsible for seeking devices that incorporate safe designs and developing procedures to support safe use.

5. Decrease complexity by reducing the number of steps in a process whenever possible (Nolan 2000). As the number of steps in a process increases, the likelihood that the process will be executed without error decreases. Periodically review all processes to determine whether they include steps that no longer provide value; all processes tend to change over time.

6. Ensure that safety initiatives address prevention, detection, and mitigation (Nolan 2000). All three are necessary to reduce harm. FMEA can assist in assessing whether they are addressed.

7. Standardize processes, tools, technology, and equipment. Variation increases complexity and the risk of error. Technology can offer great benefits but must be applied to processes that already function well. Equipment may come with features that decrease reliance on memory and thereby enhance safety, but if too many different types of equipment are in use, the risk increases that staff will make errors because buttons, switches, and other interfaces for similar functions may be located in different places. Imagine how difficult driving a rental car would be if every car manufacturer placed the gas pedal, the brake pedal, and other key controls in different locations or used a variety of designs. Many medical devices introduce those very difficulties.

8. Clearly label medications, solutions, and individual doses, including generic and trade names. Take special measures to distinguish between drugs that have similar-sounding names. (Unfortunately, healthcare organizations must add processes to address this issue because patient safety usually is not considered during the selection of drug names.)

9. Use bar coding. The Food and Drug Administration adopted bar-coding requirements for all medications in 2004, a worthy and long-overdue measure considering that supermarkets have been using bar-code readers for decades. Healthcare is shamefully behind in this regard, especially when one compares the difference in consequences between administering the wrong blood product and charging the wrong price for a grocery item. This technology will become a standard part of healthcare delivery.

10. Use forcing functions to prevent certain types of errors from occurring, but be sure to use them in a balanced manner. Staff will find ways to work around too many constraints or simple tasks that are made unnecessarily difficult. Only make things difficult that should be difficult (Norman 1988).

These elements are not new to quality improvement, industry, or, in some cases, even healthcare; yet, healthcare has not adopted them widely. As we work toward decreasing and eliminating the unintended harm that our systems cause, we must realize that our industry can, in fact, learn from industries outside of healthcare. The analogies are not perfect, for there are some distinct and important differences, but healthcare must learn from other industries if it is to achieve significant improvements in safety within our lifetime. We are privileged to work in professions that give us the opportunity to care for our fellow human beings, helping to relieve their maladies and ensuring them dignified deaths. This privilege obligates us to use every possible resource and tool at our disposal—whether created in our own industry or in others—to ensure care is delivered in the safest manner possible and never causes unintended harm. Every patient has that right.

Clinical and Operational Issues

Patient Safety Research

Many of the greatest breakthroughs in patient care have come about through research. As clinicians continue to seek improved ways of caring for their patients, research will result in new discoveries that will alter the delivery of care. Today, healthcare has best practices for many clinical conditions. Studies have demonstrated that these practices are reliable, and clinical experts agree.

Best practices include diagnostic tests for identifying disease and assessing its severity as well as interventions that improve patient outcomes. Despite the amount of knowledge that has been accumulated about these practices and the general acceptance of their validity, huge variations in their adoption and use remain a problem because they take an average of 17 years from publication of evidence to adoption (Kohn, Corrigan, and Donaldson 2000). One study found that accepted best practices for certain conditions are used in the treatment of only 50 percent of appropriate patients, at most (McGlynn et al. 2003). Failure to use a universally accepted treatment protocol is arguably a planning error, unless it is clinically contraindicated.

Limitations of Research

Research provides wonderful new knowledge, but it has some limitations. Insistence that complete and thorough research must be completed before change can take place hinders progress and the adoption of safe practices. It is also unrealistic because complete evidence for anything will never exist (Leape, Berwick, and Bates 2002). Some practices to improve patient safety make sense and do not need research studies to prove their effectiveness; they should simply be implemented. For example, how could anyone who has seen an illegible order for medication claim that we need to conduct studies about the effectiveness of computerized systems that reduce or eliminate the need for handwritten orders? Why would research need to be conducted to prove the importance of verifying a patient's identity before performing a medical intervention? Although research does provide valuable information for clinical diagnosis and treatment, we cannot research everything and should not let it become an obstacle that prevents us from adopting safer practices—especially those that do not alter **what** care is given, just **how** it is given.

Effects of Fatigue

An area that researchers have studied, in healthcare and in other industries, is the effect of fatigue on error and safety. Studies have shown that an individual who is sleep deprived demonstrates cognitive function at the ninth percentile of the overall population (Shojania et al. 2002). A person who has been awake for 24 hours often acts and makes errors similar to those of a person who is under the influence of alcohol. Despite these findings, healthcare remains one of the only high-risk professions that, until recently, did not restrict workers' hours (Leape, Berwick, and Bates 2002). In 2010, the Accreditation Council for Graduate Medical Education (the accreditation body for postgraduate medical training, or residency, programs) instituted requirements intended to address fatigue. While these are a good start, some patient-safety experts consider them inadequate. Further, no rest requirements exist for physicians who are not in training or other clinical personnel in the healthcare setting. Because many personnel work at more than one organization, no one sees the total picture. The situation is not easy to address. Given the current shortages in most clinical professions and the increasing numbers of hospitalized patients, most organizations rely on staff overtime to meet staffing levels, especially in states with mandated staffing ratios. All of these factors contribute to high workloads, increased work hours, and greater staff fatigue—circumstances that are known to contribute to the commission of errors.

Economics and Patient Safety

Healthcare is facing turbulent times, and financial pressures weigh heavily on many healthcare leaders. In addition to staffing shortages, there are concerns regarding reimbursement, malpractice coverage, regulatory requirements, and access to healthcare for the uninsured. Any healthcare CEO would agree that patient safety is important, but in actual practice it becomes a low priority in most organizations (Shojania et al. 2002). So many issues vie for attention that safety is frequently lost in the fray. Ask a hospital CEO which meeting she would be more concerned about missing—the finance committee or the patient safety committee—and she would likely choose the former.

Many factors affect healthcare, and economics is an important one (Kohn, Corrigan, and Donaldson 2000). Unsafe practices contribute to cost in many ways. Cost considerations include—but are not limited to—efficiency, increased length of stay, turnover, absorbed costs when an error or adverse event occurs, malpractice settlements, and increased premiums. The dollars lost to safety lapses every year are staggering, to say nothing of the consequences to the patients who are harmed, something that cannot always be measured in financial terms. In 2010, the US Department of Health & Human Services Office of Inspector General (OIG 2010) conducted a study of adverse events experienced by Medicare patients in US hospitals. The study found that 27 percent of beneficiaries had experienced harm. Forty-four percent of the harmful incidents were deemed preventable, and the excess cost to Medicare from adverse events was estimated at $4.4 billion annually.

Patient safety must become a priority for healthcare leaders in action as well as in word. In a safety-oriented organization, everyone takes responsibility for safety. All organizations should strive to function that way, all employees and clinicians should want to work in that kind of environment, and all patients should demand to be treated that way. We can hope that in the near future, we will be able to claim that all of healthcare has achieved the safety record that anesthesia has realized. We can hope that hospitals will be included in the list of high-reliability organizations. We must start working toward those ends so that all patients can access any part of the healthcare system confidently, without fear of harm.

Case Study: Order of Saint Francis Healthcare System

By Kathleen M. Haig and Carol Haraden

The Order of Saint Francis (OSF) Healthcare System began its journey toward safer healthcare in earnest after the release of IOM's *Crossing the Quality Chasm* report in 2001. The healthcare system operates hospital facilities, various physician office practices, urgent care centers, and extended care facilities in Illinois and Michigan. Like many organizations, OSF took the IOM report's call to action seriously and has created some of the safest systems of care in the United States.

Similar to all organizations that create transformative and lasting change, OSF employed a top-down and bottom-up improvement strategy. The corporate office and individual hospital leaders made safer care a top strategic priority. They added muscle to that declaration by tying the executive compensation package to key safety indicators. OSF also began building the robust infrastructure needed to create and sustain change at the front line. It appointed a corporate patient-safety officer and a physician change agent at the corporate office as well as patient-safety officers at each hospital site. The patient-safety officers reported directly to senior leadership, and their role was designed to allow them to work at all levels of the organization and instigate improvement driven by strategic priorities.

To kick-start its safety journey in 2001, OSF enrolled St. Joseph Medical Center in the Quantum Leaps in Patient Safety collaborative with IHI. St. Joseph Medical Center was one of 50 national and international teams that formed a learning community that would bring about unprecedented change in adverse drug event rates over the next year. An OSF team of early adopters representing administration, medical staff, nursing, and pharmacy was established and given the task of creating a strong and successful prototype. The team then used those successful changes to spread improvements throughout the organization. Leadership provided both human and financial resources and removed barriers so that the team could do its best work. OSF used the same successful process to reduce mortality and global harm rates as well, in each case beginning with a prototype team that created successful, local change that was spread throughout each hospital in the OSF Healthcare System. The combination of fully engaged leadership, a creative and committed frontline team, the expectation of organization-wide spread coupled with explicit spread plans, and the development and use of a robust measurement capability was responsible for creating the unprecedented level of safety later witnessed.

To dramatically improve adverse drug event rates, OSF determined that the following changes needed to be made:

1. Improve the safety culture and maintain a cultural survey score that demonstrates that staff have a strong belief in the importance of safe practice and experience the system of care in which they operate as respectful, empowering, and committed to learning and clear communication.

2. Develop a medication reconciliation process to ensure that patients are on the correct medications at every point in their care. OSF has implemented an electronic health record (EHR) that includes medication reconciliation in the physician and nurse work flows. OSF facilities also have a pharmacist review of discharge medications in addition to completing the medication reconciliation process. Work on this complex process continues to ensure that every patient leaves the facility with an accurate medication list every time.

3. Use FMEA to reduce risk and improve the reliability of processes. FMEA was first applied to medication dispensing. Changes implemented included automated dispensing cabinets in most OSF facilities and both bar coding and CPOE in conjunction with implementation of the EHR. Then, after a news story about a surgical fire resulting in a death in another facility in southern Illinois, OSF conducted FMEA to assess the risk potential for surgical fires. Based on the FMEA findings, gap analyses in each hospital, and a literature search of best practices, the OSF board of directors approved recommendations for implementation in each facility to reduce the risk of surgical fire.

4. Standardize the dosing and management of high-risk medications. At the start of the journey, medication events were occurring at rates that translated into the occurrence of adverse events in parts per 1,000 doses. The organization's goal was to decrease the number of adverse events so that they occurred in parts per 10,000—in other words, nearly a full year would be needed to realize the same number of adverse events that, at the time, were occurring in a month.

5. Train staff in use of SBAR. Beginning in 2004, staff at St. Joseph Medical Center were trained to communicate with physicians using SBAR supported by pocket cards and laminated "cheat sheets" posted at telephones. By 2005, more than 98 percent of nurses were using this communication model.

6. Initiate system-wide collaboratives addressing reduction in healthcare-associated infections and reduction in the percentage of elective deliveries performed before 39 weeks of gestation. OSF initiated these collaboratives in 2011.

Defining culture as "the predominating attitudes and behavior that characterize the functioning of a group or organization," OSF St. Joseph

Medical Center initiated and continues today to pursue efforts to compre-
hensively redesign its culture and care systems to reduce the rate of harm to
patients.

Reducing Adverse Events

Reducing adverse events at OSF required multifaceted changes in many
processes. No single change or small combination of changes could take
an organization to that level of safety. In 2001, OSF began by measuring
medication-related harm using the IHI Adverse Drug Event Trigger Tool.
Data indicated the hospital's adverse drug event rate was 5.8 per 1,000
doses dispensed, and a goal was set to reduce this rate to 0.58 adverse drug
events per 1,000 doses. Later, in 2004, OSF expanded the measurement to
hospital-wide adverse events using the IHI Global Trigger Tool, which it still
uses today.

OSF learned a lot about the medication harm in its system. The
organization was also concerned about its rates of reported actual errors and
potential errors. To improve these rates and the organization's learning, OSF
established an adverse-drug-event hotline. The hotline was located in the
pharmacy so that a pharmacist could check it daily for reported events and
proceed with investigations into potential causes. This solution was win–win
because the hotline identified the event for evaluation and trending, and the
staff reported easily, quickly, and anonymously and saved time by avoiding
the paperwork previously needed to complete an occurrence report. The
reporting rates of actual and potential errors improved markedly.

A key change in the reduction of adverse drug events was the use of
a medication-reconciliation process. Medication reconciliation is the act of
comparing the medications a patient has been taking with the medications
currently ordered. The reconciliation process allows the caregiver to identify
the correct medications, discover those that were missed, and identify those
that need to be continued, discontinued, or adjusted for frequency on the
basis of the patient's changing condition.

Standardization of orders based on known best practices reduced
the variability of individual clinician practices and dramatically reduced the
number of adverse drug events. In preparing to implement the EHR, a team
of system representatives, including specialty physicians and pharmacists, created more than 400 order sets covering a multitude of specialties to be used
for CPOE. The order sets were standardized across the OSF system by use
of pharmacy-based services and order sets. In 2011, each hospital had a phar-
macy-driven anticoagulation dosing program, and each ambulatory region
had an anticoagulation clinic. Renal dosing services were conducted on all
patients with a creatinine clearance of less than 50 milliliters. Development
of a perioperative beta-blocker protocol resulted in a dramatic and sustained
reduction of perioperative myocardial infarctions and realized an unexpected

benefit of reduced narcotic usage in patients receiving beta-blockers due to this protocol.

One of the most fundamental and important changes was the availability of pharmacists on the nursing units to review and enter medication orders. Pharmacists were able to look at the orders firsthand and identify potential dosing errors and drug interactions.

Cultural Changes

OSF had to transform its culture while creating remedies for care processes and high-risk medications. This work, although less evident, was essential to create and maintain a culture that could sustain and improve safety over time. It involved embedding safety into the very fabric of the organization— incorporating safety aims in the organization's mission statement, corporate strategic goals, job descriptions, and meeting agendas. The transformation involved regular communication and reminders about safety through meetings, conference calls, visits, and learning sessions. It was ever present and unrelenting.

In addition, specific changes made the importance of safety visible to frontline employees. The first change was the introduction of unit safety briefings. The staff gathered at a specified time for a five- to ten-minute review of safety concerns on the unit that day. Staff identified concerns involving equipment, medications, and care processes that posed a safety issue. The patient safety officer assigned the issues to the appropriate personnel for investigation and resolution. To close the communication loop, the issues and their resolutions were summarized and presented to staff monthly.

The second change was the institution of executive rounds. A senior leader visited a patient care area weekly to demonstrate commitment to safety by gathering information about the staff's safety concerns. The rounds also served to educate senior executives about the type and extent of safety issues in their organizations. The issues were logged into a database, owners were assigned for resolution, and a feedback loop to the staff was established.

To measure the effect of all changes on the safety culture, a survey was conducted every six months to measure the cultural climate of the staff surrounding patient-safety initiatives. The survey was a modified version of the survey developed by J. Bryan Sexton and Robert Helmreich and used by the aviation industry and NASA. Since the early days of administering this safety-culture survey, OSF has adopted the AHRQ Hospital Survey on Patient Safety. OSF has enhanced the process by setting the expectation that each hospital will evaluate the survey results, develop an action plan, assign accountability for the action steps taken, and submit the action plan to the board of directors. An update on the progress of the implementation and effectiveness of the action plan is incorporated into the annual patient safety review. To advance the culture across the continuum, OSF has added its medical office practices and nursing home to the survey process. Survey results are submitted for inclusion in the national database for benchmarking purposes.

To enhance the robustness of event investigation, a system-wide policy has been enacted specifying use of a five-step process to address serious reportable events. The five steps include signal detection, RCA, development of a corrective action plan, implementation of the corrective action plan, and follow-up monitoring of the effectiveness of the actions taken. Each action requires a measurement that must meet target before the event is recommended for closure. Additionally, the events and corrective actions are shared system-wide for learning purposes and prevention of similar future harm in other OSF facilities.

Results

OSF's hard work resulted in the following improvements:

- Medication reconciliation was introduced in the summer of 2001; by May 2003, admission reconciliation ranged from 85 percent to 95 percent, transfer reconciliation was at 70 percent, and discharge reconciliation was at 95 percent.
- The organization completed FMEAs on medication ordering and dispensing and then worked on reducing the risk at every step. The risk priority scores decreased 34 percent for ordering and 66 percent for dispensing.
- Culture survey results in the first year improved from a baseline score of 3.96 to 4.28 (out of a maximum score of 5).
- OSF's overall CPOE usage has grown to more than 75 percent.

The organization continues to work hard at making progress every day. Proof of ultimate success came in the form of the most important outcomes:

- In June 2001, the rate of adverse drug events was 5.8 per 1,000 doses. By May 2003, the rate had fallen to only 0.72 per 1,000 doses, an almost tenfold reduction in harm.
- As measured by the IHI Global Trigger Tool, OSF's overall adverse event rate was 98 adverse events per 1,000 patient days in June 2004. That rate decreased significantly to 31 adverse events per 1,000 patient days by March 2007 and fell even further, to 23.71 per 1,000 patient days, by June 2011.
- OSF's HSMR was 103 in 2002. (HSMR is the ratio of actual number of deaths to expected number of deaths, multiplied by 100. A value of 100 indicates that the actual number of patient deaths equals the expected number, whereas an HSMR above 100 means that more died

than expected, and an HSMR below 100 means that fewer died.) In 2006, OSF's HSMR had decreased to 84, indicating that 16 percent fewer patients died than expected, and in 2011, the HSMR had further decreased to 73.

In summary, OSF created a culture of improvement by embracing an organized and corporate-wide method to improve patient care. It created small prototype teams of frontline clinicians who developed robust aims and measures in support of their strategic plan to reduce harm and improve care, first in regard to adverse drug events and later in service of reducing global harm and mortality rates. The teams used various small cycle tests to adapt evidence-based care processes on their units, spread the learning and successful changes to all OSF organizations, and then hardwired those changes into their corporate system. The level of commitment and amount of work that enabled OSF to achieve its successes cannot be overstated.

Study Questions

1. Describe why common methods of reporting and measuring medical errors and adverse events underestimate actual occurrences.
2. Identify three principles to include when designing safer processes and systems, and provide a real example of each (preferably healthcare examples).
3. Explain why the perspective of the patient is the most important determinant of whether an adverse event has occurred.
4. Provide an example of an error that can occur in a healthcare process and result in patient harm. Then, describe a strategy or several strategies that would accomplish each of the following objectives:
   a. Prevent the error from resulting in patient harm
   b. Detect the error when it occurs
   c. Mitigate the amount of harm to the patient

References

Agency for Healthcare Quality and Research (AHRQ). 2012. "Patient Safety Indicators Download." Released March. http://psnet.ahrq.gov/resource.aspx?resourceID=1040.

Blendon, R. J., C. Schoen, C. DesRoches, R. Osborn, and K. Zapert. 2003. "Common Concerns Amid Diverse Systems: Health Care Experiences in Five Countries." *Health Affairs* 22 (3): 106–21.

Brennan, T. A., L. L. Leape, N. M. Laird, L. Herbert, A. R. Localio, A. G. Lawthers, J. P. Newhouse, P. C. Weiler, and H. H. Hiatt. 1991. "Incidence of Adverse Events and Negligence in Hospitalized Patients: Results of the Harvard Medical Practice Study I." *New England Journal of Medicine* 324 (6): 370–76.

Classen, D. C., R. Resar, F. Griffin, F. Federico, T. Frankel, N. Kimmel, J. C. Whittington, A. Frankel, A. Seger, and B. C. James. 2011. "'Global Trigger Tool' Shows That Adverse Events in Hospitals May Be Ten Times Greater Than Previously Measured." *Health Affairs* 30 (4): 581–89.

Findlay, S. (ed.). 2000. *Accelerating Change Today for America's Health: Reducing Medical Errors and Improving Patient Safety*. Washington, DC: National Coalition on Health Care and Institute for Healthcare Improvement.

Frankel, A., E. Graydon-Baker, C. Neppl, T. Simmonds, M. Gustafson, and T. K. Gandhi. 2003. "Patient Safety Leadership WalkRounds." *Joint Commission Journal on Quality and Safety* 29 (1): 16–26.

Gandhi, T. K., S. N. Weingart, J. Borus, A. C. Seger, J. Peterson, E. Burdick, D. L. Seger, K. Shu, F. Federico, L. L. Leape, and D. W. Bates. 2003. "Adverse Drug Events in Ambulatory Care." *New England Journal of Medicine* 348 (16): 1556–64.

Griffin, F. A., and R. K. Resar. 2009. "IHI Global Trigger Tool for Measuring Adverse Events," second edition. IHI Innovation Series white paper. Cambridge, MA: Institute for Healthcare Improvement.

Hayward, R. A., and T. P. Hofer. 2001. "Estimating Hospital Deaths Due to Medical Errors: Preventability Is in the Eye of the Reviewer." *Journal of the American Medical Association* 286 (4): 415–20.

Institute for Healthcare Improvement (IHI). 2013. "SBAR Technique for Communication: A Situational Briefing Model." Updated July 31. www.ihi.org/resources/Pages/Tools/SBARTechniqueforCommunicationASituational BriefingModel.aspx.

———. 2003. "Move Your Dot: Measuring, Evaluating, and Reducing Hospital Mortality Rates (Part 1)." IHI Innovation Series white paper. www.ihi.org/resources/Pages/IHIWhitePapers/MoveYourDotMeasuringEvaluatingand ReducingHospitalMortalityRates.aspx.

Institute of Medicine (IOM). 2001. *Crossing the Quality Chasm: A New Health System for the 21st Century*. Washington, DC: National Academies Press.

Kohn, L. T., J. M. Corrigan, and M. S. Donaldson (eds.). 2000. *To Err Is Human: Building a Safer Health System*. Washington, DC: National Academies Press.

Landrigan, C. P., G. J. Parry, C. B. Bones, A. D. Hackbarth, D. A. Goldmann, and P. J. Sharek. 2010. "Temporal Trends in Rates of Patient Harm Resulting from Medical Care." *New England Journal of Medicine* 363 (22): 2124–34.

Leape, L. L., D. M. Berwick, and D. W. Bates. 2002. "What Practices Will Most Improve Safety? Evidence-Based Medicine Meets Patient Safety." *Journal of the American Medical Association* 288 (4): 501–7.

McGlynn, E. A., S. M. Asch, J. Adams, J. Keesey, J. Hicks, A. DeCristofaro, and E. A. Kerr. 2003. "The Quality of Health Care Delivered to Adults in the United States." *New England Journal of Medicine* 348 (26): 2635–45.

Nolan, T. W. 2000. "System Changes to Improve Patient Safety." *British Medical Journal* 320 (7237): 771–73.

Norman, D. A. 1988. *The Design of Everyday Things.* New York: Doubleday.

Pronovost, P., S. Berenholtz, T. Dorman, P. A. Lipsett, T. Simmonds, and C. Haraden. 2003. "Improving Communication in the ICU Using Daily Goals." *Journal of Critical Care* 18 (2): 71–75.

Reason, J. 1997. *Managing the Risks of Organizational Accidents.* Aldershot, UK: Ashgate.

———. 1990. *Human Error.* New York: Cambridge University Press.

Sexton, J. B. 2002. "Rapid-Fire Safety Ideas Minicourse." Presented at the Institute for Healthcare Improvement 14th Annual National Forum on Quality Improvement in Health Care, Orlando, FL, December 9.

Sexton, J. B., E. J. Thomas, and R. L. Helmreich. 2000. "Error, Stress, and Teamwork in Medicine and Aviation: Cross Sectional Surveys." *British Medical Journal* 320 (7237): 745–49.

Shojania, K. G., B. W. Duncan, K. M. McDonald, and R. M. Wachter. 2002. "Safe but Sound: Patient Safety Meets Evidence-Based Medicine." *Journal of the American Medical Association* 288 (4): 508–13.

US Department of Health & Human Services Office of Inspector General (OIG). 2010. "Adverse Events in Hospitals: National Incidence Among Medicare Beneficiaries." OEI-06-09-00090. Issued November. http://oig.hhs.gov/oei/reports/oei-06-09-00090.pdf.

Weick, K. E., and K. M. Sutcliffe. 2001. *Managing the Unexpected: Assuring High Performance in an Age of Complexity.* San Francisco: Jossey-Bass.

World Health Organization (WHO). 2008. "WHO Surgical Safety Checklist and Implementation Manual." www.who.int/patientsafety/safesurgery/ss_checklist/en/.

CREATING A CULTURE OF SAFETY AND HIGH RELIABILITY

Edward A. Walker

This chapter is about change—change that is not happening fast enough. Many years have passed since the publication of the landmark Institute of Medicine (IOM) report *To Err Is Human*, a bold manifesto documenting the sad state of patient safety in American medicine (Kohn, Corrigan, and Donaldson 2000). At the time of that report's appearance, I was a practicing physician with 20 years' experience sitting in a classroom taking my first course in medical quality. Like many physicians of my generation, I knew that quality could be better and that occasionally we made mistakes; but this report shook me to the core. We were making a substantially greater number of errors than I thought possible, and many of them were serious, harmful events—so many, in fact, that medical care was beginning to be seen as one of the leading causes of death in the United States.

But how could this be true? After all of our training, our commitment to the Hippocratic oath, and the moral imperatives we all cherish to avoid harm, somehow we continue to make mistakes. Ironically, our biggest mistake has been not recognizing that we are making mistakes.

This chapter is about intentionally moving to a system of highly systematic medical care, a culture in which we prevent errors when we can, detect the errors we cannot prevent, and mitigate those that we cannot detect. This cultural transformation requires a deep understanding of the science of high reliability, changing the way we see ourselves as healthcare leaders, and acquiring the ability to influence individuals and large groups in the practice of safe and effective medical care.

Hundreds of articles and book chapters on patient safety have appeared since the IOM report, yet we do not seem to be making the progress we need toward a culture of safety and high reliability. I believe progress has lagged not because we lack information but because we are unable to understand the problem from the perspective of organizational behavior and change management. What we need for success is a thorough grounding in the science of high reliability combined with a commitment based on three organizational leadership foundations—reflective self-awareness, the art of influencing individuals, and a clear understanding of how cultures can change. This approach, which is consistent with the constructs of emotional intelligence and positivity that developed simultaneously in the years following the IOM report, will give us new ways to create and nurture cultures of safety and high reliability.

After reading this chapter, you should be a transformed, committed individual. The traditional textbook chapter format will likely not achieve that aim, but a good story might. The remainder of this chapter is a fictional narrative, in which a young, newly minted chief medical officer (CMO) approaches a senior physician mentor to ask for her help in developing a strategic patient safety plan for their hospital. In the spirit of a Socratic dialogue, the senior physician knows just the right questions to help her young colleague organize what he already knows and to supplement that knowledge with wisdom and practical influence strategies. She accomplishes this in four extended coaching sessions, each of which is based on discussion of a reading packet that focuses on a particular aspect of this transformation. This fictional story format is based on my personal experience in coaching and mentoring real leaders in the creation of highly reliable cultures of safety. Although this story is fiction, the coaching advice and educational packets are not.

You can benefit from this chapter at two levels. The first time you read it, try simply to gain an overview of the transformational issues involved in creating a culture of safety. Sometime later, I invite you to return to take a second pass and to experience the coaching vicariously by following along with the readings listed at the end of the chapter as they are discussed during the four sessions. The chapter is not a substitute for actual mentorship and coaching to create a culture of safety—you will get much farther if you do it for real. Nevertheless, you cannot lose anything by putting yourself in the shoes of this spirited CMO, thinking about your own situation and how you might make similar leaps forward in your quest for improving patient safety in your organization.

Our players in this narrative are Dr. Jeff Donovan, the new CMO of St. Joseph Medical Center, and Dr. Elizabeth Adams, a senior physician who recently arrived at the hospital. Jeff has worked at the hospital for more than ten years and has slowly risen through a variety of clinical administrative positions, serving most recently as chief of staff and medical director of the family medicine clinic. Beth has held a series of senior medical positions in other institutions but has decided to return to clinical care to focus on teaching and the development of new physician

(continued)

> *(continued from previous page)*
>
> leaders as her main passion. Jeff knows the hospital but is new to his role; Beth has the experience but is still learning the culture. Together they are setting out on an exciting coaching partnership as they come to understand and change the culture of St. Joseph.
>
> Beth has coached physician leaders before, and she has a plan. She must cover four major areas with Jeff: (1) building his self-awareness as a quality leader and fostering his personal commitment to patient safety; (2) reviewing the basic concepts of high reliability; (3) increasing his skill at influencing other physicians, both one at a time and in small groups; and (4) fostering his ability to initiate and maintain large-scale culture change. She hopes to address these areas over four extended coaching sessions by giving Jeff a series of reading packets and using the sessions to help him see the opportunities he has before him.

Prologue

"Dr. Adams?"

"Yes, I'm Dr. Adams. How can I help you?"

"Hi, I'm Jeff Donovan, the person who e-mailed you about getting some coaching in my new role as CMO here at the hospital. Several people told me you would be very helpful."

"Hello, Jeff, come on in, and please call me Beth. I was very interested in talking with you after reading your e-mail. It sounds like you have an ambitious new position, and you need some help organizing your safety and quality agenda. I'm new here, but I came from a hospital where safety and quality were well organized, so I think that the two of us together will be able to figure some of this out. I've mentored two or three other physicians in the past two years, and they seem to have done well."

"Thank you, Beth, I really appreciate this. I have to admit that when I got the e-mail describing your mentorship approach, I was initially a bit intimidated by the amount of reading and coaching time you said it would take to accomplish this transition. But as I've thought about it more, I'm beginning to see that it's the only way I can take on such a huge challenge with any chance of success."

"The articles are simply the knowledge base that we will be working with, Jeff. I think you'll come to see that patient safety is about two things: *knowing* and *influencing*. The knowing part has to do with appreciating the evidence base in the fields of high reliability and organizational behavior, but the hard work is learning how to apply that knowledge by influencing individual and culture change. Much of what we'll be talking about is the art of convincing individuals and larger groups that they need to change their behavior and summing that behavior change up into a large-scale culture change. The four reading packets address each of these areas, and we'll just take them one at a time. My plan is to send you away with a packet each time and then spend some time helping you figure out how to apply the learning to your specific situation."

"I'm feeling both excited and a bit overwhelmed; when do we get started?"

"As soon as you're ready. Take a few weeks to do some reading, and let me know when you've worked through the first packet."

> The most important ingredient in launching a successful career as a change agent for a culture of safety is having a mentor to guide the way. Many people find that one mentor is not enough—they need more of a mentorship team. A wise senior leader often provides the experiential perspective for changing people and culture and may even become an executive sponsor for the change. Sometimes, however, the most knowledgeable person about reliability and safety is not a senior leader but the director of a quality department. The key is finding the right person or persons to guide this transformation. Remember, patient safety is about knowledge plus influence.

Session One: Making the Commitment to a High-Reliability Organization

"Jeff, it's great to see you again. Let's start with the big picture. What was the most interesting thing you've learned from the first packet?"

"Well, the article by Porter and Teisberg (2007) about physicians stepping up to leadership roles[1] was excellent. Although many of my colleagues are worried about the uncertainties of what our future health system will look like, physicians will clearly have to take more of a role in directing how and where that system will develop, especially with respect to patient safety and quality. I realize that creating a patient safety culture will be a team effort, but physicians need to step up to lead because they are ultimately responsible for so many of the decisions that affect the safety of our patients. It's clear to me that only strong partnerships with our administrative colleagues will make this happen."

"That's right, Jeff. Neither physicians nor managers alone can create the high-reliability system we need to keep our patients safe. A strong sense of partnership among physicians, nurses, managers, and other members of the healthcare team will be required in this new culture that you are trying to create. The old way of doing things had the risk of compartmentalization—physicians took care of patients, and administrators took care of the business. Not enough people thought of patient safety as a shared systems responsibility, and if we learned anything since the IOM report was published, it's that medical care is a team sport, with the team being the only defense against error. We'll talk about that more next time, but for now I'm glad you're getting the shared responsibility issue."

"Yes, it's clear. My biggest surprise from the packet, however, was the *Health Affairs* article by Wachter (2010), the one that basically says that in the ten years following the IOM report, we hadn't made nearly as much progress as one might expect. If I recall correctly, the author gave an overall grade of C at the five-year point and a B– at the end of the decade. At first I found that hard to believe, but as I reflected on it, thinking about the continued patient harm events in my hospital, it began to make sense."

"How so?"

"This is part of the reason I contacted you. As I started looking around my hospital during my first year as CMO, I became really disillusioned by the average physician's overall lack of focus on safety and quality. Everybody just seems so busy, and getting them to focus on what really makes a difference is difficult. I even discussed this lack of focus with some people one-on-one, and although I couldn't find anyone who wasn't outwardly committed to patient safety and talking about it as a priority, these same people were the ones making most of the errors reported in our web-based patient safety reporting system. To be frank, I seem to have trouble getting people to feel as passionate about safety as I do."

"So why do you think that is?"

"Well, after a little more reflection it became clear. I was just like them until five years ago, when a serious patient error made me pay attention at a much deeper level. Something about the salience of that event overcame my 'business as usual' world. I sometimes worry that only a serious patient event will make all of my colleagues pay attention. I hope that's not the case."

"Good point. What did you think the *Harvard Business Review* article by Kegan and Lahey (2001) has to say about this?"

"The article was about the real reasons people don't change, and it introduced the idea of competing commitments. My understanding of a competing commitment is that people develop commitments or loyalties to values or ideas. Sometimes that commitment or loyalty is to a good thing. But if a leader comes along and requests change to a new value, the commitment to the old one may get in the way of adopting the new value, which often appears to be resistance to the new idea. Take, for example, a commitment to a total quality management efficiency process, such as Toyota Lean or Six Sigma. Most people would agree that removing waste from the system is a desirable goal, but it requires an expenditure of focus, energy, and resources that may, paradoxically, put safety and efficiency in competition with one another. I don't believe that these values are incompatible, but someone who is intensely focused on one goal may need some support to flexibly entertain both values simultaneously."

"So it sounds like you overcame your competing commitments about safety?"

"Yes. Leaders can give very mixed and conflicting messages about what is important. One day we are emphasizing finance; the next it's efficiency and productivity, then clinical outcomes, and later we move on to satisfied patients. Of course these are all important quality goals, but I think it's easy for a busy physician just to withdraw and go back to doing whatever he or she thinks is important—which could be seen as resistance to change."

"I agree. So it sounds like you need some guiding principles to help sort out all these competing values. Did any of the readings help there?"

"The two IOM reports really speak to this. *To Err Is Human* (Kohn, Corrigan, and Donaldson 2000) makes the case for error reduction, but the second report, *Crossing the Quality Chasm* (IOM 2001), provides the guide. Together they focus on using models to guide the design of systems toward safety through high reliability while balancing competing commitments. I really like the STEEEP model that the IOM offers—you know, care that is safe, timely, effective, efficient, equitable, and patient centered. The model helps sort out the problem of competing commitments so that each aspect of the model gets its appropriate amount of attention, removing the need for the domains to compete with one another. Having said that, I still feel that financial issues have prioritized efficiency at the expense of other elements of the model. I see many more projects in cost cutting than in patient safety."

"Does that surprise you?"

"Not really. Given the perils of healthcare finance these days, an emphasis on 'no margin, no mission' is understandable. Nevertheless, if the model isn't balanced across all six aspects of quality, patients are harmed in one way or another."

Quality models are essential to achieve this balance. In the absence of an overall structural quality model, individual dimensions of quality, such as efficiency, can exert undue dominance and subtract focus and resources from other aspects of quality, such as safety. Your duty as a leader is to balance the six dimensions of quality while understanding that patient safety is the most important one—the prime directive. One way to do this is to learn more about the business case for quality. High-quality care uses resources in the most efficient manner and is more cost-effective in the long run as well as safer for the patient.

"Jeff, let's move in a different direction for a moment. You spoke before about having a passion for quality, particularly patient safety, based on a personal experience. What happened?"

"It's not something I'm proud of, and I dislike talking about it, but you need to know. A few years ago, I wrote an order using an unapproved abbreviation that was misunderstood by the nurse, and the wrong drug was given to a patient. Unfortunately, this error resulted in a bad outcome, and the patient eventually died. I got help dealing with this incident, but the only thing that has ever made me feel better about it was the idea of working to prevent a similar occurrence. It shook me out of my complacency when I realized that errors could happen to me. Before then, I guess I somehow thought that only 'bad doctors' made errors, and I knew I wasn't a bad doctor. Since then, I've come to understand how easily errors can be made, how frequently they happen in the hospital, and how just a minute of inattention can result in a bad outcome. What I worry about now, as a leader, is how to create that same urgency to change—we shouldn't wait for bad things to happen to patients before we change as physicians."

"It doesn't have to be this way, Jeff. Many physicians change their practice as a result of leaders like you creating an environment where they vicariously experience the type of change required to avoid these bad outcomes. I'm sorry that you had this experience, but at the same time I'm glad that you've turned it into something positive. Stay with that positivity for a moment—it sounds like you've really changed. Can you say more about the way you would like people to be to effect this patient safety mission?"

"Something that really helped me was a lecture I heard by a professor about leadership and quality. He pointed out that unless I was willing to focus on my own leadership development first, it was unlikely that I would make an impact on the patient-safety awareness of others. He talked about three dimensions: (1) *passionate preparation*, the ability to publicly demonstrate energy and commitment to a safe patient environment; (2) *knowledge and resources*, knowing the literature and tools of patient safety; and (3) *relentless execution*, the ability to get things done and to be unstoppable. As I thought about my own journey, these three dimensions have been critical components of my own leadership development. Even though patient safety is a noble idea that everybody wants to be passionate about, the competing values we talked about before can make it difficult to stay focused. It takes self-awareness and leadership to make patient safety happen."

"Excellent, Jeff. It all starts with you. Nothing happens until the leaders of the organization realize they are role models and start walking the talk of patient safety. What are some of the things that you have done or plan to do to help people see their responsibility?"

"Well, fortunately, I've found many ways to do this. It all starts with a commitment to mindfulness about safety. The book on mindfulness by Boyatzis and McKee (2005) really confirmed what I have learned. For example,

I used to begin my day by listening to NPR as I drove to work. Now I spend that time thinking about what's important in the care of patients and what I can do to make things better. I started putting five-minute patient safety stories at the beginning of important meetings. I found these stories really focus people's attention on what is important, which then becomes a kind of expectation after a while. I also walk around the hospital a lot, talking to people about patient safety and getting their ideas. I'm surprised how often I hear about a recurring problem in one area of the hospital that seems to be the result of the subculture in that part of the facility. I have also talked with other members of the executive team and asked them to pay as much attention to patient safety as I do. You expect to hear about patient safety from the CMO, but when the chief financial officer starts talking about it, people pay attention. I guess it's a matter of increasing your personal commitment and getting everyone else to do the same."

"Once again, Jeff, it starts with you. The most common mistake I see new leaders make is to focus only on the details and miss the big picture. You can hire a consulting firm to focus on outcomes and revenue optimization, but building a culture of safety is a process very specific to an individual organization, and each organization must traverse a customized path that only its leaders can design. Now, I'm not saying that moving quickly to achieve patient-safety outcomes through measurement and error reduction isn't important, but many new leaders get lost in the weeds because they focus on individual behaviors and lose the perspective of the larger culture change. If you focus only on individual errors, you run the risk of becoming a safety enforcement officer; but when you create a culture of safety, the details take care of themselves. Once people see your transformational leadership in this area, they will be drawn to the agenda you put forward. You're creating a sustainable leadership advantage by implementing a culture of safety. Good for you!"

"The kind of leadership needed to create a culture of safety seems like a lot of work."

"Yes, it takes time, but your success depends on what kind of leader you are. *Transactional* leaders execute a series of trades and deals, constantly measuring and reminding people how to decrease error. Some of that attention to detail is necessary, but the really great leaders are also *transformational*—they create a positive vision and inspire people to create a culture of safe care. There's a strong connection between what kind of leader you are and what kind of culture you end up with. For now, don't focus on the culture part; just continue to get your own house in order. We'll tackle the big picture later. By the way, here is the second packet—we'll be focusing next time on the science of high reliability."

Beth's main point so far is that if a leader is not seen as the principal agent of a culture change, it will likely not happen. She is helping Jeff develop mindfulness, self-reflection, situational awareness, and the ability to "walk the talk" of patient-safety practice. Leaders set the tone and pace of organizations, and they do so through repeated encounters with those with whom they work. Jeff is connecting together his passion for safety, his increasing knowledge of how it is accomplished, and his relentless focus and execution on what is right for the patient. He's developing into a transformational leader.

Session Two: Designing the High-Reliability Organization

"Jeff, last time we spent a good bit of time helping you become the kind of reflective leader who will be successful as a patient safety advocate. Let's move on to another area for today. Tell me what you've learned about high reliability."

"The AHRQ (2008) report about high reliability you gave me was a bit long but very much worth the read. A high-technology, high-risk industry can only be successful when it realizes that it must also operate as a high-reliability organization (HRO). Think nuclear power or commercial aviation. HROs share five attributes that allow them to stay at the cutting edge of error reduction. First, they have what might be thought of as corporate mindfulness, always sensitive to any risks. In healthcare, this awareness clearly refers to the vigilance we need to prevent error. Second, HROs appreciate that risk is complex and that errors have no simple causal chains. Healthcare is the most complex system ever created—it never shuts down, it has a large number of interconnected parts that must work together, and it has the ability to create large amounts of harm. As we think about error causality, we need to keep this complexity in mind. Third, HROs are preoccupied with failure, using every error as a pointer to the need for root cause analyses and improvement work. Unfortunately, when we encounter medical error, we're often more concerned about litigation and blame than quality improvement. Fourth, HROs look to and respect the experts in their system, no matter where they are in the chain of command. Sometimes the respiratory tech or the medical assistant has the information or expertise we need to prevent an error, so we need to listen. Finally, HROs have resilience that allows them to adapt immediately to whatever is required. In general, medical care cultures are sluggish in how they adapt to change."

"So what kinds of individual and cultural behaviors get in the way of a medical facility becoming a true HRO?"

"Where do I begin? A true HRO is a hypercomplex organization, in which risk of error is extraordinarily high. It uses tightly coupled, well-trained teams with standardized training to prevent, detect, and mitigate errors as they occur. On these teams are individuals with highly differentiated roles, each of whom can make expertise-based decisions that the other team members respect. This design results in multiple decision makers who communicate well, each proportionally accountable for the team's success. Everyone is obsessed with accountability for an optimal outcome. The problem with medical care is that we're still too siloed and hierarchical. We're not even close to being this type of organization."

"Once again, we're a bit ahead of ourselves and way up at the culture level, which we'll take on later. So let's figure out some practical steps to overcome behavioral barriers. What do you think?"

"Well, we can start by agreeing to do standard work—doing things the same way every time. Well, not exactly every time. We want standardization, but we want to retain some flexibility to modify care when necessary. It has to do with the difference between necessary and unnecessary variance. *Necessary variance* is the customization of care that is required because of important patient differences, such as gender, medical comorbidities, and so forth. *Unnecessary variance* is simply the practice of idiosyncratic patient care methods that are largely due to physician or staff preference. An HRO has figured out how to remove the unnecessary variability and then to put standard work in place where it makes sense. In quality improvement language, it is the ability to do things right after you've figured out the right things to do. It's why Toyota Lean and Six Sigma have been so popular and effective. They promote this standard work."

"It sounds so reasonable to do things right, Jeff. Why doesn't that happen all the time?"

"I think it comes down to the competing-commitments issue again. After all, we're human beings who have habits, or comfortable ways of doing things, as well as self-interested pressures to keep things the way they are. Human factor issues are also involved—we are affected by distractions, emotional inputs, attention fatigue, and prior habits. I was particularly impressed with the effects of normalized deviance and failure tolerance."

"This is important. Tell me some more about normalization of deviance and failure tolerance."

"My understanding of normalization of deviance is that sometimes, as we come closer and closer to a danger area, our fear paradoxically decreases because we have not experienced any negative consequences. This happened at NASA as they began to launch the space shuttle at lower and lower temperatures, approaching the lower boundary of the temperature window, and the *Challenger* disaster was the outcome. In medical care, we can approach the boundary of a rule or a physiological limit where we should be drawing a line, but seeing no immediate adverse effects, we begin to relax. Failure tolerance can happen as organizations are repeatedly unsuccessful—people become used to failing, and they become demoralized about achieving higher levels of performance or just accept things the way they are. A good example of failure tolerance is ventilator-associated pneumonia (VAP). For years we've accepted VAP as an unavoidable hazard in intensive care units. It's as if someone decided that the rate is as low as we can get it, that the remaining few cases are not controllable. Then the VAP bundle arrives with its systematic approach to prevention, and the cases drop to zero."

"We'll focus on this situation more later because it's a cultural change target. Can you think of any other barriers to high reliability that you have seen in organizations?"

"Probably the biggest one is a saying I've seen attributed to Don Berwick and others, that 'every system is perfectly designed to get the results it currently gets.' It's another way of saying that the outcomes currently being generated in your hospital or clinic are the result of a cascade of system properties, many of which were not actively chosen but which conspire to achieve that outcome. No one sat down to design the system we live in, but the system properties and parameters in their current state have all been defined either actively or passively. That means that if you want a different outcome, you need to think like a systems engineer and change the system parameters to change the outcome."

"What do you know about Swiss cheese?"

"Swiss cheese? Sorry, but I'm not sure where you're going with that—oh, you mean the James Reason (2000) Swiss cheese model of system failure? Okay, here's what I know. An HRO tries to avoid error by performing standard work and implementing error barriers to achieve uniform outcomes. The Swiss cheese idea arises from the notion that no matter what kinds of barriers we choose or how many we implement, they are all still imperfect. Someday in the future, some combination of circumstances will align the imperfections, and the barriers will fail."

"So how do you get around this problem?"

"Error reduction and high reliability have three essential components: (1) the prevention of errors for which there is an engineering prevention strategy, (2) the detection of errors that cannot be prevented by using a high-reliability teamwork process, and (3) the mitigation of errors that go undetected. The Swiss cheese model reminds us that we have to think about all three of these error interactions as we design high-reliability systems. I was surprised to learn how few errors can be completely prevented through engineering. Engineering has provided some safety solutions, such as gas supply connectors on anesthesia machines that can physically prevent misconnection errors, but in general there are limitations to what engineering can do. Ultimately, most of the work in healthcare is done by people, and people are naturally error prone. So the more common issue in prevention is lowering the likelihood of an error rather than eliminating it. A good example would be the color coding of syringes on an anesthesia work table by drug class, or using 'tall man' letters to distinguish drugs with similar names, highlighting the differences in capitals."

"I agree. Prevention engineering has its limits. So the next step is...?"

"If I cannot prevent an error, I must be able to detect it. Here's where the Swiss cheese model informs us again. Humans are very good at detecting novelty and change in the environment, but we are terrible at sustained vigilance. The closest we can come to effective ongoing detection is using the diversity of a team to monitor the situation. The more the team members permit each other to point out mistakes without fear of retribution, the more likely mistakes will be found and corrected as they are actually happening or as they are about to occur. Teamwork is probably the most important part of high reliability and is the basis of important advances such as crew resource management, which exploits the high-functioning team as a sensitive detection-and-correction mechanism. It takes training and explicit permission to speak up to make such teamwork effective."

"Jeff, did you happen to look at the article—"

"Yes, Beth, I know where you're going next. You're going to ask me about the AHRQ (2014) TeamSTEPPS Program, which directly addresses this teamwork issue. I found out that TeamSTEPPS is a self-perpetuating program—training the trainer—to help groups in high-risk areas of medical care become more team focused. It was originally developed by the US Department of Defense and has been used successfully in the military, but its application in civilian healthcare has really taken off. I've already decided that some of our senior medical leaders are going to get trained in TeamSTEPPS, particularly the people in the emergency department, operating room (OR), labor and delivery, and intensive care units. It's perfect for what they need."

"Tell me what happens when the team doesn't detect an error. Even the best team will fail once in a while."

"So, the final step of the model is mitigation. What cannot be prevented is detected, and what isn't detected is mitigated. Mitigation means simply having a plan B for when an error occurs. It recognizes that an error will eventually occur and that we must know in advance what to do next to mitigate the bad outcome. The moment an error occurs is not a time for improvisation—a good team already has a backup plan. In my experience, though, this area is one where people sometimes have a sense of false security.

A good example is the OR policy and procedure we used to have here for dealing with a needle or sponge count that came up short after a surgery—to call the radiology department to do a film. It became common to call radiology whenever there was uncertainty in the count. After a while, all surgeries ended with radiographs, and people stopped worrying about the counts. As this example shows, mitigation strategies should be used as a last resort. They should never be counted on as a first-line defense. I remember another CMO telling me about a hospital that relied on radiographic screening of patients after surgery to reduce the incidence of retained objects, only to have this strategy fail on several occasions with larger patients when the object was outside the margins of the radiographic plate. No one seemed concerned about the fact that the sponge count was still in error after three counts because the team was falsely reassured by the negative radiograph."

"Okay, Jeff, I think you've got a pretty good feel for the concepts of high reliability and the importance of self-awareness for leaders in the culture change process. You can learn a lot more in this area, but you're off to a great start. Here's your third packet. The readings in this section are going to focus on influencing individuals. Sometimes your target is changing the behavior of one person, and we will take that on next."

So far, Beth has led Jeff through a reflective consideration of his own leadership readiness and confirmed his growing understanding of the science of high reliability. Why did she start with the connection between self-awareness and a culture of safety and high reliability? Transformational leaders must have a vision of safety and high reliability that is evident in their daily leadership. Part of the leader's power is the ability to inspire others to reflect on their own behavior and change the way they provide patient care. Self-knowledge and a deep understanding of the principles of high reliability are the keys to mounting a successful culture change process, and those you wish to influence must see that you have both. The next step is to acquire the skill set you need to influence others to share these attributes.

Session Three: Influencing Individuals

"Beth, before we get started today, I have to let you know I'm feeling some anxiety. My CEO and board want me to create a culture of safety. But every time we've come close to any cultural issues, you've steered me away. Furthermore, the more I think about what I have to do to create the culture of safety described in the literature, the more impossible it seems. Culture transformation is the most complex process I've ever thought about, and I don't even know where to begin."

"I understand, Jeff. At the risk of sounding like Obi-Wan Kenobi, I'm going to remind you to trust me on this. You cannot start with culture change. The way to a culture of safety is to begin as you already have—knowing the literature, understanding the process of reliability, and deeply knowing your own passion and commitment to this change. I think you're there. The next step is to think about this change as a series of one-to-one encounters, where all you're trying to do is change the behavior of one individual at a time. If you view the change process that way, the culture transformation work will feel more approachable."

"Okay, that seems reasonable. I think I can handle that for now. It also helps me make more sense of the readings you gave me this week. Actually, as a primary care physician, I have some experience changing the behaviors of individual patients. I wonder if some of the clinical models that I use are applicable to my administrative work."

"Well, let's see. Tell me what you do in the clinic."

"Most often, I work with patients who have been reluctant or repeatedly unsuccessful at stopping or changing certain behaviors, such as losing weight, smoking cessation, or making some major lifestyle change. I'm actually already familiar with the change literature on that topic. My favorite model is the Stages of Change described by DiClemente and colleagues (1991), and I use it frequently to get people to stop smoking."

"I know the model. Tell me how you might apply it to changing behaviors that affect safety and reliability."

"Well, if you recall, the model moves an individual from a precontemplative state, where he's not thinking about a change, to a contemplative state, where he is at least open to the possibility of change. For a smoker, a friend's death from cancer might move him out of denial of the health risks of smoking so that he is motivated to start considering options. Before he actually makes a choice, there is a period of preparation during which he considers the pros and cons of a range of choices. The next stage, action, results in a commitment to some form of behavior change, which is then supported in the maintenance stage by a focus on relapse prevention. The relevance of behavior change to smoking is clear to me, but I'm having trouble understanding how it relates to changing people's ideas and behaviors about safety."

"Jeff, I don't think a health-risk behavior is any different from a safety-risk behavior. Let's change the way we think about this and just do a substitution in the example you gave about smoking. The negative behavior you're trying to change is *smoking*. The positive behavior you're trying to influence is *not smoking*. You're simply trying to reinforce the desirable behavior. Let's imagine that you have a medical staff member who needs coaching with hand sanitization. Just do a step-by-step substitution in your model."

"Okay, let's see. The precontemplative smoker is not motivated to change and is in a kind of denial about the health risks. So the individual who is not systematically cleaning her hands is in a parallel kind of denial about the infection risks. What usually moves people who smoke to the contemplation stage is overcoming that denial. Sometimes a bad health outcome in a friend who smokes awakens them to the reality of their own health risk, but in many cases it's the persistent reminders I make over a series of subsequent visits. So the best time to make this kind of intervention is either when the person is feeling vulnerable because of a bad outcome or over an extended period by calling attention to the behavior frequently. So our frequent reminders at medical staff meetings about hand sanitization are probably worthwhile. My guess would be that the preparation stage really consists of increased mindfulness about the need to make hand sanitization a regular behavior and that the action stage entails setting reminders—such as alcohol pumps at the patient's room door—and empowering patients to ask providers as they enter the room if they have cleaned their hands. I can see all sorts of ways to do maintenance and relapse prevention through observational monitoring and giving results of actual performance. I imagine this would even be more powerful at the group level considering the peer pressure."

"That's right, Jeff, but again, let's not jump to the culture-change level yet. We have a bit more to explore about influencing individuals. Let's go back to a concept we discussed last time, the competing commitments issue."

"Okay, that's a bit easier to see now as well. What I'm doing is weakening the task-oriented focus of getting patient care done in an efficient manner and, instead, asking the individual to have a more balanced, mindful view of the larger set of behaviors that need to be coordinated. It's moving someone from thinking 'I need to see this inpatient efficiently so I can go to clinic' to a more mindful 'I must prepare to give care to the patient by cleaning my hands and reflectively enter the room with a care plan.' Those are two completely different mind-sets, and the second one is more conducive to high reliability. So we are changing from a commitment to efficiency and moving to a commitment to safe, reliable care."

"Very good. The challenge with competing commitments is that to instill a new behavior as a reliable action, mindfulness needs to increase and the commitment to the old behavior needs to be weakened. You mentioned something before about relapse prevention. What does your clinical work suggest as an option for that?"

"The first thing that comes to mind is weight management. My patients seem to do better when they get daily feedback—weighing themselves and recording their data—which I suppose underscores the importance of having good data systems to support safety. The problem I've faced is figuring out how to get people the data they need. The data must be personalized and related to what they're doing, actionable, and focused on the important behaviors that need to change. I'm trying to design a series of scorecards that present safety data at various levels of the medical center, tailored to the clinical setting. I'm considering how each care provider sees the clinical world and then collecting relevant key safety variables, feeding them back in the form of a monthly scorecard. I think that if I get this right, we can produce a nested system where the scorecards roll up to higher-level scorecards at the executive and board levels so that everybody sees the right data to change their behavior."

"That's an excellent idea, Jeff. Measurement is everything. If you can't measure it, you can't manage it. Organizations with strategic views of quality and safety necessarily do measurement very well. But let me go back to something you mentioned before that needs more clarification. You talked about using measurements, such as daily weighing, to change behavior, but I'm not sure you fully understand how that works. Do you know the relationship between drivers and outcomes?"

"Not sure about that one."

"When we're trying to modify an outcome, what we're really doing is modifying the behavioral driver that is producing the outcome. We usually don't modify the outcome directly. Here's an example. Say we want to lose weight, so we start thinking about calories. Two of the drivers of daily weight are calories in and calories out, both of which are measurable. But we don't directly control calories; rather, we change the behaviors that result in the number of calories in and out. Do you see that we're actually influencing eating and exercise behaviors, not calories? It's those behaviors—or drivers—that, in turn, control calories."

"So the objective is to control drivers and let the drivers control the outcomes?"

"Yes. The reason is that the drivers are controlled by other behavioral drivers in a complex, nested system. For example, if you want to eat fewer calories, you can try to force yourself to eat fewer calories, or you can focus on why you're eating as many as you currently do. Those boxes of cookies lying around the house promote snacking, and if you focus on decreasing access to snacks as a controllable behavior, the number of snacks will decrease, thus driving down your calorie intake. Brute-force focus on changing the calorie count itself is much harder than focusing on the drivers. Likewise, you can try to be vigilant about decreasing errors or you can think about the behaviors, or drivers, that lead to errors and focus on them. A good example is failure to start antibiotics before incision in the OR. You can harass people about doing it, or you can deal with the driver, which in this case is helping people remember to include it in the preoperative readiness. One hospital I worked in simply added the antibiotics start to the checklist used during the preoperative huddle or time-out, and their error rate went to zero overnight."

"I'm confused. I thought we were supposed to focus on counting things. What happened to 'if you can't measure it, you can't manage it'?"

"Okay, let's approach this explanation from a different angle. The goal is still to count things but to influence the drivers that change the counts. Let's go back to our calorie example and focus on measuring first. We can influence the number of calories we take in either by doing a direct calorie count or by managing the percentage of fat in our diet, both of which ultimately affect the number of calories in. We can also count the number of miles we walk or the number of days we attend the gym as an estimate of calories out. Now, to successfully lose weight, we really don't change calories; we change behaviors that result in changing calories. All of these behaviors must link to a countable number, and as we manage our behaviors, which are tied to calories, our weight—also a measurable outcome quantity—will change. The main point here is that individual behavior change requires quantitative feedback. If I want to change an outcome, I need to understand and modify the behavior that produces that outcome. Although it's important to give feedback about the resultant outcome, change is more likely to occur when we provide quantitative feedback on the behavioral drivers of an outcome. The calories won't change unless I focus on what I do that increases or decreases them. Making a decision to change your weight is more abstract than making a decision to increase your number of calories every day or to exercise more. You have to do it through a behavior."

"Okay, now I get it—I see the importance of this approach. I don't think I had an appreciation for the driver issue. So here's what I think you said. All outcomes need to be measurable, and to change the outcome we need to change the behavioral driver that produces that outcome."

"Very good. Now let's do a safety example."

"Hmmm. Okay, I can think of one. We recently made a significant decrease in catheter-associated bloodstream infections by standardizing our central line process. Rather than focusing on the number of infections and pneumothoraces, we focused on the behaviors that increased the likelihood of infection and error. For example, we created central line kits that made it easier to prepare a sterile field and increased the availability of portable ultrasound, which decreased the number of missed veins. As I think about applying what you just told me, I see that we were focusing on decreasing unnecessary variability among the residents by standardizing their behavior, making it easier for them to do the right thing. We did this through a combination of finding something to count, selecting the correct behavioral drivers, and figuring out how to influence those drivers."

"Good. You mentioned VAP before. What do you know about bundles?"

"I heard someone talking about bundles a few months ago. Bundles are groups of practices that have each been shown to be individually effective in the reduction of some adverse outcome, but when grouped together they take on an additional level of error reduction—the whole is greater than the sum of its parts. The one I am most familiar with is our VAP bundle. It's pretty straightforward. There is a checklist, and you are either doing each of the items or you're not. You don't get credit for the bundle unless you do all the steps. Many hospitals have gotten their VAP rates down to zero for extended periods using this technique."

"Jeff, rather than give you specific advice about individual behavior change, let's see what you know about a variety of reinforcers that are associated with changing individual physician behavior. Let's start with altruism."

"I think altruism is doing the right thing for the patient. To be honest, I've always been surprised by how powerful this value is among physicians. I don't know how many animated discussions among clinicians have come to a sudden halt when someone points out that we need to do what's best for the patient. I really like that. I think that's why the patient safety stories at the beginning of meetings are so powerful. The stories remind us of our commitment to altruism."

"Very good—I agree. What are some other reinforcers of individual physician behavior?"

"Another one that comes to mind is alignment of interests. We align interests all the time in clinical care when we negotiate with patients on aspects of treatment plans, but I think it also works well in patient safety. The competing values of other quality dimensions, particularly efficiency, sometimes compete with safety for priority. Efficient care does not have to be unsafe, but it can be if the safety component is not simultaneously addressed with the efficiency component."

"What do you know about facilitating and forcing functions?"

"I remember that from the Institute for Healthcare Improvement (IHI) physician quality white paper by Reinertsen and colleagues (2007). A facilitating function is something that makes the right thing easy to do. If the right thing is the easiest of all the options, people naturally do it, and once people try it and become familiar with it, it's more likely to become standard work. It's just a matter of making everything else more trouble than it's worth. Forcing functions are similar except that they exclude all other alternatives. They are similar to what happens on an interstate highway when, over several miles, the number of lanes are gradually reduced to accommodate a construction site. Forcing functions appear in our electronic health record (EHR) when we come to a drug interaction that forces us to make a decision about whether to proceed. The EHR prevents moving ahead until we make the decision."

"What do you think about punishment as a behavior change mechanism?"

"Well, I've never been a fan of punishment. I think it has two principal drawbacks. First, you're telling people what not to do instead of what they should do. Second, it creates resentment. I'm sure there are times when punishment is needed and appropriate as a measure of last resort, but there are other ways to bring about change. You mentioned before that you had an interest in positivity, and I think positivity can be applied in this area. You can decrease the frequency of a behavior through punishment, but a better way is to use *reciprocal inhibition*. That's the process of defining the opposite of the undesirable behavior and reinforcing it. For example, instead of punishing smoking, I can reward nonsmoking. It's a much better strategy."

"Well, Jeff, it sounds as though you paid attention to all the behavioral science lectures in medical school, and I'm sure you get plenty of practice as a family doctor. I think that's enough for today. Here's the packet for next time. Now that you have a good understanding of individual behavior change, it's time to tackle culture. This one's a bit tougher because we need to get groups of people all going in the same direction. Nevertheless, there is both an art and a science to culture change, and we'll use both to focus on creating a culture of safety in the hospital. By the way, the packet contains a culture-of-safety survey that I want you to complete between now and our next meeting. I'll be interested in what you think of the results."

Beth is now convinced that Jeff is developing good self-awareness and interpersonal influence skills, and she is going to move on to large-scale culture change. Physicians generally are exposed to mindfulness and one-to-one influence as part of their clinical training, but the ability to work at the organizational level and influence multiple groups and organizations simultaneously is an acquired skill. Strong partnerships are needed to be successful. Cultures are made up of multiple subcultures, including a variety of clinical and nonclinical disciplines. The whole group has to move as a whole, and both time and attention to the alignment of interests are required to move to a new way of doing things. Remember, the system is the way it is because the reinforcers keep it that way. Otherwise it would change by itself. So culture change starts by understanding the current status quo, how it got there in the first place, and the reinforcers that make it stay in place. The status quo is the way it is for a reason.

Session Four: Creating a Culture of Safety

"Now comes the hard part, Jeff. Most of what we've discussed so far has expanded skills that you already have developed as part of your physician training. Changing culture is a more formidable task and requires a different way of thinking. You asked me to help you develop a culture of safety here at St. Joseph, but we have to think about what that culture would look like compared to the current one. What are your thoughts about our culture as you experience it now?"

"Interesting turn of phrase, 'how I experience it now.' It reminds me that culture is largely a subjective experience, with a lot of individual perspectives. My definition of our culture is, well, my personal experience of the culture from where I sit. That's probably the most important thing to remember as we discuss culture—what I conclude is not necessarily what others would conclude, nor is it a factual statement of what the culture 'really' is, if that could even be measured."

"Rightly so. Now back to my question."

"Okay, I've been here for more than a decade since I left residency, and here is my perspective on how we do things. We tend to be a flexible, horizontal culture that is very people centered, but sometimes we get surprisingly siloed. We easily get stuck on details and forget about the big picture. Our emotional connections with each other sometimes make systematic, rational work difficult. I'd say our biggest difficulty is a kind of paradox—that thinking we are putting our patients first and giving them the best care can sometimes make standard work difficult, thus not giving them the absolute best care."

"So, the culture you have is the culture you are transforming. Where would you like it to go?"

"Well, the HRO that we need to create will build on some of our strengths and come into conflict with others. For example, standard work is about details, and I think we're pretty good at working at that level. We can use our people-centered focus to drive to good outcomes that are produced in a reliable manner. I also see that our flexibility will make change possible as we make the case for transformation. On the other hand, the ultimate need to customize everything at the final delivery point often undoes the standard work we need, and people may give themselves permission to opt out. What I'm most afraid of is people deciding that patient care cannot be done in a reliable manner because the patient's needs trump everything."

"What are some of the issues that make you feel that way?"

"We've had a few aborted attempts at standardizing care by people who were fond of Lean process improvement. They would come into a small area of the hospital and try to implement a rapid process improvement project that eventually failed as it was reabsorbed into the culture. As one of the executives once told me, 'culture eats strategy.' I can recall an OR turnover project that worked well for several weeks but then seemed to be overwhelmed by the rest of the hospital because the necessary system-level dependencies could not be sustained. For example, despite the team's enthusiasm in turning over the room, patients sometimes arrived late in the OR suite because of issues on the wards. Pharmacy was not fully on board, so preoperative medications were often late. When these Lean experiments are not carried through at a system level from a more strategic perspective, they fail to create the critical mass necessary to move the organization forward. Each failure seems to create a backlash against change and feeds the desire to protect the status quo."

"Yes, Jeff, that's usually what happens with an incremental approach. Change can be incremental and *evolutionary*, or it can be swift and *revolutionary*. We'll see later that there are appropriate circumstances for each style when it comes to creating a culture of safety. But for now, tell me more about your hospital leadership colleagues who have committed to helping you create this culture of safety."

"Just before you arrived, I made a presentation to our executive team and the board, and I feel they are more committed to this transformation than they were a year ago. The chief nursing officer (CNO) and I have a common vision of how this should come about, and we are slowly educating our colleagues that the culture change will not happen unless the entire executive team and board embrace it as a strategic priority. Even so, we still struggle sometimes in allocating the right resources and sequencing the steps necessary to prioritize this change."

"Jeff, my own personal observation has been that our CNO is equally passionate about culture change. It's good to have a natural partner who shares the same passion. I also heard that she has administered the AHRQ (2012) Patient Safety Culture instrument widely in the organization. Do you know the results?"

"It was a pretty big surprise. The staff reported the overall level of safety in the hospital to be much lower than anyone realized, and well below national benchmarks. Actually, it wasn't uniformly that way. Some areas where we have natural leadership showed strong awareness and ability with respect to safety-related performance, but other departments came up short. We're in the process of feeding the data back to the organization at the department level and facilitating discussions. Overall, I would say that most people were disappointed with where we stood against the benchmarks."

"So it sounds as though a large-scale culture change needs to happen. How do you plan to do that?"

"When I look at the overall process that has to be accomplished, I think of Malcolm Gladwell's (2000) book *The Tipping Point*. We need to reach a critical mass of concern and dissatisfaction about our current safety performance before the culture will begin to move in a positive direction. It reminds me of the chemistry courses we took in college, where we had to create activation energy to get a reaction going. The tipping point is really the instant in time when the momentum finally goes in your favor, but I'm not really sure how to get it there."

"What did you think of that little book I gave you, *Our Iceberg Is Melting* by John Kotter and Holger Rathgeber (2006)?"

"It was great. As you know, the book is a story-based version of Kotter's (1995) more scholarly article on leading change. He tells a story about a colony of penguins struggling to make a group decision about what to do as their home iceberg faces possible destruction in a coming winter storm season. He describes eight steps of change that the colony had to go through to be successful."

"Let's go through some of the steps they took, because you may find some parallels with your situation."

"The penguins had lived on this iceberg for quite some time, and it took a sense of urgency to overcome their complacency and denial that everything would be okay if they did nothing. I think that's part of the problem at our hospital—we don't have the requisite urgency about patient safety here. No one imagined the disappointing results from the Patient Safety Culture instrument, and much of it was met with denial. So the first thing we need to do is figure out a way to turn up the urgency to overcome the inertia and denial."

"Let's agree that we need to have some urgency but deal with those details later. What's the next step?"

"The protagonist penguin, Freddie, put together a group of other penguins who could help him. I think this was referred to as a *guiding coalition*—a small group of individuals with influence, skills, and the ability to organize the culture change. I think we're starting to assemble such a group here. I know that the CNO and the people from the quality office are on board, but I doubt I have enough key physician leaders. I don't know if you've met Dr. Swanson yet, but we have to get him passionate about this. When Bill Swanson wants to do something, many of the medical staff will follow because he is seen as the senior physician statesman here. I can think of four or five other physicians I would want on this committee as well, either for the same reason or because they have particular skills we need. So that would be my guiding coalition."

"What would you have that group do?"

"The most important thing they could do is develop a plan for what the change will look like. I think we spend too much time dabbling in the details of patient safety, experimenting with little projects here and there, trying out the latest measurement 'flavor *du jour*.' So the next step is to create a strategic vision of quality that involves the commitment of our board and leadership to adhering to national standards, producing meaningful and actionable data in scorecards that are usable at the clinic and bedside levels, and then managing to those results at every level of the organization. We then have to communicate this strategy widely throughout the organization and support anybody doing any part of it anywhere."

"That's correct, Jeff, and at that point you will begin to get the momentum you need. But what do you think will produce the acceleration?"

"We'll have to have some short-term wins, rewarding innovative adoption and customization of the quality and safety initiative. That means having some of our leaders demonstrate success with patient safety projects and turning those successes into best-practice heroic stories for our institution. If we do it right, we can consolidate our gains so that all of the small projects are seen as part of a larger strategic commitment to quality. I think the key is to get everybody's attention that patient safety is the new status quo."

"Many powerful subcultures in our larger culture might compete with this agenda. Any sense of the patterns?"

"The subcultures sometimes align with departments, sometimes not. Leaders and resistors are everywhere, but usually the resistance comes from people who are protecting something they value that will likely stop if the change occurs. Some of the more difficult groups are composed of people we've hired as economic engines for the medical center, who justify their idiosyncratic practice style as the price for their contribution. They just want to be left to do what they want to do the way they want to do it, and sometimes the administration isn't tough enough with them. These silo cultures can drive a lot of the larger culture because of their economic clout. Fortunately, spark plugs everywhere want to get this change done. We had to deal with similar resistance when we rolled out the EHR and used a diffusion model. In that model, we recognized that there were enthusiastic early adopters; a great middle group that needed to be gently persuaded; and the lagging, sometimes oppositional, rear guard. Each group required a different change management technique. The laggards move only when the majority of the culture just leaves them behind. They have to get on board or leave."

"Very good, Jeff. You've given a nice summary of Kotter's change model, and I think it's the right one to use. You also make good use of the Rogers (2003) diffusion model to identify the temporal sequence involved in moving the various groups forward. So it sounds like you're going to end up using a mix of sustained, evolutionary change punctuated by fast-moving, revolutionary components. Sounds good, and it's usually what works. But let's change your focus a bit for now. We've talked about the change process in general, but I'm still unclear as to what the content is going to look like. Have you thought more about that?"

"I wasn't really sure about that until you made me aware of that episode of the PBS show *Nova*, 'The Deadliest Plane Crash' (Hébert et al. 2006). That video was so moving, I think we should use it to create the sense of urgency and elicit the emotional reactions we need to make this go. I like the aviation theme for several reasons. First, it's familiar to people and they all have a stake in the outcome because they fly commercial airlines multiple times throughout the year. The transformation of commercial aviation since the 1970s is a great model on which to base healthcare change because it, too, is a comparably complex, high-risk system. I particularly like the emotional quality of that video—it gets people's attention. I tried it out in a few medical staff meetings, and the discussions were rich and meaningful. Somehow it genuinely hooks people, and they can see the parallels with medicine. Healthcare has never had a major accident to shake us into a system of high reliability, as aviation did in 1977 when those planes crashed on Tenerife."

"Tell me more about the parallels you see."

"Well, you already know the story. Basically, the most lethal accident in aviation history occurred as the result of a causal chain that unfolded as a series of minor decisions and errors summed up to a cataclysmic head-on accident between two 747s on a foggy runway, killing 583 people. What impressed me about that accident was that if attention had been paid to any single detail in the causal chain, a link would have broken, causing the chain to collapse. It's a great story about how human factors conspire with the environment to create disaster. That happens every day in the hospital. The controllers and the pilots didn't communicate well. The fog and uncertainty should have made everyone more cautious and slowed things down, but instead the urgency increased and people started shortcutting standard procedure. Again, a typical day in our hospital."

"Yes, I know the story well. So how are you going to communicate this lesson in the hospital?"

"Well, I'm committed to using the video at some of our major medical staff meetings. The CNO has agreed to do that as well. We're also asking all of the senior leaders to read John Nance's (2008) book *Why Hospitals Should Fly*."

"That's an excellent book, and I'm glad you're using it. Why do you think it's so effective?"

"First of all, Nance is a good writer, and the whole idea of approaching the topic as a novel is very creative. Most people can read the book in a few hours, and it's enjoyable to read about a senior physician leader transforming an entire hospital using aviation safety techniques. I've never met anyone who didn't think the book was worthwhile reading."

"I agree. What do you do after they're finished reading?"

"I think the important thing is to strike while the iron is hot. Turning people's passion into executable change has to be done right away. I usually get people from similar clinical areas together in small groups and start by asking them to administer the Patient Safety Culture survey again in their clinic or hospital unit. I then feed the results back to them along with the appropriate national benchmarks. This feedback usually gets them even more fired up, and then I ask them to list the three most important ways they can make their clinical areas safer. They discuss these ideas, and everyone has to leave the meeting with a commitment to change one or more of their observations."

"These are all great ideas, Jeff. Tell me more about the models you use to actually help them change the culture when they are ready to do so."

"Well, we've talked about Kotter's eight-step change model and the penguins, but some smaller changes need a more direct approach. For physicians, I like the IHI physician change model we talked about before because it was developed with medical staff in mind. I took a course a few months ago in which two books—*Switch* by Chip and Dan Heath (2010) and *Influencer* by Kerry Patterson and colleagues (2008)—were recommended by the teacher. The books are not so much change models as they are organizational behavior guides to help people understand what's going on during the process of change. They focus on leveraging influence in cultures to get small inputs to make large changes. I found both books very helpful."

"What did you think about the article on appreciative inquiry by Hart, Conklin, and Allen (2008)?"

"Sorry, Beth, I haven't gotten to that one yet."

"That's okay. Basically, it's an interesting tool based on positive psychology and social constructivism. *Positive psychology* is an approach to change that focuses on strengths and future growth rather than on weaknesses and problems. Instead of focusing on what's wrong, you build on what's right. *Social constructivism* is a pedagogic technique that theorizes that adults work and learn best when they're building something together. What I like about this model is that it combines both of these evidence-based processes into a scenario-building exercise that most people find uplifting and useful. Participants begin by thinking about past examples of effective leadership and then, in pairs, use reflective dialogue to discuss how past personal experiences with effective leadership might be applied in the current situation to move toward a positive, envisioned future. It invites people to use their previous positive experiences as a design element in a higher-quality, safer future."

"Actually, I think I participated in that kind of exercise once. It was interesting how commitment and positivity grew in the room as we told each other's leadership stories back to the group. We were able to envision a much higher-functioning organization when we pooled our experiences. I remember that the last part of the exercise was to commit to a positive change that we were willing to make in the organization. If I recall correctly, we made some of our biggest strides forward after that exercise. It hadn't occurred to me to use it specifically in the creation of a culture of safety."

"Well, there you go. You should try the exercise with that specific safety focus. It works just as well. By the way, before we lose focus on the subject of positivity, what did you think of the *Implementation Science* article by Bradley and colleagues (2009), particularly the positive deviance concept?"

"Very interesting reading. The basic idea that I remember about positive deviance is that even in a system that seems broken, one often finds a small number of individuals who are achieving the desired outcome, often through unconventional means. Positive deviance focuses on low-frequency, out-of-the-box thinking. I particularly recall the story of how an aid group in Vietnam was able to effect large-scale nutrition changes in a generally underfed population of children by focusing on a small number of kids who were adequately nourished and copying their families' feeding behaviors. The concept of positive deviance is simply that when everything seems not to be working, someone may have figured out—and is succeeding with—an innovative workaround. This is a specific example of a larger developing field known as implementation science, which seeks to understand how to make large-scale culture change in health behaviors. I don't see why we couldn't adopt some of these ideas in our culture of safety."

"By the way, we've talked a lot about error over our last two sessions, but we've said very little so far about the culture required for disclosure of error. What's your plan for that part of the culture change?"

"Fortunately, the literature on disclosure of error is growing, and I've already got some of our medical staff leaders reading and thinking about it. Some of the information is unexpected and paradoxical. For example, I used to think that disclosing error was a great way to increase the number of lawsuits in the organization, but a decade or more of research has demonstrated that it actually goes the other way. An article by Gallagher, Studdert, and Levinson (2007) has a great template for designing an error disclosure process, and our medical executive committee is currently thinking about what that process should look like. Some aspects seem to be common sense, such as telling your patients what actually happened, saying you're sorry, and inviting them to help in the process of designing profession strategies for the future. Our risk managers were a bit surprised at first when we started discussing the topic, but I think we all now have a better common understanding of how to make an effective disclosure."

"Disclosure focuses on the patient side of the error, but how do you handle the person who made the error?"

"That takes us to Just Culture (2014). The Just Culture Community was created to provide organizations with a uniform response when they fail to achieve expected outcomes and have to deal with the complex motives and behaviors of those who fail. What I like about it is that it divides failure into four categories and has a specific remedy for each. First, there are human errors and mistakes. In the Just Culture algorithm, an error is an unintentional harm—the person achieved a result other than what was intended, often through system inadequacies that allowed ambiguity. For example, before unapproved abbreviation lists started appearing, ambiguity happened a lot. The appropriate response is to focus on the system and redesign it so that the error is less likely to happen—for example, have an abbreviation policy. The second category is carelessness or at-risk behavior, where the person was inattentive to the situation that led to the error and probably needs some counseling. A resident who has a habit of providing poor transfer-of-care sign-outs is a good example. That individual needs to be counseled and put on notice. The third level involves recklessness, where the person flagrantly disregards norms and creates an error unintentionally but out of recklessness—for example, drinking while you're on trauma surgical call. Finally, some people just don't pay attention to rules and thumb their noses at authority. These last two cases demand consequences, sometimes even punishment."

"Well, Jeff, we've taken quite a journey since we started several weeks ago. How do you feel about all of our discussion, and what is your plan?"

"I'm grateful for the time you spent with me, Beth. I'm clearer about what I need to do and how to do it. Although I still have a lot more to learn about the science of high reliability, I can take care of that with some dedicated reading and focus. I feel more centered as a leader in patient safety, and I'm clear about what my priorities and commitments are and how I can be a transformation agent in the hospital. I also think the influence techniques I've used in my practice work well both for individuals and for larger groups, perhaps even for the culture at large. I was surprised to learn that organizational change is a science and that established best practices exist for changing culture at the macro level. Although I don't feel as overwhelmed as I did when we started, I still have a lot to do, and I think I'll need to meet with you periodically to fine-tune what we discussed."

"I would be delighted to continue working with you, Jeff. I think the most important thing you can do now is to write out a culture change plan that summarizes everything you've learned and prioritizes what needs to be done sooner rather than later. As we've seen, a lot of this work involves one-to-one coaching of key influence leaders in the organization, and some of this coaching can even happen over lunch. Other parts relate to what you do with our medical executive committee and with the medical staff as a whole, setting standards and outlining the envisioned future of a safety-focused culture. I agree that you need to be patient both with yourself and the culture you're trying to change. Remember, the current culture took decades to evolve into the complex system that you're trying to modify, so moving it in a different direction will take months or years. Nevertheless, you've learned that it all starts with you and the clarity of your vision as the architect of your culture of safety. When you see this vision clearly yourself, you can clearly explain and model the culture change to your physician colleagues as well as the rest of the staff, using the organizational behavior and high-reliability science concepts that you're learning. I'd say you're off to a great start, and I look forward to watching you be successful."

Epilogue: What Are You Going to Do?

I hope you are feeling a mixture of excitement and intimidation similar to what Jeff was working through. The excitement should come from the realization that you can actually move your organizational culture beyond its current configuration into a high-reliability safety culture. All you need is the passion to do it, the knowledge and resources of the sciences of high reliability and organizational behavior, and the ability to execute your vision relentlessly.

The intimidation part likely comes from your realistic assessment of the amount of work involved. These packets contain a lot of reading, and a lot of work is required to learn to apply the concepts. And that is just the beginning—transformation is not just a matter of reading a few review articles and then going out to implement the change. Leadership training—through reading, guided mentorship experience, and coaching—is the only way to make change of this magnitude possible.

What should give you courage, however, is that culture change is a team sport and that you and your leadership team will take the organization to the game together. If we followed the rest of Jeff's story, we would see that he continued to get mentorship and coaching from Beth. He would read daily and widely, not just about patient safety but about quality improvement in general. He would likely begin to attend national meetings on safety, such as the annual IHI meeting each December. He would also take courses similar to those offered by the American College of Physician Executives, the American College of Healthcare Executives, or the health administration department at his local university. He would also be part of a network of other leaders in his area working together to build their understanding of best practices in patient safety and quality. Most of all, he would build an internal leadership network that includes his fellow executives, medical and nursing staff, hospital directors and managers, and the board to join arms around this transformation of culture.

No single path leads to the destination of a culture of safety—multiple paths will get you there, but they all involve a personal leadership transformation, mastery of a well-developed literature on reliability and change, as well as the courage to make it happen—relentlessly.

Study Questions

1. Describe in detail the current level of your commitment to patient safety. Where are you in the journey that Jeff took, and what do you need to move forward?
2. Describe the characteristics of a high-reliability organization, then compare and contrast your current organization with that standard.
3. Explain the concept of competing commitments, and give examples of competing commitments in your setting.
4. Describe the use of the Swiss cheese model in error prevention and detection.
5. Pick a health-risk or safety-risk behavior and, using the Stages of Change model, describe how you would change that behavior.
6. Give two examples of modifying behavioral drivers to change behavior.
7. Define positive deviance, and give two examples of how it can be used to effect culture change.
8. Detail the workings of the Just Culture algorithm, and give an example of each of the four kinds of errors it addresses, including their remediation.

References

Agency for Healthcare Research and Quality (AHRQ). 2014. "TeamSTEPPS Curriculum Tools and Materials." http://teamstepps.ahrq.gov/abouttoolsmaterials. htm.

———. 2012. *Hospital Survey on Patient Safety Culture.* Updated June. www.ahrq. gov/qual/patientsafetyculture/hospsurvindex.htm.

———. 2008. *Becoming a High Reliability Organization: Operational Advice for Hospital Leaders.* AHRQ Publication No. 08-0022. Published April. www. ahrq.gov/hroadvice.pdf.

Boyatzis, R., and A. McKee. 2005. *Resonant Leadership: Renewing Yourself and Connecting with Others Through Mindfulness, Hope, and Compassion.* Boston: Harvard Business Review Press.

Bradley, E., L. Curry, H. Krumholz, I. Nembhard, S. Ramanadhan, and L. Rowe. 2009. "Research in Action: Using Positive Deviance to Improve Quality of Health Care." *Implementation Science* 4 (1): 25.

DiClemente, C. C., J. O. Prochaska, S. K. Fairhurst, W. F. Velicer, N. M. Velasquez, and J. S. Rossi. 1991. "The Process of Smoking Cessation: An Analysis of Precontemplation, Contemplation, and Preparation Stages of Change." *Journal of Consulting and Clinical Psychology* 59 (2): 295–304.

Gallagher, T. H., D. Studdert, and W. N. Levinson. 2007. "Disclosing Harmful Medical Errors to Patients." *New England Journal of Medicine* 356 (26): 2713–19.

Gladwell, M. 2000. *The Tipping Point: How Little Things Can Make a Big Difference.* Boston: Little, Brown.

Hart, R. K., T. A. Conklin, and S. J. Allen. 2008. "Individual Leader Development: An Appreciative Inquiry Approach." *Advances in Developing Human Resources* 10 (5): 632–50.

Heath, C., and D. Heath. 2010. *Switch: How to Change Things When Change Is Hard.* New York: Broadway Books.

Hébert, C., C. Schmidt, A. Barro, B. Vaillot, P. Crompton, P. S. Apsell, and N. Ross. 2006. "The Deadliest Plane Crash." *Nova* television series. South Burlington, VT: WGBH Boston Video.

Institute of Medicine (IOM). 2001. *Crossing the Quality Chasm: A New Health System for the 21st Century.* Washington, DC: National Academies Press.

Just Culture. 2014. Accessed January 27. www.justculture.org.

Kegan, R., and L. L. Lahey. 2001. "The Real Reason People Won't Change." *Harvard Business Review* 79 (10): 84–93.

Kohn, L. T., J. M. Corrigan, and M. S. Donaldson (eds.). 2000. *To Err Is Human: Building a Safer Health System.* Washington, DC: National Academies Press.

Kotter, J. P. 1995. "Leading Change: Why Transformation Efforts Fail." *Harvard Business Review* 73 (2): 59–67.

Kotter, J. P., and H. Rathgeber. 2006. *Our Iceberg Is Melting: Changing and Succeeding Under Any Conditions.* New York: St. Martin's Press.

Nance, J. J. 2008. *Why Hospitals Should Fly: The Ultimate Flight Plan to Patient Safety and Quality Care.* Bozeman, MT: Second River Healthcare Press.

Patterson, K., J. Grenny, D. Maxfield, R. McMillan, and A. Switzler. 2008. *Influencer: The Power to Change Anything.* New York: McGraw-Hill.

Porter, M. E., and E. O. Teisberg. 2007. "How Physicians Can Change the Future of Health Care." *Journal of the American Medical Association* 297 (10): 1103–11.

Reason, J. 2000. "Human Error: Models and Management." *British Medical Journal* 320 (7237): 768–70.

Reinertsen, J. L., A. G. Gosfield, W. Rupp, J. W. Whittington. 2007. *Engaging Physicians in a Shared Quality Agenda.* IHI Innovation Series white paper. Cambridge, MA: Institute for Healthcare Improvement.

Rogers, E. M. 2003. *Diffusion of Innovations,* fifth edition. New York: Free Press.

Wachter, R. M. 2010. "Patient Safety at Ten: Unmistakable Progress, Troubling Gaps." *Health Affairs* 29 (1): 165–73.

INFORMATION TECHNOLOGY: IMPLICATIONS FOR HEALTHCARE QUALITY

Ferdinand Velasco

The Institute of Medicine (IOM) report *Patient Safety: Achieving a New Standard for Care* (2003b) asserted that, to achieve the six aims of healthcare improvement set forth in *Crossing the Quality Chasm* (IOM 2001), "a new health care delivery system is needed—a system that both prevents errors and learns from them when they occur. This requires, first, a commitment by all stakeholders to a culture of safety, and, second, improved information systems" (IOM 2003b, 45).

In comparison with other industries, healthcare has lagged in the adoption of information technology (IT), contributing to gaps in clinical and business processes and systems that have hampered process improvement efforts. When computers first became commercially available, healthcare professionals and hospitals tended to focus on administrative and financial applications of technology—for example, support for patient registration, scheduling, and billing and for admission, discharge, and transfer transactions. Gradually, technology was introduced into ancillary clinical departments such as laboratory, pharmacy, and radiology departments. The automation greatly improved the efficiency of laboratory testing, medication dispensing, and interpretation of clinical images.

However, until recently, the delivery of actual patient care depended on paper medical records and verbal communications. The past decade has witnessed acceleration in the adoption of electronic health record (EHR) systems in hospitals and physician practices, which have helped care delivery become more reliable and efficient. This trend has been stimulated by federal efforts to promote the use of EHRs and can be seen as part of a larger effort to reform the healthcare system (Blumenthal 2009).

Just as in healthcare quality improvement, patients are increasingly playing an important role in the evolution of health IT. Many interact virtually with their care providers through personal health records (PHRs). Moreover, social media and mobile computing are growing in importance as tools for empowering people to improve their health.

Health IT Infrastructure and Information Systems

Infrastructure

Health IT has evolved significantly since the 1960s, when the first mainframe computers were acquired by hospitals to support billing and accounting functions. These large devices were housed—and still are today—in specialized facilities known as data centers. The original computers lacked the familiar interactive keyboard and user interface display, relying on input in the form of punch cards. Consequently, computing was initially performed as a batch process. With the introduction of terminals and networks, computing capability became distributed, allowing staff to conduct operations at the point of service and in real time. Subsequently, personal computers and, more recently, mobile devices such as smart phones and tablets have helped to introduce technology to serve clinical functions. The introduction of IT in clinics and physician offices followed a similar pattern but was delayed until the 1980s, when it became more affordable with the advent of personal computers and midrange machines known as servers. While this brief account of the evolution of healthcare computing may appear to be of limited historical significance, this trend—centralized to distributed, batched to real time—is being replicated in how technology affects the quality and safety of care.

Just as the technical infrastructure—the computers and the cables that connect them—of a hospital or physician practice may be thought of as a sort of "neural network" for that entity, the Internet has expanded the connections of the network to encompass multiple separate entities. First, with the introduction of regional high-speed networks, healthcare systems found it more cost-effective to move data centers to a location separate from patient care areas. More recently, the technology has been outsourced to specialized firms that manage the equipment in their own facilities, reducing the need for providers to acquire and maintain sophisticated mainframes and servers in corporate data centers. This phenomenon, in which processing capacity is viewed as a utility, is known as "cloud computing" and has been adopted in many industries. Its chief benefit is to allow IT professionals in healthcare organizations to focus on their core competency—leveraging the technology to support clinical and business needs.

Health Information Systems

Given the complexity of healthcare, the diverse array of supporting software applications is not surprising. Some of the more common systems found in a typical hospital are listed in Exhibit 13.1. This list is not intended to be an exhaustive inventory but rather provides a general sense of the variety of applications needed to sustain operations in hospitals, clinics, and physician practices. Some of these systems are found in nearly all organizations, while

Hospital Area	Systems
Financial and administrative	• Registration • Scheduling • Charge capture • Billing • Health information management
Clinical and patient management	• EHRs (inpatient, ambulatory) • Clinical information systems for clinical specialties (e.g., emergency medicine, anesthesia) • Pharmacy • Laboratory • Radiology • Case management
Data analytics	• Data warehouse • Clinical data repository • Dashboards for performance management • Registries (e.g., trauma, cancer)

EXHIBIT 13.1
Health Information Systems

others may apply only to centers providing specialized services. This chapter touches on selected examples before introducing EHR systems.

Administrative transactions—registration, scheduling, coding, billing, and accounting—remain core functions of hospital information systems. More or less, they continue to be performed the same way as they were when computers were first introduced. Increasingly, these transactions are performed by patients and clinical staff rather than by dedicated administrative personnel. As a result of their experience with self-service functions in areas such as banking, travel, and online shopping, patients have become more comfortable with similar online transactions with their healthcare providers—for example, registering for an expected newborn delivery, requesting a clinic appointment, and paying bills.

An unfortunate problem with health IT is its tendency to burden healthcare professionals with additional administrative responsibilities. As nurses and physicians spend more time performing functions such as recording patient demographic information (e.g., primary care provider, preferred pharmacy) or conducting operational functions (e.g., transferring and discharging patients), they have less time to interact with patients and with other care team members. Given the challenges associated with workforce shortages, healthcare administrators need to be attentive to the unintended consequences of this trend.

The data generated by these administrative functions have an important role in quality measurement and reporting. As discussed in Chapter 5, diagnosis and procedure codes, encounters, and even outcomes (e.g., mortality, readmission) from claims are used to compute quality and patient safety measures. Until these measures are replaced by performance measures derived directly from clinical data in EHRs, the accuracy of administrative data for evaluating healthcare quality will remain critical. Moreover, much of these data are essential for the smooth coordination of care among providers in different healthcare settings.

Ancillary clinical information systems are systems used in the support services (pharmacy, laboratory, radiology, and other departments) of hospitals and, in some cases, outpatient health centers. Commonly, these systems are not comprehensive applications but consist of an array of software solutions. For example, a pharmacy department would not typically have a single complete pharmacy information system. Instead, a more common scenario would be a combination of technologies supporting drug inventory, medication order entry and verification, clinical decision support (CDS), and dispensing. A radiology department may have separate systems for order management, digital radiography, image archiving, voice recognition, and reporting. A laboratory department may have software applications for pathology and blood banking that are distinct from other "basic" laboratory services such as chemistry and hematology.

Prior to the advent of EHRs, healthcare providers accessed information generated by these systems through printed reports or via online viewers designed for clinicians working outside of these departments. As EHR and computerized provider order entry (CPOE) systems were implemented, interfaces were established to transmit physician orders from the EHR to the ancillary systems and to transmit results from the ancillary systems to the EHR. This process allowed clinicians to rely on the EHR as a unified source of clinical information for their patients, aggregating data from multiple sources. The need for different clinical systems to communicate with each other through these interfaces has led to the emergence and widespread acceptance of messaging and terminology standards. A sample of these healthcare standards is provided in Exhibit 13.2. Health Level Seven (HL7) is the accepted standard for exchanging data between disparate clinical systems. In the United States, the American National Standards Institute is a private, nonprofit organization that oversees the development and use of these standards (Eichelberg et al. 2005).

Large healthcare organizations, especially those consisting of multiple entities, have begun to recognize the challenges of building and maintaining interfaces between different clinical systems. While standards make data exchange possible, they are not sufficient to ensure that the systems successfully communicate with each other. Establishing a point-to-point interface between two systems involves software license costs (in addition to the costs of the individual software systems) and considerable effort to ensure proper

EXHIBIT 13.2
Sample Health
IT Standards

Application	Standard
Diagnoses	International Classification of Diseases, Ninth Revision, Clinical Modification (ICD-9-CM), Volumes 1 and 2; International Classification of Diseases, Tenth Revision, Clinical Modification (ICD-10-CM)
Multiple areas of clinical vocabulary (including allergies and diagnoses)	Systematized Nomenclature of Medicine–Clinical Terms (SNOMED CT)
Procedures	Current Procedural Terminology (CPT); ICD-9-CM, Volume 3; International Classification of Diseases, Tenth Revision, Procedure Coding System (ICD-10-PCS)
Laboratory tests	Logical Observation Identifiers Names and Codes (LOINC)
Medications	National Drug Code (NDC), RxNorm
Clinical messaging	Health Level Seven (HL7)
Radiologic images	Digital Imaging and Communications in Medicine (DICOM)

coordination of the flow of data. Furthermore, upgrading one component often requires repeating this cycle of coordination and testing—albeit on a more limited scale—to prevent errors from being introduced as a result of the upgrade. Consequently, these organizations are increasingly moving to an "enterprise" approach for their IT, implementing many, if not all, software applications including the EHR and ancillary clinical systems from the same software vendor. Rather than rely on interfaces to connect numerous applications, these organizations opt for a more integrated approach. While an advantage of this option is the overall reduction in complexity, it makes the healthcare organization more dependent on a single technology provider. In addition, opting for a generic product in lieu of specialized software may entail some trade-offs in functionality.

Electronic Health Record Systems

The IOM formalized the basic concept of an EHR (sometimes referred to as an electronic medical record) in the 1991 report *The Computer-Based Patient Record: An Essential Technology for Health Care*, which was updated in 1997. The report described the primary and secondary uses of EHRs:

- Primary
  - Patient care delivery
  - Patient care management
  - Patient care support processes
  - Financial and administrative processes
  - Patient self-management
- Secondary
  - Education
  - Regulation
  - Public health and homeland security
  - Policy support

A more definitive treatment of this subject was provided in the IOM report *Key Capabilities of an Electronic Health Record System* (2003a). For health IT professionals, this IOM report represents a landmark publication, comparable in magnitude to the impact of *To Err Is Human* (Kohn, Corrigan, and Donaldson 2000) and *Crossing the Quality Chasm* (IOM 2001) for healthcare quality professionals. The report outlined the eight core functions of EHRs:

1. Health information and data storage
2. Result management
3. Order management
4. Decision support
5. Electronic communication and connectivity
6. Patient support
7. Administrative processes and reporting
8. Reporting and population health

Together, the use cases defined in *The Computer-Based Patient Record* (IOM 1991) and these eight core functions provide a framework for evaluating EHR systems that is useful to healthcare providers at various stages of adoption. An organization selecting EHR technology might use the IOM framework to draft specifications in a request for proposal, to put together a script for assessing a product demonstration or conducting a site visit, and to serve as a checklist when performing the final vendor selection. An organization that has already selected an EHR product might use the framework to develop its implementation and communication plans. One that has already deployed an EHR system might use the framework to organize how it approaches enhancement requests and opportunities for optimization. This chapter focuses on EHR use cases and functionalities especially relevant to healthcare quality.

Health Information and Clinical Documentation

The storage of health information is, arguably, the primary function of EHRs. The contents of a traditional paper-based medical record correspond to a matching component in the EHR: physician notes, vital signs, orders, medications, laboratory results, and radiology reports. To improve usability, EHR developers tend to replicate these concepts from the analog medical record in a familiar, but electronic, format. While this approach may make the transition to the digital environment easier for clinicians, it can also impair the usability of EHRs. For example, one advantage of EHRs is the ability to create a user interface for data entry separate from that used for data review. By taking advantage of this specialization, a nurse can more efficiently document vital signs in a flow sheet, while a physician reviews these data in a separate summary display. This summary display might combine relevant clinical data from different parts of the medical record—temperature, heart rate, medications, and laboratory results—and present them in a unified, logical manner. Furthermore, advanced EHRs include sophisticated search capabilities that obviate the laborious task of reviewing the charts of patients with long hospital stays and multiple encounters. EHRs limited to reproducing the paradigm of the paper record in a digital format fail to provide the benefit of these more advanced capabilities.

Capturing patient information is another element of the clinical work flow that lends itself to innovation in the EHR. Instead of merely replacing a pen with a keyboard to enter their notes, physicians are able to take advantage of structured templates to more efficiently generate this documentation. These templates can help ensure that required documentation elements are addressed, facilitate improved coding and quality reporting, and record data in a discrete manner for analytics. To capture the richness of the narrative aspect of the history of present illness, clinicians may opt to leverage speech-recognition technology to more efficiently enter free text into patient records. For nurses, interfaces with biomedical equipment automate the transfer of physiological data to the EHR.

Offsetting these benefits and the legibility of clinical notes are the unintended consequences of documentation facilitators in the EHR (Dimick 2008). One common example is the problem of *note bloat*, the tendency of some clinicians to be overly inclusive in incorporating data from other parts of the medical record in a progress note or discharge summary. The use of clinical documentation to drive coding and reimbursement has been implicated as a contributing factor. A more notorious issue is *cloning*, the misuse of tools in the EHR to copy notes entered by other clinicians. The misuse of the features available in the EHR to facilitate documentation is an unfortunate trend that demands the collective attention of healthcare leaders in the areas of quality, health information management, and IT and will receive increasing scrutiny from regulatory agencies. Ultimately, however, these behavioral issues can only be successfully addressed when clinicians themselves hold each other mutually accountable for proper documentation.

Order Management and Clinical Decision Support

Order management is an EHR function that received considerable attention in *Crossing the Quality Chasm* (IOM 2001). The landmark studies by Bates and colleagues (Bates, Leape, et al. 1998; Bates, Teich, et al. 1999) demonstrated the tremendous potential benefit of CPOE and CDS to reduce medication errors. A systematic literature review of the benefits of CDS systems conducted by Bright and colleagues (2012) showed that these systems are effective at improving healthcare process measures across diverse settings.

Osheroff and colleagues (Osheroff 2009; Osheroff et al. 2012) synthesized the body of literature on this topic and the collective experience of those involved with implementing clinical systems. Stakeholders from provider organizations, health IT vendors, federal agencies, and others are collaborating to apply decision support approaches from these guides to key care processes and outcomes. Targets include reducing hospital readmissions and controlling hypertension and asthma in the ambulatory setting. An Office of the National Coordinator for Health Information Technology (ONC) project produced tools and resources that underpin these quality improvement projects. These resources are freely available at the Clinical Decision Support Collaborative for Performance Improvement website (sites.google.com/site/cdsforpiimperativespublic/home).

CPOE often becomes a major focus of EHR projects. For physicians, CPOE can be disruptive to work flow. A poorly designed CPOE system can lead to a failed EHR implementation. Consequently, significant resources are invested in ensuring that CPOE systems are intuitive and user friendly and that physicians receive adequate training and support. When these requirements are met, the medical staff are more likely to adopt CPOE. In fact, the adoption of CPOE is a universal measure of EHR implementation success (Hudson et al. 2012).

As vital as CPOE is in engaging physicians in using the EHR, its direct contribution to patient safety is largely confined to the elimination of errors associated with transcription of handwritten physician orders in the order management system and the expedited turnaround of orders by the clinical staff and ancillary departments. Its major contribution to process improvement and patient safety is accomplished indirectly through CDS. Through such tools as order sets, alerts and reminders, and embedded references, EHRs promote adoption of evidence-based clinical practice and reduce prescribing errors that can lead to adverse drug events (Kuperman et al. 2007; Osheroff 2009; Osheroff et al. 2012).

The Leapfrog Group, a consortium of large employers, has actively promoted CPOE and CDS to improve patient safety. It has partnered with the Agency for Healthcare Research and Quality (AHRQ) to develop an evaluation tool to allow healthcare systems to test how well their CPOE systems can intercept dangerous medication errors. Although it has several limitations—its preoccupation with interruptive alerts as the principal safeguard against prescribing errors chief among them—the Leapfrog CPOE tool is the only instrument available for objectively evaluating CPOE and CDS systems (Metzger et al. 2008). Leung and colleagues (2013) studied the relationship between test scores using the Leapfrog CPOE tool and the rates of preventable adverse drug events and found a close correlation, supporting the use of the Leapfrog tool as a means of evaluating and monitoring CPOE performance after implementation.

CDS is more than the alerts triggered and displayed in a CPOE system. Examples of CDS tools include the following:

- Order sets
- Structured documentation templates
- Relevant data displays
- Clinical alerts and reminders
- Disease and drug references

CDS can play a key role in any work flow supported by the EHR: documentation, medication management, and notification of a rapid response team, among others.

Case Study: Venous Thromboembolism Prophylaxis at Texas Health Resources

An approach undertaken by a multihospital system to reduce the incidence of venous thromboembolism (VTE) illustrates the value of CDS to advance a performance improvement initiative. Recognizing the contribution of VTE to hospital mortality, Texas Health Resources established an interdisciplinary performance improvement task force, led by a hospital chief quality officer, to improve rates of VTE prophylaxis among medical and surgical patients.

The group used many of the methods described in other chapters of this book to identify opportunities for improvement. A major barrier was poor identification of patients at risk for developing VTE. In fact, VTE risk assessment was inconsistent across the system. Some hospitals had implemented formal evidence-based risk assessment tools, while others depended on physicians' subjective sense of their patients' VTE risk. Risk assessment, if done at all, was performed using paper forms and was not documented in the EHR. The committee made an early decision to standardize the assessment methodology and integrate it into the EHR. This decision not only helped to ensure a consistent practice but also provided a mechanism for monitoring clinician compliance and patient VTE risk.

To facilitate the ordering of VTE prophylaxis, changes were made to postoperative order sets in the CPOE system to include a specific section addressing VTE prevention. Surgeons encountered a "hard stop" in the process—that is, they had to either order mechanical and/or pharmacologic prophylaxis or specify a reason for not doing so. This change explicitly reminded physicians to consider ordering VTE preventive measures, and it automated the process for collecting data for surgical care improvement measures.

Finally, the group sanctioned the development and implementation of best-practice advisories for patients without VTE prophylaxis orders. Every four hours, the EHR checks for these orders for an appropriate subset of patients on the acute care census. If no order is found for a given patient, a window displays a message prompting members of the care team to place the patient on prophylaxis or to document the reason for the absence of the order.

As a result of these CDS interventions, Texas Health Resources improved the rate of VTE prophylaxis and reduced the incidence of VTE by 50 percent across the system (HIMSS 2013).

Medication Management

In addition to the benefits associated with CPOE and CDS, other forms of health IT can enhance medication management and drug safety. Bar-coded medication administration at the point of care helps ensure proper verification of the patient, drug, dose, and time. Poon and colleagues (2010) observed a 50.8 percent relative reduction in potential adverse drug events with this technology. Medication reconciliation has been recognized as an important process in care transitions to prevent adverse health outcomes (Kwan et al. 2013; Mueller et al. 2012). The Advisory Board Company (2007) report *Electronic Medication Reconciliation* provides useful guidance for leveraging health IT and employing a collaborative approach involving patients, physicians, nurses, and pharmacists to optimize medication reconciliation. Another promising area is technology to enhance long-term medication adherence for patients with chronic conditions, although additional research to demonstrate efficacy is still needed (Misono et al. 2010). Finally, the IOM (2012) has cited EHRs as a potential tool for the Food and Drug Administration to use to strengthen surveillance of new medications on the market.

Connectivity: Health Information Exchange and Patient Support

As powerful as EHRs are for supporting care delivery in an organization, their full potential is unlocked when the EHRs of separate entities are connected and are exposed to patients and providers in the community. These technologies extend the reach of EHRs beyond healthcare systems into the community and into the patient home.

The exchange of data between EHRs is accomplished through specialized technology known as health information exchange (HIE). Several different models for HIE are designed to suit different scenarios or use cases (see Exhibit 13.3). In large, integrated delivery systems, the HIE is often used to connect disparate EHR systems within the enterprise rather than convert them into a single platform. Similarly, accountable care organizations consisting of multiple partners may establish a "private" HIE to facilitate the coordination of care for their shared patient population. More loosely associated entities, such as those participating in a state or regional HIE, connect and share patient data via "public" networks. Finally, the ONC is coordinating federal efforts to exchange health information at the national level. Organizations can participate in more than one of these models.

All types of HIE depend on adherence to standards for data exchange and interoperability. A key standard is the Continuity of Care Document (CCD) specification. The CCD, which itself is part of the HL7 Clinical Document Architecture standard, specifies the structure and content of a clinical summary document. It represents a core set of pertinent administrative and clinical information associated with a patient at a particular time. The more complex HIE models used by larger or more loosely affiliated entities require a master patient identifier and record locator service to properly match individuals in a population and to transmit clinical documents faithfully.

Basing their research on 2009 data from the American Hospital Association Information Technology Survey, Adler-Milstein, DesRoches, and Jha

Model	Description	Use Cases/Examples
Point to point	Dedicated point-to-point interfaces connect participants known to each other.	Communications pushed between trusted entities (similar to fax)
Hub and spoke	Participating entities connect to a centrally managed hub that stores and forwards messages via an interface engine.	Integrated delivery systems or accountable care organizations
Central repository	This model is similar to hub and spoke, except that the data are stored and managed centrally.	Integrated delivery systems
Integrated health exchange	Participating entities respond to requests for documents.	Regional or state health information exchanges

EXHIBIT 13.3
Models for Health Information Exchange

(2011) found that only 10.7 percent of US hospitals engage in exchange of health information with unaffiliated providers. The Health Information Technology for Economic and Clinical Health (HITECH) Act, described in this chapter, is part of a federal strategy to advance the exchange of health information both regionally and nationally (Williams et al. 2012).

Case Study: Care Coordination and Population Health at Southeast Texas Medical Associates

Southeast Texas Medical Associates (SETMA) is a multispecialty medical practice in Jefferson County, Texas, located in the southeastern tip of the state. SETMA has received national recognition for its advanced use of the EHR to coordinate and manage care for its patient population. In 2005, SETMA received the Healthcare Information and Management Systems Society's Davies Award of Excellence for health IT, and in 2010, it was designated by the National Committee for Quality Assurance as a patient-centered medical home.

Shortly after implementing an EHR system in the ambulatory setting in 1999, SETMA began using its EHR to facilitate continuity of care for hospitalized patients. Clinic records were accessed to fill in information missing from the patient's admission assessment. After discharge, documentation of the hospital course was readily available during the follow-up outpatient visit. In 2000, the group established a dedicated hospital service team to provide continuous in-house coverage for its patient population.

Long before the regional hospitals implemented EHR systems, SETMA was using the EHR for its practice to produce hospital discharge summaries and to perform medication reconciliation. It subsequently adopted this approach for patients in nursing homes as well.

In 2009, the American Medical Association's Physician Consortium for Performance Improvement published the first national quality measurement set on care transitions. That year, SETMA implemented these care transition measures in its EHR. In 2013, 95 percent of SETMA patients met these criteria at the time of discharge.

In 2010, SETMA deployed a secure web-based EHR portal and an HIE to enable the seamless exchange of information between the practice, hospitals, nursing homes, and home health agencies. That same year, the group settled on the concept of a "post–hospital care summary and treatment plan" as a more comprehensive representation of the care transition model at hospital discharge. This model of a hybrid care summary and treatment plan is advanced by IT advisors and health services experts as a key strategy for reducing avoidable readmissions. Thanks, in part, to its exemplary use of health IT to support care coordination, SETMA was named by the Center for Medicare & Medicaid Services (CMS) as one of the first accountable care organizations in the Medicare Shared Savings Program.

Personal Health Records and Patient EHR Portals

Just as HIEs extend the value of EHRs to other providers, PHRs extend the reach of the EHR to consumers of healthcare. Patients can use a PHR to access their clinical information (e.g., hospital or clinic visit summaries, medications, laboratory results), browse relevant educational content, schedule an appointment with their physician, receive reminders for preventive and other health maintenance services, request prescription refills, and exchange messages securely with members of the care team. Organizations that have deployed PHRs have found them to be a key tool in engaging patients and improving their satisfaction. By interacting with their care providers through PHRs, patients become more informed about their health status and the healthcare services provided. Consequently, they are empowered to take a more active role in clinical decision making (Archer et al. 2011; Tang et al. 2006). In 2012, the federal government introduced the Blue Button program as part of an effort to encourage greater adoption of patient portals and PHRs (Austin, Hull, and Westra 2014; HealthIT.gov 2014).

Privacy and Security

One of the chief benefits of health IT is the enhanced access to clinical information. Providers are no longer limited by physical access to the patient's chart, X-rays, and other tangible artifacts. Providers can access these items anywhere they can connect to the Internet. Associated with this enhanced access, however, are concerns related to privacy and confidentiality.

Healthcare organizations implementing information systems containing patient information are obligated to ensure the integrity of that information. In addition to state laws, the Health Insurance Portability and Accountability Act (HIPAA) enacted in 1996 included provisions to address the security and privacy of health data. The HIPAA Privacy Rule (45 C.F.R. 160 and 45 C.F.R. 164 subparts A and E), which was finalized in 2000 and took effect in 2003, regulates the use and disclosure of protected health information (PHI) held by healthcare professionals and other covered entities, such as insurers and employer-sponsored health plans. A covered entity may disclose PHI to facilitate treatment, payment, or healthcare operations without a patient's express written authorization. Any other disclosures require the covered entity to obtain written authorization. The rule also authorizes individuals to request corrections to their PHI and to be notified when and to whom their health information is disclosed. The Privacy Rule covers health information maintained in any format, including paper medical records.

The HIPAA Security Rule (45 C.F.R. 160 and 45 C.F.R. 164 subparts A and C), which was issued in February 2003 with a compliance date of April 21, 2005 (or April 21, 2006, for small health plans), complements the Privacy Rule and deals specifically with PHI stored in an electronic medium. Covered entities are required to provide three classes of safeguards to ensure the security and integrity of electronic health information: administrative, physical, and technical. Examples of each are provided in Exhibit 13.4.

Recent breaches in information security, resulting in unauthorized disclosure or access to the health records of thousands of individuals, have highlighted the importance of these safeguards. Aside from the penalties associated with violations of HIPAA and other applicable regulations, healthcare professionals are entrusted with the duty and responsibility to maintain the privacy and confidentiality of personal information of those under their care.

"The Decade of Health Information Technology": The HITECH Act and Healthcare Reform

Despite the recommendations in the IOM reports and general advocacy for EHRs among quality and patient safety experts, adoption of EHRs was superficial at the turn of the twenty-first century. Jha and colleagues (2006) found that approximately 23.9 percent of physicians used EHRs in the ambulatory setting, while 5 percent of hospitals used CPOE. Jha and colleagues (2009) further studied the adoption of EHRs by hospitals and determined that fewer than 2 percent of acute care hospitals had a comprehensive EHR system and between 8 and 12 percent had a "basic" EHR system.

In his 2004 State of the Union address, President George W. Bush called for every American to have access to an EHR within ten years. This challenge launched the "decade of health information technology," a period of unprecedented federal support for the adoption of IT in the clinical domain.

While both the US Department of Defense and the Veterans Administration (VA) are exemplary in their adoption of health IT, prior to 2004 the federal government had minimal involvement in advancing EHRs in hospitals and outpatient settings. The president's speech and the establishment of the ONC in 2004 changed the situation dramatically. Created as a branch of the Office of the Secretary of the US Department of Health and Human Services (HHS), the ONC was charged with the development of a national policy and strategic road map for achieving the president's vision of widespread adoption of EHRs by 2014. Its role is to coordinate nationwide efforts to implement and adopt health IT and promote the electronic exchange of health information.

EXHIBIT 13.4

Examples of Safeguards to Ensure Health Information Security

Class	Safeguards

Administrative	• Security management process: authorizes policies and procedures to prevent, detect, contain, and correct security violations. Components of this standard include the following:
	  – Risk analysis
	  – Risk management
	  – Sanction policy
	  – Information system activity review
	• Assigned security responsibility: designates the security official responsible for development and implementation of policies and procedures related to information security
	• Workforce security: authorizes policies and procedures so that the workforce of a covered entity has appropriate access to electronic PHI and workforce members not authorized to access PHI are prevented from doing so
	• Information access management: authorizes access to PHI in a manner consistent with HIPAA requirements
	• Security awareness and training:
	  – Security reminders
	  – Protection from malicious software
	  – Log-in monitoring
	  – Password management
	• Security incident procedures: cover how security incidents such as breaches, damaged media, and stolen computers are to be addressed
	• Contingency plan: outlines the response to an emergency or other incident that damages systems containing PHI
	• Evaluation: dictates periodic, ongoing evaluation of the covered entity's security measures and safeguards
	• Business associate arrangements: require contracts with authorized third parties to create, maintain, or transmit PHI on behalf of the covered entity

Physical	• Facility access controls: require procedures to limit physical access to information systems and facilities • Workstation use: defines the proper functions that may be performed on laptops and personal computers • Workstation security: ensures that physical safeguards for computing devices are in place • Device and media controls: governs the use of electronic media containing PHI and the movement of these items within and outside a facility

Technical	• Access controls
	  – Unique user identification
	  – Emergency access procedure
	  – Automatic log-off
	  – Encryption and decryption
	• Audit controls: require mechanisms to record and evaluate access to information systems
	• Integrity: ensures that information is not damaged or altered in an unauthorized manner
	• Authentication: verifies the identity of an individual or entity seeking access to PHI
	• Transmission security: ensures the integrity of information transmitted over an electronic communications framework

Sources: HIPAA Privacy Rule (45 C.F.R. 160 and 45 C.F.R. 164 subparts A and E); HIPAA Security Rule (45 C.F.R. 160 and 45 C.F.R. 164 subparts A and C).

HITECH Act of 2009 and EHR Incentive Program

Support for health IT continued during the administration of President Barack Obama. After his election into office, the president signed into law the HITECH Act of 2009, which established a formal incentive program for the adoption of EHRs and further clarified the central role of the ONC in advancing the administration's health IT policy efforts through legislative mandate (Buntin, Jain, and Blumenthal 2010). As a result of the HITECH Act, the ONC transitioned from being a resource for supporting health IT and adopting EHRs to a federal agency with rule-making authority. To achieve its mission, the ONC established two federal advisory committees composed of industry thought leaders to further develop the national health IT policy and inform the development of EHR standards. The HITECH Act mandated three major activities of the ONC: creating a formal EHR certification program; supporting regional extension centers to assist primary care providers in local communities; and providing grants to advance health IT research, development, and learning.

Closely working with the ONC is CMS, which is charged with administering the EHR incentive program (Blumenthal 2010). Through this program, the HITECH Act allocated $17 billion in Medicare and Medicaid funding to promote the adoption and "meaningful use" of certified EHR technology to achieve health and efficiency goals. The HITECH Act specified three main components of meaningful use:

1. Use of a certified EHR in a meaningful manner, such as e-prescribing
2. Use of certified EHR technology for electronic exchange of health information to improve quality of healthcare
3. Use of certified EHR technology to submit clinical quality and other measures

CMS spelled out the meaningful use requirements more specifically through the rule-making process after receiving input from the federal advisory committees. Criteria were established for Stages 1 and 2 of meaningful use, and additional stages will be defined through subsequent regulatory activity. The meaningful use criteria for eligible hospitals and eligible professionals are available on the CMS (2014d) website.

The program was formally launched in January 2011. In the first three years, more than 334,000 eligible professionals, eligible hospitals, and critical access hospitals received more than $17.3 billion in incentive payments for achieving the criteria for demonstrating meaningful use (CMS 2014c). The distribution of incentive payments by state as of November 2013 is illustrated in Exhibit 13.5. Jha (2012) attributed the increase in physician EHR adoption (a 10 percent increase in 2011 to 35 percent of US physicians) to the

EXHIBIT 13.5
Combined Medicare and Medicaid Payments by State, 2011–2013

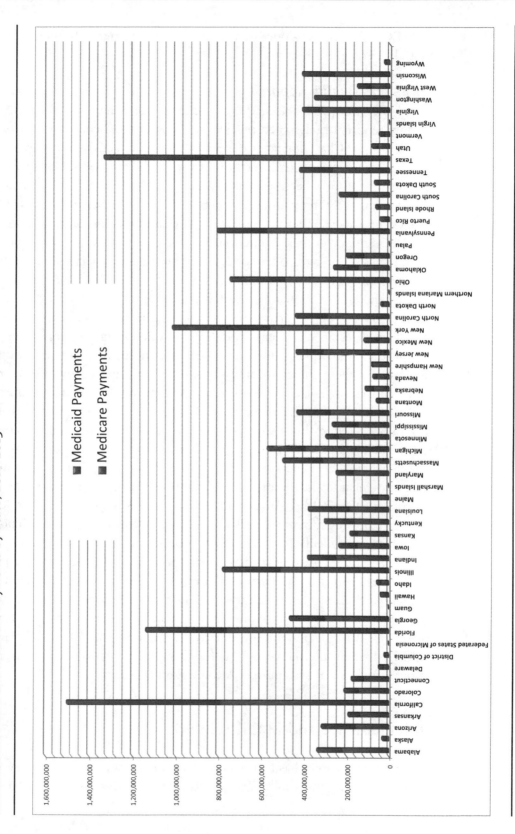

HITECH Act but cautioned that the greatest challenges of achieving meaningful use of EHRs lie ahead.

EHRs and Quality Reporting

Until the advent of EHRs, the extraction of data required for producing quality reports largely relied on two methods: manual chart abstraction and use of claims. Chart abstraction is a labor-intensive activity requiring significant human resources. A limitation of the claims method is the accuracy of billing records in reflecting clinical activity. In both cases, an added issue is the latency in the reporting of quality data. A significant delay in feedback makes the implementation of meaningful changes to clinical care more difficult. EHRs address these limitations by capturing the required data elements automatically as a by-product of care and providing clinicians and healthcare leaders with more timely feedback.

The HITECH Act established quality reporting as a core dimension of the EHR incentive program. The meaningful use framework introduces and formalizes an electronic workflow for calculating and reporting quality measures. To qualify for meaningful use incentive payments, providers must derive these clinical quality measures electronically from EHRs, registries, and HIEs. For each measure, the system must generate a numerator, a denominator, and the number of patients excluded (if applicable). CMS does not prescribe thresholds that need to be met to satisfy this meaningful use objective. In Stages 1 and 2, the only requirement is to provide to CMS the quality reports generated by the certified technology. The clinical quality measures included in the meaningful use program are available on the CMS website (CMS 2014a). In general, the measures align with other federal quality-reporting initiatives, such as the Hospital Inpatient Quality Reporting and Physician Quality Reporting System programs.

Quality indicator data derived from certified EHR systems are manually entered into a web portal established by CMS, a process referred to as *attestation*. This portal is the same one used by eligible hospitals and eligible professionals to register for the EHR incentive program and to attest to achievement of meaningful use objectives. Beginning in 2014, following an initial pilot, an alternative option for submitting clinical quality measures directly from EHR systems to CMS was made available.

Telemedicine and Mobile Health

Much of this chapter has focused on health IT in traditional clinical settings, such as hospitals and clinics. To provide more effective disease management, healthcare organizations and professionals must extend the delivery of care beyond these settings, including to patients' homes. Health IT plays an important role in this expansion of care delivery.

Telemedicine, defined as the application of telecommunications technology to provide clinical services at a distance, was first enabled by telephony and two-way radio. While telephone encounters and other interactions limited to voice continue to play an important role in patient care today, more sophisticated information and communication technology, by making video interactions and the transmission of high-resolution diagnostic images and robust clinical data possible, has substantially expanded the scope of telemedicine and its corresponding benefits. The key dimensions of this emerging field include actors (clinicians and patients), locations (clinical and nonclinical settings), and transmission synchronization. Different clinical use cases emerge from combinations of these parameters.

Interactions supported by telemedicine can be broadly separated into two modes: synchronous and asynchronous. In synchronous interaction, information is transmitted or exchanged in real time. Telephonic consultations and remote patient monitoring are examples of synchronous interaction. Examples of asynchronous telemedicine applications are teleradiology and clinical communications similar to e-mail.

The initial interest in telemedicine originated from healthcare providers in rural areas and in the military. These early applications were necessitated by barriers to access to healthcare services because of distance and limited resources. Today, even healthcare providers in densely populated areas face similar challenges. In addition, in an era of consumer-driven healthcare, patient preferences and expectations are important considerations in promoting the adoption of telemedicine. While many examples of telemedicine can have a positive impact on healthcare quality, a few illustrative use cases are discussed here.

Remote patient monitoring is a rapidly growing service. An early use case was the e-ICU concept, in which the health status of patients in intensive care units is followed by critical care specialists at a different location (Breslow 2007). Organizations that adopt this model are able to leverage limited resources to continuously monitor patients in multiple, dispersed ICU environments by creating a work environment equipped with access to vital signs, laboratory data, radiology images, medical records, and live video. From the e-ICU, the intensivist conducts audio and video interactions with the local clinicians and with the patients directly.

This technology is also applied to the home setting as a strategy to reduce hospital length of stay and avoidable readmissions and to improve the management of chronic diseases in the outpatient setting. As medical equipment used to digitally capture and record blood pressure, heart rate, weight, oxygen saturation, and point-of-care laboratory tests becomes more affordable, the equipment is increasingly being connected to PHRs and web-based portals to transmit biometric data to providers. Instead of waiting until the next office visit, a physician can routinely monitor a patient's health status, allowing issues requiring intervention to be identified in a more timely fashion. In a randomized controlled trial involving VA patients, significant improvements in HbA1c levels were achieved using home telemonitoring and active medication management for six months and were sustained for a subsequent six-month period with interventions of decreased intensity (Stone et al. 2012).

The introduction of telemedicine as part of a provider's care delivery strategy has important implications for reimbursement, professional accreditation, and the organization of the healthcare system. Does a clinic or hospital hire additional staff to perform telephonic encounters and provide remote patient monitoring, or does it partner with a third party for these services? If the latter, how is continuity of care ensured? Are these services reimbursed equitably by payers? What are the medical specialty board certification and state medical licensure requirements associated with teleconsultation services offered across state lines and national boundaries? Given the shifting nature of telemedicine as well as regional considerations, offering advice on specific approaches would be difficult. Nonetheless, telemedicine will play an increasingly transformational role in healthcare, and providers should incorporate it into the strategic planning process.

Closely related to telemedicine is the emerging area of mobile health, which refers to health IT applications residing on mobile devices such as cell phones and tablets. Although mobile health preceded the arrival of portable communication technology, the nearly universal adoption of these consumer-oriented devices has led to its rapid growth. Mobile health allows interactions between healthcare providers and patients to take place almost anywhere.

The tremendous array of mobile health applications includes robust enterprise systems originally designed for traditional computing platforms (and accessed from personal computers and laptops) that have been repurposed to run on smart phones and tablets as well as novel applications developed specifically for these devices. In fact, nearly every application of health IT discussed in this chapter has or will potentially have a mobile interface. Given the itinerant nature of care delivery, this situation is not unexpected. Healthcare workers—physicians, nurses, pharmacists, physical therapists, nutritionists, and social workers—are constantly on the move. Just as the lack of mobility associated with traditional platforms for IT has historically contributed to dissatisfaction with its poor usability in the clinical setting, the portable aspect of mobile health is its chief appeal among clinicians.

Health IT for Consumers

The ONC (2013) has provided a useful summary of applications geared toward healthcare consumers. In addition to PHRs and patient EHR portals, covered earlier in this chapter, health-related informational websites (e.g., healthfinder.gov) and peer-health websites (e.g., PatientsLikeMe.com, TuDiabetes.org) are available. The Pew Research Center published a report summarizing its research on how people are increasingly turning to these online resources (Fox 2011). The report estimates that 59 percent of all adults have looked online for health information and that 23 percent of those with chronic conditions have sought others with similar health concerns via the Internet.

Paralleling the advance of mobile health for providers is the growing popularity of mobile healthcare-related apps for consumers. Healthcare, wellness, and social networking are converging in the consumer space. Using healthcare-related apps, an individual can track food consumption, physical activity, blood sugar levels, and sleep patterns and publish this information to social networks via Twitter and Facebook. The popularity of wearable devices that wirelessly transmit data to smartphones eliminates much of the effort involved in recording these data.

Organizations, including the Mayo Clinic, are actively studying the role of social media in health and wellness (Pogoreic 2011). For example, social media sites such as Twitter have yielded insights in terms of public awareness of and community responses to outbreaks of communicable diseases and other public health threats (Chew and Eysenbach 2010). These disruptive technologies have the potential to alter the health IT landscape.

Keys to Successful Implementation and Lessons Learned

Organizational and Cultural Considerations

Successfully implementing IT in healthcare requires organizational and cultural readiness for change. A pitfall of many projects is the assumption that the technology is the central focus. In reality, the dimensions of people and process are even more important considerations. Technology should be viewed as an enabler of process improvement and innovation, rather than an end in itself (Amatayakul 2004).

In light of this insight, healthcare providers must be attentive to how their organizations are structured to ensure success. To be effective, project leadership should be based on a partnership between clinical and technology stakeholders. Project steering committees should include physicians who are in active clinical practice. A key success factor in many hospitals and health systems is formally integrating clinicians into the information services organization. These clinicians include physicians, nurses, and pharmacists with both a clinical and a technology background. An emerging role, especially in larger organizations, is the medical director of informatics or chief medical information officer (CMIO). This physician leader works closely with the medical staff and information services group to assist with the transition to EHRs and other technologies. The CMIO plays an important role in identifying the clinical informatics needs of the organization, defining requirements for information systems, and selecting, designing, and implementing these systems. The chief nursing information officer (CNIO) plays a similar role for nursing. Collectively, these individuals leverage their clinical experience to ensure that technology is introduced into the healthcare setting as smoothly as possible and is adopted by their colleagues.

The inclusion of a chapter on health IT in this book is a clear indication of its importance to healthcare quality. Accordingly, professionals and healthcare executives specializing in quality improvement and patient safety must be properly informed of and closely involved with IT initiatives in their organization. This translates into active involvement in the governance of IT initiatives; participation in project steering committees; and a collegial working relationship with the chief information officer, the CMIO, and the CNIO. Likewise, IT professionals must stay abreast of developments in the quality domain. An encouraging trend in the technology field is the introduction of such methods as Plan-Do-Study-Act (PDSA), Lean, and Six Sigma to deliver continuous quality improvement of IT services. As healthcare systems strive to become high-reliability organizations, healthcare quality and IT professionals are increasingly developing a shared vocabulary, methodology, and mind-set.

Unintended Consequences

In 2011, the IOM published a key report, *Health IT and Patient Safety: Building Safer Systems for Better Care*. Unlike previous IOM reports that tended to focus on the benefits of health IT, *Health IT and Patient Safety* was devoted to the issue of its unintended and, at times, harmful consequences. Although the potential for these consequences has been recognized for some time, this "darker" side of health IT gained significant attention through the work of Koppel and colleagues (2005). Subsequently, a number of reviews weighed in on the question of the safety of EHRs and other clinical systems. *Health IT and Patient Safety* represented the culmination of this inquiry, providing a synthesis of the relevant research and recommendations for increased transparency and accountability on the part of IT stakeholders. The IOM report concluded by articulating the following policy recommendations:

1. An action plan sponsored by HHS to engage the AHRQ to expand funding for research and education of safe practices and the ONC to implement procedures such as standardized testing to promote safe technology

2. A free exchange of information related to patient safety among health IT vendors

3. The development of measures to assess usability of information systems

4. The creation of a new health IT safety council as a voluntary consensus standards organization to evaluate criteria for assessing and monitoring patient safety

5. A requirement that all vendors publicly register and list their products with the ONC

6. Formal quality and risk management process requirements, specified by HHS, that vendors must adopt to ensure safe and usable information systems

7. A mechanism for vendors and customers to report IT–related injuries and deaths

8. The creation by Congress of an independent federal entity for investigating deaths, serious injuries, and unsafe conditions associated with health IT

In response to the IOM report, the AHRQ addressed the need to improve education on IT safety by publishing its *Guide to Reducing Unintended Consequences of Electronic Health Records* (Jones et al. 2011). As part of a series of tools intended to address the IOM's call for improved safety surveillance, the ONC chartered the ECRI Institute to publish *How to Identify and Address Unsafe Conditions Associated with Health IT* (Wallace et al. 2013). In addition, the ONC series of *SAFER Guides* outline recommended industry practices for enhancing patient safety in health IT implementations (Ash, Singh, and Sittig 2014).

Conclusion

Healthcare Reform and the Era of Accountability

With the passage of sweeping healthcare reform legislation in the form of the Affordable Care Act of 2010, care delivery models will undergo a radical makeover as payment shifts from fee-for-service reimbursement to value-based care. This transition will require greater transparency in terms of public reporting of performance data and continued expansion of the library of quality measures. Health systems and providers that invest in health IT and are able to satisfy the meaningful use criteria will be better able to cope with the challenges of accountable care.

Healthcare Quality and IT

This chapter demonstrates the parallel trajectories of the modern healthcare quality and health IT movements. Both movements can trace their origins to landmark IOM reports that called for unprecedented public and private attention to systematic gaps in the US healthcare system. Both have benefited from federal support in the form of funding for research and incentive programs. Just as pioneers in quality improvement have paved the way for all healthcare providers, innovators and early adopters of IT have set an example for others to follow. But even more remarkable than the parallels between quality and technology is their convergence. As the IOM reports have predicted, the needed transformation of healthcare delivery will come about as a result of the combined and cooperative efforts of clinicians, healthcare quality professionals, and IT workers.

Study Questions

1. Describe how health IT can facilitate care coordination.
2. Cite two examples of unintended consequences of the use of electronic documentation tools.
3. What impact has the HITECH Act of 2009 had on the adoption of EHRs?

Acknowledgment

I wish to acknowledge the assistance of Kanan Garg in the preparation of this chapter.

References

Adler-Milstein, J., C. M. DesRoches, and A. K. Jha. 2011. "Health Information Exchange Among U.S. Hospitals." *American Journal of Managed Care* 17 (11): 761–68.

Advisory Board Company. 2007. *Electronic Medication Reconciliation: Practices for Streamlining Information Transfer.* Washington, DC: Advisory Board Company.

Amatayakul, M. K. 2004. *Electronic Health Records: A Practical Guide for Professionals and Organizations.* Chicago: American Health Information Management Association.

Archer, N., U. Fevrier-Thomas, C. Lokker, K. A. McKibbon, and S. E. Straus. 2011. "Personal Health Records: A Scoping Review." *Journal of the American Medical Informatics Association* 18 (4): 515–22.

Ash, J., H. Singh, and D. Sittig. 2014. *SAFER (Safety Assurance Factors for EHR Resilience) Guides.* Office of the National Coordinator for Health Information Technology. www.healthit.gov/policy-researchers-implementers/safer.

Austin, R., S. Hull, and B. Westra. 2014. "Blue Button Movement: Engaging Ourselves and Patients." *Computers, Informatics, Nursing* 32 (1): 7–9.

Bates, D. W., L. L. Leape, D. J. Cullen, N. Laird, L. A. Petersen, J. M. Teich, E. Burdick, M. Hickey, S. Kleefield, B. Shea, V. M. Vander, and D. L. Seger. 1998. "Effect of Computerized Physician Order Entry and a Team Intervention on Prevention of Serious Medication Errors." *Journal of the American Medical Association* 280 (15): 1311–16.

Bates, D. W., J. M. Teich, J. Lee, D. L. Seger, G. Kuperman, N. Ma'Luf, D. Boyle, and L. Leape. 1999. "The Impact of Computerized Physician Order Entry on Medication Error Prevention." *Journal of the American Medical Informatics Association* 6 (4): 313–21.

Blumenthal, D. 2010. "Launching HITECH." *New England Journal of Medicine* 362 (2): 382–85.

———. 2009. "Stimulating the Adoption of Health Information Technology." *New England Journal of Medicine* 360 (15): 1477–79.

Breslow, M. J. 2007. "Remote ICU Care Programs: Current Status." *Journal of Critical Care* 22 (1): 66–76.

Bright, T. J., A. Wong, R. Dhurjati, E. Bristow, L. Bastian, R. R. Coeytaux, G. Samsa, V. Hasselblad, J. W. Williams, M. D. Musty, L. Wing, A. S. Kendrick, G. D. Sanders, and D. Lobach. 2012. "Effect of Clinical Decision-Support Systems: A Systematic Review." *Annals of Internal Medicine* 157 (1): 29–43.

Buntin, M. B., S. H. Jain, and D. Blumenthal. 2010. "Health Information Technology: Laying the Infrastructure for National Health Reform." *Health Affairs* 29 (6): 1214–19.

Centers for Medicare & Medicaid Services (CMS). 2014a. "Clinical Quality Measures (CQMs)." Updated January 16. www.cms.gov/Regulations-and-Guidance/Legislation/EHRIncentivePrograms/ClinicalQualityMeasures.html.

———. 2014b. "Combined Medicare and Medicaid Payments by State Graph." Accessed February 3. www.cms.gov/Regulations-and-Guidance/Legislation/EHRIncentivePrograms/Downloads/November2013_GraphofPaymentsbyIndividualState.pdf.

———. 2014c. "Data and Program Reports." Updated January 29. www.cms.gov/Regulations-and-Guidance/Legislation/EHRIncentivePrograms/DataAndReports.html.

———. 2014d. "Meaningful Use." Updated January 16. www.cms.gov/Regulations-and-Guidance/Legislation/EHRIncentivePrograms/Meaningful_Use.html.

Chew, C., and G. Eysenbach. 2010. "Pandemics in the Age of Twitter: Content Analysis of Tweets During the 2009 H1N1 Outbreak." *PLoS ONE* 5 (11): e14118.

Dimick, C. 2008. "Documentation Bad Habits: Shortcuts in Electronic Records Pose Risk." *Journal of the American Health Information Management Association* 79 (6): 40–43.

Eichelberg, M., T. Aden, J. Riesmeier, A. Dogac, and G. B. Laleci. 2005. "A Survey and Analysis of Electronic Healthcare Record Standards." *Association for Computing Machinery Computing Surveys* 37 (4): 277–315.

Fox, S. 2011. *The Social Life of Health Information, 2011*. Washington, DC: Pew Research Center.

Healthcare Information and Management Systems Society (HIMSS). 2013. "Menu Case Study: Reducing Venous Thromboembolism (VTE) Using Clinical Decision Support Interventions: Order Sets, Risk Assessment Calculator and Best Practice Advisories Within the Electronic Health Record." HIMSS 2013 Davies Enterprise Award Application: Texas Health Resources. http://apps.himss.org/davies/docs/2013/THR_DaviesSubmission_VTE.pdf.

HealthIT.gov. 2014. "About Blue Button." Accessed February 3. www.healthit.gov/patients-families/blue-button/about-blue-button.

Hudson, J. S., J. A. Neff, M. A. Padilla, Q. Zhang, and L. T. Mercer. 2012. "Predictors of Physician Use of Inpatient Electronic Health Records." *American Journal of Managed Care* 18 (4): 201–6.

Institute of Medicine (IOM). 2012. *Ethical and Scientific Issues in Studying the Safety of Approved Drugs*. Washington, DC: National Academies Press.

———. 2011. *Health IT and Patient Safety: Building Safer Systems for Better Care*. Washington, DC: National Academies Press.

———. 2003a. *Key Capabilities of an Electronic Health Record System*. Washington, DC: National Academies Press.

———. 2003b. *Patient Safety: Achieving a New Standard for Care*. Washington, DC: National Academies Press.

———. 2001. *Crossing the Quality Chasm: A New Health System for the 21st Century*. Washington, DC: National Academies Press.

———. (1991) 1997. *The Computer-Based Patient Record: An Essential Technology for Health Care*. Washington, DC: National Academies Press.

Jha, J. K. 2012. "Health Information Technology Comes of Age." *Archives of Internal Medicine* 172 (9): 737–38.

Jha, J. K., C. M. DesRoches, E. G. Campbell, K. Donelan, S. R. Rao, T. G. Ferris, A. Shields, S. Rosenbaum, and D. Blumenthal. 2009. "Use of Electronic Health Records in U.S. Hospitals." *New England Journal of Medicine* 360 (16): 1628–38.

Jha, J. K., T. G. Ferris, D. Donelan, C. M. DesRoches, A. Shields, S. Rosenbaum, and D. Blumenthal. 2006. "How Common Are Electronic Health Records in the United States?" *Health Affairs* 25 (6): 496–507.

Jones, S. S., R. Koppel, M. S. Ridgely, T. E. Palen, S. Wu, and M. I. Harrison. 2011. *Guide to Reducing Unintended Consequences of Electronic Health Records.* Rockville, MD: Agency for Healthcare Research and Quality.

Kohn L. T., J. M. Corrigan, and M. S. Donaldson (eds.). 2000. *To Err Is Human: Building A Safer Health System.* Washington, DC: National Academies Press.

Koppel, R., J. P. Metlay, A. Cohen, B. Abaluck, A. R. Localio, S. E. Kimmel, and B. L. Strom. 2005. "Role of Computerized Physician Order Entry Systems in Facilitating Medication Errors." *Journal of the American Medical Association* 293 (10): 1197–203.

Kuperman, G. K., A. Bobb, T. H. Payne, A. J. Avery, T. K. Gandhi, G. Burns, D. C. Classen, and D. W. Bates. 2007. "Medication-Related Clinical Decision Support in Computerized Provider Order Entry Systems: A Review." *Journal of the American Medical Informatics Association* 14 (1): 29–40.

Kwan, J. L., L. Lo, M. Sampson, and K. G. Shojania. 2013. "Medication Reconciliation During Transitions of Care as a Patient Safety Strategy: A Systematic Review." *Annals of Internal Medicine* 158 (5 Part 2): 397–403.

Leung, A. A., C. Keohan, S. Lipsitz, E. Zimichman, M. Amato, S. R. Simon, M. Coffey, N. Kaufman, B. Cadet, G. Schiff, D. L. Seger, and D. W. Bates. 2013. "Relationship Between Medication Event Rates and the Leapfrog Computerized Physician Order Entry Evaluation Tool." *Journal of the American Medical Informatics Association* 20 (e1): e85–e90.

Metzger, J. B., E. Welebob, F. Turisco, and D. C. Classen. 2008. "The Leapfrog Group's CPOE Standard and Evaluation Tool." *Patient Safety and Quality Healthcare* 5 (July/August): 22–25.

Misono, A. S., S. L. Cutrona, N. K. Choudhry, M. A. Fischer, M. R. Stedman, J. N. Liberman, T. A. Brennan, S. H. Jain, and W. H. Shrank. 2010. "Healthcare Information Technology Interventions to Improve Cardiovascular and Diabetes Medication Adherence." *American Journal of Managed Care* 16 (12, Suppl. HIT): SP82–SP92.

Mueller, S. K., K. C. Sponsler, S. Kripalani, and J. L. Schnipper. 2012. "Hospital-Based Medication Reconciliation Practices: A Systematic Review." *Archives of Internal Medicine* 172 (14): 1057–69.

Office of the National Coordinator for Health Information Technology (ONC). 2013. "e-Health." www.healthit.gov/patients-families/types-e-health-tools.

Osheroff, J. A. 2009. *Improving Medication Use and Outcomes with Clinical Decision Support: A Step-by-Step Guide.* Chicago: Health Information Management Systems Society.

Osheroff, J. A., J. M. Teich, D. Levick, L. Saldana, F. T. Velasco, D. F. Sittig, K. M. Rogers, and R. A. Jenders. 2012. *Improving Outcomes with Clinical Decision*

Support: An Implementer's Guide. Chicago: Health Information Management Systems Society.

Pogoreic, D. 2011. "Five Questions with Mayo Clinic Social Media Chief Lee Aase." *Medcity News.* Published October 18. http://medcitynews.com/2011/10/five-questions-with-mayo-clinic-social-media-chief-lee-aase/.

Poon, E. G., C. A. Keohane, C. S. Yoon, M. Ditmore, A. Bane, O. Levtzion-Korach, T. Moniz, J. Rothschild, A. B. Kachalia, J. Hayes, W. W. Churchill, S. Lipsitz, A. D. Whittlemore, D. W. Bates, and T. K. Gandhi. 2010. "Effect of Bar-Code Technology on the Safety of Medication Administration." *New England Journal of Medicine* 362 (18): 1698–707.

Stone, R. A., M. A. Sevick, R. H. Rao, D. S. Macpherson, C. Cheng, S. Kim, L. J. Hough, and F. R. DeRubertis. 2012. "The Diabetes Telemonitoring Study Extension: An Exploratory Randomized Comparison of Alternative Interventions to Maintain Glycemic Control After Withdrawal of Diabetes Home Telemonitoring." *Journal of the American Medical Informatics Association* 19 (6): 973–79.

Tang, P. C., J. S. Ash, D. W. Bates, J. M. Overhage, and D. Z. Sands. 2006. "Personal Health Records: Definitions, Benefits, and Strategies for Overcoming Barriers to Adoption." *Journal of the American Medical Informatics Association* 13 (2): 121–26.

Wallace, C., K. P. Zimmer, L. Possanza, R. Giannini, and R. Solomon. 2013. *How to Identify and Address Unsafe Conditions Associated with Health IT.* Guide prepared for the Office of the National Coordinator for Health Information Technology. Published November 15. www.healthit.gov/sites/default/files/How_to_Identify_and_Address_Unsafe_Conditions_Associated_with_Health_IT.pdf.

Williams, C., F. Mostashari, K. Mertz, E. Hogin, and P. Atwal. 2012. "From the Office of the National Coordinator: The Strategy for Advancing the Exchange of Health Information." *Health Affairs* 31 (3): 527–36.

14

LEADERSHIP FOR QUALITY

James L. Reinertsen

Leadership is essential to quality improvement, whether at the level of a small team of clinicians working to improve care for a particular condition or at the level of an entire organization aiming to improve performance on system-level measures such as mortality rates or costs per capita.

Background

A useful general definition of *leadership* is "working with people and systems to produce needed change" (Wessner 1998). Every system is perfectly designed to produce the results it gets, so if better results are to be expected, systems (and the people in them) must change. Studies of leaders and leadership have produced many theories and models of what is required to "work with people and systems to produce needed change" (Bass 2008). This complex mix of theories can be considered at two levels: individual leadership and organizational leadership systems.

Individual Leadership

This set of leadership ideas is about what people must be, and what they must know how to do, if they are to influence others to bring about needed changes. Examples of these two aspects of individual leadership are described in Exhibit 14.1. Having strong personal leadership attributes without knowing how to use them is not enough. Similarly, knowing the leadership toolbox without authentically embodying the characteristics required of leaders is insufficient for successful leadership. Both being and doing are needed, especially when the changes required for quality improvement involve reframing core values (e.g., individual physician autonomy) or remaking professional teams (e.g., the power relationships between doctors and nurses). Many improvements in healthcare will require these kinds of deep changes in values. These changes sometimes are labeled *transformational changes* to distinguish them from *transactional changes*, which do not require changes in values and patterns of behavior.

EXHIBIT 14.1
Individual
Leadership:
Being and
Doing

What Leaders Must Be (Examples)	What Leaders Must Know How to Do (Examples)
• An authentic embodiment of core values • Trustworthy: consistent in thought, word, and deed • In love with the work, rather than the position, of leadership • Someone who adds energy to a team, rather than sucks it out • Humble, but not insecure; able to say, "I was wrong" • Focused on results, rather than popularity • Capable of building relationships • Passionately committed to the mission	• Understand the system context in which improvement work is being done • Explain how the work of the team fits into the aims of the whole system • Use and teach improvement methods • Develop new leaders • Explain and challenge the current reality • Inspire a shared vision • Enable others to act • Model the way • Encourage the heart (Kouzes and Posner 2003) • Manage complex projects

Organizational Leadership Systems

The ideas and theories at this second level of leadership are not about individual leaders and what they must be and do but rather about creating a supportive organizational environment in which hundreds of capable individual leaders can thrive. This environment is at the system-of-leadership level. One way to view this level is as a complex set of interrelated activities in five broad categories:

1. *Set direction:* Every healthy organization has a sense of direction, a future self-image. A leader's job is to set that direction. The task can be thought of as something like the creation of magnetic lines of force running through the organization that pull people toward a future they find attractive and push them out of a status quo they find uncomfortable.

2. *Establish the foundation*: Leaders must equip themselves and their leadership teams with the knowledge and skills necessary to improve systems and lead change. They must choose and develop future leaders wisely and build a broad base of capable improvers throughout the organization. Often they must take the organization through a painful process of reframing values before they can set forth toward a better future.

3. *Build will*: The status quo is usually comfortable. To initiate and sustain change takes will, especially in healthcare organizations, which

seem to be highly sensitive to discord and often grind to a halt because of one loud voice opposing change. One way to build will for quality improvement is by making logical and quantitative links, including financial links, between improvement and key business goals. Will also can be greatly enhanced when boards of directors pay attention to quality and hold senior leadership accountable for performance improvement.

4. *Generate ideas*: Many healthcare quality challenges require innovation to be met successfully. Excellent organizations have well-developed systems for finding and rapidly testing ideas from the best performers, other industries, and other cultures and nations. They also find and use the thousands of ideas latent within the organization itself. Encouraging and developing ideas are key aspects of the leadership system. Ideas are particularly important for achieving depth of change.

5. *Execute change*: The best improvement ideas will fail to have much effect if they cannot be implemented across the organization. Good leadership systems adopt, teach, and use a good change leadership model and consistently execute both small- and large-scale changes. System-level measurement of performance is an important element in executing change, as is the assignment of responsibility for change to line managers rather than quality staff. This organizational system is particularly important for achieving breadth of change.

Exhibit 14.2 provides a visual representation of the leadership system with additional examples.

The model just outlined is one general version of a leadership system for quality transformation. A number of excellent organizations have established leadership systems that fit their own business contexts and missions (Tichy 2002). Any individual leader's work is set into the context of the leadership system of a specific organization. Some aspects of that leadership system (e.g., compensation, performance measurement) may support the leader's improvement work, and other aspects (e.g., human resource policies, budgeting processes, information systems) may be barriers to that work. Leaders will not achieve large-scale performance changes simply by improving their own leadership skills; they also need to work on improving the system of leadership in their organizations. Deming (2000) referred to this approach when he stated that "Workers work in the system. Leaders work on the system."

Important Leadership Concepts and Definitions

The following terms are helpful to understand when considering how to improve leadership:

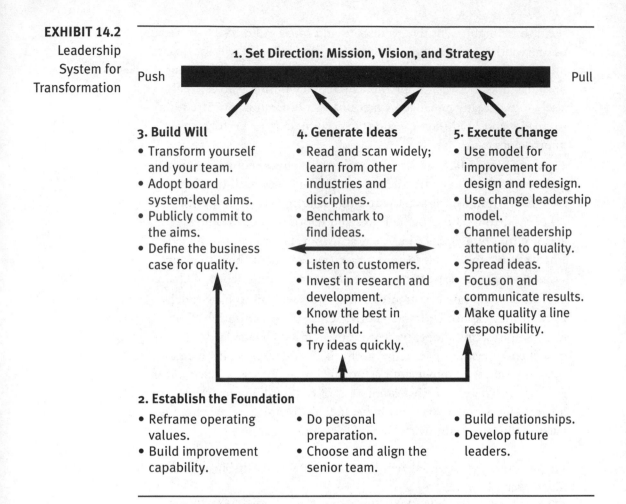

EXHIBIT 14.2
Leadership
System for
Transformation

1. Set Direction: Mission, Vision, and Strategy

Push   Pull

3. Build Will
- Transform yourself and your team.
- Adopt board system-level aims.
- Publicly commit to the aims.
- Define the business case for quality.

4. Generate Ideas
- Read and scan widely; learn from other industries and disciplines.
- Benchmark to find ideas.

- Listen to customers.
- Invest in research and development.
- Know the best in the world.
- Try ideas quickly.

5. Execute Change
- Use model for improvement for design and redesign.
- Use change leadership model.
- Channel leadership attention to quality.
- Spread ideas.
- Focus on and communicate results.
- Make quality a line responsibility.

2. Establish the Foundation
- Reframe operating values.
- Build improvement capability.

- Do personal preparation.
- Choose and align the senior team.

- Build relationships.
- Develop future leaders.

- *Leadership*: working with people and systems to produce needed change.
- *Management*: working with people and systems to produce predictable results. (Note that management is not inferior to leadership; both are important for quality. Leadership, however, is somewhat more hazardous than management because it involves influencing people to change.)
- *Governance*: the process through which the representatives of the owners of an organization oversee the mission, strategy, executive leadership, quality performance, and financial stewardship of the institution. The owner's representatives usually are structured into a board of directors or board of trustees. (In the case of not-for-profit institutions, the owner is the community—usually through a state-chartered process monitored by the state's attorney general.)
- *Technical leadership challenges*: change situations in which there is a high degree of agreement about the nature of goals as well as a high

level of certainty about how to achieve the goals (i.e., the problem has been faced before, and a method of solving it is known).

- *Adaptive leadership challenges*: change situations that require new learning, resolution of value conflicts, and resolution of deep differences in goals and methods of achieving the goals (very common in healthcare quality improvement work).

- *Boundaries of the system*: leaders must choose the boundaries of the system they wish to improve (e.g., for physicians, is the target system their individual practices, the group of physicians in which they work, the entire medical staff of the hospital, the entire community of physicians, or the entire profession?). As Deming (1995) said, "The larger the boundary chosen, the greater the potential impact, and the greater the difficulty of achieving success."

- *Change leadership*: a framework or method for planning and executing major change (Kotter 2012).

- *Leadership development*: the processes by which an organization identifies, improves, evaluates, rewards, holds accountable, and promotes leaders.

- *Transformation*: change that involves fundamental reframing of values, beliefs, and habits of behavior, along with radical redesign of care processes and systems, to achieve dramatic levels of improvement.

- *Vision*: a statement describing a future picture of the institution or care delivery system. Good visions are usually specific enough that individual staff members easily can see themselves, and what their workday would be like, in that future picture. A quality vision for a hospital, framed in terms of the Institute of Medicine's (IOM's) six dimensions of quality—to provide care that is safe, effective, patient centered, timely, efficient, and equitable—could be: "A place with no needless deaths, no needless pain, no needless helplessness, no needless delays, and no waste, for everyone we serve."

- *Mission*: a statement of the purpose of the institution; the reason it exists. This statement usually rests on the core needs of the institution's customers and on the core values of its people. In the case of hospitals, for example, a general statement of mission could be: "To cure when cure is possible; to heal, even when cure is not possible; and to do no harm in the process."

- *Strategic plan*: the organization's hypotheses about the causative relationship between a set of actions (e.g., capital investments, new structures, process redesigns, new staff capabilities) and achievement of system-level, mission-driven aims (e.g., reduced costs of care, improved levels of safety, lower mortality rates).

- *Budget*: the operational and financial expression of the strategic plan, usually for a defined period such as the next fiscal year.

Scope and Use of Leadership Concepts in Healthcare

The introduction makes obvious that effective leadership—at both the individual and the system-of-leadership levels—is essential to quality improvement. If improvement did not require people and processes to change, leadership would not be needed. However, change—often deep, transformative change—is a part of virtually every quality improvement activity, whether at the level of a small project within a department or a massive improvement effort involving entire communities. Leadership is therefore necessary.

We are tempted to think of leadership as the responsibility of those at or near the top of organizations, departments, and other structures. This hierarchical view of leadership is natural and, to a certain extent, useful. The CEO does have a larger system view and can accomplish some improvements that an individual nurse, administrator, or physician cannot. The CEO's leadership opportunities to influence the system are greater, and so are his or her responsibilities for system-level results.

To think that the term *leadership* applies only to those in formally designated senior positions of authority, however, is incorrect and often harmful. Healthcare organizations are large, complex systems and cannot be led effectively by a few senior executives. These senior leaders do not have a deep understanding of the quality issues that frontline staff face every day. Understanding and improving performance at the critical interface between clinicians and patients is work that must be done by hundreds of capable individual leaders throughout the organization, supported by a well-aligned leadership system.

Finally, there is no simple formula for successful healthcare leadership or for specific strategies that, if carried out, will result in organizational quality transformation. Care delivery systems are "complex adaptive systems" (Zimmerman, Lindberg, and Plsek 1998) and therefore behave unpredictably, in large part because of the powerful influence of the professional, community, and macrosystem (regulation, policy, markets) context of each organization and care system.

For this reason, it would be presumptuous for leaders of an organization to believe that by working alone they can transform their organization to a dramatically higher level of quality performance. The sample vision given earlier ("a place with no needless deaths . . .") describes an organization so different from the ones in which we now work that realization of the vision requires a fundamental state change, like going from water to steam. This sort of state change in healthcare will not be evolutionary but revolutionary. To put it into *Crossing the Quality Chasm* terms (IOM 2001), the gap between our current organizations and this vision is a chasm that cannot be crossed in two steps.

All of these ideas (state change, revolution, crossing a chasm) suggest that when healthcare transformation does occur, it will be an emergent event—a surprise, something that comes about in this complex adaptive system not as the result of a detailed leadership plan but because of the convergence of multiple factors, some planned and others completely unplanned. The roads that lead to that convergence could come from multiple directions. Leaders of hospitals and healthcare delivery systems can build and travel these roads, but these leaders by themselves can neither design nor build other roads that might be required. The most robust plan to achieve transformation requires healthcare leaders to work on a plan to achieve things within their control and simultaneously influence as much of their context as possible, even though that context is out of their direct control. Healthcare organizational leaders should be aware of at least four routes to the transformational surprise, only one of which (route 3) is more or less within their direct control.

Route 1: Revolution (Leadership from Below)
One critical factor in the transformation of organizations is a dramatic change in the culture of the professional workforce. The central themes of that cultural change are

- from individual physician autonomy to shared decision making,
- from professional hierarchies to teamwork, and
- from professional disengagement in system aims to "system citizenship."

Why label this route to transformation *revolution*? If these changes were to occur in the health professions, particularly in medicine and nursing, and the organizations in which those nurses and doctors worked did not change responsively, the tensions between the workforce and its organizations eventually would kindle a "peasants at the gates with torches" sort of revolution, with healthcare professionals demanding dramatic change from the leaders of healthcare organizations. This phenomenon is happening at some hospitals as the result of the many changes included in the Patient Protection and Affordable Care Act (ACA). Leaders who have not articulated a clear vision for their organization's transformation and adaptation in response to the implementation of the ACA may face significant negative backlash from both clinicians and hospital staff because many hospitals will need to profoundly change their operating structure to survive.

Route 1 is particularly important for two of the three principal strategies of the *Crossing the Quality Chasm* report: Use all the science we know, and cooperate as a system. Health leaders cannot simply wait for this cultural change to move through medicine but should be aware of it and take steps both within and outside their organizational boundaries to support and accelerate that cultural change. When possible, hospital and physician leaders should harness the energy from this slow shift in the culture of medicine and use it to drive needed changes inside their organizations. Route 1 is clearly one of the main highways to the emergent surprise called *transformation*.

Route 2: Friendly Takeover (Leadership from Outside)

The sample mission statement given earlier depicts another sort of cultural change, the impetus for which could come from outside the healthcare organizational culture: a profound shift in power from the professional and organization to the patient and family. In many ways, healthcare is already well down route 2. For example, patients and families have broken into the medical "holy of holies," the special knowledge that has defined physicians' source of professional power. They watch open-heart surgery on YouTube or other websites and bring printouts of the latest scientific articles to office visits. Patients now can see various reports on the performance of nursing homes, hospitals, and physicians. The power of information is in the hands of the public.

This shift in power is positive and needs to drive a broad range of changes, from how the aims of care plans are defined to radical redesign of how care is delivered, paid for, measured, and reported. Ultimately, this power shift to patients and families will give them as much control of their care as they wish to have. They will lead the design of their own care and make important decisions about resources. We must go down route 2 to implement a patient-centeredness strategy.

As for route 1, healthcare leaders cannot make travel down route 2 happen by themselves, but they can be aware of its importance, its necessity in the transformation of their own organizations, and its power to help leaders drive needed change. A lot of patients are driving down route 2 right now, and the job of healthcare leaders is to find them and use their energy and leadership to invite a friendly takeover of their hospitals and clinics.

Route 3: Intentional Organizational Transformation (Leadership from Above)

This route to transformation should be the one most familiar to CEOs and other senior executives. This set of leadership strategies, implemented with constancy of purpose over some years, would be likely to drive organizational transformation. To reiterate, because transformation is an emergent property of a complex adaptive system, leaders should not assume that a well-built, well-traveled route 3 will get them to the vision without some convergence from the other routes, which are not entirely within the control of leadership.

Why *leadership from above*? Route 3 contrasts with route 1 in that route 1 sees the principal drive for change coming from those working at the front lines, whereas route 3 envisions the push coming from visionary leaders who want to place their organizational change agendas at the leading, rather than trailing, edge of transformation. From a traditional hierarchical organization perspective, these leaders are from above.

Route 4: Intentional Macrosystem Transformation (Leadership from High Above)

The fourth route does not begin with diffused, perhaps even unorganized, cultural changes in professions and patients as do routes 1 and 2, nor does it arise from within healthcare delivery organizations as an intentional act of leadership. Route 4 is a way to transformation that arises out of intentional acts of policymakers, regulators, and others in positions of authority outside the healthcare delivery system. Many of the characteristics of the sample mission would be accelerated by, and perhaps even dependent on, such macrosystem changes.

For example, organizations do not naturally disclose data publicly on their performance, especially when the performance is suboptimal. Without public policy that requires disclosure, widespread transparency would not be the norm in healthcare. In general, measurement, payment, and accountability regulations that encourage and reward those who demonstrate evidence-based practices, patient centeredness, and cooperation are powerful drivers of deep organizational change. Healthcare delivery system leaders cannot design or travel this policy/regulation highway (route 4) directly, but they can influence it and harness its power to accelerate the changes they want to realize in their organizations. The role of delivery system leaders in route 4 is analogous to the military situation of "calling in fire on your own position." If such regulatory fire could be guided sensibly by what healthcare executives are learning and trying to accomplish, it might be exceptionally powerful in getting their organizations through some difficult spots on their own routes to transformation.

These routes make up the large arena for the application of leadership principles in healthcare: at the individual and system-of-leadership levels within care delivery organizations as well as in the professions, communities, and macrosystems that make up the broad context for our work. The best leaders will be able to work effectively across this arena.

Clinical and Operational Issues

Within healthcare delivery systems, some unusual quality improvement leadership challenges present themselves. These challenges are briefly described below.

Professional Silos, Power Gradients, and Teamwork

Physicians, nurses, pharmacists, and other clinicians go through separate and distinct training processes. This separation often persists in the way work is organized, information is exchanged, and improvement work is done. This *professional silo* problem is compounded by a power gradient issue—namely, that all other professionals' actions are ultimately derivative of physicians' orders. The net effect is to diminish teamwork and reduce the free flow of information, both of which are vital for safety and quality. Quality improvement leaders must be capable of establishing effective multidisciplinary teams despite these long-standing challenges.

Physician Autonomy

Physicians are taught to take personal responsibility for quality and have a highly developed attachment to individual professional autonomy. This cultural attribute can have an enormous negative effect on the speed and reliability with which physicians adopt and implement evidence-based practices. As a general rule, physicians discuss evidence in groups but implement it as individuals. The resulting variation causes great complexity in the work of nurses, pharmacists, and others in the system, and it is a major source of errors and harm. Quality improvement leaders will need to reframe this professional value. Perhaps the best way to frame it is: "Practice the science of medicine as teams, and the art of medicine as individuals" (Reinertsen 2003).

Leaders and Role Conflict in Organizations

The clinicians who work in healthcare organizations tend to see the organization as a platform for their individual work and seldom feel a corresponding sense of responsibility for the performance of the organization as a whole. As a result, they expect their leaders (e.g., department chairs, vice presidents of nursing) to protect them from the predations of the organization rather than help them contribute to the accomplishment of the organization's goals. This expectation puts many middle-management leaders in an awkward quandary. Are they to represent the interests of their departments or units to the organization, or are they to represent the interests of the organization to their departments? The answer to both questions—yes—is not comforting. Both roles are necessary, and leaders must be able to play both roles and maintain the respect and trust of their followers. This sense of role conflict is especially acute among, but not unique to, physician leaders (Reinertsen 1998).

Keys to Successful Quality Leadership and Lessons Learned

Transform Yourself

Leaders cannot lead others through the quality transformation unless they are themselves transformed and have made an authentic, public, and permanent commitment to achieving the aims of improvement. Transformation is not an accident. You can design experiences that will both transform and sustain the transformed state. Examples include the following actions:

- Personally interview a patient who has experienced serious harm in your institution, along with the patient's family members, and listen carefully to the impact of this event on that patient's life.
- Personally interview staff at the sharp end of an error that caused serious harm.
- Listen to a patient **every day**.
- Read and reread both IOM reports: *To Err Is Human* (Kohn, Corrigan, and Donaldson 2000) and *Crossing the Quality Chasm* (IOM 2001).
- Learn and use quality improvement methods.
- View and discuss the video *First, Do No Harm*[1] with your team.
- Perform regular safety rounds with your care team.

Adopt and Use a Leadership Model

Literature is replete with useful models and frameworks for leadership. Heifetz's (1994) model is particularly valuable to leaders facing adaptive leadership challenges, which tend to be marked by conflict, tension, and emotion and by the absence of clear agreement about goals and methods. Many other models are available; as leaders learn them, they often reframe the models into ones that work well for their specific situations (Joiner 1994; Kouzes and Posner 2003; Northouse 2013).

Grow and Develop Your Leadership Skills

Good leaders in healthcare engage in three activities that help them continually grow and develop as leaders:

1. *Learn new ideas and information:* Read about, talk to, and observe leaders. Take courses (including courses outside the healthcare context), and find other means of importing information.
2. *Try out the ideas:* Growing leaders take what they learn and use it in the laboratory of their practices, departments, and institutions. They use the results to decide which ideas to keep and which to discard.

3. *Reflect:* Truly great leaders tend to have maintained a lifelong habit of regular reflection on their leadership work. The method of reflection (e.g., private journaling, private meditation, written reports to peers, dialogue with mentors and coaches) is not as important as the regularity, purpose, and seriousness of the reflection.

Avoid the Seven Deadly Sins of Leadership

The following behaviors and habits are not predictive of success as a leader:

1. *Indulging in victimhood:* Leaders initiate, act, take responsibility, and approach problems with a positive attitude. They do not lapse into victimhood, a set of behaviors typified by "if only" whining about what could be accomplished if someone else would improve the information technology system, produce a new boss, or remove querulous members of the team. Leaders do not say "tell me what to do, and I'll do it." They do not join in or encourage organization bashing. To paraphrase Gertrude Stein, when one arrives at leadership, there is no "them" there. Leaders face the realities before them and make the best of their situation.

2. *Mismatching words and deeds:* The fastest way to lose followers is to talk about goals such as quality and safety and then falter when the time comes to put resources behind the rhetoric. Followers watch where their leaders deploy their time, attention, and financial resources and are quick to pick up a mismatch between words and these indicators of the real priorities in the organization.

3. *Loving the job more than the work:* As leaders rise in organizations, some become enamored of the trappings of leadership rather than of the work of improving and delivering high-quality health services. They divert their attention to signs of power and status (such as office size, reserved parking, salaries, and titles) away from the needs of their customers and staff members. This path does not lead to long-term leadership success. Leaders should be focused on doing their current job, not on getting the next job.

4. *Confusing leadership with popularity:* Leadership is about accountability for results. Leaders often must take unpopular actions and courageously stand up against fairly loud opposition to bring about positive change. In a leadership role, being respected is better than being liked.

5. *Choosing harmony rather than conflict:* In addition to popularity, leaders also are tempted to seek peace. Anger and tension, however, are often markers of the key value conflicts through which leaders must help followers learn their way. By avoiding the pain of meetings and

interactions laden with conflict or soothing it with artificial nostrums, leaders can miss the opportunity for real creativity and renewal that lies beneath many conflicts.

6. *Having inconstancy of purpose:* Nothing irritates a team more than when its leader flits from one hot idea to the next without apparent long-term constancy of aim and method. An important variant of such inconstancy is when the leader's priorities and actions vacillate because the leader is always responding to the last loud voice he or she has heard.

7. *Being unwilling to say "I don't know" or "I made a mistake":* The best leaders are always learning, and they cannot learn without recognizing what they do not know or admitting mistakes. Good leaders are secure enough to admit that they do not have the answer and are willing to bring the questions to their teams.

Case Study of Leadership: Interview with William Rupp, MD[2]

Luther Midelfort-Mayo Health System (LM), in Eau Claire, Wisconsin, although small, has gained a reputation as a successful innovator and implementer of quality and safety ideas. This fully integrated healthcare system includes a 190-physician multispecialty group practice, three hospitals, two nursing homes, a retail pharmacy system, ambulance services, a home care agency, and a partnership with a regional health plan. In a unified organizational structure with a single CEO and a single financial statement, LM provides 95 percent of all the healthcare services needed for the majority of the patients it serves.

The record of LM's quality accomplishments over the past decade is broad and deep and includes significant advances in medication safety, access to care, flow of care, nurse morale, and nurses' perception of quality. LM has been a highly visible participant in many of the Institute for Healthcare Improvement's (IHI) Breakthrough Series[3] and is now deeply involved in implementation of Six Sigma process management[4] (Nauman and Hoisington 2000) as well as the development of a culture to support quality and safety. William Rupp, MD, a practicing medical oncologist, became chairman of the LM board in 1992 and CEO of LM in 1994. He led the organization's drive to innovate in quality and safety. Dr. Rupp stepped down as CEO in December 2001. In the following interview, conducted in February 2002, he discusses the leadership challenges and lessons he learned during his tenure.

JR: Under your leadership, LM has become known as a quality leader among organizations. Are you really that good?

WR: LM is making progress in quality, although we're clearly not as good as we'd like to be. What we **are** really good at is taking ideas from others and trying them out, quickly. For example, we heard about a red/green/yellow light system for managing hospital flow and nurse staffing at a meeting I attended. We tried it out within two weeks and refined it within three months. We believed that this traffic light system was a tool for managing the flow of patients through the hospital and for directing resources to parts of the hospital that needed them. But when we tried it out, the traffic light system turned out to have little to do with managing our flow. Rather, for us, it has been an extraordinary system for empowering nurses, communicating across nursing units, improving nurse morale, and avoiding unsafe staffing situations (Rozich and Resar 2002). Our nurse vacancy rate is now **very** low. It was a great idea, but not for the purpose we originally thought.[5]

JR: How did you get interested in safety?
WR: At an IHI meeting in 1998, our leadership team heard Don Berwick talk about medication errors. We had 20 LM people at the meeting, and our reaction was, "We can't be that bad, can we?" When we came home, we interviewed some frontline nurses and pharmacists about recent errors or near misses and were amazed at the sheer number of stories we heard. So we reviewed 20 charts a week on one unit for six weeks and found that the nurses and pharmacists were right—we were having the same number of errors as everyone else. We also identified the major cause of most of the errors in our system: poor communication between the outpatient and inpatient medication record systems.

We then took our findings from the interviews and the chart reviews and went over them with the physician and administrative leadership. The universal reaction was surprise and shock, but the data were very convincing, and everyone soon agreed we needed to do something about the problem. We put a simple paper-and-pencil reconciliation system in place for in/outpatient medications, and adverse drug events decreased fivefold.[6]

JR: What was your role as CEO in driving these sorts of specific improvements?
WR: I couldn't be personally responsible for guiding and directing specific projects like the traffic light system, medication safety, and implementation of evidence-based care systems for specific diseases. But I could make sure the teams working on these problems knew that I was interested in them, and that I wanted results. I met monthly individually with the project leaders, even if only for 15 minutes, to hear about progress. And I also made sure that my executive assistant scheduled me to "drop in" for a few minutes on the meeting of each team at least once a month so that all the members of the team knew that the organization was paying attention to their work. I

know this sort of attention must be important because when specific projects didn't go well (and we had a few), they were projects to which I didn't pay this sort of attention.[7]

JR: Trying out new ideas and changes all the time must cause a lot of tension for your staff. How did you handle this?

WR: You're right—innovation and change are sources of tension. I found it exceptionally useful to have a small number of people working directly for me whose only role was to be a change agent. Roger Resar, MD, is a great example. His job was to find and try out new ideas, and when he did, I inevitably got calls from doctors, nurses, and administrators saying, "We can't get our work done with all these new ideas coming at us. Get Dr. Resar off our backs." At that point, my job was to support Roger, especially if the resistance was based simply on unwillingness to change. But I also listened carefully to the content and tone of the resistance. If I thought there really was a safety risk in trying out the idea, or if there was genuine meltdown under way, I would ask him to back down, or we might decide to try the idea on a much smaller scale.

For example, when we first tried open-access scheduling in one of our satellite offices, we didn't understand the principles well enough and the office exploded in an uproar. Rather than pushing ahead, I went to the office and said, "We really didn't do this very well. We should stop this trial. I still think open access is a good idea, but we just haven't figured out how to implement it yet." After we learned more about implementation, we tried it out elsewhere and are now successfully putting open access in place across virtually the entire system (except for the office in which the uproar occurred). I shudder to think what would have happened if we had bulled ahead.

So, I'd say my change leadership role was to push for needed change, support the change agents, listen carefully to the pain they caused, and respond.

JR: That must be a hard judgment to make—when to back down on change and when to push ahead.

WR: The right answer isn't always obvious. In some cases the decision is easy, especially when the resistance conflicts directly with a broadly supported organizational value or is in opposition to a strategic approach that the organization has adopted after a lot of debate. For example, we are now well along in our adoption and implementation of Six Sigma process management. If an administrative vice president, or a prominent physician, or a key nurse manager were to come to me and say, "This process management stuff is baloney, I'm not going to do it," my response would be to say, "Well, process management is a major strategy of this organization, and if you can't help to lead it, then you'll have to leave."

JR: How do you deal with resistance to important initiatives, such as clinical practice guidelines, if the resistance is coming from doctors?

WR: We are fundamentally a group practice. Once we have made a group decision about a care process and have designed a system for implementing that process (e.g., our insulin sliding-scale protocol or our choice of a single hip or knee prosthesis), we expect our physicians to use the protocol. We monitor protocol usage and always ask those who aren't using the protocol to tell us what's wrong with the protocol. Sometimes they point out problems with the design. But most of the time, they simply change their behavior to match the protocol. One way or another, we don't back down on our commitment to evidence-based practice of medicine.

JR: During your tenure, did you ever have to face a financial crisis? Were you ever pressured to cut back on your investment in quality and safety?

WR: In 1998–1999, we sustained financial losses for the first time in our history, due to the effects of the Balanced Budget Act. I received a lot of pressure from parts of the organization to reduce our investment in innovation and quality. They said, "Cut travel costs. Don't send the usual 20 people to the IHI National Forum." And the physicians said, "Put those physician change agents back into practice, where they can do real work and generate professional billings." I resisted both pressures. I felt that during rough times we needed more ideas, not fewer. So we sent 30 people to the IHI Forum. And we showed the doctors that for every dollar invested in change agents' salaries, we had generated ten dollars in return. The financial results have been good. Last year, we had a positive margin—3.5 percent.[8]

JR: I've heard of your work on culture change and "simple rules." What is all this about?

WR: In 1997, we realized that the rate of change in LM was not what it needed to be and that the biggest drag on our rate of improvement was our culture. We went through an organization-wide exercise in which we discussed our cultural "simple rules" with people from all levels of our organization. A leader cannot significantly change a culture until he or she can describe it and outline it on paper and the staff agrees with the description of the current culture. Only then can you begin to describe what you want a new culture to look and feel like, what you want it to accomplish for patients.

JR: What rules did you find were in place in your culture?

WR: We think the main characteristics of our old culture were embedded in six rules.

1. Success is defined by quality.
2. Physicians give permission for leaders to lead (and they can withdraw it).
3. Physician leadership means "I'm in charge."
4. Results are achieved by working hard.
5. Compliance requires consensus.
6. Conflict is resolved by compromise.

We will keep the first rule, but the others are up for redefinition. We will not get to our long-term goals if these rules define our culture. How can we reach for exceptional levels of quality if we resolve all conflicts by compromise? How can we design and implement systems of quality and safety as our primary strategy if deep in our hearts we still believe that individual effort is what drives quality?

JR: How would you sum up the main lessons you have learned about the CEO's role in leadership for quality and safety?

WR: I don't think there's a prescription that works for every CEO, in every situation. This is what I have learned from my work at LM:

- The CEO must always be strategically searching for the next good idea. On my own, I come up with maybe one good idea every two or three years. But I can recognize someone else's good idea in a flash, and my organization can get that idea implemented.
- The CEO must push the quality agenda. He or she must be seen to be in charge of it and must make it happen. There are many forces lined up to preserve the status quo, and if the CEO doesn't visibly lead quality, the necessary changes won't happen.
- The CEO doesn't make change happen single-handedly. The leader does so through key change agents, and his or her job is to protect and support those change agents while listening carefully to the pain they cause.
- This whole experience has profoundly reinforced for me the concept of a system of quality. The professional culture that focuses responsibility for quality and safety solely on individuals is dead wrong. The vast majority of our staff is doing the best they can. Asking them to "think harder next time," or telling them, "Don't ever do that again," will not work.

Conclusion

Leaders play a critical role in improvement. They create an organizational climate in which improvement teams can be effective. Leaders are responsible for the overall structures, systems, and culture in which improvement teams function. Good leaders create environments in which quality can thrive.

However, leaders do not make healthcare improvements alone. The "atomic units" of improvement are projects at the frontline or microsystem level that are carried out by nurses, doctors, and managers who know how to run rapid tests of change, measure results, respond, and then start the cycle again.

Study Questions

1. What aspects of individual leadership (being and doing) does William Rupp demonstrate?
2. Examine Exhibit 14.1 and describe the elements of this organizational leadership model evident in the LM organization.

Notes

1. For more information, see the Partnership for Patient Safety's website at www.p4ps.org.
2. William Rupp, MD (former CEO, Luther Midelfort-Mayo Health System), in discussion with the author, February 2002.
3. See IHI's website at www.ihi.org.
4. Six Sigma refers to an approach to performance improvement in which the organization's strategic goals are traced directly to certain key processes; those key processes are then managed toward a high standard of quality—3.4 defects per million opportunities, or "six sigma." For example, most hospitals' medication systems currently produce three or four medication errors per 1,000 doses, or three sigma. *Sigma* is a statistical term used to describe the amount of deviation from the norm, or average, in a population—the more sigmas, the greater the deviation (Kouzes and Posner 2003).
5. One of the most important tasks of leaders is to be on the lookout for good ideas. Leaders have more than an academic interest in ideas, however; they know that simply accumulating interesting ideas from other organizations, industries, and innovators is not sufficient. Good

leaders apply ideas to their work environment and establish ways to test many ideas on a small scale, discarding those that fail.

6. Another task of leaders is to marshal the will to take action. Data about the problem, collected in a credible fashion, can create discomfort with the status quo, often a vital factor in developing organizational will.

7. The "currency" of leadership is attention. Choosing how and where to channel attention is one of the most important tasks of leadership.

8. Healthcare leaders often state that the business case for quality is weak, in that investments in quality and safety do not produce the same kinds of business returns as investments in expensive technologies and procedures. In the case of safety, however, the professional case overwhelms concerns about the business issues; courageous healthcare leaders understand this case. When Paul O'Neill was CEO of Alcoa, he refused to allow anyone to calculate Alcoa's business returns from workplace safety improvements. He treated worker safety as a fundamental right of employment. If "first, do no harm" is a fundamental value of our profession, can healthcare leaders play dollars against patient harm?

References

Bass, B. M. 2008. *Bass and Stogdill's Handbook of Leadership*. New York: Free Press.

Deming, W. E. 2000. *Out of the Crisis*. Cambridge, MA: MIT Press.

———. 1995. *The New Economics for Industry, Government, and Education*, second edition. Cambridge, MA: MIT Press.

Heifetz, R. 1994. *Leadership Without Easy Answers*. Cambridge, MA: Belknap Press.

Institute of Medicine (IOM). 2001. *Crossing the Quality Chasm: A New Health System for the 21st Century*. Washington, DC: National Academies Press.

Joiner, B. 1994. *Fourth Generation Management: The New Business Consciousness*. New York: McGraw-Hill.

Kohn, L. T., J. M. Corrigan, and M. S. Donaldson (eds.). 2000. *To Err Is Human: Building a Safer Health Care System*. Washington, DC: National Academies Press.

Kotter, J. 2012. *Leading Change*. Cambridge, MA: Harvard Business Review Press.

Kouzes, J., and B. Posner. 2003. *The Leadership Challenge: How to Get Extraordinary Things Done in Organizations*. San Francisco: Jossey-Bass.

Nauman, E., and S. H. Hoisington. 2000. *Customer Centered Six Sigma: Linking Customers, Process Improvement, and Financial Results*. Milwaukee, WI: ASQ Quality Press.

Northouse, P. G. 2013. *Leadership Theory and Practice*. Thousand Oaks, CA: Sage.

Reinertsen, J. L. 2003. "Zen and the Art of Physician Autonomy Maintenance." *Annals of Internal Medicine* 138 (12): 992–95.

———. 1998. "Physicians as Leaders in the Improvement of Health Care Systems." *Annals of Internal Medicine* 128 (10): 833–88.

Rozich, J., and R. Resar. 2002. "Using a Unit Assessment Tool to Optimize Flow and Staffing in a Community Hospital." *Joint Commission Journal of Quality Improvement* 28: 31–41.

Tichy, N. M. 2002. *The Leadership Engine.* New York: HarperCollins.

Wessner, D. 1998. Personal communication, May.

Zimmerman, B., C. Lindberg, and P. Plsek. 1998. *Edgeware: Insights from Complexity Science for Health Care Leaders.* Irving, TX: VHA Press.

ORGANIZATIONAL QUALITY INFRASTRUCTURE: HOW DOES AN ORGANIZATION STAFF QUALITY?

A. Al-Assaf

My favorite definition of quality is simple: incremental improvement. Fulfillment of this definition, however, is a major task. The term *quality* is being transformed rapidly to *performance improvement (PI)*. Therefore, for our definition of quality, current performance must be measured as a baseline for judging whether improvement has occurred. A system also should be in place to monitor progress toward improvement on a regular, continuous basis to verify whether improvement is actually happening. This type of system requires an adequate and effective infrastructure, a process for data gathering, a process for data analysis and reporting, and a process for identifying and instituting improvements. Management must have a strong commitment to these processes, and the organization must have high intentions to improve its performance.

Quality Assurance, Quality Improvement, Quality Control, and Total Quality Management

What is the difference between quality assurance (QA), quality improvement (QI), monitoring/quality control (QC), and total quality management (TQM)? According to the quality management cycle (see Exhibit 15.1), each of these activities has certain steps that must be followed to achieve the desired objectives.

QA includes all activities related to proper planning (operational and strategic) as well as preassessment and self-evaluation. In addition, QA is the process of ensuring compliance with specifications, requirements, or standards and implementing methods for conformance. It includes setting and communicating standards and identifying indicators for performance monitoring and compliance with standards. These standards can come in different forms (e.g., protocols, guidelines, specifications). QA, however, is losing its earlier popularity because it resorts to disciplinary means and blames human error for noncompliance.

EXHIBIT 15.1
Quality
Management
Cycle

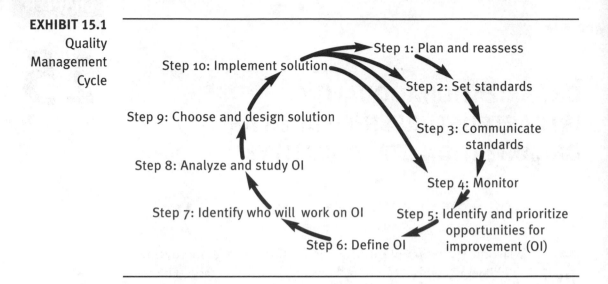

Step 1: Plan and reassess

Step 10: Implement solution

Step 2: Set standards

Step 9: Choose and design solution

Step 3: Communicate standards

Step 8: Analyze and study OI

Step 4: Monitor

Step 7: Identify who will work on OI

Step 5: Identify and prioritize opportunities for improvement (OI)

Step 6: Define OI

QC, on the other hand, is defined by Brown (2010) as "a management process where actual performance is measured against expected performance, and actions are taken on the difference." QC originally was used in the laboratory, where accuracy of test results dictates certain norms and specific (and often rigid) procedures that do not allow for error and discrepancy. Thus, an effort must be made to reduce variation as much as possible. In this stage, organizations are drafting indicators and using them to measure their performance against benchmarks.

QI efforts and processes complement QA and QC and sometimes overtake them. QI is defined as an organized, structured process that selectively identifies improvement teams to achieve improvements in products or services (Al-Assaf 1997). It includes all actions to identify gaps (opportunities for improvement), to prioritize and select appropriate gaps to study, to analyze them, and to narrow or close them.

TQM, or quality management in general, involves all the above three processes: QA, QC, and QI. It involves processes pertaining to the coordination of activities related to all or any one of the above three as well as the administration and resource allocation of these processes. Administration may include training, education, organization of committees and councils, building of infrastructure, resource acquisition and allocation, and so on. Quality management is the umbrella encompassing all processes and activities related to quality. Quality management also may encompass such terms as *continuous quality management* and *total quality leadership/improvement*.

Management Commitment

Words cannot sufficiently describe how important management commitment is to the success of quality, at least in other industries. Time and again, experts have demonstrated the value of management commitment to the quality process. Management can open doors, facilitate interventions freely, and coordinate resources easily. In most cases, management has the final say on activities and makes the final decision. Therefore, management support of activities and encouragement of professional involvement can enhance the implementation of quality in healthcare.

According to Deming (2000), if an organization does not have the commitment of top management, the odds of successful quality implementation are severely jeopardized. He further tells the prospective leader that "if you can't come, then send no one." Commitment to a cause means being involved, supportive (in words, actions, and resources), active, and participatory in that cause. Commitment also means leading the efforts, facilitating activities, participating in tasks, and providing the necessary and adequate resources to make quality improvement a reality and a success. Commitment to a process or a program means taking pride and joy in supporting it. It includes taking enthusiastic initiative to learn more about it. It certainly is not just rhetoric and verbal support, although even that is better than no support at all.

You cannot be committed without understanding what you want to commit to and for what reason. Therefore, paramount to this step are increased knowledge and awareness of the subject or field that needs your commitment. Management's unequivocal commitment to healthcare quality is difficult to procure without demonstrating results. Managers are usually quick to say, "show me that it works or it has worked." Healthcare quality must be based on data and should be driven by outcomes. With adequate planning and process design, commitment will be cultivated and positive results can be achieved.

The Role of the Coordinator of Healthcare Quality

Once commitment is achieved, the person in charge of the organization, usually the CEO, needs to identify a coordinator or director of healthcare quality. This position is usually a full-time, authoritative one and may be filled by an experienced person with leadership skills and a clinical background. A direct link is necessary between this individual and the CEO (or the CEO's designee) for maintaining credibility and authority.

This position is so important that in some organizations, CEOs themselves assume the role of quality council chairman. This approach, however, has advantages and disadvantages. A prominent person like the CEO would give instant recognition and support to the quality department. The CEO would establish commitment from day one, which sends a clear message to the rest of the organization that quality is important and everyone must concur. The disadvantage, on the other hand, is that often the CEO is not permanently appointed, meaning possible process discontinuity when the CEO resigns.

Regardless of who the QA/QI coordinator/director is, once identified this individual should be trained extensively in healthcare quality techniques and must prepare to organize the quality council. The responsibilities of the quality coordinator are numerous and include the following roles:

- Advocate and speaker for healthcare quality
- Facilitator of the quality council
- Builder of the infrastructure and necessary resources for healthcare quality
- Designated liaison with outside agencies related to quality activities
- Coordinator of strategic and operational planning for healthcare quality activities and the allocation of resources
- Developer and updater of the quality/PI program and plan documents
- Guarantor of organizational compliance with accreditation standards
- Monitor of performance measurement activities
- Member and coordinator of the organization's quality/PI committees
- Initiator of process improvement teams
- Coordinator of key quality personnel selection
- Coordinator of the healthcare quality training plan
- Facilitator of healthcare quality intervention strategies

The Role of the Quality Council

The quality council or similar entity is formed to act as the body that will direct the healthcare quality process at the facility. It works as a committee to coordinate individuals representing the different aspects of healthcare delivery, disciplines, and departments/units in the organization as they formulate policies on healthcare quality.

Organization of a quality council is not imperative but recommended. The membership of the council is important, and careful selection of these individuals should rest with the top official of the organization (CEO), supported by advice and assistance from the quality coordinator and the consultant (if any). Members should be prominent individuals representing different disciplines and units of the organization. Membership may be broadened to include other individuals from other units of the organization and may benefit from inclusion of some frontline workers.

Once members are identified, the council must develop a *charter* (a description document) that delineates roles and responsibilities. The council's role is similar to that of the quality coordinator: to give the organization a collective perspective and act as the central resource in healthcare quality matters to which the organization may refer when necessary. Also like the quality coordinator, quality council members need to be adequately prepared for their roles and should be exposed to the concept of healthcare quality and its principles at an early stage.

Mission and Vision

Once the quality council forms its charter, each member should be made aware of his or her role and responsibilities as outlined in it. Members should involve themselves actively in the revision and redrafting of the charter to reflect "ownership" in the council. The council also needs to address the development of mission and vision statements for the organization, which should reflect the desire for healthcare improvement. These statements establish the organization's constancy of purpose and serve as a constant reminder of the organization's direction as well as a map for its future. Mission and vision statements should be concise, clear, and realistic. Because they reflect the true desire of the organization, the council members should draft both statements with input from all key personnel.

A mission statement should answer the following questions:

- Who are we?
- What is our main purpose as an organization?
- Whom are we serving?
- What are the needs of those we serve, and how do we meet those needs?

Vision statements are futuristic (visionary) and should project what the organization is striving to be in the future (in three, five, or ten years).

Once these statements are finalized, the council should communicate them to the rest of the organization actively and consistently. Many organizations post their mission and vision statements online and in prominent places throughout the organization and even print them on the back of personnel business cards. In this way, all activities of the organization will be guided by the organization's mission and designed to achieve the organization's vision.

Allocation of Resources

Resources are needed for quality training and to increase healthcare professionals' awareness of the concept of healthcare quality. Additional resources are required to monitor compliance with standards; to draft, test, and enforce compliance with policies and procedures; to identify opportunities for improvement; to initiate and coordinate improvement projects; and to disseminate the concept of quality and PI at the grassroots level. Funds also should be set aside for future improvements. Some organizations use funds to acquire reference materials and create a resource library on healthcare quality. Others allocate funds to hire reviewers and quality coordinators, to publish a newsletter on quality, or to hold seminars on the subject. As incentives, funds may be allotted to offer support to units or individuals who have demonstrated substantial quality improvements.

In addition to a council, organizations also allocate resources to establish a central healthcare quality department or unit. This unit should include a number of health professionals, be headed by the quality director, and be linked directly to the CEO or her designee. This unit is responsible for setting standards (in hospitals, the standards usually are those established by The Joint Commission or the American Osteopathic Association, but organizations such as HMOs and ambulatory care facilities have a choice of accrediting organizations, each with its own standards). This unit also is responsible for communicating these standards to the rest of the organization, disseminating information related to healthcare quality, monitoring the quality of care delivered, and acting on opportunities for improvement.

The organization's CEO and board provide financial and political support to the unit and grant it broad authority to survey and monitor the performance of any healthcare or service department in the organization. The quality unit's objectives are to coordinate quality for the entire organization—supported by direct input and participation of every unit—and to institutionalize and ensure sustainability of quality.

Organizational Structure

What is the organizational structure of this quality unit? To answer this question, one should outline the main and customary functions of this unit and then decide where to place the unit in the organization's hierarchy. One also should consider the support this unit should receive from the organization's committee structure.

This unit's responsibilities may include the following functions:

- Initiate planning for quality initiatives
- Set organizational standards for quality (including the development of essential policies and procedures and ensuring proper documentation of processes and activities in the organization)
- Communicate standards to the organization's employees
  - Organize seminars to increase awareness
  - Disseminate information on standards
  - Discuss mechanisms for compliance with standards
  - Deliver workshops and lectures on standards

- – Provide training on quality skills and methods
- Monitor compliance with standards
  - – Identify measurable indicators of performance
  - – Collect data on indicators
  - – Analyze data on indicators
  - – Perform periodic audits
  - – Review medical records
  - – Review care processes retrospectively
  - – Measure outcomes of patient care
  - – Measure satisfaction of customers, employees, patients, and providers
  - – Collect data on patient complaints and concerns
  - – Assist in meeting accreditation standards
  - – Review and update policies and procedures
  - – Identify and draft new policies and procedures
- Identify opportunities for improvement in care and services
- Initiate and coordinate improvement projects
- Facilitate performance and productivity measurement and improvements
- Facilitate and provide guidelines for proper and adequate documentation of essential processes and activities, including medical record entries, risk management, patient safety issues, staff education and training, and personnel files
- Coordinate all committees related to quality and PI
- Identify and acquire necessary resources for quality and PI
- Develop the organization's quality program document and annual plan
- Evaluate the organization's quality program annually
- Develop the annual quality report for the organization's board of directors
- Coordinate all functions and activities related to the optimum use of resources
- Coordinate all functions and activities related to the prevention, control, and management of risks to the organization's customers—both internal and external
- Coordinate an effective system for credentialing and recredentialing the organization's practitioners
- Act as liaison with all of the organization's units to facilitate the improvement of their performance

The quality unit should have access to the data the organization collects on patient care and the services the organization provides internally and externally. It therefore should work closely with the organization's information technology unit.

The organizational structure of quality units varies considerably. There is also variation in who reports to this unit and to whom this unit should report. Traditionally, it has been placed under the medical staff affairs section of the organization, although many organizations have recently moved it to a higher level, where it reports directly to the CEO. In some organizations, both administrative and clinical functions report to the unit, whereas in other organizations only the clinical functions do. Some hospitals add more, including infection control, utilization, case management, risk management, and credentialing.

Other functions of this unit usually are handled through the informal structure of the organization (i.e., the committees). Again, there is considerable variation as to which committees belong to quality and which belong to medical staff affairs. In general, however, the credentialing, peer review and clinical services management, utilization and case management, patient safety, risk management, infection control, and medical record review committees usually report to the quality unit. In addition, the organization's quality council (or similar entity) is directly related to the quality unit (although it does not report to it), and the quality unit staff usually coordinate the quality council's activities. Other committees—such as pharmacy, therapeutics, facility management, and information technology—may be a part of the quality structure.

Increasing Awareness of Healthcare Quality

Healthcare quality is a concept that has different facets, principles, skills, techniques, and tools. A vast amount of literature has been written about it. Therefore, early on, the members of the quality council should participate in a seminar on healthcare quality. This seminar should be followed by intellectual discussions with a designated facilitator on the application of this concept to the organization, taking into consideration the available resources, the culture, and the current healthcare status and structure. A similar activity should be organized to present healthcare quality to other key personnel to obtain further support and to increase dissemination of the concept. Certainly, the facilitator's services could be used to present a number of short sessions with other key personnel and middle managers to discuss healthcare quality. These sessions, to be repeated at least annually, should be attended by at least the quality coordinator and some members of the quality council and can serve as focus group sessions to gather feedback on quality implementation and applications in healthcare. Information and feedback gathered at these sessions can be used in the next planning phase at the operational level and in launching improvement projects and initiatives.

Mapping Quality Improvement Intervention

In collaboration with the quality council and with information collected during the planning phase, the quality coordinator may identify areas in the system where opportunities for improvement exist. Identified areas should be selected carefully to include the projects that require the least amount of resources yet have the highest probability of success and benefit a large population. Examples of such projects include

- improving the reception area of the organization;
- improving the aesthetics of the organization;
- improving the timeliness of tests and services to patients;
- identifying and improving patient safety in areas such as infections, falls, complications, and medication errors;
- initiating a campaign to improve reporting on sentinel events and their management efforts;
- selecting a few areas that receive numerous complaints from external customers and trying to improve them;
- initiating a campaign to promote health awareness to the public; and
- leading an informational campaign on improvement initiatives with participation of all units.

Of course, the council is not limited to these projects. It can identify other opportunities for quality improvement and initiate improvements with an interdisciplinary team from the affected departments. When a project is completed, the quality council should analyze the lessons learned and prioritize services and organizational areas for further implementation of improvements. For example, services selected for intervention could be those that are

- high volume,
- problem prone,
- high risk,
- high impact, or
- high cost.

On the other hand, other criteria used for selection of venues and units for intervention may include

- availability and accessibility of necessary data,
- size and homogeneity of the "study" population,
- simplicity of the infrastructure,
- definition and focus of the proposed intervention,
- stability and supportiveness of leadership,
- level of need for improvement,
- ability to complete the intervention with available resources,
- willingness of health professionals to participate, and
- feasibility of demonstrating improvements.

Using these criteria, the quality council will be able to choose the specific area or service and decide what resources are needed to implement the intervention. The use of objectivity in selecting a system or an area for intervention is crucial to successful outcomes.

Quality/PI Program Document

One of the most important documents the quality unit must develop is the program description document, which is required for accreditation of the organization. An organization that lacks this document never will be accredited.

This document should provide a description of the different activities of the quality unit and an outline of the scope of work in which this unit or the organization's quality program is engaged. It also should describe the functions of the different individuals and committees associated with the quality program. This document should serve as the basis for evaluating the organization's quality performance. The following list provides suggestions for the outline of a program description document.

Quality Program Document

- Purpose of document
- General program description and overview
- Statements of mission, vision, and values of the organization and the quality unit
- Goals and objectives of the quality program
- Strategies for PI
- Organizational structure supporting PI
- Formal structure
- Committee structure
- Roles and responsibilities of the PI program (narrative of roles and responsibilities of each of the following)

- Board of directors
- CEO and executive team
- Quality council
- Quality/PI unit
  - Quality director
  - Quality coordinators
  - Quality reviewers/specialists
- Quality committees
- Project teams
- Departmental, section, and other unit leaders
- Staff responsibilities and involvement in PI
- Scope of work and standards of care and service
- Authority and accountability
- Reporting mechanisms
- Criteria for setting priorities on PI monitors and projects
- List of indicators for monitoring PI
- Methods of monitoring compliance with standards and measuring performance
- Confidentiality of information
- Mechanism/model for improvement interventions
- Education and awareness activities on quality/PI
- Rewarding results program
- Annual evaluation of QI/PI
- Audits and reviews
- Credentialing and recredentialing
- Peer review
- Utilization management
- Risk management and patient safety

This document should be reviewed, rereviewed, and approved at least once annually by appropriate staff of the QA unit.

Evaluation, Monitoring, and Continuous Quality Improvement
Evaluation
The 1990s were dubbed the "period of performance measurement." Providers, consumers, and purchasers were looking for ways to satisfy one another through measuring and reporting on care outcomes. Several third-party organizations attempted to produce certain measures to report on these care outcomes. As a result, a number of national indicators were developed and

are now in use by healthcare organizations. Report cards are being assembled on the nation's healthcare organizations. Benchmarking efforts are under way to identify and emulate excellence in care and services. All these activities are being carried out in an effort to measure and improve performance in healthcare. In the international arena, the World Health Organization (WHO) organized and facilitated a number of activities related to quality assessment, performance improvement, and outcomes measurements (see work coordinated by the Centers for Medicare & Medicaid Services [CMS] at www.cms.gov and by the Agency for Healthcare Research and Quality at www.qualitymeasures.ahrq.gov). A large number of countries and institutions participated in these activities and initiatives. In the end, all agreed that an organized mechanism is needed to account for quality and continuous measurement and to improve performance in healthcare organizations (see 2000 WHO report on health systems rankings at www.who.int/whr/2000/en/whr00_en.pdf).

Performance measurement includes the identification of certain indicators for performance. Data are collected to measure those indicators and then compare current performance to a desired performance level. Several systems of measurements and indicators already have been developed. The Healthcare Effectiveness Data and Information Set is one example (www.ncqa.org/tabid/59/Default.aspx) of a system of measurements and indicators. This set has 75 measures, primarily for preventive health services, against which organizations can measure their performance, compare their performance with that of their peers, and trend their progress toward improvement. Other systems include the US Public Health Service Healthy People 2010 and 2020 list of indicators (www.healthypeople.gov), The Joint Commission's ORYX clinical indicator system for hospitals (www.jointcommission.org/facts_about_oryx_for_hospitals/), the Canadian Council on Health Services Accreditation hospital indicators (www.accreditation.ca/), and the CMS QISMC indicator system for managed care (www.cms.gov).

Monitoring

Monitoring is based on specific and measured indicators related to standards. It is a process of measuring variance from standards and initiating processes to reduce this variance. Monitoring is a necessary step for proper selection and consideration of quality improvement projects and studies. It also can provide the organization with an indication of the status of care and services provided.

In advanced healthcare systems, elaborate and comprehensive systems of monitoring have been developed that use the patient's medical record for the abstraction of specific data, which in turn are fed into a central database for analysis and monitoring. Each organization then receives a periodic report showing aggregate data of national healthcare indicators compared to their specific set of data for the same indicators. Variance from the mean is then studied and acted on using the QA/QI process described earlier.

Continuous Quality Improvement

Improvements are not one-time activities. When a team has worked on a process and improvement has been accomplished, it should not abandon this process and move on to the next one. Improvement is itself a process, and a process is continuous. Monitoring should continue, and improvements should be initiated every time they are needed. Once compliance has been achieved, incremental improvements in the standards also are important. If high or even perfect compliance with a specific standard has been documented, upgrading this standard is the next step to take. Otherwise, the organization will stay in the status quo and further improvement will not occur.

Challenges, Opportunities, and Lessons Learned for Sustaining QA/QI

A Quality Culture

Establishing a quality culture is the next milestone. A hospital that combines high-quality standards with a quality culture institutionalizes quality. Institutionalization is achieved when appropriate healthcare quality activities are carried out effectively, efficiently, and on a routine basis throughout a system or an organization (Brown 1995). It is a state of achievement whereby healthcare quality is practiced and maintained without additional outside resources. In such a state, expertise is available within and commitment is fully integrated and maintained.

A quality environment or culture is achieved when quality activities become day-to-day activities. Such activities are not separate from the normal activities carried out daily by the system and its personnel. It is a state in which each employee is aware of the quality concept, believes in it, practices its principles, and makes it part of his or her responsibility and not the responsibility of a department or another individual. In such a culture, each individual is responsible for his or her task's own quality structure, process, and outcome. Employees make every effort at that level to ensure that the processes of QA are maintained (i.e., planning, standard setting, and monitoring). Employees also practice QI—they identify variance from standards and select opportunities for improvements to be acted on individually or in collaboration with others. A quality culture empowers employees to achieve their goals, which are in turn aligned with the organization's mission and vision statements.

Lessons in Institutionalization

- *Planning* for quality should be done systematically and thoroughly. Delineation of responsibility, identification of scope of involvement, allocation of resources, and anticipation for the change should be completed before activities in QA or QI begin.

- Securing *commitment* from management is helpful and can make the process of implementation move rapidly. The involvement of top managers in early planning activities is essential.

- Develop a *policy* for quality at the central level as early and as solidly as possible. A policy that is well prepared and developed in collaboration with senior staff will have a much better chance of survival, even with its expected high turnover.

- Identification of a *leader* or *champion* (local cadre) to lead this movement is highly recommended. A local person with authority, credibility, enthusiasm, and interest can be an asset to the acceleration of healthcare quality implementation. This individual can act as facilitator and cheerleader for healthcare quality initiatives.

- Organization of a steering committee or *council* of local or internal representatives gives the healthcare quality process credibility, sustainability, and momentum.

- Formation of the *structure* for healthcare quality should be gradual, cautious, and based on progress and understanding of the concept and practice. Early formation of large committee and council structures may shift the focus to the organization and away from the actual mission of healthcare quality, which is improvement. At the beginning of implementation, staff should concentrate more on learning and understanding the concept and then practice it daily to achieve positive results. Too many committees with too many meetings and tasks distract from the focus on expected goals.

- Always have an *alternative plan* in case one is slowed down because of staff changes. Do not rely on a single individual when trying to implement healthcare quality effectively. Train a number of individuals, and prepare several qualified staff members simultaneously. This practice will allow for wider selection of coordinators and will enhance sustainability efforts.

- Prepare to answer questions related to *incentives* for staff to participate. As long as healthcare quality activities are not required as integral parts of their jobs, employees will question their role in participation. A system of employee rewards and recognition based on healthcare quality achievements is necessary.

- *Document improvements* by measuring pre- and post-status. Always have quantitative data available for comparisons and measurements of effectiveness. Calculation of cost savings is useful in measuring efficiency. Providing measurable parameters gives credibility and sustainability to the process of healthcare quality.

- Actively *disseminate achievements* and healthcare quality awareness information to as many individuals in the system as possible. Make sure participation is voluntary and open to everyone as opportunities for improvement are identified. Do not make it a private club. Keep everybody informed and involved as much as possible.

- Resist the temptation of *expansion* to other regions or sectors early. Building an effective process in one area is more important than starting several incomplete processes in different locations and areas. Keep the implementation process focused.

- Always keep *adequate funding* available for the development of new projects and activities not originally planned. Doing so also will give you the flexibility of shifting additional funds to areas where improvements are taking place more effectively. Adequate funds will increase the likelihood of sustainability.

- Finally, encourage and foster an environment of *learning, not judgment*. In particular, rely on data and facts in making judgments. Avoid the antiquated disciplinary method of management.

Remember that, according to Deming (2000), "Every system is perfectly designed to meet the objectives for which it is designed." Therefore, ensuring that the quality infrastructure is designed effectively is essential, and monitoring its performance regularly is even more important.

Case Example

It was only 8 pm when Jerry, an intern, wheeled the new electrocardiogram (EKG) machine into Ms. Smith's room, but Jerry could sense he was in for another sleepless night. Ms. Smith, who was 68 years old, had been admitted earlier in the day for an elective cholecystectomy. She now appeared acutely ill. She was pale and sweaty, her pulse was 120, her respiration was shallow and rapid, and her blood pressure was 90/60.

Jerry quickened his attempts to obtain the EKG. He momentarily considered asking a nurse for help but reasoned that the night shift would not have received any more training on the use of these new EKG machines than he had.

He had read an article in the hospital's weekly employee newspaper that the new EKG system was great. It featured a computerized interpretation of the cardiogram, which was tied to data banks containing previous EKGs on every patient. The chief of cardiology spearheaded the effort to purchase the system, believing it would provide sophisticated EKG interpretations during off hours and solve growing data storage problems. Technicians operated the EKG machines during the day, but they had long since gone home.

After affixing the EKG electrodes to the patient, Jerry looked at the control panel. He saw buttons labeled STD, AUTO, RUN, MEMORY, RS, and TIE. Other buttons, toggles, and symbols were attached, but Jerry had no clue as to what they meant. He could not find an instruction manual. "Totally different from my old favorite," Jerry thought as he began the process of trial and error. Unfortunately, he could not figure out how to use the new machine, and after 15 minutes he went to another floor and fetched his favorite machine.

"Admitted for an elective cholecystectomy," Jerry remarked to himself on reading the EKG, "and this lady's having a massive heart attack! She came to the floor at 4 pm; I hadn't planned to see her until 9 pm!" He gave some orders and began looking through the chart to write a coronary care unit transfer note.

Jerry's eyes widened when he came across the routine preoperative EKG, which had been obtained at 1 pm using the new computerized system. It had arrived on the floor four hours earlier, along with Ms. Smith. It showed the same abnormalities as Jerry's cardiogram, and the computer had interpreted the abnormalities appropriately.

Jerry returned to Ms. Smith's room. On direct questioning, she volunteered that her chest pain had been present since late morning, but she didn't want to bother nurses or physicians because they appeared too busy.

Jerry then discussed the case with the cardiac care unit team. They decided with some regret that Ms. Smith would not qualify for thrombolytic therapy (an effective treatment for myocardial infarction) because the duration of her symptoms precluded any hope that it would help her. They initiated conservative therapy, but Ms. Smith's clinical condition steadily deteriorated overnight, and she died the next morning.

Jerry reflected on the case. Why had he not been notified about the first abnormal tracing? He called the EKG lab and found that a technician had noticed the abnormal cardiogram coming off the computer. However, he assumed the appropriate physicians knew about it and, in any event, did not feel it was his duty to notify physicians about such abnormalities.

Jerry assumed the new EKG system would notify him about marked abnormalities. When Jerry first read about the new system, he thought it would serve a useful backup role in the event he did not have time to review EKGs himself until late in the evening.

1. What is the main problem in this scenario?

2. What should be done about it?
3. How should this hospital organize for quality?

Study Questions

1. If you were assuming the chief executive position in a hospital and the chief quality officer position was vacant, what type of person would you seek to fill the position? Background? Experience?
2. How do accreditation and adherence to standards mix with quality/performance improvement activities? Is there an optimal percentage of time a group should spend on one or the other?
3. What are the cultural barriers and enablers to achieving a successful quality improvement program?

References

Al-Assaf, A. 1997. "Strategies for Introducing Quality Assurance in Health Care." In *Quality Assurance in Health Care: A Report of a WHO Intercountry Meeting*, edited by A. Surabay and A. Indoren, 33–49. New Delhi, India: World Health Organization.

Brown, J. A. 2010. *The Healthcare Quality Handbook*. Glenview, IL: National Association for Healthcare Quality.

Brown, L. D. 1995. "Lessons Learned in Institutionalization of Quality Assurance Programs: An International Perspective." *International Journal of Quality in Health Care* 7 (4): 419–25.

Deming, W. E. 2000. *Out of the Crisis*. Cambridge, MA: MIT Press.

Suggested Reading

Al-Assaf, A. 2001. *Health Care Quality: An International Perspective*. New Delhi, India: World Health Organization–SEARO.

———. 1998. *Managed Care Quality: A Practical Guide*. Boca Raton, FL: CRC Press.

———. 1997. "Institutionalization of Healthcare Quality." *Proceedings of the International Association of Management* 15 (1): 55–59.

Al-Assaf, A. F., and J. A. Schmele. 1993. *The Textbook of Total Quality in Healthcare*. Delray, FL: St. Lucie Press.

Juran, J., and K. F. Gryna. 1988. *Juran's Quality Control Handbook*. New York: McGraw-Hill.

Nicholas, D. D., J. R. Heiby, and T. A. Hatzell. 1991. "The Quality Assurance Project: Introducing Quality Improvement to Primary Health Care in Less Developed Countries." *Quality Assurance in Health Care* 3 (3): 147–65.

IMPLEMENTING QUALITY AS THE CORE ORGANIZATIONAL STRATEGY

Scott B. Ransom and Elizabeth R. Ransom

The changing paradigm of competition in healthcare in the twenty-first century has resulted in an increased premium placed on implementing change focused on improving healthcare quality. While many of the initiatives described in this book are well supported in the literature, make sense conceptually, and appear to be practical approaches that can be implemented, identifying organizations that have successfully executed a strategy that focuses on lasting improvement in healthcare quality remains a challenge.

Volumes have been written about the value of quality improvement frameworks, such as continuous quality improvement, for healthcare. Organizations and foundations such as the Institute of Medicine (IOM), the Leapfrog Group, the Institute for Healthcare Improvement, the National Quality Forum (NQF), the National Commission for Quality Long-Term Care, the Brookings Institution, the Commonwealth Fund, the Robert Wood Johnson Foundation, the RAND Corporation, and the Center for Health Transformation have focused their energy and resources on improving healthcare quality. These organizations have engaged numerous experts and have spent countless hours and millions of dollars to critically examine and encourage quality. In addition, prestigious awards such as the Malcolm Baldrige National Quality Award have been offered as a way to encourage quality.

Despite these continuing efforts, the US healthcare system faces more challenges related to quality improvement than ever before. Improvement is selectively occurring; for example, Chassin and colleagues (2010) highlighted that in 2009, 98.3 percent of eligible patients with acute myocardial infarction received a beta-blocker at hospital discharge, compared with 87.3 percent of such patients in 2002. But the tidal wave of quality improvement efforts has unfortunately resulted in only minimal improvements in the US healthcare system, and the quality of healthcare that Americans receive has remained largely unchanged. Conservative estimates are that hospitalized patients experience 380,000 to 450,000 preventable adverse drug events (ADEs) each year (Weiss and Elixhauser 2013). ADEs are, overall, the most common nonsurgical adverse events that occur in hospitals.

The question of value has become a recurring theme in the challenge for improvement. In 2009, the United States was in the lowest quartile of OECD (Organisation for Economic Co-operation and Development) countries for life expectancy at birth even though the United States continues to far outpace all other countries in health expenditures (Fineberg 2012). This poor value proposition highlights the need for health system redesign and improvement (Christensen, Grossman, and Hwang 2009).

Implementing a culture that has quality improvement at its core is an important goal for organizations that want to better serve patients, gain the support of healthcare providers, stay ahead of government regulations, meet the demands of consumers for transparent information on quality and cost, and gain a competitive advantage in the marketplace. However, only a few of these quality improvement efforts have been successful, while a large number have not resulted in the sustainable quality improvements that the leaders who designed the change had hoped for.

Incorporating quality as a central element of an organization's culture and strategy must begin with leadership from the board of trustees, the CEO, and the executive team. Despite best intentions, developing a focus on improving quality is a challenge for most healthcare organizations because of the many internal competing agendas; the rapidly changing competitive environment shaped by providers, employees, and policymakers; and the often underappreciated impact of organizational culture on quality improvement efforts. Healthcare providers confront nearly daily conflicts that can disrupt a quality focus—for example, declining revenues and market share, union difficulties, electronic health records, Health Insurance Portability and Accountability Act requirements, review by The Joint Commission, malpractice concerns, employee recruitment and retention, physician relations, and community expectations. While every governing board member and CEO voice support for improving the quality of healthcare, only the rare board and senior leader are able to establish a culture that supports the execution of a sustainable strategy that will result in improved quality of care.

Successful organizations have visionary leaders who are willing to take calculated risks and who approach their journey to quality with a realization that the first step is to establish an organizational culture that will support this excursion. The starting point for this effort is leadership that is aligned with and fully supports a cultural perspective of quality. One tool to align individual goals of the provider with those of the organization is the use of quality measures specific to the individual physician (Ofri 2010).

Many of these leaders have expanded their view of quality to include a more balanced vision that reflects the ideas embedded in the performance management tool developed by Kaplan and Norton (2001) called the balanced scorecard. While some healthcare providers have fully embraced this tool, others have more loosely used the ideas of the balanced scorecard to shape their strategy. The balanced scorecard approach includes the perspective of the patient and family, internal processes such as use of clinical pathways, learning and growth opportunities that focus on employees, and financial performance. By adopting this broader and more balanced view, these organizations reflect an understanding of the wide range of interdependent factors that they must address on their journey to implementing a change strategy that focuses on quality of care (Blumenthal 2012). Leaders in these organizations continue to ask financial questions about market share, margins, and the quality implications of choices such as purchasing a multimillion-dollar da Vinci robot to maintain the cutting edge of surgical innovation. In addition, they raise questions related to the satisfaction of their internal and external customers and ask what business processes must be implemented to improve and sustain quality. Deliberately making this broad range of organizational measures the primary focus is essential to creating a culture of quality. This approach helps to ensure not only that the journey toward quality improvement is grounded in financial metrics but also that the organization develops the capabilities and skills that will be needed to carry out the quality improvement strategy.

The role of leadership and the interdependence of the elements of an organization with a performance excellence culture are best described by the Baldrige National Quality Program (2013) criteria for performance excellence. Exhibit 16.1 presents a slightly modified version of the Baldrige framework that includes the all-encompassing role of culture in creating and sustaining performance excellence. As the exhibit suggests, the change toward quality starts with leaders who create and drive a system of excellence that will bring about sustainable results.

Sharing a road map for change is helpful as senior leadership starts to manage organizational change. Kotter (1995, 1996) suggested a practical and useful change process that can serve as a guide for the leadership team starting the quality improvement journey. The following eight-stage change process, modified from Kotter's (1996) seminal work *Leading Change*, serves as a realistic and viable framework to guide leaders who are managing a change to quality. The eight steps are as follows:

1. Unfreezing the old culture
2. Forming a powerful guiding coalition
3. Developing a vision and strategy
4. Communicating a vision and strategy
5. Empowering employees to act on the vision and strategy
6. Generating short-term wins
7. Consolidating gains and producing more change
8. Refreezing new approaches in the culture

EXHIBIT 16.1
Baldrige
Performance
Excellence
Framework

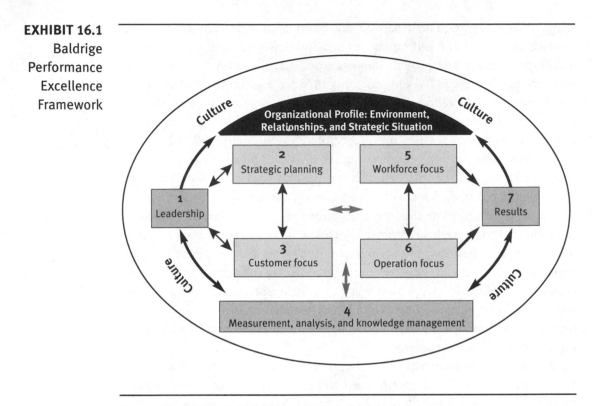

Source: Adapted from Baldrige National Quality Program (2013).

Implementing Quality in Healthcare Organizations

Unfreezing the Old Culture

The time to repair the roof is when the sun is shining.

—John F. Kennedy

Leaders establish the vision and set direction. The essential trait of leadership is the courage to set a direction. The transition to a high-performance healthcare organization requires a leader to define a culture that has quality at its core and to establish clear and specific expectations for employees involved in the quality journey. This step is the most difficult because of the influence of culture on employee behavior and the desire of some employees to resist change and impede progress.

Organizational culture comprises values, underlying assumptions, behaviors, ceremonies, symbols, language, and activities that are learned and shared by a group. Culture is like an iceberg: Some elements of culture, such as management information systems, organizational structure, and behaviors that employees are encouraged to follow, are more visible—that is, above the waterline; but like the underwater part of an iceberg, the more significant elements of culture are those that are less visible. These elements include shared values and behaviors that influence employees and persist over time (Kotter and Heskett 1992). Culture contributes significantly to employees' identification with a strategy and helps with the success or failure of executing the strategy. The role of culture is often overlooked or minimized by leaders who tend to focus on highly visible changes, such as improved financial performance, new service lines, or employee layoffs; however, it is critical to link individual employee contributions and culture to the shifting mission of the organization (Bohmer and Lee 2009). The real changes in behavior that will hold the new culture in place over the long term are the elements of culture that are below the waterline and take years to change.

Before this process can begin in earnest, the leader must motivate employees to change. To help transform behaviors, the leader must "raise leadership accountability and consistency . . . change behavior . . . and continue to move the culture to one of excellence" (Ballard 2014, 12). The first step is for leaders to clearly define and communicate the idea that the status quo is no longer acceptable. This task is not easy, especially if the organization is not in a financial crisis. Although numerous conflicts occur in the typical healthcare organization, the movement toward quality is easier when conflict is minimal and the financial strength of the organization is sound. In reality, most organizations prefer to stand pat when times are good or make only superficial changes to give an appearance of improvement. Rare is the leader who can effectively communicate a sense of urgency about an opportunity or a potential crisis without creating a sense of fear or resistance among employees. More often than not, the urgency of change is brought about by weakening financial performance, employee discontent, or declining dominance in the marketplace. Unfreezing the cultural iceberg and transforming the organization must start with making employees understand that changing the organization to embrace quality is required for growth and survival (IOM 2010).

High-performing organizations spend time on what is important, and if quality is the desired focus, leaders must create a sense of urgency that will move people from the comfort of the status quo to a new culture that reflects the values of quality (Volpp, Lowenstein, and Asch 2012). Changing culture without a sense of urgency is possible, but change is more easily obtained if leadership identifies some real or perceived sense of urgency. As an example, the leaders of Baptist Health Care recognized that the system could not compete in its marketplace by outspending its competitors and that it had to change because its flagship hospital was losing market share. In their search for ways to regain market dominance, the leaders examined many options but eventually embraced quality, which started the organization on a successful journey to winning the coveted Malcolm Baldrige National Quality Award and, in the process, regaining its competitive advantage (Griffith and White 2011).

Strong leadership is required to unfreeze the old culture and transition the organization to one that focuses on high value (Gabow, Halvorson, and Kaplan 2012). These culture changes may be facilitated through a shift in the development of healthcare professionals to better match what hospitals and society need (Aretz 2011). Although a greater emphasis on interprofessional teams may assist in this cultural transition, achieving the much-needed transformation to higher-quality and lower-cost healthcare delivery ultimately requires engaging physicians and leveraging professionalism (Conway and Cassel 2012).

Forming a Powerful Guiding Coalition

You can accomplish anything in life, provided you do not mind who gets the credit.

—Harry S. Truman

"Leaders get the right people on the bus (and the wrong people off the bus) and set the direction," says Jim Collins (2001, 13), author of *Good to Great*. Creating a strategy for quality improvement requires a team because no single leader can drive a sustainable change without the rest of the leadership on the bus and in the correct seat. The organization's change effort will determine what skills are needed in specific leadership positions. Senior leaders must coach, promote, or hire the right people who clearly understand the urgency, see the need to change, and have the correct set of skills essential to guide and support the change. At this stage of the journey, a few key leaders may need to be asked to get off the bus or change seats because they are unwilling to embrace the shift to the new culture or do not have the required skills. If, for example, a hospital CEO realizes that the market position of the hospital is challenged by lower reimbursements that negatively affect margins and quality, all of the senior leaders must clearly accept the threat and the strategy to address this threat. Leadership that is responsible for communicating this challenge in a troubled organization must recognize the feelings and perspectives of employees. Atchison and Bujak (2001) provide the following insight about this situation:

> Individuals go through a predictable progression in working with an organization. First, an egocentric position, do I have a job—am I going to get fired? Only when that issue is worked out can the employee progress to a role-centric situation, what is my job—where is my desk? If the person has a good grasp on her role then a mission-centric situation develops, what can I do to help—let's do good for the organization?

The first step is moving senior leadership to a mission-centric position. The leadership team must first clearly understand their job and expected objectives as the journey to quality improvement begins (Lee 2012). Thus, the CEO must ensure that the leaders understand the expectations for their performance and then must provide effective and timely feedback on their behavior. Senior leaders, including the board of directors, must be held accountable for their performance, which requires the tenacity, focus, and skills essential to what Gardner and colleagues (2011) have called *authentic leadership*. This common understanding about expectations and accountability helps to create what Kotter (1995) labeled the *guiding coalition* that has the responsibility for leading the change effort. The members of the team must have the desire, knowledge, and skills to support the vision, to direct change, and to deal with resistance, and they must be passionate about quality. The role of the guiding coalition is to help the organization develop a shared understanding of the vision and the goal to move toward a new organizational culture based on quality.

Executives must include key clinical leaders and staff in the guiding coalition. While executives can prod and support change, the real drivers of improving clinical care are physicians, nurses, and other clinical staff. Executives may attempt to inspire a shared vision through effective communication and finding common ground, but key clinical leaders must lead improvement initiatives in patient care areas.

A guiding coalition should include a healthy dose of innovative thought to inspire change. Creating innovation within the guiding coalition is critical, and fortunately the science of innovation seems to be evolving (Dyer, Gregersen, and Christensen 2009). In fact, Christensen, Grossman, and Hwang (2009) refined an approach for disruptive innovation that may serve as a framework for creating a guiding coalition with the skills necessary for transformation.

But perhaps the most critical asset that the team members must have is trust in each other. Without trust, true teamwork will never be achieved and the strategy will fall short of its goals.

Developing a Vision and Strategy

A great hockey player skates to where the puck is going to be.
—Wayne Gretzky

Establishing a vision and creating a new strategic direction is an exercise that allows everyone in the organization to understand what the future will look like and what they will have to do to achieve the future state. Most for-profit organizations create a vision and a strategy that focus on improving profits, which is only one element of the balanced scorecard. In contrast, most not-for-profit organizations have tended to focus on the opportunity to pursue a mission-oriented existence without great concern for fiscal stability and strength. In the increasingly competitive healthcare market, most not-for-profits now recognize that without a margin, there is no mission. This view reflects a more balanced perspective of what is needed for success (McCarthy et al. 2009).

In a world where a significant number of healthcare organizations continually face financial pressures, the trade-off between bottom line and quality has a predictable result. The organization in financial straits does not focus on quality but emphasizes a positive bottom line, which may compromise improvement and lead to a less competitive position (Joynt and Jha 2012).

The critical step that will get the organization out of this downward spiral starts with a leader who creates a succinct and inspiring vision that will transform the organization into a focused one that will be attractive to employees, have achievable goals, and allow for the range of individual interests. A simple and effective way to think of vision is that it answers the question, what do we want to be? The vision statement should motivate employees to move in a common direction and give them a clear sense of the future. For a vision to have this effect, the statement must also reflect the essence of the mission and values of the organization. Vision, values, and mission are the bedrock of any strategy and must be aligned and totally integrated into the organizational culture.

An effective strategy must be built on the organization's vision, values, and mission and describe what activities are needed to implement the strategy. These activities can be referred to as goals that should answer the question, what do we expect to achieve? Tactical initiatives clarify how the goals are to be accomplished and answer the question, how will we accomplish our goals? An organization must excel at these activities if it is to successfully implement the strategy. Porter (1996, 64) supports the critical importance of these activities when he argues that "the essence of strategy is in activities— choosing to perform activities differently or to perform different activities than rivals."

The final elements of an effective strategy are the metrics that answer the question, how do we know that we are there? As the adage suggests, "what gets measured gets done." The failure to develop a few key metrics that will drive the change and then consistently measure the organization's performance on those metrics is one factor contributing to the break between strategy and performance. Metrics are critical to adjusting strategy and serve to reinforce new behaviors and processes. Healthcare can sometimes drown in metrics, but knowing the few areas to measure that will directly drive the strategy and motivate employee behavior is critical. Fewer metrics are usually better.

Key stakeholders need to be fully involved in selecting the metrics and determining how they will be monitored. Although involving stakeholders makes the process more time consuming, it will help to ensure their ownership of the strategy and the efforts to measure progress. Engaging clinical staff in this step is imperative. Physicians and other providers will support efforts to measure quality if they have real commitment and involvement from the beginning. If physicians and other providers are involved from the beginning, they will be a better translator of the process to other providers. In particular, physicians need to understand how their practice style or behavior will be affected by the proposed quality improvement initiatives. Physicians will support change, but like most employees, they are often skeptical at first. As suggested previously, change will occur when physicians understand the inadequacy of the current behavior or process. Physicians often have divergent views based on past personal experience. A physician who has participated in a similar, but failed, quality improvement program will be reluctant to spend time or lend support to measuring some aspect of clinical care and may see the initiative as a waste of time. Physicians also often have financial conflicts of interest in working on these projects. These conflicts can be direct, such as in the case of the internist who is paid for every day the patient is admitted to the hospital while the hospital receives a fixed payment based on a diagnosis-related group. The hospital that attempts to limit length of stay may present a direct conflict with the physician. The senior leaders need to understand that the private-practice physician is an independent businessperson and sees the hospital only as a place to admit patients. Hospital committee work and time spent on improvement initiatives take away from time the physician can spend seeing patients and earning money for the private practice. Providing medical services that offer a revenue stream is how the private physician practice survives. The leadership team must understand these direct and indirect conflicts when targeting physicians' participation in improvement and change programs.

Strategy must be an integral part of a strategic management system that includes three additional processes: resource allocation to support the strategic initiatives, action plans, and a communication plan. The alignment of these elements is essential if the strategy is to be successful. Perhaps the biggest challenge for organizations that do not have a strategy focus is to distinguish between strategic planning and other types of planning, such as operational planning. "Improving operational effectiveness is a necessary part of management, but it is not strategy" (Porter 1996, 78). Strategy has more of an external focus. As Porter (1985, 1) advocates, "competitive strategy is the search for a favorable competitive position in an industry, the fundamental arena in which competition occurs." The strategic planning process involves deciding what to do rather than how to do it and therefore must look beyond organizational boundaries. Understanding opportunities in the external environment that match internal strengths is the starting point of a solid strategy.

Communicating a Vision and Strategy

Think like a wise man but communicate in the language of the people.
—William Butler Yeats

A vision and strategic plan are the cornerstone of a transformation change but will not successfully drive the change if only a few select employees understand and hear the message. The vision and strategy will help to galvanize employees only if the message is effectively communicated. Senior leadership must manage the communication of the vision and strategy. Communicating the transformation to a culture of quality requires that senior leadership convey this message over and over in both their words and their actions. Personal meetings with credible messengers have the best chance to build rapport and credibility with key individuals. Committee discussions can be effective, but the key leaders need to be enthusiastic supporters of the change before the meeting begins. The process of effective change implementation can be very time consuming. Presenting new initiatives to a group may appear to be more time efficient; however, unless key people see and support the information before the group meeting, the initiative is unlikely to move forward. Similarly, letters, phone calls, newsletters, bulletin board messages, and e-mail tend to be ineffective in moving projects forward. These impersonal methods of communication can be beneficial as an information source for employees, but the real work must be done through one-on-one and small-group discussions to explain the initiative to supervisors who will help move the change forward with the employees who report to them.

Leaders who are effective in communicating the change must eliminate the "we versus them" mentality and work toward expanding the guiding coalition. Medical staff members are not a homogenous group and therefore cannot be represented by a common voice. Elected leaders commonly assume that the physicians agree with both the vision and the strategic direction. In reality, support must be tested through direct and open discussions with individuals on the medical staff. Although the chief of staff may have clout, other practicing physicians do not necessarily recognize this individual as their representative.

Effective communication also depends on a clear understanding of terminology and language. The increasing specialization of healthcare can impair effective communication about quality improvement efforts. Physicians are science oriented, value autonomy, and focus on patients, whereas administrators are business oriented, value collaboration, and focus on the organization (Dye and Sokolov 2013, 9). Frequently, words used by an administrator to communicate quality improvement may not convey the intended message to the physician. For example, an experiment was conducted with the leadership team of a large health system comprising more than 40 hospitals nationwide. The leadership team consisted of all site CEOs and chief medical officers. Each member of the team was asked to write ten words that describe or support the term *quality healthcare*. Fewer than 25 percent of the group used three or more of the same terms to describe quality healthcare. In fact, 60 percent of the group had just one of the same terms in common. Although everyone in the room was an expert in leading his or her hospital, the group had inconsistent definitions of healthcare quality. This simple experiment shows the difficulty of effective communication of even basic concepts to healthcare workers.

Leaders rekindle passion and commitment while changing behavior, which in turn advances the culture (Ballard 2014, 12). There is no substitute for communicating change toward a new vision clearly, simply, and through multiple forums (Kotter 1996). Leadership by example is perhaps the most powerful communication tool, and senior leadership and all members of the guiding coalition must consistently model the desired change.

Empowering Employees to Act on the Vision and Strategy

One does not "manage" people. The task is to lead people. And the goal is to make productive the specific strengths and knowledge of each individual.

—Peter F. Drucker

The ultimate success of a strategy is measured by how well it is executed. The research of Mankins and Steele (2005) "suggests that companies on average deliver only 63 percent of the financial performance their strategies promise." Leaders often look first to areas such as poor planning or lack of clear priorities as factors that affect the successful execution of their strategy. These barriers may play a significant role in strategy implementation, but they are not the most basic factors that influence the execution of a new strategy. Often overlooked are that "individuals usually have their own passions that drive them" and that "the results achieved by empowering people throughout their organizations with passion and purpose are far superior to what can be accomplished by getting them to be loyal followers" (George 2007, 180, 184). Although a crisis can be used to empower people, building a culture that supports these values takes time, and time is often what an organization in crisis does not have.

Many excellent strategies have failed to be successfully executed because senior leadership does not entrust employees with the responsibility and authority to make the decisions that need to be made on a day-to-day basis. In implementing a new strategy, leaders often make the critical mistake of acting as though the implementation process can be centrally controlled. A lack of appreciation for the important role other employees play in implementing the new strategy may result from leaders' lack of trust in and respect for anyone who is not in the executive suite. No leadership team can transform an organization to one that has a culture of quality without ultimately empowering employees. Bill George (2007), in his book *True North*, suggests that effective leaders use the following six approaches at different times and in different ways to empower employees:

1. *Showing up:* Take the time to be there for employees.
2. *Engaging a wide range of people:* Share work, family, personal, and career concerns with these people.
3. *Helping teammates:* Offer suggestions or assist them with their concerns.
4. *Challenging leaders:* Ask people why they made particular decisions and engage them in a discussion to help them become better leaders.
5. *Stretching people:* Assess people and give them assignments that will help them develop and grow.
6. *Aligning everyone around a mission:* Show people how their existing passion and drive can be fulfilled within the organization's mission.

The ability to successfully create a new culture of quality and implement a strategy to reinforce this culture requires sensitivity to organizational history, to the resistance of employees to change, and to the need to empower people through passionate leadership and clear, repeated communication of the new vision.

Generating Short-Term Wins

Victorious warriors win first and then go to war, while defeated warriors go to war first and then seek to win.

—Sun Tzu

Establishing a culture that will focus on quality as the core objective is a process that takes time. As with any change that occurs slowly, people need to see that their efforts are contributing to the change and helping to make a difference. "Not all wins are equal. In general, the more visible victories are, the more they help the change process" (Kotter and Cohen 2002, 128). If wins are not identified and shared, the risk that the change effort will lose momentum increases. Creating and celebrating a win is similar to learning a new sport such as golf. Hardly anyone would play golf if they had to wait until they could finally shoot par. Rather, lessons that help the beginning player hit greens with greater regularity or reduce the number of slices per round provide encouragement.

A similar need for positive reinforcement applies to people involved in a transformational effort. Employees need feedback and recognition to let them know that their efforts pay dividends and that leadership cares about their efforts. As successes are noted, the benefit of the effort becomes more widespread and the desire to accelerate the change grows. Putting a spotlight on the wins helps to reinforce the success of the transformation effort to the guiding coalition and demonstrates to the doubters that the change efforts are working. The wins that are celebrated must be central to the change efforts and be seen as genuine by employees. A critical challenge for leadership is to keep the sense of importance high in the organization. Short-term wins play a critical role in helping to keep the urgency level high and building the momentum. Without leadership keeping a sense of urgency in front of them, employees can easily stop short of executing the change to quality.

Consolidating Gains and Producing More Change

The good-to-great companies understand a simple truth: Tremendous power exists in the fact of continued improvement and the delivery of results. Point to tangible accomplishments—however incremental at first—and show how these steps fit into the context of an overall concept that will work.

—Jim Collins

The process of effective change implementation takes years and is a time-consuming task for leadership and the guiding coalition. People have an instinctive resistance to change, and doubters continue to exist in the organization for months into the change process. These doubters will vocalize their concerns that leadership is "going too fast" or ask how they can focus on learning new skills with everything else they already have to do. If leadership lets these voices muffle the change effort, all the gains made can be reversed quickly because the new behaviors that will create a culture of quality have not fully materialized.

This stage is characterized by relying more on the employee empowerment efforts discussed previously, which will result in expanding the guiding coalition to include an even larger group of employees. At this stage, the training and process efforts that contributed to the short-term wins should be leveraged to focus on larger projects with wider organizational impact. The celebration of continued successes will contribute to changing employee behaviors that will help solidify the change and minimize resistance. Leadership must pay special attention to ensure that, during this stage, the performance expectations are realistic and achieved. Mankins and Steele (2005) contend that "unrealistic plans create the expectations throughout the organization that plans simply will not be fulfilled. Then, as the expectations become experience, it becomes the norm that performance commitments won't be kept." This backward slide is described by Mankins and Steele (2005) as an "insidious shift in culture," and they note that "once it takes root it is very hard to reverse."

Refreezing New Approaches in the Culture

The biggest impediment to creating change in a group is culture.
—John P. Kotter

One vital purpose of the process is to unfreeze the old culture and refreeze a new culture that has new behaviors and approaches at its core that support quality. Culture matters because it drives employees who are responsible for executing strategy. The key to solidifying the new culture is to measure the success of the strategic goals and share the data throughout the organization. Sharing data in a transparent way will help to drive the change to quality and reinforce the new behaviors that brought about the positive results.

The challenge for the leadership team and the guiding coalition is to decide just how detailed and precise the information has to be to support the change and anchor the new culture. Information paralysis is a common problem in healthcare organizations. Despite the promise of data from powerful management systems, the effective leader must act on trends rather than wait for statistical significance. Achieving statistical significance for critical management decisions may take years. An executive who waits for perfect information may impede the change process and damage the organization's competitive position.

One must know what to measure. While the powerful data systems in most hospitals can churn out reams of data, only a few pieces of information are useful to implementing improvement. Michael Lewis (2003), in his book *Moneyball*, presents the story of how the Oakland A's achieved championship baseball seasons despite having one of the lowest-salaried teams in the major leagues. The manager of the team found that the traditional measures of batting average and home runs were not necessarily the most important measures correlated to winning baseball games; he understood that on-base percentage was far more important. With this new way of thinking, the A's were able to recruit less-expensive players who could consistently get on base, which helped win games. This simple story demonstrates the importance of knowing the critical few measures that will drive change. Healthcare leaders can learn from this baseball story to look at their data in a different way. By identifying the right measures to achieve the organizational vision, executives can better lead the organization to success.

In making informed decisions, the executive must consider the effect of those decisions from all perspectives. A decision to improve financial performance may have a downstream effect on clinical quality or patient satisfaction. Similarly, a program to improve patient satisfaction may have a negative effect on the bottom line. The effective executive must quickly understand the implications of these decisions and act accordingly. Waiting for statistically significant information is not operationally feasible in the highly competitive healthcare environment. As executives ponder options and conduct further studies to make the best decision, the competitor may act quickly and eliminate the window of opportunity.

Case Study: An Academic Medical Center's Journey to Quality

Because changing culture takes a long time, this case study highlights several steps in one institution's journey. While significant changes have occurred, the road is still long and treacherous; however, the institution's journey provides a glimpse of the significant effort and conflicts inherent in a transformation effort.

The University of North Texas Health Science Center at Fort Worth (UNTHSC) is one of nine public health–related institutions in Texas. The medical school, which was chartered as the Texas College of Osteopathic Medicine (TCOM), accepted its first students in 1970. In addition to TCOM, UNTHSC includes a physician assistant program, a new physical therapy program, a new college of pharmacy, a graduate school of biomedical sciences, a school of public health, a school of health professions, and UNT Health, the entity responsible for the clinical practice. UNTHSC, which became part of the University of North Texas System in 1999, had 1,949 students, 410 full-time and 851 part-time and adjunct faculty, and approximately 1,400 staff in 2013. UNTHSC cultivated a successful research culture that has resulted in a steady growth in research funding and in 2012 received approximately $48 million in extramural research support. UNT Health has approximately 240 physicians, who see patients in 39 clinics throughout the county as well as in the patient care center located on campus. Nearly 600,000 patient encounters occurred in 2012. Revenues in 2012 for UNT Health were in the region of $85 million. UNTHSC has long-standing ties to the community and actively supports such annual events as the Cowtown Marathon and the delivery of educational outreach programs in local school districts that are designed to encourage young adults' interest in health and science. As a result of its research activity, the institution gained in state and national stature, and in the area of medical education, TCOM has been ranked among the *U.S. News & World Report*'s top 50 medical schools in primary care education since 2002, with 2013 rankings of 15th in rural medicine, 15th in geriatrics, and 20th in family medicine. The other side of this coin is a state institution that had faced a decade of challenges—namely, the vicissitudes of state funding, a physician practice plan that struggled with declining reimbursements, increased competition, and the closing of its primary teaching hospital.

From 2006 to 2012, the institution experienced what most would consider radical and positive change. The number of students grew from 1,000 to nearly 2,000, the number of academic programs expanded from five to ten, the clinical practice went from a money-losing enterprise with 185,000 patient encounters annually to a reliable money maker with nearly 600,000 patient encounters annually, extramural research funding expanded from $20 million to $48 million, and the number of faculty grew from 190 to 410. These dramatic gains were experienced as state funding was cut by more than 30 percent and the National Institutes of Health (NIH) faced unprecedented budgetary pressures, resulting in decreased research grant funding across the country.

This case study outlines the institution's road map to transformation.

Unfreezing the Old Culture

Against this backdrop, UNTHSC hired a new president in the summer of 2006. The search committee was charged with identifying a transformational leader who could effectively leverage the strengths of UNTHSC and address the challenges that the institution faced. As required by state law, the new president was an osteopathic physician, but in contrast to previous presidents, he also had master of public health and master of business administration (MBA) degrees. In addition, the new president had a broad foundation of experiences as an active clinician, a successful researcher with a significant track record of obtaining NIH and other extramural funding, an author with a significant publication history including more than 100 articles and 9 books, a leader who had implemented clinical improvement in previous executive and consulting roles, and a national presence who had held leadership roles in professional organizations, including as the president of the American College of Physician Executives.

He arrived on the campus in July 2006 and was presented with a strategic plan that the leadership had just developed over the past ten months. Prior to assuming the presidency, he had gained an understanding of UNTHSC, but once on campus he was able to learn about the overall operation of UNTHSC firsthand and in greater depth. The urgency to learn more about the academic, clinical, research, and community missions of UNTHSC was a function of the upcoming legislative session that was to start in January 2007 and his mandate from the search committee to lead UNTHSC in a new direction. During this biennial legislative session, the school's budget for the next two years would be determined. The recently completed strategic plan and the rapidly approaching legislative session created a perfect stage for him to launch his change effort.

As a result of his discussions with key leaders, faculty, and staff on the UNTHSC campus, the chancellor of the UNT system, Board of Regents members, and community leaders and extensive review of the institution's academic, research, clinical, and financial picture, he came to understand why business as usual was not working and what areas had to change. Enrollment concerns facing the institution, the continued challenges of declining reimbursements for healthcare, increasing competitive pressures in the healthcare marketplace, increased demands for accountability, growing concerns about declining federal funding for research, and new research models that were driving funding agencies such as the NIH all suggested that a new strategy was needed. The board members and the system chancellor had recognized many of these issues and therefore had chosen to hire a transformational leader who could guide the change process. Convincing some of the UNTHSC senior leadership, faculty, and staff of this view posed the first challenge of many that he would face over the months ahead.

The change effort required discussing more candidly than in the past such realities as enrollment trends, challenges facing UNT Health, and the need for measuring performance and holding leadership accountable. Addressing these and other opportunities required a new focus. His new focus was anchored by a commitment to four areas: (1) excellence in everything UNTHSC did, (2) goals determined and executed by a strategic map, (3) budgets dedicated to priorities set forth in the strategic plan, and (4) accountability by measuring results. Holding people accountable by measuring results had not been common practice at UNTHSC. To support this commitment with reliable, timely, and accurate data, the Office of Strategy and Measurement (OSM) was established in place of the previous Institutional Planning and Performance Improvement department. The OSM was responsible for collecting, analyzing, and reporting internal and external data in support of the newly refined strategy map and metrics and the new external reporting requirements.

The institution had developed strategic plans in the past but had no track record of execution. The new president acted quickly in working with the management team to refine the previously developed strategic plan into one that spoke to execution. The plan was refined over two months with the input of stakeholders across the institution in an effort to align the institutional plan to school-specific plans, department plans, and specific individual employee expectations.

With the change process barely two months old, the sense of urgency and the need for change were—as the new president had anticipated—still not fully appreciated by all stakeholders, and the pace of change caught many administrators, faculty, and staff off guard. The Board of Regents approved the strategy map in early September, which solidified the reasons for change and the sense of urgency. As would be expected, this radically different approach was embraced by some, ignored by others, and aggressively attacked by several. The individuals who had the most to lose quickly responded and attacked the plan and the new president. The negative reaction to the new approach was fully expected and was required to unfreeze the low-performing and stagnant culture.

Forming a Powerful Guiding Coalition

Recognizing that the president's executive team, other key leaders (e.g., department chairs, unit heads), and most faculty and staff had not yet fully embraced the sense of urgency and the need for change, the president took significant actions. First, he completely restructured his office by moving a number of staff to different positions on the campus, hired a new executive director who had an MBA degree, and consolidated some responsibilities among senior leaders, which resulted in one senior administrator's decision to retire. This reorganization of the administration was both symbolic and practical.

Next, he established strategic thinking councils (STCs). Each council represented one of the five mission-centric areas of the strategic map: Administrative, Academic, Research, Clinical, and Community Engagement. Each STC comprised key stakeholders from all levels of the organization and from across the campus. The STCs also included the president, the executive director, and the vice president for strategy and measurement. The STCs met monthly and were charged with examining issues that affected their area of the strategic plan and getting input from and providing feedback to other interested persons on the campus. The involvement of the president in each STC allowed the STCs to convey a consistent message about the sense of urgency and the need for change.

In fall 2006, these councils addressed concerns and listened carefully as employees described long-standing issues that fit under the rubric "we have always done things that way." Empowered to act by the president, the STCs challenged the status quo and examined approaches and solutions that reflected the drive toward excellence. As team members saw their ideas change how things got done, the members of the STCs began to appreciate how their ideas could directly affect the existing bureaucracy. This process created a culture in which more and more people participated in the change effort because they knew their ideas would be acted on. These efforts not only had the desired effect of challenging the status quo but also helped to make many members of the STCs better understand the president's message regarding the need to change and the slowly evolving shared vision of the future.

To enlarge the guiding coalition, the president established the leadership team, which comprised the executive team and all academic and non-academic department heads. A specific purpose of creating this group was to ensure that the vision and message of change was correctly communicated beyond the executive team and to provide a direct line of communication between these leaders and the president about their concerns and issues. The first meeting of the leadership team was a one-day program that was held off campus. This program used an outside facilitator, and the agenda was designed to clarify the reasons for the sense of urgency, the pace of change, the vision, the strategic direction, and the critical role the leaders would play in executing the new strategy. Perhaps the most significant event that occurred during this meeting was the playing of a video that showed the chancellor formally introducing the president to the public as a transformational leader. Sharing this video allowed the president to reinforce his vision of the institution becoming a top ten health science center, his sense of urgency, and his passion to create a high-performing academic health science center. Few members of the leadership team left the meeting without a clearer sense of the need to change and a better sense of how the vision would act as the guiding light for the journey.

Coinciding with these efforts, the president's executive team had been meeting monthly to discuss operational and strategic issues as well as the upcoming legislative session. Although the sense of the importance of change became clearer with each meeting, more needed to be done to help the executive team better understand the need to change and move toward a culture of excellence. The president, working with each team member, developed a written set of performance expectations with stretch targets. These performance expectations also included appropriate team goals that helped to reinforce the dependency among executive team members. Having written performance expectations was a new experience for most team members and initially met with some skepticism about the attainability of the targets and the value of the approach. These performance expectations wove accountability into every activity of the executive team. As a result of this effort to set expectations and other activities that required the executive team to address changes that were required to move forward, a member of the executive team announced his resignation from UNTHSC. This announcement demonstrated to the campus community that the president was serious about change, and it caused many senior leaders and faculty to carefully examine if they were on the right bus.

This accountability needed to extend beyond the executive team to the entire campus community. The level of transparency was a significant shift in culture and contributed to the belief of all stakeholders that business would be done in a very different way. Holding people accountable moved beyond the executive team when the evaluation process for faculty and staff was reenergized. Each faculty and staff member was required to be evaluated using standardized forms developed by either a committee of faculty or the human resource department. This process met with varying levels of resistance but clearly sent the message that accountability extended to every employee at UNTHSC and that business as usual was not acceptable.

As the legislative session approached, the executive team built a legislative agenda around a new program called the Health Institutes of Texas (HIT). The thought behind HIT was that chances for funding would be increased if a unique bench-to-bedside program could be developed to address the unmet health needs of Texans. The second purpose behind HIT was to create a new organizational structure built around core research programs conducted by interdisciplinary research teams. This model would leverage the strengths of faculty from different schools, thereby breaking down the traditional culture of research, a move that was being encouraged by the NIH.

Some members of the leadership team and most faculty and staff perceived the pace of change to be very fast. However, few members of the executive team could argue with the fact that the efforts had contributed to expanding the guiding coalition, building trust, and sending the message that senior leadership was encouraging new ways of doing business. One remaining challenge was that more faculty and staff needed to understand the impact of these efforts to create a new culture of excellence, but the good news was that more senior leaders, faculty, and staff were getting on the bus.

The journey resulted in a strong guiding coalition. The guiding coalition included the engagement of most key executives and the majority of employees, but establishing the coalition was not easy. While many employees voluntarily transitioned to the new approach, others strongly resisted. This process resulted in a significant turnover of leadership and faculty. Between 2006 and 2012, 9 of 18 members of the executive team were hired from outside the institution, and several others were recruited from lower levels in the organization. Further, of the 190 faculty members at the beginning of the journey, only 90 remained. This turnover allowed the institution to recruit 320 new faculty with diverse talents and experiences from across the country. This influx of faculty and leadership was critical to unfreezing the old culture.

The president met with all new faculty and staff at the beginning of their employment. In biweekly group meetings in his office, he told the institution's story and conveyed the need for all to engage and inspire transformational change. This personal connection helped engage most new employees that were interested in creating a top institution; however, the expectation of change and the expectation of accountability was a difficult transition for others. Overall, these processes established a strong guiding coalition from across the institution supporting radical change and rapid improvement.

Developing a Vision and Strategy

While the president focused on sharing his sense of urgency with the executive and leadership teams, a process was also underway to refine the newly developed strategic plan that would ultimately drive the change process. The strategy map was polished with input from leadership, faculty, and staff and resulted in a new vision—"to become a top ten health science center." In addition to the focused vision, the mission statement and values were clarified so that they were in alignment and in support of the vision. The strategy map had five mission-centric areas that were crucial to the mission of UNTHSC since its inception. One major difference in the strategic plan was that for the first time, each mission-centric area had specific and focused goals, tactical initiatives, and metrics. The metrics were developed with input from the appropriate stakeholders and the executive team. This process ensured that the managers who would be held accountable for the metrics had ownership of the target. Measurement with accountability meant that for the first time, the strategic plan was not a document that would be dusted off once a year and used as a prop to support a senior leader's presentation. Senior leaders, deans, and vice presidents recognized that performance now mattered. All senior leaders understood that they were going to be held responsible for the success or failure of their respective schools or units.

To help convey the importance of the change and accountability, each senior leader was held responsible for creating a strategy map and action plans that would be in alignment with the UNTHSC strategy map for his or her area of responsibility. The president requested strategy maps and action plans from all academic and nonacademic schools and departments. The development of strategy maps for each area of the institution required stakeholders to think not just about what they wanted to do but about how they would accomplish the activity and how they would measure their success. The development of strategy maps was accomplished in the context of a new strategic management system (SMS) that was built around the president's new focus and directed particular attention to programs that would be determined and executed on the basis of the strategy and budgets that were dedicated to planned priorities. This new SMS also included a focus on action and communication plans.

After using the SMS for four years, most of the chairs, deans, and vice presidents had an appreciation for the process of improvement; however, few of the department chairs and managers actually carried the approach to the level of individual faculty or employees. The SMS was therefore changed to include all employees of the institution. Specifically, the SMS aligned the institutional goals and metrics to that of the school, the department, and the individual employee. As part of an annual review and goal-setting exercise, each employee received goals, expectations, metrics, and compensation aligned with his or her department's goals and budgets, which were aligned with those of the school and the institution. This process better aligned the transformational effort and allowed even quicker gains.

Communicating a Vision and Strategy

Communicating the vision and strategy relied heavily on the efforts of the president, the executive team, and the newly formed leadership team. The efforts to effectively communicate the vision and strategy had so far relied mostly on the president, the executive team members, the members of the STCs, and to a lesser extent the newly formed leadership team. In addition to the meetings held with these groups, the president and other senior leaders had numerous meetings with key individuals to explain the vision and strategy. Some of these meetings were formal, whereas some occurred in the hallway or on the elevator. No opportunity was overlooked to beat the drum of change.

A number of approaches were used to engage faculty and staff. Starting on his arrival on campus, the president scheduled town hall meetings with all faculty and staff every three months. These meetings took place after each Board of Regents meeting and provided the president the opportunity to share what was presented at the most recent meeting and to answer any questions that faculty and staff had about campus activities. Normally, three meetings were scheduled during the day to accommodate the various schedules of faculty and staff. Particular attention was paid to setting a time that would work for clinical faculty and staff. These meetings always included a presentation on the quarterly metrics, progress that had been made on the new strategy, and the rapidly evolving new master plan for the campus. The employee questions were often provocative and reflected a growing interest in the change efforts. One effect of these meetings was that they helped to communicate the new vision and strategy and often addressed the latest rumor dealing with the change. In addition, video recordings of the town hall meetings were placed on the intranet along with all quarterly metrics to highlight the progress made at the institution. The posting of all metrics every quarter was met with resistance. Although most leaders enjoyed the posting of favorable metrics that highlighted the achievement of various goals, these same leaders strongly resisted the posting of metrics that did not meet goals or indicated poor progress. The president insisted that all metrics would be published every quarter whether they demonstrated success or failure. The posting of the institution's performance on the intranet and publicly on the Internet was an additional method to promote transformation and engagement from key executives and faculty.

An additional communication effort revolved around the remake of the *Campus Connection*, which was the main communication vehicle for the campus. This online publication focused on critical issues that affected the campus community, such as the campus master plan, and generally included a column by the president. Key leaders selectively highlighted the vision and strategy in many of the issues, and with each issue a growing number of faculty and staff became regular readers.

Leaders who are effective in communicating a change must eliminate the "we versus them" mentality and work toward expanding the guiding coalition, especially when dealing with medical staff. The UNTHSC physicians were not a homogenous group and therefore could not be represented by a common voice. The president was careful not to assume that the physicians would agree with both the vision and the strategic direction. He engaged physicians and their key leaders in direct and open discussion about the new direction and vision for UNTHSC and the expectations he had about their clinical, educational, and research roles.

Recognizing the importance of changing the culture, the president decided in early spring 2007 to use the Denison Organizational Culture Survey (Denison and Mishra 1995) to assess the UNTHSC culture. TCOM and the School of Public Health had used the survey in the past, but it had never been given to all faculty and staff. This survey examines four elements of culture, with three indexes for each area: (1) mission, which includes vision, goals and objectives, and strategic direction; (2) involvement, which examines empowerment, team orientation, and capability development; (3) adaptability, which includes change creation, customer focus, and organizational learning; and (4) consistency, which includes core values, agreement, and coordination and integration. Not surprisingly, the overall results showed room for improvement, but the area that had the highest results was mission, with vision having the highest score. The next highest element was consistency, with core values having the highest score. The Denison survey results were communicated to all faculty and staff, and departments were challenged to examine the opportunities the results presented in their areas. The data demonstrated that the message of the vision was taking hold but much work remained to create the new culture.

The Denison survey was used in every odd-numbered year since the beginning of the transformation effort. In addition, an employee satisfaction survey was completed every even-numbered year. These tools helped measure the institution's progress in engagement and provided evidence of progress. Similarly, a student satisfaction survey was completed each year starting in 2007. These surveys were conducted with an expectation of explicit improvement based on the results. Each executive was responsible for developing and executing a plan to support better employee and student satisfaction. Six months later, the president discussed the progress of the plan with executives in each major unit of the institution and requested feedback to improve the process. This personal engagement proved the president's engagement and interest in the employees' and students' opinions and perspectives. In addition, this process required that each executive follow through on the plan knowing that the president would learn the truth from the employees and students without any filters.

In addition to the internal transformation effort, an effort to brand UNT Health was designed to create an identity in the community for the clinical services provided by the UNT Health physicians. This campaign included the institution's first-ever billboards and new marketing collateral, such as a physician directory. This marketing campaign coincided with a focus on conducting patient satisfaction surveys and improving patient satisfaction and access to care by creating a call center. These quality improvement efforts all linked directly to the vision of becoming a top ten health science center and demonstrating excellence in everything UNTHSC did. The other obvious benefit was that this branding effort benefited the clinicians who were central to the success of driving change in clinical care.

Efforts ranging from an annual UNTHSC golf tournament and the Campus Pride Campaign to the restructuring of the UNTHSC Foundation Board and the revision of the faculty bylaws were done in a deliberate way that engaged stakeholders, which helped to ensure that the new vision and direction were effectively communicated. All of these communication efforts were coordinated by the newly expanded and reenergized marketing and communications department, which prior to the president's arrival had only minimal staff and budget support. As the marketing and communication team gained momentum, the message of change became clearer, and more and more people, both inside and outside of the organization, started to hear and understand the message.

Empowering Employees to Act on the Vision and Strategy

Executing the strategy depended on getting faculty and staff to feel empowered to act on the vision and strategy. The previous culture had relied heavily on centralized control, specifically in the area of finance and budgeting. In addition, the majority of the faculty were highly motivated and productive individuals who enjoyed working in higher education because this environment allowed them to exercise a level of professional freedom rarely found in other work situations. All the efforts had been designed to align everyone around the vision and strategy, but one critical element was missing: Those who had the greatest impact on implementation—department chairs and unit heads—had no real control or accountability over their budgets.

The president, with the support of the executive team and the budget office, changed who would manage and be accountable for the departmental budgets. These budgets, which had traditionally been controlled by the deans or vice presidents, became the responsibility of each department chair and unit head. This process required significant changes in how the budget accounts were set up and reported. During this shift in responsibility, the president made the decision to eliminate deficit spending in all accounts. This long-standing practice, which was part of the old culture, had helped to deflect accountability. The change challenged many senior leaders to learn new financial skills and helped to cement the values of transparency and accountability that were central to the new culture. The change paved the way for the additional financial accountability and responsibility that was shifted to senior leaders during the fiscal year 2008 budgetary process, which occurred in summer 2007. These additional change efforts paid big dividends among many chairs and department heads, but doubters remained in the organization.

A performance-based compensation plan was subsequently implemented to engage faculty. The plan gave each faculty member an opportunity to highlight their personal goals and the alignment to the goals of the institution. Compensation was directly linked to contributions in teaching, research, clinical care, and administration. This performance-based compensation plan met with resistance from several faculty members. Without fail, the least productive faculty members resisted the approach, while the most productive faculty members quietly supported the new program. As the least productive earned lower salaries and the most productive saw increases in their salaries, the faculty that experienced salary reductions responded in one of three ways: (1) some expanded their contributions to result in high compensation, (2) some earned lower salaries and continued to complain that the process was not "fair," and (3) others sought employment at other institutions or retired. This compensation approach provided a means to align goals and empower faculty to contribute to the institution in meaningful ways. While the process of implementation was a challenge, the results were predictable.

Generating Short-Term Wins

By spring 2007, the wave of change was evident across the campus, and the time had come to celebrate some of the success that had been achieved. Because the change was less than eight months old, identifying specific improvements was difficult even though a number of activities that were underway had broad-based support. While the Denison survey results dealing with vision and values were encouraging, change that affected the everyday lives of faculty, staff, and students had also become evident.

The president and the executive team created an annual Employee Appreciation Day. The day included a catered picnic-style lunch with various games and activities as well as the distribution of a specially designed T-shirt to every employee. In addition, the president, along with a few other key executives, visited every major unit on campus to say "thank you" to all employees in their own work area. Although it did not celebrate a specific win, the Employee Appreciation Day championed the most important asset of UNTHSC—namely, its faculty and staff in their efforts to create a culture with the vision of becoming a top ten health science center at its core. The lunch, which was served by the executive team and became a tremendous success, demonstrated the value that leadership placed on the importance of faculty and staff. The other significance of the Employee Appreciation Day, especially for the members of the expanded guiding coalition, was that faculty and staff began to see that their efforts to change to a new culture that valued transparency, accountability, and excellence were truly appreciated. During the campus visits and lunch and for weeks afterward, faculty and staff regularly expressed their appreciation to the president and senior leaders and endorsed the efforts to improve UNTHSC. As successful as this appreciation day was, the real work of solidifying the new culture and executing the strategic direction still had a long way to go.

Consolidating Gains and Producing More Change

The foundation had been created to collect, analyze, and share information about the strategy map and metrics. The president recognized early in the process that reliable and transparent data were essential to refreeze the new culture, drive the change process, and support new behaviors. The metrics established for each mission-centric area were deliberately limited to three or fewer critical measures. These metrics were seen as being measurable, were accepted by the executive team as credible indicators of the success or failure of the strategy, and were understandable to all stakeholders. The metrics were far from perfect but represented a balance of what was "good enough" information to drive the change process and what was obtainable and measurable.

When the measures were originally established, some members of the team felt that more was better, and this view was prevalent in the strategy maps that were developed at the school and department levels. Because the entire strategic management process was new to so many people, the team decided not to let the perfect be the enemy of the good when the strategy maps and corresponding metrics were being developed. A great effort went into ensuring alignment of the strategy maps and metrics whenever possible. Realistic stretch targets were set for all the metrics, and the executive team, which had the responsibility to ensure that the targets were obtained, generally felt comfortable with the targets. The metrics were collected and reported on a quarterly basis, and the president shared them with the Board of Regents and, during the quarterly town hall meetings, with all faculty and staff. The results were posted on the intranet and also on a Quality Wall maintained on the campus. The effect of setting targets, holding people accountable for achieving results, and sharing information in a transparent way was seen as very positive. This effort contributed to establishing new patterns of behaviors that would help to drive the change process toward the goal of becoming a top ten health science center.

Refreezing New Approaches in the Culture

By the end of 2012, UNTHSC had established a path toward greater organizational excellence and had created a new, high-performance culture. With a solid foundation for the new culture, UNTHSC has made steady progress toward becoming a top ten health science center, and several rankings indicate that the institution is getting closer to achieving its goal. Refreezing these new behaviors and processes will depend on continued commitment by the board of directors and at all levels of the leadership team.

Study Questions

1. In the case study, what steps did the president take to unfreeze the old culture?
2. How should the leadership team in the case study build a sense of trust that will support the vision of becoming a top ten health science center?
3. What activities could the executive team in the case study initiate that would empower more of the faculty and staff to act on the strategy?
4. In the case study, what critical steps need to be taken to refreeze the new culture, and who should be responsible for those steps?

References

Aretz, H. T. 2011. "Some Thoughts About Creating Healthcare Professionals That Match What Societies Need." *Medical Teacher* 33 (8): 608–13.

Atchison, T. A., and J. S. Bujak. 2001. *Leading Transformational Change: The Physician–Executive Partnership*. Chicago: Health Administration Press.

Baldrige National Quality Program. 2013. *Health Care Criteria for Performance Excellence, 2013–2014*. Gaithersburg, MD: Baldrige National Quality Program.

Ballard, D. J. 2014. *Achieving STEEEP Health Care: Baylor Health Care System's Quality Improvement Journey*. Boca Raton, FL: CRC Press.

Blumenthal, D. 2012. "Performance Improvement in Health Care—Seizing the Moment." *New England Journal of Medicine* 366 (21): 1953–55.

Bohmer, R. M. J., and T. H. Lee. 2009. "The Shifting Mission of Health Care Delivery Organizations." *New England Journal of Medicine* 361 (6): 551–53.

Chassin, M. R., J. M. Loeb, S. P. Schmalz, and R. M. Wachter. 2010. "Accountability Measures—Using Measurement to Promote Quality Improvement." *New England Journal of Medicine* 363 (7): 683–88.

Christensen, C. M., J. H. Grossman, and J. Hwang. 2009. *The Innovator's Prescription: A Disruptive Solution for Health Care.* New York: McGraw-Hill.

Collins, J. 2001. *Good to Great: Why Some Companies Make the Leap . . . and Others Don't.* New York: HarperBusiness.

Conway, P. H., and C. K. Cassel. 2012. "Engaging Physicians and Leveraging Professionalism: A Key to Success for Quality Measurement and Improvement." *Journal of the American Medical Association* 308 (10): 979–80.

Denison, D. R., and A. K. Mishra. 1995. "Toward a Theory of Organizational Culture and Effectiveness." *Organization Science* 6 (2): 204–23.

Dye, C. F., and J. J. Sokolov. 2013. *Developing Physician Leaders for Successful Clinical Integration.* Chicago: Health Administration Press.

Dyer, J. H., H. B. Gregersen, and C. M. Christensen. 2009. "The Innovator's DNA." *Harvard Business Review* 87 (12): 60–7, 128.

Fineberg, H. V. 2012. "A Successful and Sustainable Health System—How to Get There from Here." *New England Journal of Medicine* 366 (11): 1020–27.

Gabow, P., G. Halvorson, and G. Kaplan. 2012. "Marshaling Leadership for High-Value Health Care: An Institute of Medicine Discussion Paper." *Journal of the American Medical Association* 308 (3): 239–40.

Gardner, W. L., C. C. Cogliser, K. M. Davis, and M. P. Dickens. 2011. "Authentic Leadership: A Review of the Literature and Research Agenda." *Leadership Quarterly* 22 (6): 1120–45.

George, B., with P. Sims. 2007. *True North.* San Francisco: Jossey-Bass.

Griffith, J. R., and K. R. White. 2011. *Reaching Excellence in Healthcare Management.* Chicago: Health Administration Press.

Institute of Medicine (IOM). 2010. *The Healthcare Imperative: Lowering Costs and Improving Outcomes: Workshop Series Summary.* Washington, DC: National Academies Press.

Joynt, K. E., and A. K. Jha. 2012. "The Relationship Between Cost and Quality: No Free Lunch." *Journal of the American Medical Association* 307 (10): 1082–83.

Kaplan, R. S., and D. P. Norton. 2001. *The Strategy-Focused Organization.* Boston: Harvard Business School Press.

Kotter, J. P. 1996. *Leading Change.* Boston: Harvard Business School Press.

———. 1995. "Leading Change: Why Transformation Efforts Fail." *Harvard Business Review* 73 (2): 58–67.

Kotter, J. P., and D. S. Cohen. 2002. *The Heart of Change.* Boston: Harvard Business School Press.

Kotter, J. P., and J. L. Heskett. 1992. *Corporate Culture and Performance.* New York: Free Press.

Lee, T. H. 2012. "Care Redesign—a Path Forward for Providers." *New England Journal of Medicine* 367 (5): 466–72.

Lewis, M. 2003. *Moneyball*. New York: Norton.

Mankins, M. C., and R. Steele. 2005. "Turning Great Strategy into Great Performance." *Harvard Business Review* 83 (7): 64–72, 191.

McCarthy, D., S. K. H. How, C. Schoen, J. C. Cantor, and D. Belloff. 2009. *Aiming Higher: Results from a State Scorecard on Health System Performance*. New York: The Commonwealth Fund.

Ofri, D. 2010. "Quality Measures and the Individual Physician." *New England Journal of Medicine* 363 (7): 606–7.

Porter, M. E. 1996. "What Is Strategy?" *Harvard Business Review* 74 (6): 61–78.

———. 1985. *Competitive Advantage: Creating and Sustaining Superior Performance*. New York: Free Press.

Volpp, K. G., G. Lowenstein, and D. A. Asch. 2012. "Choosing Wisely: Low-Value Services, Utilization, and Patient Cost Sharing." *Journal of the American Medical Association* 308 (16): 1635–36.

Weiss, A. J., and A. Elixhauser. 2013. "Characteristics of Adverse Drug Events Originating During the Hospital Stay, 2011." Agency for Healthcare Research and Quality, Healthcare Cost and Utilization Project Statistical Brief #164. Issued October. www.hcup-us.ahrq.gov/reports/statbriefs/sb164.pdf.

IMPLEMENTING HEALTHCARE QUALITY IMPROVEMENT: CHANGING CLINICIAN BEHAVIOR

Valerie Weber and Jaan Sidorov

Today's healthcare environments are increasingly complex and require the ability to nimbly respond to rapidly changing conditions. Healthcare leaders must possess the ability to implement change throughout organizations to react to the evolving healthcare environment, improve the quality of care provided, and create and sustain improvements for the benefit of patients. In the field of healthcare quality, often the lack of both leadership for change management and an appropriate focus on implementation has slowed progress. What steps can a leader take to ensure that a new initiative succeeds? What are the best practices for introducing new quality improvement endeavors? An understanding of the evidence base for change management is an essential component of the healthcare leader's tool kit.

Understanding Change Management in Healthcare

Healthcare has undergone a more dramatic technological explosion in the past few decades than perhaps any other industry, yet healthcare organizations have not reacted with the same speed and agility to improve quality processes and decrease error that organizations in other industries, such as airlines, manufacturing, and financial services, have demonstrated. Although healthcare has made remarkable strides in improving quality and patient safety, organizations in many healthcare settings still approach patient care using the same traditional practice paradigms that have been in place for decades, despite their tendency to be inefficient and error prone. The ability to manage change is the distinguishing feature of the successful healthcare organization—and the successful healthcare leader—in the twenty-first century.

No matter how well a system or solution is conceived, designed, and executed, it will fail if people do not embrace it. Conversely, no matter how poorly a system or solution is conceived, designed, and executed, it will succeed if people want it to work (Shays 2003). Accordingly, the ultimate goal of the change leader is to create well-designed solutions that will gain wide acceptance.

Diffusion of Innovations and Other Change Theories

How do some new ideas in healthcare, such as a new drug or treatment, gain broad acceptance, whereas other ideas that present an equally strong—or even stronger—case for change never catch on? An often-cited example in healthcare is the use of laparoscopic surgery. Within a few years of its invention, it became widely used, and it is now considered the standard approach for most routine surgery. However, simpler innovations with a robust evidence base, such as the use of beta-blockers and aspirin after myocardial infarction, still demonstrate variability (Margulis et al. 2011). Similarly, the benefits of hand hygiene have been known since the mid-1800s, yet most healthcare organizations struggle with hand-washing compliance, resulting in an elevated rate of hospital-acquired infections (Gould et al. 2007).

The science of *innovation diffusion* focuses on the rate at which change spreads and can help to explain these differences. Innovation diffusion theories center on three basic themes: (1) the attributes of the innovation itself and how it is perceived, (2) the characteristics and behaviors of adopters, and (3) the context in which the innovation is introduced (Glanz, Rimer, and Viswanath 2008). The first theory of innovation diffusion states that certain intrinsic characteristics of an innovation and how an innovation is perceived are important predictors of the rate at which the innovation will spread. The features that lead certain innovations to spread more quickly than others are relative advantage, compatibility, complexity, trial-ability, and observability (Rogers 2003).

- *Relative advantage* is the degree to which the innovation is seen as better than the convention it replaces. The greater the perceived relative advantage of an innovation, the more rapid its rate of adoption will be. In medicine, the decision to adopt a new idea usually results from a risk–benefit calculation made by the individual physician. For example, most physicians make the decision to try a new medication by weighing its efficacy against the need for monitoring, potential side effects, and cost. A physician is more likely to prescribe a new medication if it is cheaper, is easier for the patient to take (e.g., once a day as opposed to multiple doses), is safer, or requires less monitoring.
- *Compatibility* is the degree to which potential adopters perceive the innovation as being consistent with their past experiences, values, and needs. Trying a new drug that is similar to one a physician has tried with success in the past is less risky than trying a different one. A plethora of drugs on the market are those that were released in the

same drug class once the initial drug in the class was deemed effective and was frequently prescribed. These drugs are easy to introduce successfully into the market because of this compatibility factor.

- *Complexity* is the perception of the difficulty of the innovation's application. Conversely, the simpler the change is, the more likely it is to take root. To employ another medication example, physicians are unlikely to try a new drug if they must write a letter to a pharmacy benefits manager for approval for a formulary exception. This requirement would make trying the new drug more complex and would make its use less likely.

- *Trial-ability* implies that the innovation can be used on a trial basis before the decision is made to adopt it, which enhances the perception that trying the innovation carries low risk. Availability of a medication to physicians in a trial form (pharmaceutical sampling) has been widely used to increase the use of a new drug.

- *Observability* is the ease with which a potential adopter can view others trying the change first. Pharmaceutical companies, in marketing new drugs to physicians and patients, use the observability and trial-ability concepts extensively. The use of in-office pharmaceutical samples decreases complexity, increases trial-ability and observability, and allows for compatibility once the physician experiences success with the new drug.

Multiple studies have analyzed how some of the above characteristics relate to the adoption of new medical evidence or recommended clinical guidelines. In addition to showing that adoption correlates with the strength of the evidence presented in the guidelines, these studies show that new guidelines are more easily adopted for acute health problems than for chronic ones. In addition, compatibility of the recommendation with existing values, decreased complexity of the decision-making needed, and decreased organizational change needed to follow the recommendation all increase the likelihood of guideline adoption (Francke et al. 2008; Glanz, Rimer, and Viswanath 2008).

Social science helps explain how individual characteristics of the members of a social group aid the spread of an innovation. Rogers's (2003) theory of innovation diffusion explains that any innovation within a social group is adopted over time in a process termed *natural diffusion*. Individuals generally form their reaction toward an innovation by observing peers who are already using the innovation, and therefore the decision to innovate is a mental process that begins with knowledge of the innovation, proceeds with forming an opinion about the innovation, involves the decision to adopt or reject the new idea, then requires acting on its implementation, and concludes with the confirmation of the decision to innovate.

A few adopters, whom Rogers termed *innovators* and who are excited by change and cope well with uncertainty, generally initiate the change process. They often perform a gatekeeping role for the introduction of new ideas into a system. Although this role is important, the rest of the group generally regards innovators as somewhat radical; therefore, innovators do not help the majority of the group to enact an innovation but rather are the first to introduce it.

The next, and most important, individuals to adopt an innovation are the *early adopters*. This group includes the opinion leaders. Others look to these individuals for guidance about the innovation. They often are the informal leaders and decrease uncertainty about the innovation by networking with their peers. Identifying and engaging the opinion leaders in a change initiative is a key strategy of successful change leaders.

Innovations generally begin to spread when members of the *early majority*, hearing from satisfied adopters of the new idea, begin to create a critical mass for change. The *late majority* eventually will follow the lead of others after increasing pressure from their peers. The *laggards*, the last group of individuals in a system to adopt, remain suspicious of change agents and innovations. They tend to be socially isolated and resist change efforts. These groups tend to be represented in a social group over a normal distribution (see Exhibit 17.1).

EXHIBIT 17.1
Rogers's Adopter Categories Based on Degree of Innovativeness

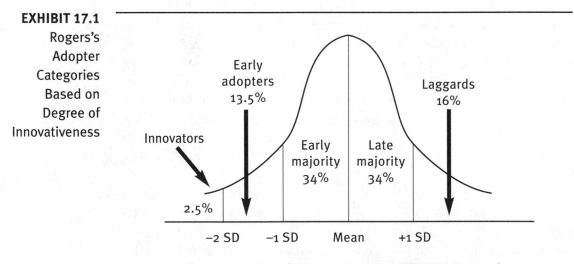

Time to Adoption (Standard Deviations [SD] from Mean)

The rate of diffusion of innovations has much to do with organizational context—that is, the characteristics of an organization's culture that tend to support (or discourage) innovation and its spread. Clear goal setting; strong support from physicians, nurses, and administrative staff; and the use of high-quality feedback data are important factors contributing to success (Cheater et al. 2005).

Healthcare-Specific Research

The innovation diffusion processes pertain to any social group reacting to a new innovation. But what data exist to demonstrate that these tenets hold true with groups of clinicians? To implement changes in healthcare, we must understand how and why physicians and other healthcare workers change. Hand washing was mentioned previously as a relatively simple behavior that has been markedly difficult to establish as part of routine practice in all healthcare settings. A survey of 120 doctors and nurses in hospitals and skilled nursing facilities showed multiple barriers to compliance, including problems of knowledge and attitudes (lack of conviction, questioning of the evidence), organizational problems (workload, lack of time), and social context (disruption of usual routines) (Pittet 2000). A behavioral study targeted at general practitioners in London showed that behavior change rarely had a single trigger but rather was caused by an accumulation of evidence that change was possible, desirable, and worthwhile. These cues came from educational interactions in some cases, but more often from contact with professional colleagues, particularly those who were especially influential or respected. When enough of these cues accumulated, the behavior would change. On the basis of this "accumulation model," the study's authors (Armstrong, Reyburn, and Jones 1996) theorized that only a limited number of changes could be made over a fixed amount of time—on average, three to four changes over a six-month period.

At other times, though, changes occurred abruptly when an immediate challenge arose; Armstrong, Reyburn, and Jones (1996) termed this phenomenon the *challenge model of change*. One particularly strong source of influence was the practitioner's personal experience of a drug or an illness. Another was a clinical disaster, or a negative outcome that changed the practitioner's prescribing behavior abruptly. A patient's experience with a particularly serious or life-threatening side effect could cause a physician to discontinue a medication's use.

The *continuity model of change* (Armstrong, Reyburn, and Jones 1996) describes how sometimes practitioners change readily on the basis of a level of preparedness for a particular change (e.g., the provider was waiting for a more acceptable treatment because of the current treatment's difficulty of use or cost). The strongest reinforcer of continuing change is patients' feedback. A patient's positive report reinforces the behavior change; conversely, a negative result, such as a major side effect, is often enough to stop the experiment. In the initial stages of the change, high risk of reverting to the original prescribing pattern exists.

Although many clinicians espouse evidence-based medicine—which emphasizes the importance of proving effectiveness in large numbers of patients—most physicians in the London study seemed to base their prescription changes on the results of a few initial experiments with a small number of patients (Armstrong, Reyburn, and Jones 1996). Most changes required a period of preparation through education and contact with opinion leaders. Educational efforts were necessary, but by no means sufficient, to produce the needed change on a lasting basis.

Physicians often fail to comply with best practices. One study analyzed self-reports by physicians explaining why in particular instances, after chart review, they did not follow best practices for diabetes, such as screening for microalbuminuria, hyperlipidemia, and retinopathy. Reasons included inadequate oversight ("it slipped through the cracks"), systems issues, and patient nonadherence, but in a surprising number of cases, physicians made a conscious decision not to comply with the recommendation (Mottur-Pilson, Snow, and Bartlett 2001).

Leading Change

Change in organizations cannot occur in the absence of skilled leadership. Many believe that leadership is entirely about creating change. John Kotter, in his classic *Harvard Business Review* article "What Leaders Really Do," writes: "Leadership . . . is about coping with change. . . . Leading an organization to constructive change begins by setting a direction—developing a vision of the future (often the distant future) along with strategies for producing the changes needed to achieve that vision" (Kotter 2001, 86). Managers create order and predictability, whereas leaders establish direction and motivate and inspire people. Although both management and leadership are necessary, change depends on skilled leadership. As Kotter states, leaders "don't make plans, they don't solve problems, they don't even organize people. What leaders really do is to prepare organizations for change and help them cope as they struggle through it" (Kotter 2001, 85).

Reinertsen (1998, 834) describes leaders as "initiators" who "define reality, often with data." Leaders develop and test changes; persuade others; are not daunted by the loud, negative voices; and are not afraid to think and work outside their immediate areas of responsibility. Similarly, Kotter (1996) proposed a road map to create change that includes establishment of a sense of urgency, creation of a guiding coalition, creation of a vision, effective communication of the vision, and creation of short-term wins to show that success can be achieved (see Exhibit 17.2).

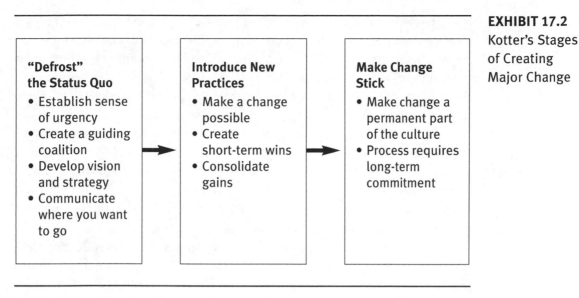

EXHIBIT 17.2
Kotter's Stages
of Creating
Major Change

Source: © Joint Commission Resources: "Effecting and Leading Change in Health Care Organizations." *Joint Commission Journal on Quality Improvement* Volume 26 (7): 388–399, 2000. Reprinted with permission.

Leaders of change need to remove structural barriers to ensure that the required changes are possible. For example, if time resources are an issue, it may be necessary to dedicate a percentage of key employees' time to direct quality initiatives or to restructure reward and incentive systems to promote quality improvement.

Although physician leadership in quality and patient safety efforts is critically needed in healthcare organizations, many organizations unfortunately do not have an appropriate structure to support these efforts or enough physicians with training and experience in leading quality improvement (Pronovost et al. 2009).

Reducing Variation: The Example of Clinical Practice Guidelines

Large variations in standards of care exist for many healthcare conditions. Studies, most notably the Dartmouth Atlas Project, have demonstrated that higher healthcare expenditures in Medicare populations have not resulted in better quality, increased access to services, improved satisfaction, or better health outcomes (Fisher et al. 2009). Ample evidence indicates, however, that quality can be readily achieved by reducing variation. The clinical practice guideline movement was born from this concept in the last decades of the twentieth century.

Since the 1980s, the knowledge base required to practice high-quality medicine has increased dramatically. Each month, thousands of articles in the medical literature can result in practice changes. The clinical practice guideline movement aims to translate and condense the medical literature into concise statements meant to change practice. This translation is especially important when one considers the constantly changing evidence base needed for best practice. By 2011, more than 3,700 practice guidelines existed across 39 countries (Institute of Medicine 2011). Although this movement continues, observations show that its basic mission has seen limited success. Because of a lack of attention to implementation, clinical guidelines often are not translated into action.

During the development of most guidelines, the sponsoring body, often a national specialty organization, synthesizes the data from the literature. Experts review the quality of the evidence and then collate the information into guidelines. Although these guidelines are widely available, most practitioners do not use them in everyday practice. Why not? A number of possible reasons have been proposed.

First, some qualities of the guidelines themselves may influence their adoption by clinicians. In the implementation of disease management strategies, clinicians insist that the strategies must (1) be simple, (2) be practical, and (3) not increase their or their staff's workload. The less complicated the guideline is, the more compatible the recommendations are with existing beliefs or values, and the easier the guideline is to use, the more likely it is to be adopted. Other variables—such as the characteristics of the healthcare professional (age and country of training in particular), characteristics of the practice setting, and use of incentives and imposed regulations—also can influence a guideline's adoption. Other barriers to guideline implementation include physician knowledge (e.g., lack of awareness and familiarity), attitudes (e.g., lack of agreement, self-efficacy, and outcome expectancy; inertia of previous practice), and behavior (Francke et al. 2008).

Patient characteristics—most notably comorbidities, complexity, and age—may also affect guideline uptake (Durso 2006). Physician factors also affected adherence to guidelines; most notably, the more experience the physician had in treating the condition, the less likely the physician was to follow the guideline (Simpson, Marrie, and Majumdar 2005).

Active Implementation Strategies

As previously noted, changes in medical practice are sometimes rapid and dramatic, such as with the replacement of many open surgical procedures with laparoscopic procedures in the span of just a few years, and sometimes slow to proceed, such as with the use of beta-blockers for patients after myocardial infarction. Continuing medical education (CME) is most often used to attempt to improve the dissemination of new medical knowledge, yet this approach has usually been shown to have little effect on performance or health outcomes (Grimshaw et al. 2002) or, at best, a modest effect (Grimshaw et al. 2006). In particular, most studies that used only printed materials failed to demonstrate changes in performance or health outcomes, a finding that also has been associated with the distribution of guidelines. Strategies using live activities, especially those that involve multiple instructional techniques, have demonstrated more positive results (Davis and Galbraith 2009).

More active strategies of diffusing medical knowledge have also shown more promise. The use of opinion leaders—locally influential physicians whose opinions hold sway with their peers—has been shown to be effective in improving outcomes (Grimshaw et al. 2001). A comprehensive review of strategies employing the use of opinion leaders alone or in combination with other strategies has shown that the recruitment of these leaders to disseminate information via local implementation of clinical practice guidelines can successfully promote evidence-based practice (Flodgren et al. 2011).

A strategy termed *academic detailing*, which involves outreach visits to a practice site by opinion leaders, has been found to be effective in accelerating the dissemination of best practices. This strategy is modeled on the methods used by pharmaceutical sales representatives, who train physicians or pharmacists to deliver one-on-one education or feedback sessions. Evidence from controlled trials shows that academic detailing alters prescribing and improves adherence to clinical guidelines (Chhina et al. 2013). These studies suggest that, although the content of the guidelines is indeed important, the mode of presentation of the guidelines is critical to their acceptance. Guidelines distributed by low-impact methods—such as mass mailings—were not accepted as well as guidelines distributed through proven methods such as academic detailing and the use of opinion leaders (Flodgren et al. 2011; Grol and Grimshaw 2003).

The use of reminders involves interventions (manual or computerized) that prompt the healthcare provider to perform a clinical action. Examples include concurrent or intervisit reminders to professionals regarding follow-up appointments or enhanced laboratory reports, or administrative systems that can prompt these reminders. These methods are moderately effective, particularly for prevention (vaccination or cancer screening). A review of more than 100 trials showed that about 75 percent had substantial improvements (Grol and Grimshaw 2003).

Audit and feedback systems provide clinicians with information comparing their practices and outcomes with those of other physicians in their group or an external benchmark. The use of these methods has resulted in decreased laboratory ordering (Ramoska 1998) and more appropriate drug-prescribing behavior (Schectman et al. 1995). A recent systematic review of 140 studies that used audit and feedback to change clinician behavior showed overall moderate effects (Ivers et al. 2012). This review further found that feedback may be more effective when baseline data are low, when the feedback comes directly from the supervisor or a valued peer, when it is given in both written and verbal forms, when it includes specific targets, and when it is repeated on more than one occasion (Ivers et al. 2012). Other authors note that effects of audit and feedback strategies are likely to vary with the intensity of the audit and feedback intervention, the appropriateness of the data, and how the feedback was delivered (Foy et al. 2005).

Administrative interventions that control test ordering have been shown to be effective in various settings. For example, evidence shows that simple modifications to laboratory order forms or changes to funding policy decrease the use of certain laboratory studies (Liu et al. 2012). Other strategies that have shown some degree of effectiveness include the expanded use of the role of pharmacists or nurses to assist physicians with test ordering or guideline adherence as well as the use of multiprofessional teams to tackle diagnoses such as mental health, geriatric care, or cancer (Grol and Grimshaw 2003).

The use of multifaceted interventions—including combinations of audit and feedback, reminders, academic detailing, and opinion leaders—has demonstrated changes in professional performance and, less consistently, changes in health outcomes. A systematic review of interventions intended to change clinician behavior found that 62 percent of interventions aimed at one behavioral factor were successful in changing behavior, whereas 86 percent of interventions targeted at two or more behavioral factors reported success (Solomon et al. 1998). Although a clear dose–response relationship between the number of interventions and the effect size appears not to exist, two or more different intervention strategies used together appear to increase the success of the intervention overall (see Exhibit 17.3). More recent trials confirm the utility of multifaceted interventions (Döpp et al. 2013).

The 100,000 Lives Campaign, sponsored and implemented in a variety of hospital systems by the Institute for Healthcare Improvement from 2004 through 2006, provides a robust example of how combined implementation strategies can improve performance. The campaign led efforts that focused on improving patient safety in hospitals, including the prevention of ventilator-associated pneumonia, the prevention of catheter-associated sepsis, and other initiatives. In this program, an interdisciplinary team, led by physician opinion leaders with multidisciplinary representation, first obtained data on performance and communicated the shortfalls within the organization (audit and feedback). Using Plan-Do-Study-Act (PDSA) cycles and other well-established implementation strategies, the team then worked to create sustained changes. The program was successful in many organizations, and many US hospitals have adopted its interventions as their expected standards of care (Berwick et al. 2006). This effort was followed by the 5 Million Lives Campaign between 2006 and 2008,

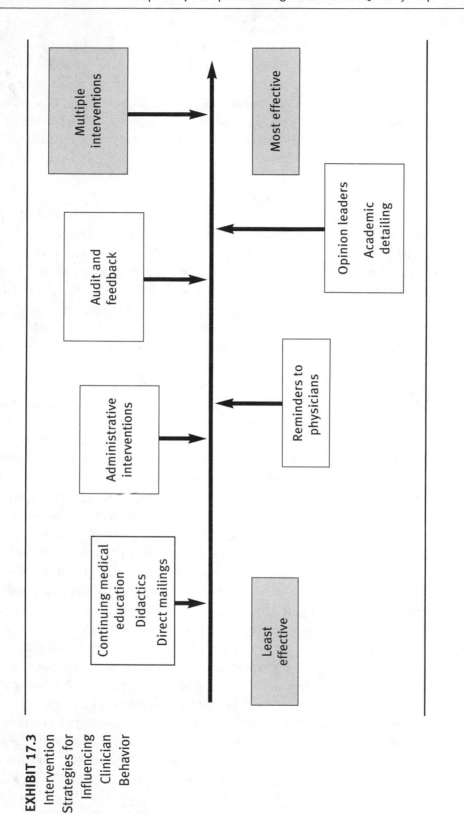

EXHIBIT 17.3
Intervention
Strategies for
Influencing
Clinician
Behavior

which focused on additional measures of quality among participating hospitals. More recently, Honigfeld, Chandhok, and Morales (2011) reported outcomes from the Educating Practices in the Community Program of the Child Health and Development Institute of Connecticut. This successful program combines the use of academic detailing, audit and feedback, and enabling team strategies to improve care for a broad range of pediatric health conditions.

Decision Support/Informatics

The use of reminder systems has long been suggested as a method of increasing clinicians' adherence to guidelines. Many early studies used manual chart-review strategies that provided reminders to physicians during their patient office visits. Such strategies included chart stickers or tags, medical record checklists, flow sheets, and nurse-initiated reminders. Patient-directed reminders, including letters, telephone calls, and questionnaires, also have been used. Many of these interventions have proven effective; however, limitations of these efforts center on their cost and labor-intensive nature and the inability to sustain them over time.

Information technology and electronic health records (EHRs), which have been widely introduced into clinical settings, have held promise for improved compliance with guidelines and quality indicators. Computerized reminder systems began to appear in the early 1990s. Early trials showed significant performance differences in both ambulatory care (McPhee et al. 1991) and hospital settings (Dexter et al. 2001; Durieux et al. 2000). Other studies have shown that the use of informatics-based interventions can improve the use of statin drugs for the secondary prevention of coronary disease (Lester et al. 2006) and can reduce polypharmacy and falls in the elderly (Weber, White, and McIlvried 2008). A systematic review of 100 controlled trials of computerized clinical decision support demonstrated that performance improved in 64 percent of the studies (Garg et al. 2005). The strongest effects were seen for drug dosing and prescribing systems and for reminder systems for ordering tests or preventive services.

More recent work has failed to support the premise that EHRs and decision support can independently result in large gains in healthcare quality. Romano and Stafford (2011) analyzed data on 255,402 US ambulatory clinic visits from 2005 to 2007. Seventeen percent of these visits included the use of an EHR that offered clinical decision support. Using several previously developed quality indicators, the authors assessed the relationship of EHRs and clinical decision support to the provision of better care and found no consistent association. Another major study (Zhou et al. 2009) linked two data sources—a statewide survey of physicians' use of EHRs and claims data reflecting quality-of-care indicators over a four-year period. For all six clinical conditions analyzed, the study found no difference in performance between physicians using an EHR and those using a paper record. Other recent studies, however, have demonstrated benefits consistent with earlier findings. For example, Cebul and colleagues (2011) analyzed data for more than 27,000 adults with diabetes seen at 46 practices from July 2009 to June 2010 and found that diabetes care standards were significantly higher at clinics with EHRs than at those with paper records.

These mixed data suggest that EHRs can be an important ingredient in enhancing the quality of care but are not alone sufficient if they are not rooted in an environment where quality of care is emphasized and systems exist to improve care. For EHRs to live up to their promise, much work remains to be done to understand which uses of the EHR improve care the most, taking into account issues such as the preservation of work flows and physician autonomy (DesRoches et al. 2010). Much work on the interface of chronic disease management and information technology focuses on the use of computerized chronic disease registries, which shifts the attention from what occurs in individualized patient visits to strategies that allow for enhanced management of populations. For example, many EHRs identify patients with important conditions, such as diabetes, hypertension, asthma, or congestive heart failure. Patients whose care does not conform to best-practice guidelines can be targeted for various interventions by nonphysicians operating under a protocol or standing orders under physician supervision, or, alternatively, the registry information can be fed back to the physicians for action. Such approaches have demonstrated improvements in chronic disease management (Weber et al. 2008).

Checklists

A safety checklist is a "list of action items, tasks or behaviours arranged in a consistent manner, which allows the evaluator to record the presence or absence of the individual items listed" (Hales et al. 2008, 24). Safety checklists have attracted interest as a means to standardize and thus improve care. Long used in other industries, such as aviation, checklists have been shown to reduce errors—particularly in the surgical setting, where the use of checklists has reduced postoperative death rates and complications (de Vries et al. 2010; Haynes et al. 2009). Surgical checklist changes have included the use of a "time out" prior to surgery to correctly identify the patient, confirm the operative site, and ensure the timely administration of prophylactic antibiotics. Checklists have also been applied at the time of hospital discharge to decrease medication errors and address other safety issues (Halasyamani et al. 2006).

Disease and Population Health Management

Disease management has been instrumental in motivating physicians to conform to best practices. *Disease management* can be defined as any program devoted to the care of populations characterized by the presence of a chronic disease. This type of program, which began in earnest in the 1990s, has evolved to include wellness, prevention, and other care coordination services in a broader suite of offerings in what has been dubbed *population health*. Most of these programs have been designed by third parties, such as managed care organizations and investor-owned service providers, to reduce costs through increased conformity, reduced variation, and greater involvement of patients in their own care. The underlying business case for population health management is to improve health outcomes while simultaneously lowering healthcare use and costs.

Underlying much of this approach to care is an explicit belief that the most effective method of changing physician behavior is to make "doing the right thing" the path of least resistance by removing the responsibility for the guideline from the physician and sharing the management of chronic diseases with an expanded healthcare team composed of nonphysician health professionals, such as nurses and pharmacists. Such programs have proven effective in improving outcomes and reducing costs of chronic diseases such as diabetes (Sidorov et al. 2002), congestive heart failure (Rich et al. 1995), dementia (Vickrey et al. 2006), and asthma (Bolton et al. 1991). Characteristics of such programs include population risk assessment (a method of identifying the population of patients with the most pressing care needs), outreach, and recruitment, followed by education, engagement in self-care, personalized one-on-one case management when necessary, and targeted health promotion or disease prevention activities (Care Continuum Alliance 2012). Barriers to the use of such programs include lack of financial and staffing resources as well as cultural issues that emerge when physician practices evolve to a more team-based method of disease management. As with any implementation, adequate attention to physician buy-in as well as administrative support and involvement are crucial.

Financial Incentives

In the aftermath of the Institute of Medicine's (2001) publication of *Crossing the Quality Chasm*, the government and employers—which are responsible for paying the large majority of US healthcare costs—wanted to accelerate the pace of change in healthcare by reducing variation, attacking unnecessary costs, and increasing quality. One approach has been the introduction of significant financial incentives that reward physicians and provider organizations for delivering high-quality medical care. The payers and many policymakers hoped that this approach could "move the dial" by stimulating improvements in performance. Yet empirical studies of the effect of direct quality incentives on physician performance have shown an inconsistent effect (Campbell et al. 2009; Conrad et al. 2006; Petersen et al. 2006). For example, in one report (Lindenauer et al. 2007), changes in 14 quality measures were monitored over two years during a Centers for Medicare & Medicaid Services (CMS) pay-for-performance demonstration project. Although pay-for-performance hospitals outperformed control hospitals, improvements after adjusting for baseline performance and hospital characteristics were modest, ranging from 2.6 to 4.1 percent. Another review of 128 studies undertaken between 1990 and 2009 found that pay for performance had some positive effects on clinical effectiveness and on access to and equity of care without widespread unintended consequences (Van Herck et al. 2010). A recent analysis using Medicare data to compare outcomes among 252 hospitals participating in the Premier Hospital Quality Incentive Demonstration found no evidence that the program affected mortality (Jha et al. 2012). Yet despite any skepticism, the implementation of pay for performance has quickly outstripped the evidence, and such programs are widely in use nationally (Cromwell et al. 2011).

Concerns about such programs include whether they would prompt physicians to "game" a pay-for-performance system by either not caring for sicker or economically disadvantaged populations or, alternatively, cherry-picking healthier patients who would improve a provider's overall performance. This concern has significant implications for vulnerable underserved populations with multiple health problems or psychiatric diagnoses, which could theoretically put providers at a significant economic disadvantage, and especially for patient groups disproportionately represented among hospitals and healthcare providers that are less well financed (Werner et al. 2011). Whether pay for performance will have enough of an effect on quality to justify the early enthusiasm for the model and its subsequent widespread implementation remains to be seen.

The New Wave: Medical Homes and Accountable Care Organizations

Other new care models have emerged in an attempt to deliver higher-quality, cost-effective care. The patient-centered medical home (PCMH) model promotes the use of organized primary care teams to expand the traditional one-on-one model of care to a coordinated team that provides extended care, particularly to patients with complex medical conditions or chronic diseases. Supporters of the PCMH note that it can increase access to primary care, promote a longitudinal relationship with a provider and the provider's team, leverage health information technology to include disease registries, and drive greater care coordination. This model includes financial incentives to reward the team for these elements, including a monthly per-patient care management fee, pay-for-performance incentives, and sharing of any cost savings brought about by the model. PCMH models have been tested in demonstration projects in Colorado, North Carolina, Pennsylvania, Wisconsin, Utah, North Dakota, and Vermont and have demonstrated reductions in hospitalizations, emergency department visits, and total costs per patient (Cassidy 2010).

The concept of accountable care organizations (ACOs) was set forth in the Affordable Care Act of 2010. ACOs consist of a group of providers (which may combine physicians, hospitals, and other elements of the healthcare system) who would be jointly accountable for both providing care (including quality improvements) and reducing spending for a defined population of patients. This concept has taken shape as commercial insurers have begun to form ACO contracts with provider groups (Shields et al. 2010). Pending further evaluation of the outcomes of ACO implementation, it is unclear whether the healthcare system as currently configured is ready to meet the considerable organizational requirements of ACOs, including advanced health information technology and expertise in care coordination, to name just a few. Outside of major cities, most healthcare is still provided by small one- and two-physician offices and community hospitals, which simply may not be ready to take the needed jump demanded by such models (McClellan et al. 2010).

Addressing the Cost of Implementation

Information about how implementation of many of the health system reforms described in this chapter will affect health resources is lacking. As a result, one barrier to implementation may be the perception that the value gained is not worth the cost. Efforts to change physicians' clinical behavior should be in accord with administrative and reimbursement policies. For example, if an organization asks physicians to spend more time identifying and treating depression and at the same time pressures them to see more patients, depression care is unlikely to improve. If the structure of the healthcare system, in particular its reimbursement structure, runs counter to medical guidelines, even the best guidelines will not be implemented successfully.

It is necessary to distinguish between treatment cost-effectiveness (i.e., the incremental costs and benefits of a treatment) and policy cost-effectiveness (the cost in relation to treatment cost-effectiveness and the cost and magnitude of the implementation method needed to enact the change). Having to invest resources to change physician behavior imposes an additional cost on treatment cost-effectiveness.

Policy cost-effectiveness will remain attractive only when effective but inexpensive implementation methods exist or if large health gains per patient exist for a high-prevalence disease. For example, the use of angiotensin-converting enzyme inhibitors for heart failure is considered cost-effective at $2,602 per life year gained. Estimates of successful implementation of academic detailing programs used in the United Kingdom by the National Health Service, which had a significant effect at a small cost per patient ($446 per life year gained), allowed the intervention to retain its cost-effectiveness. However, the cost of academic outreach to promote a reduction in the use of newer classes of antidepressants in favor of less-expensive tricyclic antidepressants is not economical because the outreach cost per patient exceeds the cost saved from behavioral change. Thus, the cost and efficacy of the implementation method must be added to the cost-effectiveness of the treatment to make a policy decision (Mason et al. 2001).

Goetzel and colleagues (2005) reviewed the literature reporting cost–benefit data for disease management programs. Their analysis showed that disease management programs focusing on congestive heart failure save more money than they cost, even in the short run—likely because they prevent avoidable hospital readmissions for congestive heart failure, one of the most prevalent inpatient hospital admission diagnoses in the United States. Mixed results were found when considering programs directed at diabetes, depression, and asthma, suggesting that such programs may cost more than the savings they generate, at least in the short term.

Whether quality improvement initiatives make financial sense for an organization is a complex consideration. A healthcare organization operating under a global payment structure is likely to benefit from a strategy that reduces utilization or hospital admissions. A health system that receives reimbursement under fee-for-service plans or relies on diagnosis-related group payments from Medicare would lose money from a program that reduces hospital admissions. Successful chronic care programs have been discontinued because financial incentives did not exist to support the expense of such programs. In the ambulatory setting, increased utilization of ambulatory resources for unreimbursed chronic disease management results in decreased revenue per visit in a capitated managed care setting, while substituting in-person visits with telephonic management by nursing personnel would be financially disadvantageous in a fee-for-service model.

Thus, to create a favorable business case for quality improvement initiatives, the savings or increased revenue from improved care must accrue to the organization paying for the improvements. External incentives are likely to become increasingly important in driving quality improvement and the use of clinical guidelines and chronic disease models.

Keys to Successful Implementation and Lessons Learned

The preceding discussion addressed specific tools that improve dissemination of healthcare quality initiatives. This section summarizes key steps in the successful implementation of such initiatives.

1. *Focus on high-impact interventions.* What disease processes are most prevalent in your population? Hypertension, diabetes, and obesity top the list for most adult populations. What is your goal? If your goal is to reduce avoidable hospital readmissions, a focus on large-volume, high-impact conditions such as congestive heart failure can show improvements and cost savings in the short term through well-proven strategies.

2. *Assess how you are performing now.* To know what to focus on, you need to know your current performance relative to benchmarks. Initially, the baseline metrics that are furthest from benchmarks are easiest to correct (the so-called low-hanging fruit). Keep in mind the Pareto principle, or 80/20 rule, recognizing that you will expend the greatest amount of effort trying to accomplish that final 20 percent.

3. *For every hour spent discussing the content of the initiative, spend four hours planning its implementation.* Your practice guideline will not improve care in your organization unless it is used. Emphasizing the structural or developmental phase without adequate attention to implementation is a sure recipe for failure. Use proven implementation methods, not merely passive education and dissemination, and use multiple interventions simultaneously.

4. *Determine who needs to change.* Analyze which individuals in the organization must respond to the proposed change and what barriers exist. Invest in the innovators and early adopters. Know who your opinion leaders are, and enlist them as your champions. Spend little time with the laggards, recognizing that in an era of constrained resources, change leaders must direct efforts at those who are on board or coming aboard.

5. *Do a cost–benefit analysis.* Weigh the costs of implementation, taking into account the implementation method, against both the costs of inaction and the gains of a successful result. Too often, leaders fail to factor in the cost of a change early enough in the process. As a result, a great deal of work is done in an area that will not be sustainable over the long term. As described previously, the party expending the resources generally must be the same party reaping the financial benefits of the change.

6. *Enlist multidisciplinary teams.* Teams should consist of individuals who actually do the work, not the formal leadership. For example, an

office redesign project should include representation from the front desk personnel, administrative assistants, nursing staff, and operational leadership, not just physicians.

7. *Think big, but start small.* The old saying "Rome wasn't built in a day" applies here. Projects that are too ambitious may be harder to build momentum for—you need to achieve an early short-term gain to keep the bosses on board and silence the naysayers. Is your real goal to convert your practice from a traditional scheduling scheme to an open-access scheduling system? Start with a small project—either piloting this idea with one physician or working on a smaller, related project—before redesigning the entire system.

8. *Once you have defined your goal, construct a timeline and publicize it.* Teams sometimes spin their wheels forever without accomplishing anything. This timeline will give the team accountability to keep moving along in the process. You can change milestones midstream—flexibility is important—but procrastination cannot be an excuse.

9. *Communicate the change effectively.* Many initiatives have failed because the changes were poorly communicated. Make use of multiple and informal forums—everything from meetings to e-mails to watercooler conversations. Make sure your vision can be clearly articulated in 30 to 60 seconds. If the new way is transparent, seems simple, and makes sense, it will be easier to spread.

10. *Back up talk with actions.* Leaders should not be exempt from following the new path, and they also must be perfect role models of the new process. Do you want to implement open access in your practice? Do it yourself first. Have you reconstructed a new patient identification process to reduce the chance of wrong-site surgery? Follow it yourself 100 percent of the time.

11. *Celebrate successful change.* Hold system-wide meetings highlighting how your new medication error reduction system is reducing errors. Ensuring that everyone in your organization is aware of the success makes change less threatening the next time around. Moreover, publishing and speaking outside your organization about your successes can spread successful techniques externally. In exchange, from others, you may learn successful approaches to apply in your organization.

12. *Create a culture of continual change within your organization.* Successful organizations and industries understand that their survival depends on a continual reinvention of themselves—continuous quality improvement. Many experiencing the ongoing change will ask, "Are we almost there yet?" The answer is *no*. Organizations should strive continuously for a state of perfection, which they may approach but likely will never reach. Exhibit 17.4 summarizes common pitfalls encountered in the change process.

EXHIBIT 17.4
Common
Implementation
Pitfalls

- Lack of attention to implementation
  - Overemphasis on guideline development
  - No knowledge of effective implementation strategies
- Involvement of the wrong people
  - Lack of recognition of informal leadership
  - Failure to enlist opinion leaders
- Failure to commit adequate resources to the implementation process
  - Lack of commitment of time and staffing
  - Lack of visible leadership support
- Inadequate communication
  - Message too complex
  - Lack of establishing a sense of urgency
- Implementation too costly/failure to assess cost-effectiveness
  - Program too expensive or incentives misaligned
- Competing crises or uncontrollable factors in the external environment

Case Studies

Case 1: A Good Strategy at the Wrong Time

A large East Coast academic medical center was located in a highly competitive market. A number of managed care organizations in the marketplace were asking the organization to negotiate contracts that placed a significant degree of risk on the organization. An early experiment showed this approach to be very costly to the organization.

To prepare for this wave of risk contracting, the CEO and chief quality officer embarked on a major endeavor to make quality the driving force of the organization. They believed that a strategy of providing the best care with assistance from disease management programs throughout the organization's practice network would allow the organization to engage in full-risk capitation, earn the organization a competitive advantage of offering the best quality, and thus help the organization negotiate favorable contracts in the healthcare marketplace.

The program addressed deviations from best practice in the care of high-volume chronic conditions, such as congestive heart failure, diabetes, and asthma. Clinical champions—well-known physicians respected by their peers—led teams in designing outpatient clinical guidelines according to evidence-based best practices. The multipronged effort included educational strategies, academic detailing in individual physician practices, clinical decision support with prompts and reminder systems, and office-based coordinators to disseminate the guidelines.

At its peak, the department responsible for the program contained three medical directors, employed 70 persons, and enrolled more than

14,000 patients in 28 specific programs. It was successful in demonstrating improved outcomes in asthma care, including reduced hospitalizations and emergency department visits, as well as improved compliance with best practices in congestive heart failure and asthma care. The program was successful because of its intense focus on implementation. Particularly effective was the focus on the use of opinion leaders and clinical champions as well as the use of multiple interventions to increase physician enrollment and buy-in. In addition, the system's leadership communicated a strong mandate for quality improvement and disease management, and the programs had strong physician leadership. Initial programs in high-impact areas were able to demonstrate short-term wins.

However, the organization began suffering financial losses, and the entire program was abruptly dismantled during a round of consultant-driven expense reduction. The expected rush to full-risk capitation never occurred, and the organization's emphasis on quality did not seem to garner it a special place in the crowded marketplace. In reality, the party incurring the cost was not the party obtaining the financial benefit. The insurers and managed care organizations benefited financially from the program, but the health system paid the expense. Thus, the cost of the program was not sustainable over time.

Case 2: A Novel Approach

An integrated healthcare delivery system implemented a disease management effort that emphasized both short- and long-term goals. The system included two acute care hospitals, a large academic physician group practice, and a health maintenance organization (HMO). The leadership of the disease management effort established goals to drive the process; these goals included improving the quality of patient care (appealing to the providers in the group practice), decreasing the variation in care (appealing to health system leadership, who realized that decreased variation means increased cost efficiency), and decreasing long- and short-term utilization by health plan members (appealing to the HMO by decreasing medical loss ratios). These goals formed a viable financial model, and each stakeholder gained ownership in the success of the endeavor.

Physicians actively engaged in the group practice led the disease management program, although the program was centered in the HMO. These leaders were respected clinicians and continued to practice at the grassroots level, helping to sell the program to peers and creating instant credibility for the program.

The model began with the target population and sought strategies to affect this group. High-prevalence, high-impact areas were chosen, including tobacco cessation, asthma, diabetes, congestive heart failure, hypertension, and osteoporosis. Each area was rolled out individually. Strategies for this mix of conditions offered both short-term (decreased hospitalizations for asthma and congestive heart failure) and long-term (decreased lung disease from smoking, decreased complications from diabetes) gains. The implementation team included physicians, case management nurses, information systems, triage systems, physician office staff (e.g., nurses, medical records personnel, scheduling coordinators), and patients themselves.

The implementation plan included the following strategies:

- Place health plan–employed care coordination nurses in local physician offices to coordinate care and assist primary care physicians and their staff.
- Establish evidence-based guidelines by employing nationally recognized basic guidelines and engaging opinion leaders from the academic group practice to review and disseminate the data.
- Enroll all members of a population in the program and allow them to opt out if they choose.
- Stratify patients according to risk and target the highest-risk members of the population first, thereby achieving early successes.
- Use regional case managers to help oversee management of difficult or high-acuity cases.
- Use timely electronic decision support to allow providers a greater opportunity to follow guidelines. (Providers were given up-front input on the content, and each new intervention was pilot tested on a small group.)
- Promote member self-management, allowing the patient—the true consumer of the service—to become a stakeholder.
- Provide frequent member and provider education in multiple media and forums, including regional group sessions, face-to-face contact, and print and electronic active and passive communication.
- Maintain an active data acquisition and processing department to measure progress, fine-tune procedures, and recognize successes.

The health plan had approximately 250,000 members in more than 1,200 primary care providers' offices. These physicians included those employed by the health system and those contracted by the health plan. The disease management program employed more than 70 full-time-equivalent professionals, with more than two-thirds in direct patient care at the point of service. The health plan received "excellent" accreditation status from the National Committee for Quality Assurance (NCQA), and NCQA and the American Diabetes Association recognized the disease management program for excellence and innovation. The program realized tangible positive results, including increased quality of care, decreased variation in practice, decreased cost to the system, and decreased utilization for the health plan.

Why did this disease management system succeed? First, it used a step-wise approach (think big, but start small), and pilot projects were launched before large-scale rollouts. Attainable goals were set using high-impact diseases, outcomes were measured, and successes were celebrated. Second, all constituencies were stakeholders in the change process. The program took a global, multifaceted approach to implementation, involving as many different resources and tools as possible. It enlisted thought leaders from each affected area and used innovative approaches to implement, maintain, publicize, and remediate processes. Most important, the downstream cost savings produced by the program accrued directly to the health system that financed the programs, allowing for sustainability over the long term (i.e., the party bearing the cost of the program directly benefited).

Case 3: System Implementation of Clinical Office Redesign

An integrated health system in the mid-Atlantic region, heeding complaints from referring physicians and patients regarding access issues, joined a collaborative initiated by the Institute for Healthcare Improvement called the Idealized Design of Clinical Office Practices. This initiative centered on multiple facets of office practice, including access (the ability to get into the system), interaction (the experience of the patient in the system), reliability (the practice of state-of-the-art medicine), and vitality (financial sustainability). This healthcare system chose to focus its early efforts on redefining access as a means of gaining market share, increasing patient satisfaction, and enhancing clinical and financial performance. The system began with implementation in two practice sites and employed rapid-spread methods for implementing successful processes across multiple sites. Lessons learned from these early sites were then used to spread the process to the entire system and medical center specialty departments.

The deployment model included a team of dedicated, trained staff to support the rollout. The staff were trained in change management and quality improvement and taught local leadership how to lead the practice through these changes. Local teams took ownership of the process and tailored it to fit their needs. The support team worked with the sites for eight to ten weeks to assist with team formation, facilitate team leadership, introduce data collection tools, and encourage change. The team also provided periodic follow-up support and review. Positive early prototype results incited interest throughout the system practices. Rolling, scheduled spread then occurred across community practice sites, followed by sites at the medical center. These sites were able to markedly improve access, demonstrate improved patient satisfaction, and increase market share.

This model included the following key components of a successful rollout:

- Visible support from leadership
- Demonstration of short-term successes with early results from the prototype sites
- Use of multidisciplinary, local teams
- Structural support for the teams
- Active communication of the process through multiple forums
- Development of a structured timeline for the rollout
- Accountability at the local leadership level
- Celebration of successes both locally and nationally

The success of this initiative has been a model for other quality improvement initiatives in the organization.

Conclusion

This chapter reviewed practical methods of leading healthcare organizations through change. US healthcare needs substantial improvement in care delivery; for healthcare leaders, mastery of skills that will contribute to effective quality improvement is critical. Further research on the use of informatics, pay for performance, and other strategies is needed to expand our knowledge and discover additional methods of inducing change in the healthcare system.

Study Questions

1. You are the medical director for a practice network. You would like to improve diabetes care for the patients in your network. You have an EHR system that allows you to identify patients with this condition and receive reports of the patients' performance on specific quality indicators. Outline your plan to improve diabetes care for your population.
2. Your hospital has learned that patients with a diagnosis of congestive heart failure are readmitted 28 percent of the time. You have received notification that CMS is no longer going to reimburse hospitals for readmissions within 30 days. Outline a strategy to tackle this quality problem.

3. You are the lead cardiac surgeon in a large group. The hospital's chief medical officer informs you that the outcome data for coronary artery bypass surgery are going to be made public on a state website. You obtain the data for wound infection rates and discover that your group's rate is double the state average. What steps would you take to correct this problem?

References

Armstrong, D., J. Reyburn, and R. Jones. 1996. "A Study of General Practitioners' Reasons for Changing Their Prescribing Behavior." *British Medical Journal* 312 (7036): 949–52.

Berwick, D. M., D. R. Calkins, C. J. McCannon, and A. D. Hackbarth. 2006. "The 100,000 Lives Campaign: Setting a Goal and a Deadline for Improving Health Care Quality." *Journal of the American Medical Association* 295 (3): 324–27.

Bolton, M. B., B. C. Tilley, J. Kuder, T. Reeves, and L. R. Schultz. 1991. "The Cost and Effectiveness of an Education Program for Adults Who Have Asthma." *Journal of General Internal Medicine* 6 (5): 401–7.

Campbell, S., D. Reeves, E. Kontopantelis, B. Sibbald, and M. Roland. 2009. "Effects of Pay for Performance on the Quality of Primary Care in England." *New England Journal of Medicine* 361 (4): 368–78.

Care Continuum Alliance. 2012. *Implementation and Evaluation: A Population Health Guide for Primary Care Models.* Published October. www.carecontinuum alliance.org/pdf/I-E-Document.pdf.

Cassidy, A. 2010. "Patient-Centered Medical Homes." *Health Affairs*/Robert Wood Johnson Foundation health policy brief. Issued September 14. www.rwjf.org/content/dam/farm/reports/issue_briefs/2010/rwjf66043.

Cebul, R. D., T. E. Love, A. K. Jain, and C. J. Herbert. 2011. "Electronic Health Records and Quality of Diabetes Care." *New England Journal of Medicine* 365 (9): 825–33.

Cheater, F., R. Baker, C. Gillies, H. Hearnshaw, S. Flottorp, N. Roberston, E. J. Shaw, and A. D. Oxman. 2005. "Tailored Interventions to Overcome Identified Barriers to Change: Effects on Professional Practice and Health Care Outcomes." *Cochrane Database of Systematic Reviews* 3: CD005470. DOI: 10.1002/14651858.CD005470.

Chhina, H., V. M. Bhole, C. Goldsmith, W. Hall, J. Kaczorowski, and D. Lacaille. 2013. "Effectiveness of Academic Detailing to Optimize Medical Prescribing Behavior of Family Physicians." *Journal of Pharmacy & Pharmaceutical Sciences* 16 (4): 511–29.

Conrad, D. A., B. G. Saver, B. Court, and S. Heath. 2006. "Paying Physicians for Quality: Evidence and Themes from the Field." *Joint Commission Journal of Quality and Patient Safety* 32 (8): 443–51.

Cromwell, J., M. G. Trisolini, G. C. Pope, J. B. Mitchell, and L. M. Greenwald (eds.). 2011. *Pay for Performance in Health Care: Methods and Approaches.* RTI Press Publication No. BK-002-1103. Published March. www.rti.org/rtipress.

Davis, D., and R. Galbraith. 2009. "Continuing Medical Education Effect on Practice Performance: Effectiveness of Continuing Medical Education: American College of Chest Physicians Evidence-Based Educational Guidelines." *Chest* 135 (3 Suppl.): 42S–48S.

DesRoches, C. M., E. G. Campbell, C. Vogeli, J. Zheng, S. R. Rao, A. E. Shields, K. Donelan, S. Rosenbaum, S. J. Bristol, and A. K. Jha. 2010. "Electronic Health Records' Limited Successes Suggest More Targeted Uses." *Health Affairs* 29 (4): 639–46.

de Vries, E. N., H. A. Prins, R. M. Crolla, A. J. den Outer, G. van Andel, S. H. van Helden, W. S. Schlack, M. A. van Putten, D. J. Gouma, M. G. Dijkgraaf, S. M. Smorenburg, M. A. Boermeester, and SURPASS Collaborative Group. 2010. "Effect of a Comprehensive Surgical Safety System on Patient Outcomes." *New England Journal of Medicine* 363 (20): 1928–37.

Dexter, P. R., S. Perkins, J. M. Overhage, K. Maharry, R. B. Kohler, and C. J. McDonald. 2001. "A Computerized Reminder System to Increase the Use of Preventive Care for Hospitalized Patients." *New England Journal of Medicine* 345 (13): 965–70.

Döpp, C. M., M. J. Graff, S. Teerenstra, M. W. Nijhuis-van der Sanden, M. G. Olde Rikkert, and M. J. Vernouij-Dassen. 2013. "Effectiveness of a Multifaceted Implementation Strategy on Physicians' Referral Behavior to an Evidence-Based Psychosocial Intervention in Dementia: A Cluster Randomized Controlled Trial." *BMC Family Practice* 14 (1): 70.

Durieux, P., R. Nizard, P. Ravaud, N. Mounier, and E. Lepage. 2000. "A Clinical Decision Support System for Prevention of Venous Thromboembolism: Effect on Physician Behavior." *Journal of the American Medical Association* 283 (21): 2816–21.

Durso, S. C. 2006. "Using Clinical Guidelines Designed for Older Adults with Diabetes Mellitus and Complex Health Status." *Journal of the American Medical Association* 295 (16): 1935–40.

Fisher, E., D. Goodman, J. Skinner, and K. Bronner. 2009. "Healthcare Spending, Quality, and Outcomes: More Isn't Always Better." Dartmouth Atlas Project topic brief. Issued February 27. www.dartmouthatlas.org/downloads/reports/Spending_Brief_022709.pdf.

Flodgren, G., E. Parmelli, G. Doumit, M. Gattellari, M. A. O'Brien, J. Grimshaw, and M. D. Eccles. 2011. "Local Opinion Leaders: Effects on Professional Practice and Health Care Outcomes." *Cochrane Database of Systematic Reviews* 8: CD000125. DOI: 10.1002/14651858.CD000125.pub4.

Foy, R., M. P. Eccles, G. Jamtvedt, J. Young, J. M. Grimshaw, and R. Baker. 2005. "What Do We Know About How to Do Audit and Feedback? Pitfalls in Applying Evidence from a Systematic Review." *BMC Health Services Research* 5 (July 13): 50.

Francke, A. L., M. C. Smit, A. J. E. de Veer, and P. Mistiaen. 2008. "Factors Influencing the Implementation of Clinical Guidelines for Health Care Professionals: A Systematic Meta-review." *BMC Medical Informatics and Decision Making* 8 (1): 38. DOI: 10.1186/1472-6947-8-38.

Garg, A. X., N. K. Adhikari, H. McDonald, M. P. Rosas-Arellano, P. J. Devereaux, J. Beyene, J. Sam, and R. B. Haynes. 2005. "Effects of Computerized Clinical Decision Support Systems on Practitioner Performance and Patient Outcomes: A Systematic Review." *Journal of the American Medical Association* 293 (10): 1223–38.

Glanz, K., B. K. Rimer, and K. Viswanath (eds.). 2008. *Health Behavior and Health Education: Theory, Research, and Practice*, fourth edition. San Francisco: Jossey-Bass.

Goetzel, R. Z., R. J. Ozminkowski, V. G. Villagra, and J. Duffy. 2005. "Return on Investment in Disease Management: A Review." *Health Care Financing Review* 26 (4): 1–19.

Gould, D. J., J. Chudleigh, N. S. Drey, and D. Moralejo. 2007. "Measuring Handwashing Performance in Health Service Audits and Research Studies." *Journal of Hospital Infection* 66 (2): 109–15.

Grimshaw, J., M. Eccles, R. Thomas, G. MacLennan, C. Ramsay, C. Fraser, and L. Vale. 2006. "Toward Evidence-Based Quality Improvement: Evidence (and Its Limitations) of the Effectiveness of Guideline Dissemination and Implementation Strategies 1966–1998." *Journal of General Internal Medicine* 21 (Suppl. 2): S14–S20.

Grimshaw, J. M., M. P. Eccles, A. E. Walker, and R. E. Thomas. 2002. "Changing Physicians' Behavior: What Works and Thoughts on Getting More Things to Work." *Journal of Continuing Education in the Health Professions* 22 (4): 237–43.

Grimshaw, J. M., L. Shirran, R. Thomas, G. Mowatt, C. Fraser, L. Bero, R. Grilli, E. Harvey, A. Oxman, and M. A. O'Brien. 2001. "Changing Provider Behavior: An Overview of Systematic Reviews of Interventions." *Medical Care* 39 (8, Suppl. 2): II-2–II-45.

Grol, R., and J. Grimshaw. 2003. "From Best Evidence to Best Practice: Effective Implementation of Change in Patients' Care." *Lancet* 362 (9391): 1225–30.

Halasyamani, L., S. Kripalani, E. Coleman, J. Schnipper, C. van Walraven, J. Nagamine, P. Torcson, T. Bookwalter, T. Budnitz, and D. Manning. 2006. "Transition of Care for Hospitalized Elderly Patients: Development of a Discharge Checklist for Hospitalists." *Journal of Hospital Medicine* 1 (6): 354–60.

Hales, B., M. Terblanche, R. Fowler, and W. Sibbald. 2008. "Development of Medical Checklists for Improved Quality of Patient Care." *International Journal for Quality in Health Care* 20 (1): 22–30.

Haynes, A. B., T. G. Weiser, W. R. Berry, S. R. Lipsitz, A. H. Breizat, E. P. Dellinger, T. Herbosa, S. Joseph, P. L. Kibatala, M. C. Lapitan, A. F. Merry, K. Moorthy, R. K. Reznick, B. Taylor, A. A. Gawande, and Safe Surgery Saves Lives Study Group. 2009. "A Surgical Safety Checklist to Reduce Morbidity and Mortality in a Global Population." *New England Journal of Medicine* 360 (5): 491–99.

Honigfeld L., L. Chandhok, and M. Morales. 2011. "Using Academic Detailing to Change Child Health Service Delivery in Connecticut." Farmington, CT: Child Health and Development Institute of CT. www.chdi.org/ourwork-signature-epic.php.

Institute of Medicine. 2011. *Clinical Practice Guidelines We Can Trust*. Report brief. Released March 23. www.iom.edu/Reports/2011/Clinical-Practice-Guidelines-We-Can-Trust/Report-Brief.aspx.

———. 2001. *Crossing the Quality Chasm*. Washington, DC: National Academies Press.

Ivers, N., G. Jamtvedt, S. Flottorp, J. M. Young, J. Odgaard-Jensen, S. D. French, M. A. O'Brien, M. Johansen, J. Grimshaw, and A. D. Oxman. 2012. "Audit and Feedback: Effects on Professional Practice and Healthcare Outcomes." Cochrane Database of Systematic Reviews 6: CD000259. DOI: 10.1002/14651858.CD000259.pub3.

Jha, A. K., K. E. Joynt, E. J. Orav, and A. M. Epstein. 2012. "The Long-Term Effect of Premier Pay for Performance on Patient Outcomes." *New England Journal of Medicine* 366 (17): 1606–15.

Kotter, J. P. 2001. "What Leaders Really Do." *Harvard Business Review* 79 (11): 85–96.

———. 1996. *Leading Change*. Cambridge, MA: Harvard Business School Press.

Lester, W. T., R. W. Grant, G. O. Barnett, and H. C. Chueh. 2006. "Randomized Controlled Trial of an Informatics-Based Intervention to Increase Statin Prescription for Secondary Prevention of Coronary Disease." *Journal of General Internal Medicine* 21 (1): 22–29.

Lindenauer, P. K., D. Remus, S. Roman, M. B. Rothberg, E. M. Benjamin, A. Ma, and D. W. Bratzler. 2007. "Public Reporting and Pay for Performance in Hospital Quality Improvement." *New England Journal of Medicine* 356 (5): 486–96.

Liu, Z., A. Abdullah, G. Lewis, G. Kelter, C. Naugler, and L. Baskin. 2012. "An Intervention to Reduce Laboratory Utilization of Referred-Out Tests." *Laboratory Medicine* 43 (5): 164–67.

Margulis, A. V., N. K. Choudhry, C. R. Dormuth, and S. Schneeweiss. 2011. "Variation in Initiating Secondary Prevention After Myocardial Infarction by Hospitals and Physicians, 1997 Through 2004." *Pharmacoepidemiology and Drug Safety* 20 (10): 1088–97.

Mason, J., N. Freemantle, I. Nazareth, M. Eccles, A. Haines, and M. Drummond. 2001. "When Is It Cost-Effective to Change the Behavior of Health Professionals?" *Journal of the American Medical Association* 286 (23): 2988–92.

McClellan, M., A. N. McKethan, J. L. Lewis, J. Roski, and E. S. Fisher. 2010. "A National Strategy to Put Accountable Care into Practice." *Health Affairs* 29 (5): 982–90.

McPhee, S. J., J. A. Bird, D. Fordham, J. E. Rodnick, and E. H. Osborn. 1991. "Promoting Cancer Prevention Activities by Primary Care Physicians: Results of a Randomized, Controlled Trial." *Journal of the American Medical Association* 266 (4): 538–44.

Mottur-Pilson, C., V. Snow, and K. Bartlett. 2001. "Physician Explanations for Failing to Comply with 'Best Practices.'" *Effective Clinical Practice* 4 (5): 207–13.

Petersen, L. A., L. D. Woodard, T. Urech, D. Daw, and S. Sookanan. 2006. "Does Pay-for-Performance Improve the Quality of Health Care?" *Annals of Internal Medicine* 145 (4): 265–72.

Pittet, D. 2000. "Improving Compliance with Hand Hygiene in Hospitals." *Infection Control and Hospital Epidemiology* 21 (6): 381–86.

Pronovost, P. J., M. R. Miller, R. M. Wachter, and G. S. Meyer. 2009. "Perspective: Physician Leadership in Quality." *Academic Medicine* 84 (12): 1651–56.

Ramoska, E. 1998. "Information Sharing Can Reduce Laboratory Use by Emergency Physicians." *American Journal of Emergency Medicine* 16 (1): 34–36.

Reinertsen, J. L. 1998. "Physicians as Leaders in the Improvement of Health Care Systems." *Annals of Internal Medicine* 128 (10): 833–38.

Rich, M. W., V. Beckham, C. Wittenberg, C. L. Leven, K. E. Freedland, and R. M. Carney. 1995. "A Multidisciplinary Intervention to Prevent the Readmission of Elderly Patients with Congestive Heart Failure." *New England Journal of Medicine* 333 (18): 1190–95.

Rogers, E. M. 2003. *Diffusion of Innovations*, fifth edition. New York: Free Press.

———. 1995. "Lessons for Guidelines from the Diffusion of Innovations." *Joint Commission Journal on Quality Improvement* 21 (7): 324–28.

Romano, M. J., and R. S. Stafford. 2011. "Electronic Health Records and Clinical Decision Support Systems: Impact on National Ambulatory Care Quality." *Archives of Internal Medicine* 171 (10): 897–903.

Schectman, J. M., N. K. Kanwal, W. S. Schroth, and E. G. Elinsky. 1995. "The Effect of an Education and Feedback Intervention on Group-Model and Network-Model Health Maintenance Organization Physician Prescribing Behavior." *Medical Care* 33 (2): 139–44.

Shays, E. M. 2003. "Helping Clients to Control Their Future." *Consulting to Management* 14 (2): 1–7.

Shields, M. C., P. H. Patel, M. Manning, and L. Sacks. 2010. "A Model for Integrating Independent Physicians into Accountable Care Organizations." *Health Affairs* 30 (1): 161–72.

Sidorov, J., R. Shull, J. Tomcavage, S. Girolami, N. Lawton, and R. Harris. 2002. "Does Diabetes Disease Management Save Money and Improve Outcomes? A Report of Simultaneous Short-Term Savings and Quality Improvement

Associated with a Health Maintenance Organization–Sponsored Disease Management Program Among Patients Fulfilling Health Employer Data and Information Set Criteria." *Diabetes Care* 25 (4): 684–89.

Simpson, S. H., T. J. Marrie, and S. R. Majumdar. 2005. "Do Guidelines Guide Pneumonia Practice? A Systematic Review of Interventions and Barriers to Best Practice in the Management of Community Acquired Pneumonia." *Respiratory Care Clinics of North America* 11 (1): 1–13.

Solomon, D. H., H. Hashimoto, L. Daltroy, and M. H. Liang. 1998. "Techniques to Improve Physicians' Use of Diagnostic Tests: A New Conceptual Framework." *Journal of the American Medical Association* 280 (23): 2020–27.

Van Herck, P., D. De Smedt, L. Annemans, R. Remmen, M. B. Rosenthal, and W. Sermeus. 2010. "Systematic Review: Effects, Design Choices, and Context of Pay-for-Performance in Health Care." *BMC Health Services Research* 10: 247.

Vickrey, B. G., B. S. Mittman, K. I. Connor, M. L. Pearson, R. D. Della Penna, T. G. Ganiats, R. W. Demonte Jr, J. Chodosh, X. Cui, S. Vassar, N. Duan, and M. Lee. 2006. "The Effect of a Disease Management Intervention on Quality and Outcomes of Dementia Care: A Randomized, Controlled Trial." *Annals of Internal Medicine* 145 (10): 713–26.

Weber, V., F. Bloom, S. Pierdon, and C. Wood. 2008. "Employing the Electronic Health Record to Improve Diabetes Care: A Multifaceted Intervention in an Integrated Delivery System." *Journal of General Internal Medicine* 23 (4): 379–82.

Weber, V., A. White, and R. McIlvried. 2008. "An Electronic Medical Record (EMR)–Based Intervention to Reduce Polypharmacy and Falls in an Ambulatory Rural Elderly Population." *Journal of General Internal Medicine* 23 (4): 399–404.

Werner, R. M., J. T. Kolstad, E. A. Stuart, and D. Polsky. 2011. "The Effect of Pay-for-Performance in Hospitals: Lessons for Quality Improvement." *Health Affairs* 30 (4): 690–98.

Zhou, L., C. S. Soran, C. A. Jenter, L. A. Volk, E. J. Orav, D. W. Bates, and S. R. Simon. 2009. "The Relationship Between Electronic Health Record Use and Quality of Care Over Time." *Journal of the American Medical Informatics Association* 16 (4): 457–64.

HEALTHCARE QUALITY IN THE ENVIRONMENT AND EMERGING TRENDS

THE QUALITY IMPROVEMENT LANDSCAPE

Kimberly D. Acquaviva and Jean E. Johnson

The healthcare quality improvement landscape in the United States is dynamic—continuously evolving as both established and new organizations cultivate the seeds of change. Understanding the roles of these organizations is foundational to understanding these quality improvement initiatives and, perhaps more important, to anticipating the future direction of quality improvement in the United States. Public and private entities play significant roles in a complex network of quality improvement efforts, many of which overlap. The means by which these organizations influence quality is varied, with some influencing quality through the accreditation process, others by developing measures of quality, and still others by advocating for the integration of quality improvement into the US healthcare system.

Organizations approach quality improvement from differing perspectives depending on their mission as well as the needs and desires of key stakeholders. Purchasers and insurers strive to link quality and cost containment in an effort to create more value for each dollar spent on healthcare. Healthcare providers work to improve patient care and mitigate risk through internal quality improvement and the use of quality measures. Patients—the ultimate stakeholder of all these organizations—expect (and are beginning to demand) to know more about the quality of care delivered by their providers. Policymakers require data to drive evidence-based policy decisions related to healthcare. This chapter examines the organizations that play a major role in shaping the quality improvement landscape, details important trends in quality improvement, and provides an overview of quality initiatives in specific healthcare settings.

Quality Improvement Organizations

The quality improvement landscape is complex, with multiple organizations playing overlapping and, at times, divergent roles. The interactions between these organizations may be collegial or contentious depending on the issue under discussion, but almost without exception, the interactions are dynamic. Exhibit 18.1 illustrates the roles of these organizations and demonstrates

EXHIBIT 18.1
Roles of
Organizations
in the Quality
Improvement
Process

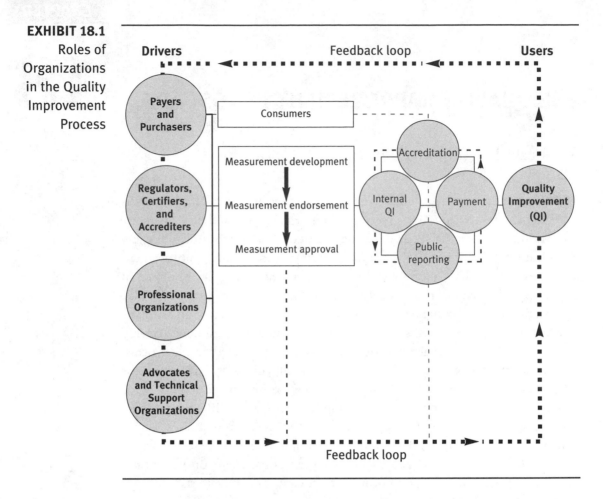

that consumers are involved in the quality improvement feedback loop and will likely be more involved in the future. The illustration includes organizations that create quality-related incentives through payment; those that are involved in the measurement process, including development, review, endorsement, and approval of quality measures; and those that use the measures. While many organizations are involved in quality improvement, Exhibit 18.2 describes the roles of the major organizations that have quality at the center of their mission.

Drivers of Quality

Several forces dictate the national quality agenda. These drivers (payers; purchasers; regulators, certifiers, and accreditors; professional organizations; and advocacy and technical support organizations) directly or indirectly shape and advance the national quality agenda.

EXHIBIT 18.2
Organizations with a Major Role in Quality by Type

Type	Name of Organization	Mission	Website
Business groups	National Business Group on Health	• National voice of *Fortune* 500 employers concerned about cost and quality to find solutions to important health issues	www.businessgrouphealth.org
	National Business Coalition on Health	• Organization of employer-based healthcare coalitions to improve quality through value-based purchasing	www.nbch.org
	Pacific Business Group on Health (50 businesses)	• Regional coalition to improve the quality and availability of healthcare, moderate costs through value-based purchasing, use quality measurement and improvement, and engage consumers	www.pbgh.org
	Leapfrog Group	• Mobilizes employer purchasing power to improve care through access to health information, and rewards good care	www.leapfroggroup.org
Federal agencies	Centers for Medicare & Medicaid Services	• Major governmental agency that purchases and pays for care, regulates care through certification and licensure processes for providers receiving Medicare and Medicaid funds, provides consumer information, and conducts demonstration projects	www.cms.gov
	Center for Medicare & Medicaid Innovation (CMS Innovation Center)	• Aims to transform Medicare, Medicaid, and the Children's Health Insurance Program through improvements in the healthcare system	innovation.cms.gov
	Agency for Healthcare Research and Quality	• Improves the quality, safety, efficiency, and effectiveness of healthcare through research and by providing guidelines and other tools to educate and support providers and consumers	www.ahrq.gov
	Institute of Medicine	• Independent, nonprofit organization that works outside of government to provide unbiased and authoritative advice to decision makers and the public	www.iom.edu
	US Preventive Services Task Force	• Makes evidence-based recommendations on clinical preventive services	www.uspreventiveservicestaskforce.org
Accrediting organizations	The Joint Commission	• Supports performance improvement in healthcare organizations	www.jointcommission.org
	National Committee for Quality Assurance	• Accredits health plans and other organizations, develops quality measures, and educates policymakers about quality issues	www.ncqa.org

(Continued)

EXHIBIT 18.2
Organizations with a Major Role in Quality by Type *(continued)*

Type	Name of Organization	Mission	Website
Alliances	AQA Alliance (formerly known as the Ambulatory Care Quality Alliance)	• Reviews and approves measures for use in ambulatory care; supports public reporting of measures	www.aqaalliance.org
	Measures Application Partnership	• Reviews and aligns performance measures in support of public- and private-sector programs as well as federal reporting and rule-making efforts	www.qualityforum.org/map/
	Nursing Alliance for Quality Care	• Advances the highest quality, safety, and value of consumer-centered healthcare for all individuals—patients, their families, and their communities	www.naqc.org
	Physician Consortium for Performance Improvement	• American Medical Association–sponsored group that reviews and approves use of measures	www.ama-assn.org/go/PCPI
	Association of American Medical Colleges	• Supports "the entire spectrum of education, research, and patient care activities conducted by . . . member institutions" (medical schools, health systems, teaching hospitals, and academic and scientific societies)	www.aamc.org
Public–private partnerships	National Quality Forum	• Sets national priorities and goals for performance improvement, endorses national consensus standards for measuring and publicly reporting on performance, and promotes the attainment of national goals through education and outreach programs	www.qualityforum.org
Professional organizations	Institute for Healthcare Improvement	• Aims to reduce needless deaths, pain, and waiting; accelerates the measurable and continual progress of healthcare systems throughout the world using the six aims of the IOM	www.ihi.org
	Institute for Patient- and Family-Centered Care	• Advances the understanding of patient- and family-centered care in healthcare settings	www.ipfcc.org
Foundations	National Patient Safety Foundation	• Awards small grants, serves as a resource for knowledge and public awareness, and enhances culture of patient safety	www.npsf.org
	Robert Wood Johnson Foundation	• Supports regional initiatives in quality; supports measure development and communication strategies targeted to communities	www.rwjf.org
	California HealthCare Foundation	• Aims to improve the care of chronically ill individuals and create incentives to improve care	www.chcf.org
	Commonwealth Fund	• Supports independent research on healthcare issues and awards grants to improve health-care practice and policy	www.commonwealthfund.org

Payers

The entities that have the greatest influence on improving quality are those that pay for care. One of the largest and most powerful of these entities is the Centers for Medicare & Medicaid Services (CMS). With healthcare costs reaching an estimated $2.8 trillion in 2012 and the federal government's share of costs projected to increase almost 14 percent in 2014, CMS is deeply vested in making sure that Medicare and Medicaid enrollees get the best care for each dollar spent (Cuckler et al. 2013).

CMS has driven the accreditation process for all settings and has emerged as a major driver linking financial incentives to improving quality. Because of its role as the largest single healthcare payer in the United States, CMS has the power to catalyze quality improvement through financial incentives, such as the voluntary reporting programs that provide incentives in the form of additional Medicare payment.

As a result of the passage of the Affordable Care Act (ACA), the Center for Medicare & Medicaid Innovation (referred to hereafter as the Innovation Center) was established "to move quickly to identify, test, and spread delivery and payment models to help providers improve care while cutting costs" (CMS 2012b). Because the Innovation Center was established by Congress, its mandate includes both robust financial support and an unprecedented degree of flexibility in testing and evaluating care delivery and payment/reimbursement models (CMS 2013a). In its first year of operation, the Innovation Center launched 16 initiatives (Exhibit 18.3).

Purchasers

Businesses (purchasers) and health plans have been able to affect quality through financial incentives similar to those of CMS. As healthcare costs continue to rise, purchasers and health plans are looking to quality improvement to help control costs and maximize return on investment. Coalitions of large businesses that provide health insurance benefits to employees have also provided leverage to improve quality through the development of measures and system changes. Many states, regions, and even cities have business groups on health. The National Business Coalition on Health (2014), an organization of 52 employer-based healthcare coalitions (representing 7,000 employers and more than 25 million employees), works to enhance value-based purchasing of healthcare services. A similarly named but separate organization, the National Business Group on Health (2013), established the Institute on Health Care Costs and Solutions (and the leadership committees that it comprises) in 2001 to address evidence-based health benefits, consumer engagement, and payment and delivery reform. Business coalitions at the regional level play a significant role in influencing policy to improve health and control costs as well. The Pacific Business Group on Health (2013) represents 60

EXHIBIT 18.3
Center for Medicare & Medicaid Innovation Initiatives

Initiative	Description	Start Date	Length	Total Funding
Primary Care Transformation				
Comprehensive Primary Care Initiative Demonstration	Public–private partnership to enhance primary care services, including 24-hour access, care plans, and care coordination	2012	Four years	$322 million
Federally Qualified Health Center (FQHC) Advanced Primary Care Practice Demonstration	Care coordination payments to FQHCs in support of team-led care, improved access, and enhanced primary care services	November 1, 2011	Three years ending on October 31, 2014	$49.7 million
Multi-payer Advanced Primary Care Practice Demonstration	State-led, multipayer collaborations to help primary care practices transform into medical homes	Phased in starting July 1, 2011	Three years	$283 million
Independence at Home	Home-based care for patients with multiple chronic conditions	Summer 2012	Three years	$15 million
Bundled Payments for Care Improvement				
Bundled Payment for Care Improvement Initiative	Episodic payments around inpatient hospitalizations to incentivize care redesign	2012	Three years	$118 million
Accountable Care Organizations				
Pioneer Accountable Care Organization (ACO) Model	Experienced provider organizations taking on financial risk for improving quality and lowering costs for all of their Medicare patients	January 2012	Three years (with optional two-year extension)	$77 million
Accelerated Development Learning Sessions	Public opportunities to learn from leading experts about successful ACO development	June 2011	Three sessions completed	$1.5 million
Advanced Payment Accountable Care Organization Model	Prepayment of expected shared savings to support ACO infrastructure and care coordination	April 1, 2012, or July 1, 2012	Payments end June 2014	$175 million
Physician Group Practice Transition Demonstration	A precursor to the Medicare Shared Savings Program; rewards physician groups for efficient care and high quality	January 1, 2011	Up to three years	$500,000 in administrative costs

(Continued)

EXHIBIT 18.3

Center for Medicare & Medicaid Innovation Initiatives *(continued)*

Initiative	Description	Start Date	Length	Total Funding
Medicare/Medicaid Enrollees				
State Demonstrations to Integrate Care for Medicare-Medicaid Enrollees	Assistance to help states engage stakeholders in redesigning care for Medicare/Medicaid enrollees	April/May 2011	18 months (with extension option)	$15 million
Financial Alignment Model Demonstrations	Opportunity for states to implement new care and payment systems to better coordinate care for Medicare/Medicaid enrollees	January 2013	Three years	To be determined
Capacity to Spread Innovation				
Partnership for Patients	National campaign targeting a 40% reduction in hospital-acquired conditions and a 20% reduction in 30-day readmissions	April 12, 2011	Ongoing	$500 million
Innovation Advisors Program	Training healthcare providers from around the country in achieving the Institute for Healthcare Improvement's Triple Aim	January 2012	Ongoing	$5.9 million
Health Care Innovation Challenge	A broad appeal for innovations with a focus on developing the workforce for new care models	March 30, 2012	Three years	$1 billion
Other				
Medicaid Emergency Psychiatric Demonstration	Expanding access to inpatient psychiatric services for Medicaid beneficiaries	Spring 2012	Three years	$75 million
Medicaid Incentives for Prevention of Chronic Diseases Program	Collaborating with states to test the effectiveness of preventive services in Medicaid	Sites awarded September 13, 2011	Five years	$100 million

Source: CMS (2012b).

purchasers that spend a combined $12 billion a year for healthcare coverage for more than 3 million individuals in California.

The Leapfrog Group is another organization representing the business sector's concern about quality and the cost of hospital care. Chartered in 2000, the Leapfrog Group gained considerable attention when it identified four practices that would create a "leap" in quality and patient safety. These practices are "computer physician order entry; evidence-based hospital referral; intensive care unit (ICU) staffing by physicians experienced in critical care medicine; and the Leapfrog Safe Practices Score" (Leapfrog Group 2014). As hospitals improve their quality, the Leapfrog Group members provide financial rewards.

Regulators, Certifiers, and Accreditors

CMS is the executive branch agency that has regulatory control over much of the healthcare system—particularly hospitals, nursing homes, home care, hospice care, and some aspects of outpatient care. Regulations are a powerful tool to influence quality and serve to operationalize legislation. CMS influences quality through the development of standards, survey instruments, and interpretive guidelines (guidance on interpreting regulations). An example of the regulatory influence of CMS is its nursing home survey requirements, which are federally mandated and are conducted by state survey agencies. In addition, through "deemed status" CMS has recognized The Joint Commission as the accreditor of hospitals, with CMS maintaining its regulatory force through the requirements for payment. Accrediting bodies that certify providers as being safe and competent have a significant impact on quality. Several certifying boards are now integrating questions about quality improvement into their exams to highlight the importance of being knowledgeable and engaged in quality improvement.

Professional Organizations

Organizations representing the entire spectrum of health professionals are embracing quality improvement through the development of educational initiatives, tools for providers to use in practice, and certification programs to recognize competence in specific areas. For instance, professional organizations have used seminars, workshops, webinars, and other means to make their members more aware of the need to improve quality. The American Nurses Association (ANA) developed the National Database of Nursing Quality Indicators, in which more than 2,000 hospitals report nursing-sensitive measures (ANA 2014), and the American Medical Association (AMA) developed measures for ambulatory care through its sponsorship of the Physician Consortium for Performance Improvement (AMA 2014). Professional organizations have also been key partners in consortia that include an array of stakeholders involved in reviewing, endorsing, and approving the use of measures for different settings. Boards of medicine, nursing, and allied health professionals play a major role through certification and licensure programs and by establishing standards for entry into practice as well as continued competence.

Advocacy and Technical Support Organizations

Organizations that provide advocacy and technical support related to healthcare quality play an important role in the quality improvement landscape. In fulfillment of its mission to improve the safety of patients, the National Patient Safety Foundation (2013) identifies and creates a core body of knowledge, identifies pathways to apply the knowledge, develops and enhances the culture of receptivity to patient safety, and raises public awareness and fosters communications about patient safety. The Institute for Healthcare Improvement (IHI) has worked to engage healthcare providers, as well as stakeholders and the general public, to improve the quality of care and reduce the number of needless deaths and medical errors. IHI has promoted the Plan-Do-Study-Act (PDSA) method of quality improvement and has created collaboratives to bring providers together to work on projects related to a specific area. (The IHI campaigns are discussed in a case study later in this chapter.)

Quality improvement organizations (QIOs) evolved from the Medicare Utilization and Quality Control Peer Review Program created by statute in 1982. The primary function of QIOs is to improve the quality of care and efficiency of the health system for Medicare beneficiaries. CMS oversees the work of the QIOs and reports annually to Congress on the QIOs' impact. CMS has contracts with QIOs covering all 50 states, the District of Columbia, Puerto Rico, and the US Virgin Islands.

Another group of supporting organizations is philanthropic foundations that focus on quality and provide a catalyst for innovative quality initiatives. For instance, the Robert Wood Johnson Foundation has a team focused on developing and funding programs to improve quality. The foundation has supported initiatives to improve quality, such as Transforming Care at the Bedside, an initiative to reengineer nursing care in medical-surgical units in hospitals. It also funded Rewarding Results, which supported programs providing incentives to improve care, and has invested in regional projects to improve care through Aligning Forces for Quality. The California Health-Care Foundation has funded projects to improve care, such as pay-for-performance initiatives, and has explored ways to improve the quality of chronic illness care. The Commonwealth Fund (2014) sponsors programs that focus on healthcare delivery system reform, tracking health system performance, increasing healthcare access, and identifying practice innovations.

Quality Measure Development Process

Measure Development

The major developers of quality measures are the National Committee for Quality Assurance (NCQA), the Agency for Healthcare Research and Quality (AHRQ), the AMA, the ANA, and The Joint Commission. NCQA continues to add and delete measures from the Healthcare Effectiveness Data and Information Set (HEDIS) database, and it develops measures for other programs, such as the Diabetes Recognition Program (NCQA 2013a). In addition, NCQA (2014) has developed measures to recognize patient-centered medical homes (PCMHs). AHRQ (2013) has developed the Consumer Assessment of Healthcare Providers and Systems (CAHPS) survey for hospital, outpatient, nursing home, and home health settings. The AMA (2014) has developed measures as part of the Physician Consortium for Performance Improvement. The ANA (2014) developed the National Database of Nursing Quality Indicators (NDNQI), which comprises measures of hospital nursing care. In 1997, The Joint Commission (2013) developed the ORYX measures, which integrate patient outcome measures into the accreditation process. Other national organizations have developed measures specific to their specialty and stakeholder groups.

Measure Endorsement

The National Quality Forum (NQF) was born from a recommendation in 1998 by the President's Advisory Commission on Consumer Protection and Quality in the Health Care Industry (1998) established by President Clinton. NQF was chartered in 1999 and provides scientific review and endorsement of measures for public reporting purposes. CMS recognizes NQF as a voluntary national consensus standard–setting organization adhering to the guidelines established by the National Technology Transfer and Advancement Act of 1996 and Office of Management and Budget Circular A-119, which allows CMS to use these standards rather than create an entity with a similar function within CMS. NQF is a membership organization with a broad array of stakeholders who participate in the review and endorsement of measures. NQF works to create a coherent approach to measurement and reporting at the national level.

Measure Approval

A relatively new phenomenon is the emergence of consortia that bring stakeholders together to review performance measures to ensure that the measures are science-based, important measures of quality. The first consortium formed was the Hospital Quality Alliance (HQA). Founded in 2002 by the Association of American Medical Colleges (AAMC), the American

Hospital Association (AHA), and the Federation of American Hospitals (FAH), HQA worked closely with CMS to review and approve measures for hospital reporting. HQA (2011) encompassed a broad array of stakeholders, including consumers, purchasers, health plans, and providers. The consortium continues its efforts today under the name Optional Public Reporting. Another consortium is the AQA alliance, formerly known as the Ambulatory Care Quality Alliance. Initiated in 2004 by the American Academy of Family Physicians, the American College of Physicians, America's Health Insurance Plans, and the AHRQ to work collaboratively on performance measurement and reporting issues in ambulatory care, this consortium includes consumers, purchasers, physicians, health insurance plans, and representatives from more than 100 different organizations. AQA works closely with CMS to adopt appropriate measures for ambulatory care (AQA 2010).

Measure Use

Quality measures have four primary uses: (1) for internal quality monitoring and improvement, (2) for accreditation, (3) as a basis for incentive payments to improve care, and (4) for public reporting. The first use primarily enables health professionals to improve care, while the other three uses are primarily related to holding providers accountable.

The first use of quality measures—internal monitoring and improvement—helps providers and institutions track specific measures to improve care and is related to professional and personal commitments to care as well as institutional expectations. Although quality measures have long been used for internal monitoring and reporting, providers have not been able to compare themselves easily to others because the data elements and collection instruments have not been synchronized. Collecting and reporting the same data using the same specifications helps organizations and providers understand how they perform compared to other organizations and enables them to identify opportunities for focused quality improvement efforts. For example, if the rate of preventable falls is significantly higher in Facility X than in similar organizations, the data indicate that Facility X should be able to reduce the number of preventable falls. This example also demonstrates how providers can use quality improvement processes to decrease their exposure to risks as a result of preventable incidents.

The second of these uses—accreditation—is carried out by organizations such as The Joint Commission for hospitals and NCQA for health plans. The Joint Commission accredits nearly all of the hospitals in the United States and has an international accrediting arm, Joint Commission International. The Joint Commission (2013) developed the ORYX system, which consists of a core set of measures used in the hospital accreditation process. NCQA uses the HEDIS measures for accreditation of health plans. Accreditation began in the early 1990s with the initial set of HEDIS measures. HEDIS includes 75 measures representing eight "domains of care" (NCQA 2013b). More than 90 percent of US health plans use HEDIS (NCQA 2013c).

The third use of quality measures—as a basis for incentive payments to improve care—is used by payers to create incentives for the provision of high-quality care. The CMS pay-for-performance projects, as well as health plans' use of measures to reward the provision of high-quality care, depend on valid and reliable measures as a basis for payment decisions.

The fourth use of quality measures—public reporting—entails reporting of uniform data by provider type (e.g., hospitals), which allows consumers to compare institutions on the basis of the same data. Organizations such as CMS, The Joint Commission, the Leapfrog Group, and NCQA provide the public with information obtained from their quality measures. The Hospital Compare and Nursing Home Compare websites sponsored by CMS are examples of this use. The NCQA Health Plan Report Card is another example. Findings from The Joint Commission accreditation results are also available online.

Trends in Quality Improvement

Impact of Federal Legislation on Quality

Several pieces of legislation—including the American Recovery and Reinvestment Act, the Health Information Technology for Economic and Clinical Health (HITECH) Act's funding for the Office of the National Coordinator for Health Information Technology to push healthcare providers into the electronic age, and the far-reaching ACA—have greatly influenced quality improvement. These acts have made a significant contribution to improving several important aspects of quality, including value-based purchasing, electronic health records (EHRs), consumer information, and the establishment of a national healthcare quality strategy.

Value-Based Purchasing

The ACA, while having a significant focus on access to healthcare, is largely about value-based purchasing. With the cost of healthcare estimated to increase from $2.6 trillion in 2010 to $4.6 trillion in 2020 and to consume nearly 20 percent of the gross domestic product in 2020, value-based purchasing is viewed as critical to the health of the US economy (Keehan et al. 2011). Preventing the overuse, underuse, and inappropriate use of healthcare is seen as essential for both quality and cost. The federal government has a large stake in cost and quality. A seminal report issued by the US Department of Health & Human Services (HHS) Office of Inspector General (OIG

2010) found that 13.5 percent of Medicare enrollees experienced an adverse event while hospitalized, and an additional 13.5 percent experienced a harmful event during their hospitalization. The report concluded that 44 percent of adverse or harmful events could have been prevented and more than $320 million could have been saved.

Defining value as high-quality healthcare at the lowest cost assumes that the appropriate care is delivered in an efficient and effective manner. The ACA includes requirements for quality measurement coupled with cost controls to stimulate more efficient models of care. While pay for performance is being introduced in many countries, it is a complicated issue. Evidence suggests that pay for performance can have a positive effect on the quality of care in both hospital and outpatient settings. For instance, the CMS Premier Hospital Quality Incentive Demonstration (HQID) project experienced an 18.6 percent increase in its overall quality score over six years (Premier 2012a). In addition, reports have demonstrated improved care of patients with diabetes and those with hypertension (Bernacki et al. 2012; Cheng, Lee, and Chen 2012; Petersen et al. 2009; Petersen et al. 2011).

Even though reports have demonstrated positive effects of pay for performance, particularly in improving care, other reports provide a mixed picture of value-based purchasing (Chen, Lee, and Kuo 2012; Eijkenaar 2012; Petersen et al. 2011; VanLare, Moody-Williams, and Conway 2012). Concerns about pay for performance include several significant issues. One concern is that providers, hospitals, and other healthcare organizations that provide care for largely underserved minority populations and see very ill patients may score lower on reported measures (Jha, Orav, and Epstein 2011; Ryan 2013). Possible adverse effects also include concerns that physicians working in areas with a large minority population may receive reduced payments and that health plans may avoid patients who could cause them to have lower quality scores and poorer outcomes reported to the public (Casalino and Elster 2007). In response to this concern, CMS noted that hospitals and other providers serving minority populations would receive reimbursement based on improvements within the institution or practice rather than in comparison to others (VanLare, Moody-Williams, and Conway 2012). In addition, risk adjustment in reported measures would be needed to avoid penalizing physicians and institutions that care for sicker patients. If providers encounter a financial penalty for taking care of sicker patients, physicians will find it more difficult to accept these patients. While a strong move toward developing aggregated measures of care is in progress, it will take time for these measures to be fully vetted and useful in measuring the quality of care and determining reasonable payment for care of patients with multiple chronic diseases. A final concern is that practices and health organizations may focus their attention on the diseases that are measured, to the exclusion of other important aspects of healthcare.

The mixed results of the impact of value-based purchasing are related to the complex challenge of tailoring the payment to the specific type of care. One size does not fit all. Different payment levels may be effective for different settings and different populations within those settings. Also, sustaining long-term change may be difficult and potentially costly. Practices may become accustomed to getting incentive payments, and if benchmarks are raised and they no longer receive the incentive payment, the program may have a negative effect. While CMS began its focus on value-based purchasing by providing incentives for reporting quality measures, payment incentives in the future will be linked to actual care outcomes based on performance on select measures.

Value-based purchasing is also integrated in the move toward accountable care organizations (ACOs). CMS defines ACOs as "groups of doctors, hospitals, and other health care providers, who come together voluntarily to give coordinated high quality care to their Medicare patients" (CMS 2013b). The focus on ACOs is intended to improve the quality of care as well as to lower costs. The ACO model includes an embedded incentive payment in the form of revenue sharing as part of the savings that can be achieved. However, savings must be accompanied by hitting quality benchmarks. ACOs require providers to share in the financial risk of the plan, rather than place the financial risk on insurers as occurs in a traditional managed care model. CMS has two programs underway: the Shared Savings Program and the Pioneer ACO Model program. The Pioneer program is aimed at high-functioning health systems that can take on great financial risk in exchange for the potential of a greater financial reward. The initial set of Pioneer projects included 32 health systems (CMS 2012c).

While the ACA strongly promotes the ACO model, concerns about the success of ACOs include the challenges inherent in managed care models and the limited incentives available through the revenue-sharing program. Measures will need to be developed to assess the quality of ACOs in addition to the quality of individual participant organizations and individual providers (Devers and Berenson 2009).

In addition to the federal government's focus on value, private insurers are instituting programs that link quality and payment to create more efficient systems of care. An increasing number of private insurers are following CMS's policies on value-based purchasing and are implementing value-based purchasing for physician, hospital, long-term, hospice, and other types of care. No longer can providers expect payment for services from private insurers without accountability. In the time since the AHRQ developed and disseminated information for payers on implementing pay-for-performance and other valued-based approaches (Dudley and Rosenthal 2006), pay-for-performance programs such as Medicare's Premier Hospital Quality

Incentive Demonstration have yielded mixed results, with low-performing hospitals realizing slower gains in quality scores than higher-performing hospitals (Ryan, Blustein, and Casalino 2012).

Electronic Health Records

Health systems have been slow to fully adopt EHRs primarily because of cost and complexity. Other industries have far surpassed healthcare in the implementation of electronic systems for data collection, monitoring, and quality improvement. To support the implementation of EHRs, the federal government invested more than $19 billion through the HITECH Act of 2009 to help institutions and outpatient practices adopt EHRs. The reason for the support of EHRs is to improve the quality of care. Regionalized EHRs can provide up-to-date information about patient status regardless of where the patient is, enabling providers to make informed decisions about care, coordinate care across settings, and continually improve care. The HITECH grants funded Regional Extension Centers (RECs) intended to assist primary care providers and institutions providing services to traditionally underserved populations (HHS 2011). The results of these efforts have been impressive: As of November 2013, more than 334,000 healthcare providers were participating in and receiving payment from the Medicare and Medicaid EHR Incentive Programs (CMS 2014b). Institutions that receive federal support must commit to using the EHRs meaningfully—that is, using the EHRs to collect and report data and to use the data to improve care and control costs.

The government supports the use of information technology to create more efficient and effective systems of care. Providers are required to meet several performance standards referred to as *meaningful use criteria*. Meaningful use criteria will be implemented in three stages. The first stage includes the development of the initial measures that providers need to report and processes for implementation of incentive programs. As part of the first stage, 15 core measures and 10 menu measures are being collected, of which 5 measures are required to be reported. In the second stage (launched in 2014), providers must meet either 17 core objectives plus 3 menu objectives or 20 core objectives. When the final stage rolls out in 2016, additional requirements will be added that focus on patient safety, quality, and decision-support tools (ONC 2014).

Consumer Information

Increasingly, efforts are being made to give consumers useful information in making choices about their healthcare. As consumers pick up more healthcare costs by paying a greater share of the cost of health insurance, higher deductibles, and higher copayments, they have more reason to be value conscious. A landmark study supports the contention that consumer sensitivity to costs reduces use of healthcare services with few adverse effects (Brook et al. 1984). In addition, consumers are increasingly using information about quality of services through sources such as Angie's List, *Consumer Reports*, and Consumers' Checkbook. Blogs also serve as sources of information about products and services. Consumers provide ratings when purchasing items online. To make informed decisions, consumers must know about both cost and quality. The reason for informing consumers about quality as well as cost is to have consumers drive demand on the basis of value. While this economic concept is straightforward, providing information about healthcare that is valid and reliable and that consumers find useful in making an informed decision has been a challenge. Consumers rarely know the cost of care before a service is delivered, and only in the last decade has providing information about quality been attempted. The exception in the availability of cost information is in retail clinics, where the costs of visits and procedures are publicly posted.

To support efforts to make information about quality of care available to consumers, CMS has created websites that inform consumers about the quality of care in nursing homes, home care, hospitals, and dialysis facilities (HHS 2013b). The Hospital Compare and Nursing Home Compare sites are informative and widely visited. CMS continues to look for ways of organizing information to make it easy for consumers to interpret. For instance, to help consumers choose a high-quality nursing home, Nursing Home Compare provides a rating of quality using one to five stars, with five stars designating the highest quality (HHS 2013a). Hospital Compare includes general information (including CAHPS results) and information on medical conditions and surgical procedures (Exhibit 18.4). The scores are a numeric rating of the percentage of times that an event happened, such as the percentage of patients who reported that their pain was always well controlled. The website includes regional and national data for comparison.

Determining what information is useful to consumers is an ongoing effort. The AHRQ and others have identified specific recommendations about publicly reported quality information (Hibbard and Sofaer 2010a, 2010b). These findings summarize the key aspects of how reports can be made more useful to consumers, such as by providing meaningful information, illustrative examples, and context for measures. These reports and studies have noted that publicly reported measures are useful but complicated, and many variables go into decisions about where to seek healthcare (Dafny and Dranove 2008; Faber et al. 2009; Hafner et al. 2011; Mazor and Dodd 2009; Mazor et al. 2010). Public reporting of information will continue to move forward in both informing consumer choice and providing incentives for providers to provide better care.

National Quality Strategy

A driving force promoting an integrated approach to improving healthcare quality is the strategic road map for quality that HHS initiated as required

Condition	Measures
Acute myocardial infarction	• Average number of minutes before outpatients with chest pain or possible heart attack who needed specialized care were transferred to another hospital • Average number of minutes before outpatients with chest pain or possible heart attack got an ECG • Outpatients with chest pain or possible heart attack who got drugs to break up blood clots within 30 minutes of arrival • Outpatients with chest pain or possible heart attack who got aspirin within 24 hours of arrival • Heart attack patients given fibrinolytic medication within 30 minutes of arrival • Heart attack patients given PCI within 90 minutes of arrival • Heart attack patients given aspirin at discharge • Heart attack patients given a prescription for a statin at discharge
Heart failure	• Heart failure patients given discharge instructions • Heart failure patients given an evaluation of left ventricular systolic (LVS) function • Heart failure patients given ACE inhibitor or ARB for left ventricular systolic dysfunction (LVSD)
Pneumonia	• Pneumonia patients whose initial emergency room blood culture was performed prior to the administration of the first hospital dose of antibiotics • Pneumonia patients given the most appropriate initial antibiotic(s)
Surgical Care Improvement Project	• Outpatients having surgery who got an antibiotic at the right time (within one hour before surgery) • Surgery patients who were given an antibiotic at the right time (within one hour before surgery) to help prevent infection • Surgery patients whose preventive antibiotics were stopped at the right time (within 24 hours after surgery) • Patients who got treatment at the right time (within 24 hours before or after their surgery) to help prevent blood clots after certain types of surgery • Outpatients having surgery who got the right kind of antibiotic • Surgery patients who were taking heart drugs called beta blockers before coming to the hospital, who were kept on the beta blockers during the period just before and after their surgery • Surgery patients who were given the right kind of antibiotic to help prevent infection • Heart surgery patients whose blood sugar (blood glucose) is kept under good control in the days right after surgery • Surgery patients whose urinary catheters were removed on the first or second day after surgery • Patients having surgery who were actively warmed in the operating room or whose body temperature was near normal by the end of surgery

EXHIBIT 18.4
Hospital Compare Measure Set for Timely and Effective Care

(Continued)

EXHIBIT 18.4
Hospital
Compare
Measure Set
for Timely and
Effective Care
(continued)

Condition	Measures
Emergency department throughput	• Average time patients spent in the emergency department, before they were admitted to the hospital as an inpatient • Average time patients spent in the emergency department, after the doctor decided to admit them as an inpatient before leaving the emergency department for their inpatient room • Average time patients spent in the emergency department before being sent home • Average time patients spent in the emergency department before they were seen by a healthcare professional • Average time patients who came to the emergency department with broken bones had to wait before receiving pain medication • Percentage of patients who left the emergency department before being seen • Percentage of patients who came to the emergency department with stroke symptoms who received brain scan results within 45 minutes of arrival
Preventive care	• Patients assessed and given influenza vaccination • Patients assessed and given pneumonia vaccination
Children's asthma care	• Children who received reliever medication while hospitalized for asthma • Children who received systemic corticosteroid medication (oral and IV medication that reduces inflammation and controls symptoms) while hospitalized for asthma • Children and their caregivers who received a home management plan of care document while hospitalized for asthma
Stroke care	• Ischemic stroke patients who got medicine to break up a blood clot within 3 hours after symptoms started • Ischemic stroke patients who received medicine known to prevent complications caused by blood clots within 2 days of arriving at the hospital • Ischemic or hemorrhagic stroke patients who received treatment to keep blood clots from forming anywhere in the body within 2 days of arriving at the hospital • Ischemic stroke patients who received a prescription for medicine known to prevent complications caused by blood clots before discharge • Ischemic stroke patients with a type of irregular heartbeat who were given a prescription for a blood thinner at discharge • Ischemic stroke patients needing medicine to lower cholesterol, who were given a prescription for this medicine before discharge • Ischemic or hemorrhagic stroke patients or caregivers who received written educational materials about stroke care and prevention during the hospital stay • Ischemic or hemorrhagic stroke patients who were evaluated for rehabilitation services

(Continued)

Condition	Measures
Blood clot prevention and treatment	• Patients who got treatment to prevent blood clots on the day of or day after hospital admission or surgery • Patients who got treatment to prevent blood clots on the day of or day after being admitted to the intensive care unit (ICU) • Patients who developed a blood clot while in the hospital who **did not** get treatment that could have prevented it • Patients with blood clots who got the recommended treatment, which includes using two different blood thinner medicines at the same time • Patients with blood clots who were treated with an intravenous blood thinner, and then were checked to determine if the blood thinner was putting the patient at an increased risk of bleeding • Patients with blood clots who were discharged on a blood thinner medicine and received written instructions about that medicine
Pregnancy and delivery care	• Percent of newborns whose deliveries were scheduled too early (1–3 weeks early), when a scheduled delivery was not medically necessary

EXHIBIT 18.4
Hospital Compare Measure Set for Timely and Effective Care *(continued)*

Source: CMS (2014c).

under Section 3011 of the ACA. The National Health Care Quality Strategy and Plan requires the inclusion of provisions for: "1) agency-specific plans and benchmarks; 2) coordination among agencies; 3) strategies to align public and private payers; and 4) alignment with meaningful use of health information technology (IT)" (HHS 2010). To achieve these goals, three aims were developed (AHRQ 2014):

1. *Better care:* Improve the overall quality by making healthcare more patient centered, reliable, accessible, and safe.
2. *Healthy people/healthy communities:* Improve the health of the US population by supporting proven interventions to address behavioral, social, and environmental determinants of health in addition to delivering higher-quality care.
3. *Affordable care:* Reduce the cost of quality healthcare for individuals, families, employers, and government.

Toward the fulfillment of these aims, HHS identified six priority areas (AHRQ 2014):

1. Making care safer by reducing harm caused in the delivery of care
2. Ensuring that each person and family is engaged as partners in care
3. Promoting effective communication and coordination of care

4. Promoting the most effective prevention and treatment practices for the leading causes of mortality, starting with cardiovascular disease

5. Working with communities to promote wide use of best practices to enable healthy living

6. Making quality care more affordable for individuals, families, employers, and governments by developing and spreading new healthcare delivery models

AHRQ was charged with implementing the plan, which will require continued involvement of stakeholders including providers, consumers, purchasers, and payers. The implementation of this plan will require active participation of all parties along with continued efforts regarding quality measurement and reporting as well as incentives for providing high-quality care.

Trends and Initiatives in Specific Healthcare Sectors

Ambulatory Care

Quality improvement efforts have begun to focus more intensely on ambulatory care. Quality improvement in ambulatory care settings has been challenging because of the numerous and varied practices and the inability to obtain critical quality data. The uptake of EHRs in ambulatory care practices has enabled the quality movement to go forward. The Tax Relief and Health Care Act of 2006 mandated CMS to establish the Physician Quality Reporting System (PQRS). Reporting by eligible individual professionals was initially voluntary, with providers receiving incentive payments for reporting. This arrangement will evolve into value-based purchasing, in which providers have to meet certain quality benchmarks to receive incentive payments (CMS 2014f). Some examples of nonphysician professionals deemed eligible by CMS are nurse practitioners, physician assistants, clinical social workers, registered dietitians, and physical therapists (CMS 2013c).

Patient care delivery systems have been evolving toward a PCMH model since the 1960s. The American Academy of Pediatrics developed the concept of a "medical home" in 1967 to organize healthcare delivery to meet the needs of chronically ill children (Kilo and Wasson 2010). In the 1990s, the IHI called for the development of primary care models, and the IOM (1996) issued its report on the future of primary care. However, primary care received little attention between the mid-1990s and 2012.

As policymakers, purchasers, and payers look for ways to create efficiencies throughout the system, a strong primary care system continues to be an important part of managing cost and quality. Demonstration projects have shown a variety of benefits of PCMHs, including reduced hospitalizations and readmissions, better management of chronic illnesses, and improved patient satisfaction (Grumbach and Grundy 2010; Reid et al. 2010). Even though the PCMH can improve the quality of care, the National Demonstration Project analyzed data from 36 diverse family practice sites and concluded that the PCMH model would be viable on a large scale only if the healthcare system underwent significant reforms, particularly in regard to financing (Crabtree et al. 2010). The passage of the ACA in 2010 provided numerous elements to support the PCMH movement, including reimbursement strategies, community coordination, innovation, and evidence-based practice and quality improvement initiatives (Safety Net Medical Home Initiative 2010). An example of support provided through the ACA is the Multi-Payer Advanced Primary Care Practice Demonstration intended to evaluate benefits of PCMHs, such as reducing costs, improving the quality of care, increasing patient decision making, and providing better access to underserved populations (CMS 2010).

NCQA has a substantial role in supporting PCMH quality improvement through its recognition program. The program associates scores on the Physician Practice Connection–Patient Centered Medical Home (PPC-PCMH) survey with the assignment of a rating between one and three, with three being the highest achievable (Solberg et al. 2011). PCMH practices have an incentive to secure NCQA PPC-PCMH recognition because it facilitates enhanced reimbursement from public and private payers (NCQA 2014). In 2010, NCQA recognized PCMHs that are led by advanced practice registered nurses (APRNs) in states that allow APRNs to provide the full range of primary care and to practice independently (Scudder 2011).

Hospitals

In 2003, CMS and the Premier healthcare alliance initiated the Premier HQID project. The main purpose of the demonstration was to assess the effect on quality of incentive payments to hospitals. This project first required the reporting of data, and then it linked payment to quality (Premier 2012a, 2012b). The reported events became known as "never" events and are now referred to as *serious reportable events*.

Several pieces of legislation have aimed to improve quality and control the costs of hospital care. The Deficit Reduction Act of 2005 created an incentive program for hospitals to report quality measures (CMS 2012a). This program also established the principle that CMS would not pay for treatment of preventable hospital-acquired conditions (CMS 2012a).

The ACA authorized several value-based purchasing policies for hospitals. These provisions followed a significant history of quality improvement efforts and value-based purchasing policies for hospitals. The policies, in general, provide guidance on payment for serious reportable events, institute incentive payments for hitting benchmarks for quality improvement, and establish payment rates related to hospital readmission. For fiscal year 2013, the maximum payment reduction is 1 percent, for FY 2014 it is 2 percent, and for FY 2015 and thereafter it is capped at 3 percent (AAMC 2013). Results from the demonstration showed that hospitals improved performance on the required quality measures for which they received incentive payments (Premier 2012a). The 18.6 percent increase in overall quality score was accompanied by incentive payments of $60 million over six years (Premier 2012a). The measures required for reporting include process, outcome, and Hospital Consumer Assessment of Healthcare Providers and Systems (HCAHPS) measures.

Nursing Homes

Quality monitoring and improvement in the nursing home industry have been deeply rooted in the regulatory process. Because of the frailty and vulnerability of the population served as well as historic issues related to quality of care, nursing homes have been the target of many sustained efforts to monitor and improve care. In the early 1980s, the nursing home industry developed quality improvement programs such as the Quest for Quality program offered by state nursing home organizations. At the same time, standards for care were established and used as the basis for the survey process. Nursing home quality is monitored by state agencies and includes reporting of data as well as site visits. The survey process includes information about staffing, patient outcomes, and fire safety. A move to focus on outcomes of care has taken place. In the early 2000s, CMS began the national Nursing Home Quality Initiative to provide consumers and providers with information regarding the quality of care in nursing homes through publicly reported data from the nursing home survey. (See the discussion of Nursing Home Compare earlier in this chapter.) Exhibit 18.5 provides a list of the measures. In the time since CMS launched the Quality Indicator Survey project using a phased approach in 2005, the initiative has spread nationwide, and surveyors of long-term care programs now use a software program called ASE-Q to carry out computer-assisted surveying (CMS 2014a).

Nursing homes are unique in having a standardized, federally required assessment for every resident in a CMS-certified facility. The Minimum Data Set (MDS) is an instrument that includes information about resident function and major health problems and risks and that generates a plan of care based on the assessment. Every resident in every certified facility undergoes the same assessment, thus providing patient-level data that are useful in monitoring quality of care (CMS 2012d).

Measure Type	Measure
Long-Stay Quality Measures	• Percentage of long-stay residents experiencing one or more falls with major injury • Percentage of long-stay residents with a urinary tract infection • Percentage of long-stay residents who self-report moderate to severe pain • Percentage of long-stay high-risk residents with pressure ulcers • Percentage of long-stay low-risk residents who lose control of their bowels or bladder • Percentage of long-stay residents who have/had a catheter inserted and left in their bladder • Percentage of long-stay residents who were physically restrained • Percentage of long-stay residents whose need for help with daily activities has increased • Percentage of long-stay residents who lose too much weight • Percentage of long-stay residents who have depressive symptoms • Percentage of long-stay residents assessed and given, appropriately, the seasonal influenza vaccine • Percentage of long-stay residents assessed and given, appropriately, the pneumococcal vaccine • Percentage of long-stay residents who received an antipsychotic medication
Short-Stay Quality Measures	• Percentage of short-stay residents who self-report moderate to severe pain • Percentage of short-stay residents with pressure ulcers that are new or worsened • Percentage of short-stay residents assessed and given, appropriately, the seasonal influenza vaccine • Percentage of short-stay residents assessed and given, appropriately, the pneumococcal vaccine • Percentage of short-stay residents who are newly administered antipsychotic medications

EXHIBIT 18.5
Nursing Home Quality Measures

Source: CMS (2014d, 2014e).

As with hospitals and ambulatory care, a push for value-based purchasing is taking place in nursing homes. The Nursing Home Value-Based Purchasing Demonstration project rewards nursing homes that perform well in four areas: nurse staffing, patient outcomes as measured by the MDS, appropriate hospitalizations, and performance on surveys. Nursing homes that score in the top 20 percent on these measures within each state are eligible for bonus payments (CMS 2009).

Home Health Care

Beginning in 1999, CMS (2011b) began to require Medicare-certified home health agencies to complete a standardized health assessment for each client using the Outcome and Assessment Information Set (OASIS). This requirement has evolved, and core measurement elements were revised as clinical and empirical research became available. The objective was to provide home health agencies with essential measurement elements that can be modified on the basis of clinical judgment, rather than produce a comprehensive assessment instrument (CMS 2011b). As with many data collection processes, the information has several uses. OASIS provides aggregate patient data as well as care planning information that links to the patient data. This information provides the basis for quality monitoring and improvement. Exhibit 18.6 provides an overview of the process and outcome measures as well as a list of the potentially avoidable events.

The Home Health Quality Improvement (HHQI) National Campaign was initiated to focus on improving home care. Stakeholders moving the campaign forward include the Visiting Nurse Associations of America, AHRQ, and the National Association for Home Care and Hospice. The campaign's multipronged efforts include disseminating best practices and providing educational resources (HHQI 2013).

Case Studies

Case Study: Premier Hospital Quality Incentive Demonstration Project

In early 2003, the CMS Premier HQID project began tracking process and outcome measures for healthcare delivery in five clinical areas using more than 30 nationally standardized quality indicators. The five clinical areas were acute myocardial infarction, isolated coronary artery bypass graft, heart failure, pneumonia, and hip and knee replacement. A sixth area, surgical care improvement, was added in the fifth year of the demonstration project.

In the HQID project, hospitals received a composite quality score (CQS) for each clinical area. Hospitals participating in the project received financial incentives depending on their performance in each clinical area. During the fourth year of the demonstration, participating hospitals became eligible for additional financial rewards based on either exceptional performance, significant improvement, or sustained attainment of the median overall CQS benchmark. For each of the clinical areas, hospitals scoring in the top 20 percent received a Top Performance Award and an additional

Measure Title	Measure Description
Emergent Care for Injury Caused by Fall	Percentage of patients who need urgent, unplanned medical care due to an injury caused by fall
Emergent Care for Wound Infections, Deteriorating Wound Status	Percentage of home health episodes of care during which the patient required emergency medical treatment from a hospital emergency department related to a wound that is new, is worse, or has become infected
Emergent Care for Improper Medication Administration, Medication Side Effects	Percentage of home health episodes of care during which the patient required emergency medical treatment from a hospital emergency department related to improper medication adminis-tration or medication side effects
Emergent Care for Hypo/hyperglycemia	Percentage of home health episodes of care during which the patient required emergency medical treatment from a hospital emergency department related to hypo- or hyperglycemia
Development of Urinary Tract Infection	Percentage of home health episodes of care during which patients developed a bladder or urinary tract infection
Increase in Number of Pressure Ulcers	Percentage of home health episodes of care during which the patient had a larger number of pressure ulcers at discharge than at start of care
Substantial Decline in 3 or More Activities of Daily Living	Percentage of home health episodes of care during which the patient became substantially more dependent in at least three out of five activities of daily living
Substantial Decline in Management of Oral Medications	Percentage of home health episodes of care during which the patient's ability to take medicines correctly (by mouth) got much worse
Discharged to the Commu-nity Needing Wound Care or Medication Assistance	Percentage of home health episodes of care at the end of which the patient was discharged, with no assistance available, needing wound care or medication assistance
Discharged to the Com-munity Needing Toileting Assistance	Percentage of home health episodes of care at the end of which the patients was discharged, with no assistance available, need-ing toileting assistance
Discharged to the Com-munity with Behavioral Problems	Percentage of home health episodes of care at the end of which the patient was discharged, with no assistance available, demonstrating behavior problems
Discharged to the Com-munity with an Unhealed Stage II Pressure Ulcer	Percentage of home health episodes of care at the end of which the patient was discharged with a stage II pressure ulcer that has remained unhealed for 30 days or more while a home health patient

EXHIBIT 18.6
Home Health Quality Measures— Potentially Avoidable Events

Source: CMS (2011a).
Note: Measures collected from the Outcome and Assessment Information Set (OASIS).

incentive payment, while hospitals demonstrating quality improvement per-centage gains in the top 20 percent of all participating hospitals received an Improvement Award and an additional incentive payment. The Attainment Award provided an incentive payment to hospitals that attained the median

EXHIBIT 18.7
Centers for Medicare & Medicaid Services Hospital Inpatient Quality Reporting Measures

Topic	Fiscal Year 2014 Payment Determination
Acute Myocardial Infarction (AMI)	1. AMI-1: Aspirin at arrival [SUSPENDED]. 2. AMI-2: Aspirin prescribed at discharge. 3. AMI-3: ACEI/ARB [Angiotensin Converting Enzyme Inhibitor or Angiotensin II Receptor Blocker] for left ventricular systolic dysfunction [SUSPENDED]. 4. AMI-5: Beta-blocker prescribed at discharge [SUSPENDED]. 5. AMI-7a: Fibrinolytic (thrombolytic) agent received within 30 minutes of hospital arrival. 6. AMI-8a: Timing of Receipt of Primary Percutaneous Coronary Intervention (PCI). 7. AMI-10: Statin Prescribed at Discharge.
Heart Failure (HF)	1. HF-1: Discharge instructions. 2. HF-2: Evaluation of left ventricular systolic function. 3. HF-3: Angiotensin Converting Enzyme Inhibitor (ACEI) or Angiotensin II Receptor Blocker (ARB) for left ventricular systolic dysfunction.
Pneumonia (PN)	1. PN-3b: Blood culture performed in the emergency department prior to first antibiotic received in hospital. 2. PN-6: Appropriate initial antibiotic selection.
Surgical Care Improvement Project (SCIP)	1. SCIP INF-1: Prophylactic antibiotic received within 1 hour prior to surgical incision. 2. SCIP INF-2: Prophylactic antibiotic selection for surgical patients. 3. SCIP INF-3: Prophylactic antibiotics discontinued within 24 hours after surgery end time (48 hours for cardiac surgery). 4. SCIP INF-4: Cardiac surgery patients with controlled 6 a.m. postoperative serum glucose. 5. SCIP INF-6: Appropriate Hair Removal [SUSPENDED]. 6. SCIP INF-9: Postoperative urinary catheter removal on postoperative day 1 or 2 with day of surgery being day zero. 7. SCIP INF-10: Surgery patients with perioperative temperature management. 8. SCIP Cardiovascular-2: Surgery Patients on a Beta Blocker prior to arrival who received a Beta Blocker during the perioperative period. 9. SCIP INF-VTE-1: Surgery patients with recommended Venous Thromboembolism (VTE) prophylaxis ordered. 10. SCIP-VTE-2: Surgery patients who received appropriate VTE prophylaxis within 24 hours pre/post surgery.
Mortality Measures (Medicare Patients)	1. Acute Myocardial Infarction (AMI) 30-day mortality rate. 2. Heart Failure (HF) 30-day mortality rate. 3. Pneumonia (PN) 30-day mortality rate.
Patient Experience of Care	1. HCAHPS survey.
Readmission Measure (Medicare Patients)	1. Acute Myocardial Infarction 30-day Risk Standardized Readmission Measure. 2. Heart Failure 30-day Risk Standardized Readmission Measure. 3. Pneumonia 30-day Risk Standardized Readmission Measure.

(Continued)

Topic	Fiscal Year 2014 Payment Determination
AHRQ Patient Safety Indicators (PSIs), Inpatient Quality Indicators (IQIs), and Composite Measures	1. PSI 06: Iatrogenic pneumothorax, adult. 2. PSI 11: Post-Operative Respiratory Failure. 3. PSI 12: Post-Operative PE [pulmonary embolism] or DVT [deep vein thrombosis]. 4. PSI 14: Postoperative wound dehiscence. 5. PSI 15: Accidental puncture or laceration. 6. IQI 11: Abdominal aortic aneurysm (AAA) mortality rate (with or without volume). 7. IQI 19: Hip fracture mortality rate. 8. Complication/patient safety for selected indicators (composite). 9. Mortality for selected medical conditions (composite).
AHRQ PSI and Nursing-Sensitive Care	1. Participation in a Systematic Database for Cardiac Surgery. 2. Participation in a Systematic Clinical Database Registry for Stroke Care. 3. Participation in a Systematic Clinical Database Registry for Nursing Sensitive Care. 4. Participation in a Systematic Clinical Database Registry for General Surgery.**
Healthcare-Associated Infections	1. Central Line Associated Bloodstream Infection. 2. Surgical Site Infection.* 3. Catheter-Associated Urinary Tract Infection.**
Hospital-Acquired Condition Measures	1. Foreign Object Retained After Surgery. 2. Air Embolism. 3. Blood Incompatibility. 4. Pressure Ulcer Stages III & IV. 5. Falls and Trauma (Includes: Fracture, Dislocation, Intracranial Injury, Crushing Injury, Burn, Electric Shock). 6. Vascular Catheter-Associated Infection. 7. Catheter-Associated Urinary Tract Infection (UTI). 8. Manifestations of Poor Glycemic Control.
Emergency Department Throughput	1. ED-1: Median time from emergency department arrival to time of departure from the emergency room for patients admitted to the hospital.* 2. ED-2: Median time from admit decision to time of departure from the emergency department for emergency department patients admitted to the inpatient status.*
Prevention: Global Immunization Measures	1. Immunization for Influenza.*
Cost Efficiency	2. Immunization for Pneumonia.* 3. Medicare Spending per Beneficiary.**

Sources: 42 C.F.R. 412, 413, and 476; 76 Fed. Reg. 51628–51629 (August 18, 2011).

Notes: Fiscal year (FY) 2014 payment determination reflects retirement of four measures, suspension of data collection for four measures, and adoption of three new measures. Single asterisks indicate measures finalized in the FY 2011 Inpatient Prospective Payment System/Long-Term Care Hospital Prospective Payment System final rule for the FY 2014 payment determination. Double asterisks indicate additional measures adopted in this final rule for FY 2014 payment determination.

CQS two years in a row (Premier 2012a). In each of years five and six of the demonstration project, $12 million was budgeted for these financial incentives, with 60 percent of the funds going to the Top Performance Award and Improvement Award recipients and the remainder of the funds going to the Attainment Award recipients (Premier 2012b).

While financial incentives were an important aspect of the HQID quality improvement approach, HQID used more than just incentives to stimulate improvements in quality: Financial penalties were an equally important aspect of the HQID strategy. Hospitals whose scores in year four fell below the tenth-decile threshold were penalized via a 2 percent decrease in the Medicare payment they would receive in year six for each of the HQID clinical areas (Premier 2012b). The results from the first six years of the HQID project are impressive: The 216 participating hospitals demonstrated an average increase of 18.6 percent in overall quality, provided care to more than 2.7 million patients under the demonstration project, and reported data on almost 1 million clinical quality measures (Premier 2012a). The measures tracked by HQID are detailed in Exhibit 18.7.

Case Study: Hospital Public Reporting

In 2002, HHS recognized the leading organizations in the hospital industry (specifically the AHA, the FAH, and the AAMC) for supporting voluntary reporting by hospitals as part of the CMS efforts to provide public information about hospital quality of care. At the urging of CMS, these organizations formed the National Voluntary Hospital Reporting Initiative, which came to be known as the HQA. The initial set of voluntary measures included ten measures related to three disease areas: acute myocardial infarction, heart failure, and pneumonia. These measures were part of a database that was intended to be made available to consumers on the Hospital Compare website. However, fewer than 500 hospitals reported data in 2003. An incentive to report data was introduced into the 2003 Medicare Prescription Drug, Improvement, and Modernization Act, which stipulated that hospitals failing to report data would have a 0.4 percent reduction in their Medicare annual payment update (APU) for FY 2005. To get the full APU, hospitals had to sign up with the Quality Improvement Organization Clinical Warehouse. By 2007, the measure set had expanded to 21 measures, including five measures of surgical care. Hospitals that failed to report data received a reduction of 2.0 percent of the APU. The following year, CMS required the reporting of 24 measures, including the HCAHPS survey of patient experiences.

In December 2011, HQA transferred its quality measurement activities to the Measures Application Partnership (MAP). At the time of the transfer, HQA had compliance levels of 95 percent or higher for almost all of the 10 core measures identified at its inception. The decision to transfer the quality measurement process from HQA to the MAP stemmed from provisions of the ACA in which the National Quality Forum was called on to convene the MAP to advise HHS with regard to performance measures for reporting and payment purposes (HQA 2011).

Throughout its existence, HQA worked closely with CMS to review and approve measures for hospital reporting. This relationship played a vital role in creating a public–private partnership that involves representatives of the providers affected by reporting requirements. The participation of HQA in the measure approval process provided the mechanism for bringing hospitals to the table as decision makers and working with CMS to get public reporting projects underway. The push by CMS for the public reporting of data was balanced by HQA's efforts to ensure that the product of the reporting was an honest appraisal of the quality of hospital care related to specific health problems. The work of the MAP is expected to build on those efforts.

Case Study: Institute for Healthcare Improvement Campaigns

The IHI initiated a campaign in 2004 to save 100,000 lives. In response to an IOM report estimating that nearly 100,000 lives are lost annually in hospitals from medical errors (Kohn, Corrigan, and Donaldson 2000), IHI partnered with the ANA, the Centers for Disease Control and Prevention (CDC), the National Business Group on Health, the AMA, the Leapfrog Group, and The Joint Commission, among others, to launch the 100,000 Lives Campaign (IHI 2006). The campaign swiftly claimed impressive results—an estimated 122,000 lives saved—but some scholars have questioned the calculations underlying this claim (Wachter and Pronovost 2006). Regardless of the exact number of lives saved, however, the 100,000 Lives Campaign successfully united hospitals and health systems in a collective commitment to improving quality and generated considerable excitement among providers as well as the media.

Several key factors were instrumental in the success of the 100,000 Lives Campaign, the most significant of which was having a credible organization with committed, highly visible, and highly respected people in healthcare promoting the campaign. Another key factor was IHI's development of the structure and process for participants to learn from one another and reinforce change. As part of the promise to create change, participating hospitals were required to provide data as evidence of outcomes achieved, thus further strengthening (and exemplifying) the organizational commitment of participants in this groundbreaking initiative.

The 100,000 Lives Campaign helped lay the groundwork for a campaign with a different focus. The 5 Million Lives Campaign focused on reducing the incidence of medical harm to hospitalized patients, currently estimated to be 15 million incidents of harm each year. With the powerful slogan "Do

No Harm," this two-year campaign (2006–2008) built on lessons learned from the 100,000 Lives Campaign. Along with the ambitious goal of preventing 5 million instances of medical harm, the 5 Million Lives Campaign sought to increase the number of providers committed to quality improvement who are appointed to the boards of hospitals and health systems (IHI 2013).

By the time the campaign ended in December 2008, 18 states had more than 90 percent of their hospitals enrolled. A 70 percent reduction was observed in the incidence of pressure ulcers in participating New Jersey hospitals, and participating hospitals in Rhode Island decreased central-line-associated bloodstream infections by more than 40 percent (IHI 2013). Despite these impressive results, IHI acknowledged that it was not possible to determine whether hospitals participating in the campaign were actually able to prevent 5 million instances of harm (IHI 2013).

The IHI campaigns exemplify quality improvement efforts that use evidence to identify high-priority areas on which to focus, change individual provider behavior, and mobilize public action for policy change. The IHI campaigns demonstrated sophistication, with clear objectives and a powerful call to action. Yet, for a campaign to be deemed a success, success needs to be operationally defined at the outset so that a clear relationship between goals, activities, and measurable outcomes is evident. This goal requires understanding the target audience, identifying desired actions, and providing clear strategies for implementation. IHI defined the goal—saving 5 million lives from medical harm—and defined the 12 target areas, but it failed to execute a nationwide outcome data collection effort of similarly ambitious scope. This observation should not be seen as a negative reflection on IHI's efforts in the 5 Million Lives Campaign but rather as an indication of the need for more robust investment in similar initiatives so that evaluation of outcomes can be carried out in as rigorous a manner as possible.

Experience gained during the first campaign provided insight as to which implementation strategies would be most effective. Part of the campaign's success lay in its simple message—a message that echoes and builds on the "do no harm" charge given to physicians since the time of Hippocrates. The slogan engages both providers and media and serves as a clear message to consumers that participating provider hospitals are committed to protecting their patients from medical harm.

Case Study: Chronic Care Initiative

The economic burden of chronic illness in the United States is expected to significantly increase as the population ages (CDC 2012). To begin addressing this issue, the Medicare Prescription Drug, Improvement, and Modernization Act of 2003 authorized a demonstration project to evaluate chronic care improvement programs. This program was first known as the Voluntary Chronic Care Improvement Program and in 2007 was renamed the Medicare

Health Support program. The program sought to improve the quality of care provided to Medicare enrollees with chronic illness, improve enrollees' satisfaction with care, and hit targets for savings. Payment to participating organizations (called Medicare Health Support Organizations, or MHSOs) was based on a pay-for-performance model in which monthly fees were paid, but organizations were required to meet specified standards to keep all the funds. If a participating organization failed to meet the standards, the organization was required to pay back a portion of the Medicare payments.

The first phase of the program was initiated with the selection of eight chronic care improvement MHSOs that began operations in 2005. Each organization was required to have a designated contact person to facilitate communication with enrollees and the other healthcare providers, provide self-care education to enrollees, educate healthcare providers about relevant clinical information, and educate enrollees to effectively use monitoring technologies to provide relevant information to healthcare providers. Participating organizations were required to report specific data to CMS to facilitate the comparison of enrollees in the intervention program to those in a control program. In Phase I, CMS identified beneficiaries using claims data in the geographic areas of the participating organization. Each enrollee was randomly assigned to an intervention or control group, with those assigned to the intervention group given the option to refuse to participate.

The Phase I report to Congress in 2008 noted that "to date, this is the largest randomized experiment in disease management ever conducted" (McCall et al. 2008, 70). The results showed modest improvements in measures of quality of care but minimal differences in health outcome measures. Among the eight participating MHSOs (each of which reported on five quality-of-care measures), 40 percent of the 40 total measures demonstrated some level of improvement. Yet, these improvements in quality of care did not translate into improvement in health outcomes. The eight MHSOs each reported on 15 health outcome measures, none of which demonstrated statistically significant decreases in the growth rate for emergency department visits, hospital readmissions, or hospitalizations (McCall et al. 2008). The starkest failure of the pilot, however, was its inability to control costs. As the evaluators asserted to Congress (McCall et al. 2008, 79):

> The Medicare Health Support authorizing legislation states that if the results of the independent evaluation indicate that a program (or the components of such a program) improves clinical quality of care and beneficiary satisfaction, and achieves targets for savings, the program (or its components) may be expanded to additional geographic areas. None of the MHS pilot programs at the mid-point of the pilot have yet to meet the three statutory requirements to improve clinical quality of care and beneficiary satisfaction and achieve budget neutrality with respect to their fees.

In short, "none of the 8 MHSOs achieved gross savings rates that were statistically different from zero" and "the lack of financial success was uniform across five broad disease groups" (McCall et al. 2008, 70).

Conclusion

The ACA provides the potential for significant impact on healthcare quality strategies for business, accrediting agencies, organizations, and providers across the United States. The momentum of national strategies to improve healthcare quality is sustained by public and private funding and by the development of policies that support measurement, public reporting, and accountability. The enhanced role of consumers in healthcare also represents a substantial societal change. Consumers are positioned at the center of the quality improvement process and are recognized as significant stakeholders in the advancement of healthcare delivery systems. Innovation and collaboration will continue to be a priority for quality improvement efforts as new care delivery and value-based purchasing models are explored to support integration across healthcare sectors. The challenge for the future will be to continually incorporate new evidence into quality improvement practice as data emerge from scientific research.

Study Questions

1. Discuss how passage of the ACA has changed or will change the quality of services delivered to the consumer, the ultimate stakeholder in healthcare services.

2. Construct an evidence-based timeline of future quality improvement activities and legislative initiatives. Include levers such as value-based purchasing, the role of QIOs, consumer demographics, business groups, accreditors, and the HITECH Act.

3. Discuss the impact that trends in federal quality improvement initiatives will have on healthcare delivery in the state in which you reside. What federal legislative initiatives are controversial in your state or have a high degree of support? Why?

4. Compare and contrast the mandated quality improvement reporting activities and nonmandated, judgment-driven reporting activities in the health sectors discussed in this chapter. In your opinion, what are the pros and cons of each approach?

References

Agency for Healthcare Research and Quality (AHRQ). 2014. "About the National Quality Strategy." Accessed January 4. www.ahrq.gov/workingforquality/about.htm.

———. 2013. "About CAHPS." Accessed December 20. https://cahps.ahrq.gov/about-cahps/index.html.

Ambulatory Quality Alliance (AQA). 2010. "AQA Strategic Plan." Approved October 28. www.aqaalliance.org/files/AQA_Strategic_Plan_10282010.pdf.

American Medical Association (AMA). 2014. "Physician Consortium for Performance Improvement." Accessed January 4. www.ama-assn.org/ama/pub/physician-resources/physician-consortium-performance-improvement.page.

American Nurses Association (ANA). 2014. "National Database for Nursing Quality Indicators." Accessed January 4. www.nursingquality.org/About-NDNQI#quality-data.

Association of American Medical Colleges (AAMC). 2013. "Selected Medicare Hospital Quality Provisions Under the ACA." Accessed December 19. www.aamc.org/advocacy/medicare/153882/selected_medicare_hospital_quality_provisions_under_the_aca.html.

Bernacki, R. E., D. N. Ko, P. Higgins, S. N. Whitlock, A. Cullinan, R. Wilson, V. Jackson, C. Dahlin, J. Abrahm, E. Mort, K. N. Scheer, S. Block, and J. A. Billings. 2012. "Improving Access to Palliative Care Through an Innovative Quality Improvement Initiative: An Opportunity for Pay-for-Performance." *Journal of Palliative Medicine* 15 (2): 192–99.

Brook, H. R., J. E. Ware, W. H. Rogers, E. B. Keeler, A. R. Davies, C. A. Sherbourne, G. A. Goldberg, K. N. Lohr, P. Camp, and J. P. Newhouse. 1984. *The Effect of Coinsurance on the Health of Adults: Results from the Rand Health Insurance Experiment.* Report No. R-3055-HHS. Santa Monica, CA: The Rand Corporation.

Casalino, L. P., and A. Elster. 2007. "Will Pay-for-Performance and Quality Reporting Affect Health Care Disparities?" *Health Affairs* 26 (3): w405–w414.

Centers for Disease Control and Prevention (CDC). 2012. "Chronic Diseases and Health Promotion." Updated August 13. www.cdc.gov/nccdphp/overview.htm.

Centers for Medicare & Medicaid Services (CMS). 2014a. "CMS Quality Indicator Survey/ASE-Q." Accessed January 4. www.cms.gov/Medicare/Provider-Enrollment-and-Certification/SurveyCertificationGenInfo/Downloads/QIS-Brochure.pdf.

———. 2014b. "EHR Incentive Programs: Data and Program Reports." Accessed January 4. www.cms.gov/Regulations-and-Guidance/Legislation/EHRIncentivePrograms/DataAndReports.html.

———. 2014c. "Measures Displayed on Hospital Compare." Accessed January 4. www.medicare.gov/hospitalcompare/Data/Measures-Displayed.html.

———. 2014d. "Nursing Home Compare: Why Quality Measures Are Important to You (Long-Stay Resident)." Accessed January 4. www.medicare.gov/NursingHomeCompare/Data/Long-Stay-Residents.html.

———. 2014e. "Nursing Home Compare: Why Quality Measures Are Important to You (Short-Stay Resident)." Accessed January 4. www.medicare.gov/NursingHomeCompare/Data/Short-Stay-Residents.html.

———. 2014f. "Physician Quality Reporting System." Accessed January 4. www.cms.gov/Medicare/Quality-Initiatives-Patient-Assessment-Instruments/PQRS/?gclid=CIm4gLfk5bsCFbFxOgod7DQAyQ.

———. 2013a. "About the CMS Innovation Center." Accessed December 19. http://innovation.cms.gov/About/index.html.

———. 2013b. "Accountable Care Organizations (ACO)." Updated March 22. www.cms.gov/ACO/.

———. 2013c. "Physician Quality Reporting System: List of Eligible Professionals." Updated November 14. www.cms.gov/Medicare/Quality-Initiatives-Patient-Assessment-Instruments/PQRS/Downloads/PQRS_List-of-Eligible Professionals_022813.pdf.

———. 2012a. "Hospital-Acquired Conditions Overview." Updated September 20. www.cms.gov/HospitalAcqCond/.

———. 2012b. "One Year of Innovation: Taking Action to Improve Care and Reduce Costs." Published January 26. http://innovation.cms.gov/Files/reports/Innovation-Center-Year-One-Summary-document.pdf.

———. 2012c. "Pioneer Accountable Care Organization Program: General Fact Sheet." Updated September 12. http://innovation.cms.gov/Files/fact-sheet/Pioneer-ACO-General-Fact-Sheet.pdf.

———. 2012d. "Research, Statistics, Data and Systems: Minimum Data Sets 2.0 Tool and Public Reports." Updated March 8. www.cms.gov/MinimumDataSets20/.

———. 2011a. "Home Health Quality Measures—Potentially Avoidable Events." Revised August. www.cms.gov/HomeHealthQualityInits/Downloads/HHQIOutcome-AvoidableEvent-Process-Measures.zip.

———. 2011b. *Outcome and Assessment Information Set (OASIS-C) Process-Based Quality Improvement (PBQI) Manual.* Revised December. www.cms.gov/Medicare/Quality-Initiatives-Patient-Assessment-Instruments/HomeHealthQualityInits/downloads/HHQIProcessBasedQualityImprovementManual.pdf.

———. 2010. "CMS Introduces New Center for Medicare and Medicaid Innovation, Initiatives to Better Coordinate Health Care." Press release issued November 16. www.cms.gov/Newsroom/MediaReleaseDatabase/Press-Releases/2010-Press-Releases-Items/2010-11-16.html.

———. 2009. "Nursing Home Value-Based Purchasing Demonstration: Fact Sheet." Released August. www.cms.gov/DemoProjectsEvalRpts/downloads/NHP4P_FactSheet.pdf.

Chen, P. C., Y. C. Lee, and R. N. Kuo. 2012. "Differences in Patient Reports on the Quality of Care in a Diabetes Pay-for-Performance Program Between 1 Year Enrolled and Newly Enrolled Patients." *International Journal for Quality in Health Care* 24 (2): 189–96.

Cheng, S. H., T. T. Lee, and C. C. Chen. 2012. "A Longitudinal Examination of a Pay-for-Performance Program for Diabetes Care: Evidence from a Natural Experiment." *Medical Care* 50 (2): 109–16.

Commonwealth Fund. 2014. "Programs." Accessed January 4. www.commonwealthfund.org/Grants-and-Programs/Programs.aspx.

Crabtree, B. F., P. A. Nutting, W. L. Miller, K. C. Stange, E. E. Stewart, and C. R. Jean. 2010. "Summary of the National Demonstration Project and Recommendations for the Patient-Centered Medical Home." *Annals of Family Medicine* 8 (Suppl. 1): S80–S90.

Cuckler, G. A., A. M. Sisko, S. P. Keehan, S. D. Smith, A. J. Madison, J. A. Poisal, C. J. Wolfe, J. M. Lizonitz, and D. A. Stone. 2013. "National Health Expenditure Projections, 2012–22: Slow Growth Until Coverage Expands and Economy Improves." *Health Affairs* 32 (10): 1820–31.

Dafny, L., and D. Dranove. 2008. "Do Report Cards Tell Consumers Anything They Don't Know Already? The Case of Medicare HMOs." *Rand Journal of Economics* 39 (3): 790–821.

Devers, K., and R. A. Berenson. 2009. "Can Accountable Care Organizations Improve the Value of Health Care by Solving the Cost and Quality Quandaries?" Robert Wood Johnson Foundation and Urban Institute. Published October. www.urban.org/uploadedpdf/411975_acountable_care_orgs.pdf.

Dudley, R. A., and M. B. Rosenthal. 2006. *Pay for Performance: A Decision Guide for Purchasers.* AHRQ Publication No. 06-0047. Rockville, MD: Agency for Healthcare Research and Quality.

Eijkenaar, F. 2012. "Pay for Performance in Healthcare: An International Overview of Initiatives." *Medical Care Research and Review* 69 (3): 251–76.

Faber, M., M. Bosch, H. Wollersheim, S. Leatherman, and R. Grol. 2009. "Public Reporting in Healthcare: How Do Consumers Use Quality-of-Care Information? A Systematic Review." *Medical Care* 47 (1): 1–8.

Grumbach, K., and P. Grundy. 2010. *Outcomes of Implementing Patient Centered Medical Home Interventions: A Review of the Evidence from Prospective Evaluation Studies in the United States.* Washington, DC: Patient-Centered Primary Care Collaborative.

Hafner, J. M., S. C. Williams, R. G. Koss, B. A. Tschurtz, S. P. Schmaltz, and J. M. Loeb. 2011. "The Perceived Impact of Public Reporting Hospital Performance Data: Interviews with Hospital Staff." *International Journal for Quality in Health Care* 23 (6): 697–704.

Hibbard, J., and S. Sofaer. 2010a. *Best Practices in Public Reporting No. 1: How to Effectively Present Healthcare Performance Data to Consumers.* AHRQ Publication No. 10-0082-EF. Rockville, MD: Agency for Healthcare Research and Quality.

———. 2010b. *Best Practices in Public Reporting No. 2: Maximizing Consumer Understanding of Comparative Quality Reports: Effective Use of Explanatory Information.* AHRQ Publication No. 10-0082-1-EF. Rockville, MD: Agency for Healthcare Research and Quality.

Home Health Quality Improvement (HHQI). 2013. "Welcome to the HHQI National Campaign." Accessed December 20. www.homehealthquality.org/hh/default.aspx.

Hospital Quality Alliance (HQA). 2011. "Press Release: HQA Recaps Accomplishments, Readies Measures Review Transfer." Press release issued December 13. www.fah.org/fahcms/Documents/On%20The%20Record/Hospital%20Quality%20Alliance/HQA%20Press%20Releases/HQA_Announcement.pdf.

Institute for Healthcare Improvement (IHI). 2013. "Overview: Protecting 5 Million Lives from Harm." Accessed December 20. www.ihi.org/offerings/Initiatives/PastStrategicInitiatives/5MillionLivesCampaign/Pages/default.aspx.

———. 2006. "Overview of the 100,000 Lives Campaign." Accessed December 20, 2013. www.ihi.org/offerings/Initiatives/PastStrategicInitiatives/5MillionLivesCampaign/Documents/Overview%20of%20the%20100K%20Campaign.pdf.

Institute of Medicine (IOM). 1996. *Primary Care: America's Health in a New Era.* Washington, DC: National Academies Press.

Jha, A. K., E. J. Orav, and A. M. Epstein. 2011. "Low-Quality, High-Cost Hospitals, Mainly in South, Care for Sharply Higher Shares of Elderly Black, Hispanic, and Medicaid Patients." *Health Affairs* 30 (10): 1904–11.

Joint Commission. 2013. "Facts About ORYX for Hospitals (National Hospital Quality Measures)." Issued September. www.jointcommission.org/assets/1/6/ORYX_for_Hospitals.pdf.

Keehan, S. P., A. M. Sisko, C. J. Truffer, J. A. Poisal, G. A. Cuckler, A. J. Madison, J. M. Lizonitz, and S. D. Smith. 2011. "National Health Spending Projections Through 2020: Economic Recovery and Reform Drive Faster Spending Growth." *Health Affairs* 30 (8): 1594–605.

Kilo, C. M., and J. H. Wasson. 2010. "Practice Redesign and the Patient-Centered Medical Home: History, Promises, and Challenges." *Health Affairs* 29 (5): 773–78.

Kohn, L. T., J. M. Corrigan, and M. S. Donaldson (eds.). 2000. *To Err Is Human: Building a Safer Health System.* Washington, DC: National Academies Press.

Leapfrog Group. 2014. "Fact Sheet." Accessed January 4. www.leapfroggroup.org/about_leapfrog/leapfrog-factsheet.

Mazor, K. M., J. Calvi, R. Cowan, M. E. Costanza, P. K. Han, S. M. Greene, L. Saccoccio, E. Cove, D. Roblin, and A. Williams. 2010. "Media Messages About

Cancer: What Do People Understand?" *Journal of Health Communication* 15 (Suppl. 2): 126–45.

Mazor, K. M., and K. S. Dodd. 2009. "A Qualitative Study of Consumers' Views on Public Reporting of Healthcare-Associated Infections." *American Journal of Medical Quality* 24 (5): 412–18.

McCall, N., J. Cromwell, C. Urato, and D. Rabiner. 2008. *Evaluation of Phase I of the Medicare Health Support Pilot Program Under Traditional Fee-for-Service Medicare: 18-Month Interim Analysis. Report to Congress.* Published October. www.cms.gov/reports/downloads/MHS_Second_Report_to_Congress_October_2008.pdf.

National Business Coalition on Health. 2014. "About NBCH." Accessed January 4. www.nbch.org/About-NBCH.

National Business Group on Health. 2013. "Institute on Health Care Costs and Solutions (IHCCS)." Accessed December 26. www.businessgrouphealth. org/about/hccs.cfm.

National Committee for Quality Assurance (NCQA). 2014. "Patient-Centered Medical Home Recognition." Accessed January 4. www.ncqa.org/Programs/Recognition/PatientCenteredMedicalHomePCMH.aspx.

———. 2013a. "Diabetes Recognition Program (DRP)." Accessed December 26. www.ncqa.org/Programs/Recognition/DiabetesRecognitionProgramDRP. aspx.

———. 2013b. "HEDIS & Performance Measurement." Accessed December 26. www.ncqa.org/HEDISQualityMcasurement.aspx.

———. 2013c. "HEDIS and Quality Compass." Accessed December 26. www.ncqa. org/HEDISQualityMeasurement/WhatisHEDIS.aspx.

National Patient Safety Foundation. 2013. "Mission and Vision." Accessed December 26. www.npsf.org/about-us/mission-and-vision/.

Pacific Business Group on Health. 2013. "About the Pacific Business Group on Health." Accessed December 26. www.pbgh.org/about.

Petersen, L. A., T. Urech, K. Simpson, K. Pietz, S. J. Hysong, J. Profit, D. Conrad, R. A. Dudley, M. Z. Lutschg, R. Petzel, and L. D. Woodard. 2011. "Design, Rationale, and Baseline Characteristics of a Cluster Randomized Controlled Trial of Pay for Performance for Hypertension Treatment: Study Protocol." *Implementation Science: IS* 6 (October 3): 114.

Petersen, L. A., L. D. Woodard, L. M. Henderson, T. H. Urech, and K. Pietz. 2009. "Will Hypertension Performance Measures Used for Pay-for-Performance Programs Penalize Those Who Care for Medically Complex Patients?" *Circulation* 119 (23): 2978–85.

Premier. 2012a. "CMS/Premier Hospital Quality Incentive Demonstration." Accessed February 23. www.premierinc.com/p4p/hqi/.

————. 2012b. "Overview of CMS Hospital Quality Incentive Demonstration Project Payment Method." Accessed February 23. www.premierinc.com/quality-safety/tools-services/p4p/hqi/payment/project-payment-year6.jsp.

President's Advisory Commission on Consumer Protection and Quality in the Health Care Industry. 1998. *Quality First: Better Healthcare for All Americans.* Darby, PA: Diane Publishing.

Reid, R. J., K. Coleman, E. A. Johnson, P. A. Fishman, C. Hsu, M. P. Soman, C. E. Trescott, M. Erikson, and E. B. Larson. 2010. "The Group Health Medical Home at Year Two: Cost Savings, Higher Patient Satisfaction, and Less Burnout for Providers." *Health Affairs* 29 (5): 835–43.

Ryan, A. M. 2013. "Will Value-Based Purchasing Increase Disparities in Care?" *New England Journal of Medicine* 369 (26): 2472–74.

Ryan, A. M., J. Blustein, and L. P. Casalino. 2012. "Medicare's Flagship Test of Pay-for-Performance Did Not Spur More Rapid Quality Improvement Among Low-Performing Hospitals." *Health Affairs* 31 (4): 797–805.

Safety Net Medical Home Initiative. 2010. *Health Reform and the Patient-Centered Medical Home: Policy Provisions and Expectations of the Patient Protection and Affordable Care Act.* Published October. www.safetynetmedicalhome.org/sites/default/files/Policy-Brief-2.pdf.

Scudder, L. 2011. "Nurse-Led Medical Homes: Current Status and Future Plans." *Medscape News.* Published May 27. www.medscape.com/viewarticle/743197.

Solberg, L., S. Asche, P. Fontaine, T. Flottemesch, L. Pawlson, and S. Scholle. 2011. "Relationship of Clinic Medical Home Scores to Quality and Patient Experience." *Journal of Ambulatory Care Management* 34 (1): 57–66.

US Department of Health & Human Services (HHS). 2013a. "Nursing Home Compare." Accessed January 15. www.medicare.gov/nursinghomecompare/.

————. 2013b. "Quality Care Finder." www.medicare.gov/Quality-Care-Finder/.

————. 2011. "Over 100,000 Primary Care Providers Sign Up to Adopt Electronic Health Records Through Their Regional Extension Centers." News release issued November 17. www.hhs.gov/news/press/2011pres/11/20111117a.html.

————. 2010. *National Health Care Quality Strategy and Plan.* Issued September 9. www.hhs.gov/news/reports/quality/nationalhealthcarequalitystrategy.pdf.

US Department of Health & Human Services Office of Inspector General (OIG). 2010. *Adverse Events in Hospitals: National Incidence Among Medicare Beneficiaries.* Published November. http://oig.hhs.gov/oei/reports/oei-06-09-00090.pdf.

US Department of Health & Human Services Office of the National Coordinator for Health Information Technology (ONC). 2014. "How to Attain Meaningful Use." Accessed January 4. www.healthit.gov/providers-professionals/how-attain-meaningful-use.

VanLare, J. M., J. Moody-Williams, and P. H. Conway. 2012. "Value-Based Purchasing for Hospitals." *Health Affairs* 31 (1): 249.

Wachter, R. M., and P. J. Pronovost. 2006. "The 100,000 Lives Campaign: A Scientific and Policy Review." *Joint Commission Journal on Quality and Patient Safety* 32 (11): 621–27.

ACCREDITATION: ITS ROLE IN DRIVING ACCOUNTABILITY IN HEALTHCARE

Diane Storer Brown and Kevin Park

The Affordable Care Act (ACA) of March 2010 created a healthcare reform law for the United States in an effort to improve the quality and safety of healthcare. The healthcare industry had well documented the need for improvements; however, fragmentation and variation in the healthcare delivery system made widespread accountability for improvement challenging. This chapter examines accreditation in both its past and prospective roles in driving accountability in the healthcare delivery system.

Background and Terminology

Accountability and *healthcare* are terms that are frequently found together in current literature. Accountability is defined as "an obligation or willingness to accept responsibility or to account for one's actions" (Merriam-Webster 2014). Accountability in healthcare has been driven by three major forces: the marketplace, regulation, and professionalism. In healthcare, the parties that may seek accountability include those directly affected by health services (patients) and those who directly or indirectly pay for the services (insurers, employers, employees, or taxpayers). This chapter refers collectively to this group of interested parties as *the public*.

Accountability can be achieved by informal, subjective means or through the exchange of information using a formal set of metrics. One mechanism that has been used to create accountability is accreditation. *Accreditation* is a process by which an entity external to the organization providing goods or services evaluates that organization against a set of predetermined requirements or desirable attributes and publicly attests to the results.

The term *certification* often is used to denote a similar process, except that certification more often is used in reference to the determination of an individual's (rather than an organization's) competency, to the government's determination of an organization's eligibility to participate in a government program, or to an organization's ability to provide evidence-based care to a specific population. The use of the words *accreditation* and *certification* may differ by organization, so professionals and students need to be careful to use the terms correctly in reference to the specific organization's programs. Although organizational accreditation or certification—as contrasted with licensure—is usually thought of as voluntary, the decision to seek accreditation can be truly optional, linked to participation in an insurance program, required for licensure by government at the federal or state level, or required by customers. Throughout the world, either private-sector bodies or government agencies provide organizational accreditation and certification; in the United States, private-sector bodies provide organizational accreditation, and either private-sector or government agencies provide certification. In contrast, *licensure* is always the domain of government, is nearly always mandatory, and requires that organizations meet certain legally defined requirements to practice or exercise a certain activity.

Regulation and Accreditation

A major reason for the genesis of accreditation or private-sector certification is professionals' desire to define adherence to professional norms and standards in the delivery of services at both individual and organizational levels. Organizations that provide accreditation and certification services may be created and governed by trade associations or professional societies within the field or by independent business organizations. However, regulatory and market forces also have a strong influence on the presence of accreditation. Regulatory forces, including licensure and federal or state regulations or mandates, and the justice system, including malpractice litigation, urge professional groups to offer accreditation—both to encourage adherence to standards of performance beyond those required by licensure and as an alternative to additional regulatory control. Some see the implicit delegation of a portion of accountability to accreditation as a manifestation of the self-monitoring that society has historically granted—and expected—through the implicit and explicit contracts it establishes with healthcare professionals.

Market forces also play a role in accreditation, as purchasers (governmental or private sector) either encourage accreditation or require it as a prerequisite for inclusion in the insurance programs they offer. Thus, in most situations, accreditation exists where both a professional drive to set and maintain standards and either regulatory or market pressures that support accreditation as an alternative to regulatory oversight by state or federal agencies are present. For example, in the United States, the Centers for Medicare & Medicaid Services (CMS), as a governmental payer through the Social Security Act, requires minimum compliance with process standards for hospitals, skilled nursing facilities, home health agencies, hospice programs, critical access hospitals, comprehensive outpatient rehabilitation facilities, laboratories, and ambulatory surgical centers. This compliance may be assessed by a state health agency or other appropriate state agency (or the appropriate local agencies). The *Code of Federal Regulations* (42 C.F.R. 488) provides regulation so that certain providers may elect to be reviewed by private accreditation organizations that CMS has preapproved as having standards and survey procedures that at a minimum are equivalent to CMS or state surveyors (this is known as deemed status). CMS posts in the *Federal Register* the names of accreditation agencies that have been approved and provides a list of organizations and their contact information for hospitals, home care and hospice agencies, and ambulatory surgery centers (CMS 2013a).

Documented evidence of the value of accreditation is emerging in the healthcare literature nationally and internationally. After many years in which public proclamations that an organization is vested in providing the infrastructure for quality patient care were taken on face value, evidence-based literature on accreditation has begun to emerge. The most extensive review of the value of accreditation was published by Accreditation Canada (Nicklin 2013). The review addresses the fact that accreditation is an integral part of healthcare services in more than 70 countries as either a voluntary measure or a government-mandated requirement; however, the science of accreditation is still under development. Accreditation Canada provides a list of accreditation benefits based on an extensive international literature review (Nicklin 2013):

- Provides a framework to help create and implement systems and processes that improve operational effectiveness and advance positive health outcomes
- Improves communication and collaboration internally and with external stakeholders
- Strengthens interdisciplinary team effectiveness
- Demonstrates credibility and a commitment to quality and accountability
- Decreases liability costs; identifies areas for additional funding for healthcare organizations and provides a platform for negotiating this funding
- Mitigates the risk of adverse events
- Sustains improvements in quality and organizational performance
- Supports the efficient and effective use of resources in healthcare services
- Enables ongoing self-analysis of performance in relation to standards
- Ensures an acceptable level of quality among healthcare providers
- Enhances the organization's understanding of the continuum of care
- Improves the organization's reputation among end users and enhances their awareness and perception of quality care

- Promotes capacity building, professional development, and organizational learning
- Codifies policies and procedures
- Promotes the use of ethical frameworks
- Drives compliance with medication reconciliation
- Decreases variances in practice among healthcare providers and decision makers
- Provides healthcare organizations with a well-defined vision for sustainable quality improvement initiatives
- Stimulates sustainable quality improvement efforts and continuously raises the bar with regard to quality improvement initiatives, policies, and processes
- Leads to the improvement of internal practices
- Increases healthcare organizations' compliance with quality and safety standards
- Enhances the reliability of laboratory testing
- Improves patients' health outcomes
- Provides a team-building opportunity for staff and improves their understanding of their coworkers' functions
- Promotes an understanding of how each person's job contributes to the healthcare organization's mission and services
- Contributes to increased job satisfaction among physicians, nurses, and other providers
- Engenders a spillover effect, whereby the accreditation of one service helps to improve the performance of other service areas
- Highlights practices that are working well
- Promotes the sharing of policies, procedures, and best practices among healthcare organizations
- Promotes a quality and safety culture

Accreditation Canada (Nicklin 2013) also identified that the literature was lacking in a number of areas and that further research was required to better understand the value of accreditation. The report specifically noted the following deficits:

- Collecting data through accreditation; ensuring completeness and accuracy
- Emphasizing uniformity and adherence to standards over an individual organization's performance and innovation
- Demonstrating, through research, a strong link between accreditation status and client outcomes
- Achieving "soft" results—increased comprehensiveness is necessary

- Ensuring consistency in surveyors' approach
- Reducing the workload of the accreditation process
- Involving physicians and patients in quality improvement and healthcare accreditation
- Establishing other methods for assessing and ensuring quality (e.g., information technology, performance measures)

Few studies have attempted to draw causal inferences about the direct influence of accreditation on patients' health outcomes, so further research is warranted.

The Accreditation Process

Accreditation is based on the premise that it is possible both to define attributes critical (either required or highly desirable) to the quality and safety of a healthcare product or service and to create a method to measure whether a threshold of performance has been achieved. Critical attributes can be defined for both administrative and clinical activities, and they can be based on expert opinion, consensus (of providers or multiple stakeholders), or research studies (qualitative or quantitative studies). These attributes are published as requirements or standards with which the organization must demonstrate compliance. The requirements or standards vary in content and rigor among accrediting agencies, which becomes a consideration for organizations when choosing an accreditation agency.

Measurement can involve a combination of methods, including on-site observation (announced or unannounced), review of policies, review or abstraction of data from administrative or clinical records, surveys, and interviews with provider staff or patients (see Exhibit 19.1). Many accreditation programs rely on on-site observation and review of reports and policies as the primary source of standard compliance measurement. However, the accreditation industry is shifting to more electronic review in advance of on-site survey activity as technology has improved the capability to transport large volumes of confidential information securely.

Following the measurement phase, an analysis of all data collected is translated into an accreditation decision. The decision usually includes an overall assessment of the entity (organization or service) as a whole that reflects either a full accreditation decision or a decision with limitations or restrictions that the organization must resolve for full accreditation. Decisions may also include assessment of specific components, functions, or services of the larger entity that may require additional follow-up by the organization to demonstrate full compliance and to establish a full accreditation decision.

To complete the process, the accrediting body shares information concerning the results of the evaluation or accreditation decision with both the evaluated organization and interested parties such as consumers, patients,

EXHIBIT 19.1
Potential
Sources of
Data for Use in
Accreditation

Data Source	Description
Observation	Direct observation of structures or processes used by an entity, or tracing of a patient's individual care from entry (or admission) through exit (or discharge), covering all aspects of the organization's care delivery system
Interviews	Structured and unstructured interviews with consumers or patients, frontline staff, managers, and organizational leaders
Audit	Verification of the integrity and accuracy of organizational data, including data collection and reporting processes
Document review	On-site or electronic remote review of written documentation, including reports, policies, medical records, investigations of adverse events, or responses to formal complaints
Surveys	Collection and analysis of data from surveys of those using the services (e.g., consumers, patients, practitioners) or those supplying the services (e.g., nurses, doctors, pharmacists, therapists, vendors)
Derived information	Collection and analysis of data contained in either paper or electronic form, which may be used in required performance metrics, required state reporting, claims (e.g., office visits; laboratory, pharmacy, or other services), reports on clinical processes (e.g., laboratory results), or publications

purchasers, and government agencies who have requested the accountability. The level of detail that the accrediting body shares with the evaluated organization and outside groups varies. Published information ranges from a simple list of organizations that received accreditation (with no indication of organizations that did not apply or applied but failed to be accredited) to relatively detailed information on comparative performance, including performance on specific subsets of the requirements. The accredited organization often receives more in-depth information that can be used internally to prioritize activities to improve quality and safety. The implicit expectation is that the accredited organization will use this feedback to improve.

The duration of a survey and the composition of the survey team for on-site or remote review of documents vary greatly and are typically determined by the size and complexity of services offered by the organization. Surveys may include a presurvey phase conducted remotely, an on-site survey phase, and a postsurvey follow-up phase for deficiency resolution. Between review cycles (typically two- to three-year cycles), accrediting agencies may also have intracycle monitoring requirements that require submission of data, self-assessments, or attestations of process completion. In addition, if performance measures are included in the accreditation process, these measures may be assessed annually and organizations' accreditation status recalculated annually as well. The accrediting agency charges a fee to the accredited organization on a sliding scale that reflects the size and complexity of the organization and the number of surveyor hours or days required for the review. Costs for survey preparation, hosting the survey team for the on-site survey process, intracycle monitoring, and fees assessed for the regular survey cycle are also factors considered as organizations choose an accreditation agency.

Use of Accreditation in Healthcare

Insurers

Before the emergence of health maintenance organizations (HMOs), insurers were regulated primarily though state insurance laws. Through the 1980s, accountability for HMOs, which emerged in the late 1970s and early 1980s and combined insurance with varying degrees of oversight of clinical delivery functions, remained largely within an insurance regulatory framework. Accountability for care in HMOs that employed physicians or ran hospitals was subject to the same licensing and accreditation standards as those of other hospitals and physicians. Initially, HMO functions related to utilization or quality management or contractually imposed controls on physicians or other providers received little or no oversight.

Not motivated by these limited regulatory requirements, HMO accountability instead grew in response to market forces, specifically pressures from the purchasers of healthcare for more detailed information on the quality of services provided by HMOs. One manifestation of this pressure was the creation of voluntary accreditation processes by such organizations as the National Committee for Quality Assurance (NCQA), URAC (formerly known as the Utilization Review Accreditation Commission), and the Accreditation Association for Ambulatory Health Care (AAAHC). Accreditation may encompass an entire health plan's operations or may focus on a specific function within the health plan, such as disease management or pharmacy management. For some accrediting bodies for health plans, *certification* denotes review and approval of a part of an organization's operations and *accreditation* denotes review and approval of the entire organization.

Although some large employers (e.g., Ford, Boeing) have historically required health plan accreditation, in the past relatively few other employers have. With the increased regulation and emphasis on accountability and quality that began in the latter half of the 2000s and intensified with the passage of the ACA in 2010, 48 states, the District of Columbia, and the Federal Employee Plan have begun to recognize private accreditation as fulfilling part or all of HMO licensure requirements (URAC 2013).

In addition, CMS has issued rules that allow HMOs and preferred provider organizations (PPOs) to substitute deemed status by CMS-approved accrediting bodies for most CMS requirements related to the Medicare Advantage program. Because the accreditation process for Medicare HMOs and PPOs overlaps significantly with the distinct Medicare Stars Quality rating system that rewards plans for excellence in healthcare quality and health plan operations, more and more Medicare managed care organizations are seeking accreditation.

New programs are continually being assessed for the possibility of accreditation. For example, patient-centered medical homes (PCMHs), in which a small group of primary care and specialist providers are responsible for a cohort of patients, can become accredited, although only a small percentage of them have undergone the accreditation process. In addition, accreditation programs for accountable care organizations (ACOs), which are medical groups or independent practice associations that serve similar functions to PCMHs but on a larger scale and with a wider scope, have also been developed. Six organizations have enrolled in NCQA's (2014a) ACO accreditation program as early adopters: Billings Clinic, the Children's Hospital of Philadelphia, Crystal Run Healthcare, Essentia Health, HealthPartners, and Kelsey-Seybold Clinic. NCQA expects many additional ACOs to seek accreditation.

NCQA was one of the early pioneers of health plan accreditation. Both health plans and private purchasers' demands for accountability strongly influenced NCQA's early development. As a result, NCQA became an independent nonprofit organization in 1990 and has evolved to include directors on its board from consumer, purchaser, provider, and other healthcare sectors.

As a prime example of the accreditation process, NCQA accreditation has changed in important ways. Initially the focus of accreditation was primarily on internal organizational operations. Standards were applied in key operational areas such as utilization management (UM). An example from the 2014 set of standards (NCQA 2014d) is UM 5:

5. Timeliness of UM Decisions (UM 5)

Does the organization use time frames specific to the clinical urgency of a situation when it makes coverage decisions?

Does the organization notify members and practitioners of coverage decisions within the required time frames?

This standard is one of the 15 standards that relate to utilization management in the set of NCQA accreditation standards for managed care plans. This approach is paralleled in other accreditation programs. In the URAC accreditation process, an example standard in the utilization management area is titled "P-UM 1-Independent Review Process."

Where NCQA has differed from other health plan–accrediting bodies is in the development and implementation of a set of clinical performance measures, the Healthcare Effectiveness Data and Information Set (HEDIS). The goal was to create a reliable, feasible, and standard set of clinical performance measures that would provide useful information on quality for purchasers and consumers. HEDIS includes more than 100 performance measures or submeasures, many of which are specified for use at both plan and physician office practice levels.

In 1999, NCQA began to incorporate performance on selected HEDIS measures as an integral and substantial portion of the overall accreditation score, representing a major change in accreditation practice. NCQA accreditation also includes performance on Consumer Assessment of Healthcare Providers and Systems (CAHPS), a survey of member satisfaction with care and health plan operations. A list of measures included in 2014 accreditation is provided in Exhibit 19.2.

NCQA (2014b) reports its accreditation decisions on a public website—Health Care Quality Report Cards—as *excellent, commendable, accredited, provisional, interim,* or *denied.* The website also includes plan-specific information about performance on accreditation standards and HEDIS measures grouped in five categories understandable to consumers (Access and Service, Qualified Providers, Staying Healthy, Getting Better, and Living with Illness).

In summary, for managed care organizations (both HMOs and PPOs), the market—driven primarily by private purchasers, Medicare, and state Medicaid agencies—has played a larger role in the evolution of accountability than it has in the physician or hospital sectors.

Providers Across the Continuum
Hospitals
Accountability for hospital quality in the United States has relied primarily on regulation and accreditation, both of which are highly influenced by professionalism and professionals. Hospital licensure is codified in laws at the state level and usually is overseen by state-appointed medical or hospital boards, the majority of whose members are physicians. However, the federal government, in its role as the largest purchaser of hospital care in the United States through the Medicare program, has played the most prominent government role in defining hospital accountability. The 1964 legislation that created the program required hospitals participating in Medicare to undergo a federal regulatory review and certification by the organization now called CMS. As an alternative to federal review, the legislation allowed hospitals to participate in Medicare through deemed status based on accreditation by a private body, specifically the Joint Commission on Accreditation of Hospitals (now

EXHIBIT 19.2
Measures Included in NCQA Accreditation in 2014

Measure	Product			Source
	Commercial	Medicare	Medicaid	
Adult BMI Assessment	•	•	•	HEDIS
Antidepressant Medication Management (Both Rates)	•	•	•	HEDIS
Appropriate Testing for Children with Pharyngitis	•		•	HEDIS
Appropriate Treatment for Children with Upper Respiratory Infection	•		•	HEDIS
Avoidance of Antibiotic Treatment with Acute Bronchitis	•		•	HEDIS
Breast Cancer Screening	•	•	•	HEDIS
Cervical Cancer Screening	•		•	HEDIS
Childhood Immunization Status (Combination 2)	•		•	HEDIS
Chlamydia Screening in Women (Total Rate)	•		•	HEDIS
Cholesterol Management for Patients with Cardiovascular Conditions (LDL-C Screening Only)	•	•	•	HEDIS
Claims Processing	•			CAHPS
Colorectal Cancer Screening	•	•		HEDIS
Comprehensive Diabetes Care (Eye Examination, LDL-C Screening, Hemoglobin A1c Testing, Medical Attention for Nephropathy)	•	•	•	HEDIS
Comprehensive Diabetes Care—HbA1c Poorly Controlled (>9.0%)	•	•	•	HEDIS
Controlling High Blood Pressure	•	•	•	HEDIS
Customer Service	•		•	CAHPS
Flu Vaccinations for Adults Ages 18–64	•			CAHPS
Flu Vaccinations for Adults Ages 65 and Older		•		CAHPS
Follow-Up After Hospitalization for Mental Illness (7-Day Rate Only)	•	•	•	HEDIS
Follow-Up for Children Prescribed ADHD Medication (Both Rates)	•		•	HEDIS
Getting Care Quickly	•	•	•	CAHPS

(Continued)

EXHIBIT 19.2
Measures Included in NCQA Accreditation in 2014 *(continued)*

Measure	Product			Source
	Commercial	**Medicare**	**Medicaid**	
Getting Needed Care	•	•	•	CAHPS
Glaucoma Screening in Older Adults		•		HEDIS
How Well Doctors Communicate	•	•	•	CAHPS
Medical Assistance with Smoking and Tobacco Use Cessation (Advising Smokers and Tobacco Users to Quit)	•	•	•	CAHPS
Osteoporosis Management in Women Who Had a Fracture		•		HEDIS
Persistence of Beta-Blocker Treatment After a Heart Attack	•	•		HEDIS
Pharmacotherapy Management of COPD Exacerbation (Both Rates)	•	•	•	HEDIS
Pneumococcal Vaccination Status for Older Adults		•		CAHPS
Prenatal and Postpartum Care (Both Rates)			•	HEDIS
Prenatal and Postpartum Care (Postpartum Rate Only)	•			HEDIS
Rating of All Health Care	•	•	•	CAHPS
Rating of Health Plan	•	•	•	CAHPS
Rating of Personal Doctor	•	•	•	CAHPS
Rating of Specialist Seen Most Often	•	•	•	CAHPS
Use of Appropriate Medications for People with Asthma (Total Rate)			•	HEDIS
Use of High-Risk Medications in the Elderly (Rate 1)		•		HEDIS
Use of Imaging Studies for Low Back Pain	•		•	HEDIS
Use of Spirometry Testing in the Assessment and Diagnosis of COPD	•	•	•	HEDIS
Weight Assessment and Counseling for Nutrition and Physical Activity for Children/Adolescents (Total of All Ages for Each of the Three Rates)	•		•	HEDIS

Source: Data from NCQA (2014e).

known as The Joint Commission). The legislation invited other organizations to also apply for deeming status, and in 1965 the American Osteopathic Association's Healthcare Facilities Accreditation Program (HFAP) was also approved. Not until 2008 was another accreditation agency approved—Det Norske Veritas (DNV) Healthcare's National Integrated Accreditation for Healthcare Organizations (NIAHO)—and most recently, the Center for Improvement in Healthcare (CIHQ) was approved in 2013.

The majority of hospitals in the United States are accredited. The Joint Commission (2013a), the most mature of the accrediting organizations, is also by far the largest with more than 4,000 general, children's, long-term acute, psychiatric, rehabilitation, and specialty hospitals. DNV (2014) has accredited more than 500 hospitals since 2008 and listed 352 accredited hospitals on its website at the beginning of 2014. HFAP (2014) listed more than 200 accredited hospitals on its website at the beginning of 2014; the number of CIHQ-accredited hospitals is not yet known. The National Center for Health Statistics (2012b) reports that healthcare expenditures amount to $2.6 trillion annually (17.9 percent of the gross domestic product), with 40.1 percent of expenditures paid through public funds and 31.4 percent of the expenditures attributed to hospital care. The financial viability of most hospitals depends on their ability to participate in the Medicare program. In their distrust of direct government oversight and yet with a need to participate in Medicare, most hospitals seek accreditation by The Joint Commission (Greenberg 1998). In addition, 46 states and one territory license hospitals on the basis of attainment of accreditation by The Joint Commission.

Accreditation agencies base their evaluations of hospitals on published standards. To meet deemed status requirements, the agencies are preapproved by CMS to ensure that their standard foundation meets or exceeds the Conditions of Participation for Hospitals (42 C.F.R. 482) and the State Operations Manual: Survey Protocol, Regulations, and Interpretive Guidelines for Hospitals (CMS 2014) and that the survey process includes unannounced on-site surveys at least every 36 months. For accreditation to be granted, hospitals must be in compliance with the CMS conditions. If a hospital is found to be out of compliance with the CMS conditions during the survey, CMS requires an on-site follow-up survey to ensure that compliance has been achieved. The agency standards for accreditation vary, however. Exhibit 19.3 outlines the chapters of each organization's accreditation standards for comparison. The intracycle monitoring process also varies among the agencies, ranging from triennial surveys (HFAP) to annual self-assessments (The Joint Commission) or annual surveys (DNV). The Joint Commission has also been on the forefront of public transparency by including on its website not only the organizations' accreditation status but also their comparative performance with respect to discrete National Patient Safety Goals and quality goals based on ORYX data (e.g., acute myocardial infarction, heart failure,

EXHIBIT 19.3 Accreditation Standard Chapter Comparison

The Joint Commission	HFAP	DNV NIAHO	CIHQ
• Environment of Care • Emergency Management • Human Resources • Infection Prevention and Control • Information Management • Leadership • Life Safety • Medication Management • Medical Staff • National Patient Safety Goals • Nursing • Performance Improvement • Provision of Care, Treatment, and Services • Record of Care, Treatment, and Services • Rights and Responsibilities of the Individual • Transplant Safety • Waived Testing	• Section One: The Accreditation Process • Section Two: Organizational Management • Administration of the Organizational Environment • Allied Health Practitioners • Medical Staff • Required Committees • Other Required Activities • Medical Disaster Committee (Function) • Joint Advisory Committee (Function) • Medical Records Committee (Function) • Mortality Review Committee (Function) • Pharmacy & Therapeutics Committee (Function) • Library Committee (Function) • Tissue Audit Committee (Function) • Transfusion Review Committee (Function) • Tumor Evaluation Committee (Function) • Infection Control Committee	• Human Resources Management • Section Three: Support Services • Infection Control • Materials Management • Professional Medical Library • Medical Records (Health Information) Services • Physical Environment Services • Quality Assessment—Improvement • Organ Procurement • Section Four: Patient Diagnostic and Therapeutic Services • Multidisciplinary Patient Assessments and Plans of Care • Nursing Department • Respiratory Care Services • Cardiovascular Services • Diagnostic Radiology and Radiation Therapy Services • Emergency Services • Endoscopic Services • Laboratory Services • Nuclear Medicine Services	• Nutritional Services • Pharmacy Services/Medication Use • Physical Rehabilitation Services/Integrated Mutidisciplinary Program • Physical Rehabilitation Services/Physical Therapy • Physical Rehabilitation Services/Occupational Therapy • Physical Rehabilitation Services/Speech Therapy • Physical Rehabilitation Services/Audiology Services • Psychiatric Hospital/Unit—Non-Distinct Part, Non-PPS Excluded Units • Distinct Part Psychiatric Unit/Prospective Payment System Excluded Unit • Substance Abuse Services • Special Care Units • Surgical Services • Outpatient Surgical Services • Outpatient Services • Swing Beds

DNV NIAHO	CIHQ
• Quality Management System • Governing Body • Chief Executive Officer • Medical Staff • Nursing Services • Staffing Management • Medication Management • Surgical Services • Anesthesia Services • Laboratory Services • Respiratory Care Services • Medical Imaging • Nuclear Medicine Services • Rehabilitation Services • Emergency Department • Outpatient Services • Dietary Services • Patient Rights • Infection Prevention and Control • Medical Records Service • Discharge Planning • Utilization Review • Physical Environment • Organ, Eye and Tissue Procurement	• Governance & Leadership • Quality Assessment & Performance Improvement • Medical Staff • Human Resources • Managing the Care Environment • Infection Prevention & Control • Emergency Preparedness • Utilization Review • Patient Rights • Medication Management • Management of the Medical Record • Use of Restraint & Seclusion • Targeted Patient Quality & Safety Practices • Anesthesia Services • Dietary (Nutrition) Services • Discharge Planning Services • Emergency Services • Laboratory Services • Organ, Tissue & Eye Procurement • Nuclear Medicine Services • Nursing Services • Operative & Invasive Services • Outpatient Services • Radiology Services • Rehabilitation Services • Respiratory Services • Psychiatric Hospitals • Long-Term Care Services

Sources: CIHQ (2014); DNV (2012); HFAP (2011); Joint Commission (2013b).

community-acquired pneumonia, pregnancy and related conditions, surgical infections, childhood asthma care, additional national standardized core measures for other diseases and conditions).

Nursing Homes

Nursing home accreditation has been limited, largely because of the dominance of state Medicaid programs (Medicare accounts for less than 10 percent of nursing home expenditures) and self-pay (private pay) as the means of financing nursing home care. The National Center for Health Statistics' (2012b) most recent data list nursing home care as 3.2 percent of healthcare expenditures. CMS (Medicare and Medicaid) and the states (Medicaid) have developed an extensive set of regulatory standards and a government survey and certification program to enforce nursing home regulations. Given the less-than-adequate quality of nursing home care and, in some instances, outright abuse of patients in nursing homes in the past, most public advocacy groups have been strongly opposed to allowing deemed status out of fear that the largely for-profit nursing home industry would try to lower current regulatory standards. Thus, no legislation authorizes CMS or states to allow deemed status in Medicare or Medicaid for private accrediting bodies to substitute for governmental survey and certification of nursing homes. The Joint Commission and others offer accreditation to nursing homes, but few apply because the deemed status and market benefits are not present.

Home Health Care

Home health care and hospice agencies may be the fastest-growing segments of the continuum of care as healthcare reform encourages providers to design and deliver models of care that are more patient centered. The National Center for Health Statistics (2007a, 2007b) reported 1.5 million patients enrolled in home health care (average enrollment of 315 days) and 1 million discharges from hospice care (average enrollment of 65 days). CMS has granted deeming status to several accreditation agencies for home care, including the Accreditation Commission for Health Care, Community Health Accreditation Program, and The Joint Commission. It is not clear what percentage of the agencies are accredited, but The Joint Commission (2013b) states on its website that 7,000 agencies are accredited with it, and the Community Health Accreditation Program (2014) website states that 8,300 agencies are accredited with it.

Ambulatory Care

Accreditation of ambulatory care and ambulatory surgery practices is growing. The emergence of large regional or national for-profit entities providing imaging (magnetic resonance imaging, mammography), renal dialysis, cancer treatment, and other services—combined with purchasers', insurers', and the public's growing recognition of the wide variation in the quality and cost of ambulatory care services—has prompted a number of programs and entities to offer accreditation of ambulatory care programs. Some examples include accreditation of office-based surgery (e.g., by the AAAHC, the American Association for Accreditation of Ambulatory Surgery Facilities, The Joint Commission) and imaging centers (e.g., by the American College of Radiology, The Joint Commission), but none of these activities has achieved close to universal acceptance, even when deemed by CMS, with the exception of the deemed accreditation of mammography centers by the American College of Radiology.

Accreditation has been most widespread in renal dialysis, where the dominance of Medicare as a payer and the creation of deemed status for some parts of the program by CMS have created close to universal accreditation of programs. However, most insurers, including Medicare, have few, if any, requirements other than licensure for ambulatory care sites (e.g., physician groups, individual offices) to participate in their programs even though the National Center for Health Statistics (2012a) reports 1.2 billion visits annually (averaging four visits per person), accounting for 21.2 percent of healthcare expenditures (National Center for Health Statistics 2012b). A notable and ultimately unsuccessful attempt at ambulatory care accreditation was the American Medical Accreditation Program, created by the American Medical Association to offer accreditation to physician office practices. A lack of regulatory and market incentives from the public and private sectors and the concern of some specialty boards that a physician's office accreditation would be redundant alongside board certification of the individual physician appear to have been major factors in the program's demise.

The Future of Accreditation: Challenges and Changes

If accreditation is to remain an important part of ensuring accountability, it will need to evolve in response to market forces, specifically the evolution of the healthcare system with healthcare reform. The current accreditation system is segmented, or conducted within silos across the continuum of care, as each healthcare provider decides whether and from which organization to seek accreditation. One of the most important challenges to accreditation is the proliferation of new accreditation services and products and the types of organizations that provide them.

For example, most of the growth in hospital revenues since the mid-1990s has been in ambulatory and ancillary services; some hospitals now receive the majority of their income from services other than inpatient care.

This movement also has given rise to myriad outpatient facilities that provide some components of inpatient services, such as urgent care centers, ambulatory surgery centers, and office-based surgery sites. An accreditation process for hospitals that focuses largely on inpatient standards would not address this new reality, nor would it address the handoffs that occur as patients transition across the continuum of services. Services such as disease management, mental health benefits management, and pharmacy benefits management may be provided through contracts with separate entities—entities for which no system of accountability for quality and safety exists. The current accreditation model that focuses on hospitals or individual providers across the continuum, even if it addresses delegated functions, does not capture these activities and sites fully. The ACA includes a number of policies to help physicians, hospitals, and other caregivers improve the safety and quality of patient care across care transitions. It is hoped that delivery system reforms, by linking payments to outcomes, will help improve the health of individuals and communities in addition to slowing cost growth. As the ACA is implemented, and as providers across the continuum of care must increasingly work together, accreditation models will also need to develop across the continuum. Although The Joint Commission will accredit multiple programs within an organization together, the accreditation is linked to the individual program that aligns with CMS reimbursement models and deeming status for the individual programs.

Accreditation will need to evolve quickly toward a more flexible, multientity, performance-based process to serve both the public interest and that of these new organizations. Accreditation also will need to address issues related to coordination of services for patients and data sharing among the increasingly fragmented entities involved in healthcare. The US Department of Health & Human Services (HHS 2014) released preliminary outcomes from the Medicare reform, which appears to have helped doctors, hospitals, and other providers better coordinate care for Medicare patients through ACOs. ACOs create incentives for healthcare providers to work together to treat an individual patient across care settings, including doctors' offices, hospitals, and long-term care facilities. The Medicare Shared Savings Program will reward ACOs that lower the growth in healthcare costs while meeting performance standards on quality of care and putting patients first. Accreditation models are being explored to align with the ACO model. NCQA (2014a) has already published one program for ACO accreditation.

Another factor that continues to gain momentum is public demand for information that allows comparison of individual clinicians, clinical groups, hospitals, and health plans regarding clinical quality and cost. The need for quality measurement data to use as the basis for payment in the growing number of pay-for-performance programs has further accelerated the demand for this information (Cromwell et al. 2011). Reliance on structure and process standards to provide a decision on accreditation for a single organization can provide only limited meaningful information to consumers or purchasers. In other words, although this information helps to differentiate between accredited and nonaccredited organizations, it is less helpful in differentiating accredited organizations with respect to specific services or programs. This lack of differentiation is especially evident in the hospital sector, where virtually all hospitals are accredited.

Given the costs of information gathering and the low fiscal margins in virtually all sectors of healthcare, accrediting organizations and others will need to find ways to reduce the number of redundant standards and measures and the cost of data collection. Without these developments, efforts to enhance accountability at the provider level are likely to result in redundant and dysfunctional evaluations—and unnecessary costs—and to increase the resistance of those being evaluated. On the other hand, in the health plan sector, the ACA and other reforms have created financial incentives for insurers to pursue accreditation as part of a strategy to improve healthcare quality.

As noted, NCQA now includes performance measures as part of health plan accreditation and reports information on accreditation of HMOs and PPOs at multiple levels of performance. Likewise, as noted, The Joint Commission reports comparative data on its website that are more useful to the public and purchasers in selecting healthcare provider organizations, especially at the hospital or large group level. However, because of issues with small sample size (especially within a given health plan), information on clinical performance measures—although already collected at the individual physician level for some measures—cannot be reported reliably for most measures at the physician level. In addition, the system in which a physician provides care can influence the physician's patient outcomes (Fung et al. 2010). Pennsylvania's release of surgeon-specific mortality data demonstrated that some surgeons who operated in multiple hospitals had better-than-average (statewide) results in one hospital and worse-than-average results in another hospital. Thus, collection of the depth and quantity of information necessary to prepare reports that are reliable and valid at the physician small group or individual physician level will pose a formidable challenge.

Nevertheless, with the increasing demand for value-based purchasing—purchasing healthcare services on the basis of quality and safety, not just costs—interest in measuring performance in physician offices has increased. The Medicare Physician Group Practice Demonstration, the first pay-for-performance initiative for physicians under Medicare, provides incentive payments to providers to improve the quality and the cost efficiency of healthcare services (CMS 2011). Accurate measures of quality are instrumental to the success of the program. Accreditation cannot play a central role in accountability in the future unless it can provide the public (purchasers, insurers, consumers, patients) with reliable and valid comparative information on quality and safety.

Other groups not tied directly to accreditation have created report cards of various types. Most of these report cards rely on consumer surveys of varying reliability or validity. Few use random samples or have large enough sample sizes to offer valid comparisons between entities. Some larger HMOs rate providers, and others furnish basic demographic information about physicians in their clinical networks. In another effort, the Pacific Business Group on Health and the Integrated Healthcare Association created a more sophisticated set of measures to rate providers in relation to their managed care organization membership; this set included physician group practice information for larger physician groups in the California market (Damberg 2009).

Although some large purchasers are able to use current information on HMO quality as part of their purchasing decisions, most consumers feel overwhelmed by the number of sites and are distrustful of conflicting report cards or ratings. The result is that consumers still rely largely on word-of-mouth information from friends, relatives, coworkers, or their physicians in making healthcare choices.

The long-term hope for more effective accreditation and information about quality depends on enhancement of information technology use in healthcare. The wide availability of web-enabled data collection eventually may enable accreditation based on real-time measurement of a rich array of clinical structure, process, and outcome performance measures that also can be used for quality monitoring, rather than on retrospective measures or survey-assessed compliance with standards alone.

Accreditation Sets the Bar Too Low
Issue
Accreditation, especially when it is a prerequisite for participating in large insurance programs such as Medicare, must be constructed to set a basic level of acceptable quality that encompasses the minimal level required by law and regulation. If the threshold is set too far above this minimal level, many or most providers will not be able to achieve accreditation, thus reducing the information about them that enables consumer choice and adversely affecting access for many consumers. Most important, the fewer organizations enrolled in the accreditation process, the less influence accreditation has on improving the quality and safety of care. On the other hand, if the threshold is set too close to the regulatory minimum, providers with serious quality defects may gain access to the insurance program and patients will receive less protection from harm. This dilemma is similar to that seen in licensing and has led some

to see accreditation as a basic floor of requirements that everyone doing business in a given area should achieve. Thus, if regulatory requirements are considered the minimum level of performance that must be achieved to remain in business, accreditation could be described as a basic level of quality and safety that should be achieved.

Where accreditation is optional, providers who do not attempt to achieve accreditation avoid the cost of accreditation and the risk of not passing. With no pressure to participate, a high threshold could discourage providers from seeking accreditation because the risk of failure is far worse than not being evaluated at all. In a competitive environment with multiple accrediting bodies to choose from, purchasers or consumers may or may not distinguish one body's accreditation from that of another even though their standards are very different. A move by one accrediting body to raise standards may be seen by its competitor(s) as an opportunity to gain market share by retaining a lower standard. When neither strong pressure from state regulation nor incentives (e.g., differential payment or selection) from private purchasers exist to push standards to high levels, provider organizations may move to the easiest accreditation program or drop accreditation altogether. Anecdotal information suggests a growing trend in the hospital industry of hospitals not seeking accreditation and relying on state agency oversight for CMS participation.

Finally, the governance of many accrediting organizations is a concern. As noted previously in this chapter, accreditation traditionally has been a bridge between professionalism and regulation. In many instances, professionals have created accrediting bodies to drive quality assessment and improvement and to reduce the need for direct government regulation. Many accrediting organizations emanate from professional groups themselves. Although involvement of those within the profession is important in setting credible standards, if the interests of other stakeholders—particularly consumers—do not balance this involvement, the accrediting organization may refrain from setting standards that could disadvantage members of the professional organization that controls or strongly influences it. Accrediting bodies given deemed status by the federal government must act in the interest of the public.

Analysis and Response

Given these disparate forces, the decision on where to set the threshold of acceptable performance can be challenging. The problem of setting the bar too low often resolves itself over time because nearly all accreditation programs implement new standards and requirements that periodically raise the bar. Even more important in terms of raising the bar over time are the inclusion of quality improvement standards that emphasize demonstration of improvement on clinical measures, the relative performance of an entity on clinical measures as part of its accreditation score, and the incremental inclusion of specific patient safety goals in the accreditation process.

The decision on where to set the "passing" level may be even more problematic to the degree that accrediting bodies are strongly influenced or controlled by the providers they accredit or, in contrast, by those that advocate higher quality but are not willing to pay more to attain it. One approach to addressing this challenge is to seek broad input from those being accredited and those desiring accountability through formal groups such as multi- and single-stakeholder advisory councils. Structuring the accrediting body's board of directors or committees that have decision-making authority so that they are representative of all the relevant stakeholder groups is also helpful in addressing this challenge. In addition, the accrediting body's collaboration with other multistakeholder groups, such as the National Quality Forum, helps to create stakeholder buy-in.

Empirically, the environmental landscape can cause standards to tighten. For HMOs and PPOs, accreditation is seen not as a competitive advantage but as a minimum requirement. Partly in response to increased interest in accreditation, beginning with the 2011 reporting year NCQA began to tighten the scoring of its performance measures. Although this scoring adjustment is not projected to reduce the number of accredited organizations, it will reduce the number of organizations that receive the highest levels of accreditation (excellent and commendable), thereby differentiating the top performers from the remaining organizations.

An important factor in the usefulness of accreditation is the careful determination of a standard's importance and evidence base. Good standards must be based on a carefully structured determination of what evidence can be found and documented to support a conclusion that compliance with the standard in question is critical to good quality and safety. In the case of endpoint outcomes, any endpoint seen as important and desirable by those with an interest in the action should be a standard. However, a more formal, consensual process is valuable in determining the scope and definition of critical outcomes. Although outcomes often are considered the most desirable type of requirement or standard, numerous instances exist in which outcomes are not measurable, are so infrequent (e.g., death from wrong-site surgery), or are so remote in time (e.g., myocardial infarction from untreated hypertension) that using a process or structural standard as a proxy is more desirable. Any standard—and its corresponding metric based on a structure, a process, or an intermediate outcome—must be linked to some desired outcome. Structural or process standards can relate to either administrative or clinical systems.

In the administrative realm, few, if any, experimental studies suggest links to health outcomes, and most links rely on face validity (including laws) and expert opinion (e.g., Baldrige National Quality Award criteria for managing and improving quality; advisory group expert advice on the role of organizational leadership in improving safety). To avoid meaningless and burdensome administrative standards, careful dialogue and review by experts external to the staff of the accrediting body are critical. In clinical services, evidence should come from experimental studies (e.g., studies on safe practices and infection-control procedures such as hand washing) and, when possible, from randomized controlled trials (e.g., the guideline that HbA1c levels in diabetics should be lower than 9.0).

To transform standards into information about an organization's performance, accreditation must include some metric or verification process to ensure that the organization has met the required standards and criteria. Few means of gathering data exist (see Exhibit 19.1). Historically, accreditation has included only structural or process standards measured by reviews of documentation, interviews with patients or staff, or observation of certain processes. Because this type of review is subjective, the reviewers' levels of expertise, experience, and survey training were crucial for valid measurement.

Since 1999, in assessing health plan accreditation NCQA has included scores of plans' relative performance on measures of clinical processes or intermediate outcomes (HEDIS) and on surveys of patient experience of care (CAHPS). Since 2001, The Joint Commission has included similar measures of intermediate and physiological outcomes in the ORYX measures that hospitals use, and CAHPS results from hospitals to survey the patient experience. Relative performance on these measures was included in a subset called "accountability measures" within The Joint Commission accreditation standards beginning in 2012. Four criteria for use in selecting which measures to include in accreditation decisions have been identified (Chassin et al. 2010): (1) a strong evidence base shows that the care process leads to improved outcomes; (2) the measure accurately captures whether the evidence-based care process has, in fact, been provided; (3) the measure addresses a process that has few intervening care processes that must occur before the improved outcome is realized; and (4) the implementation of the measure has little or no chance of inducing unintended adverse consequences.

Clinical performance measures and patient experience-of-care surveys, especially when used for public accountability, are, in most cases, based on higher levels of scientific evidence than on-site reviews of structures or processes are. This scientific evidence links them directly to final outcomes (e.g., survival, quality of life). Thus, clinical performance measures and patient experience-of-care surveys provide a view of quality unavailable in reviews of structures and administrative processes alone. In addition, if these performance measures are collected from a sufficient sampling frame and reported in a timely manner, those being evaluated can use them as internal quality improvement measures. Thus, the potential exists for performance measures to serve as an effective and efficient means for both external reporting and internal quality improvement purposes. If a measure is not useful for internal quality improvement because it measures a process or an outcome that is not under the control of the measured entity, the measure is probably not relevant as an accountability measure either. Accountability must be based on the ability to control—at least in part—the things for which one is held accountable.

External measurement of outcomes may be the ultimate goal in most instances, but in some areas, such as safety, structural or process measures of risk reduction are necessary even if the undesirable outcome never occurs. Rare adverse or sentinel events may happen even when the infrastructure is in place to prevent such events, which makes it difficult to judge quality even in accredited organizations. Verification of structural or process elements critical to quality and safety remains a part of accreditation. In addition, because of coding and reporting problems, insufficient sample sizes, or a lack of robust electronic information systems, reliable or valid performance measures on many aspects of quality are currently impossible or prohibitively expensive to collect. Thus, metrics other than performance measures still play a central and critical role in providing accountability for quality.

Accreditation Fails to Provide Critical Information Needed for Either Consumer Choice or Quality Improvement
Issue
In the past, most accreditation decisions have been reported as pass/fail or, in many instances, as a list of the organizations that received accreditation, with no reporting of those that attempted and failed or those that did not even attempt accreditation. Although this pass/fail information can be considered as meeting the basic intent of accreditation (to ensure that a basic floor—beyond the minimum—has been met), most accreditation processes now include a rich set of information that can be used for comparison or choice. Moreover, the scoring or determination of achieving a threshold is not an exact science. Reasonable individuals can disagree on which requirements are most critical or should contribute most to the scoring. Finally, the level of data publicly reported may reflect the relative influence of those who want to limit external reporting and those who want more public accountability.

Analysis and Response
In most traditional forms of accreditation, the only information provided to those outside the entity being accredited was whether the entity received accreditation. In some cases, this information did not include whether a group had been evaluated but was denied accreditation. In some cases, such as airline safety, public knowledge that a given airline, airplane, and pilot are

certified may be enough, but where personal services are involved, a reasonable argument can be made that the public needs more detailed information. Although accreditation itself is an important differentiation from nonaccredited status, consumer and payer demand for more in-depth information about quality in healthcare has increased.

CMS (2013b) now publishes performance data on its Quality Care Finder website, which includes data on hospitals, nursing homes, home health agencies, dialysis centers, physicians, and Medicare plans. Both the number of metrics submitted and the number of organizations submitting data have progressively increased. For hospitals, some of the same measures are reported by both CMS and The Joint Commission on their public websites, allowing the public to compare performance on a number of metrics. Although the data are now publicly available, consumers may still find it challenging to sift through all of the metrics and interpret the information provided to make decisions on where to seek healthcare based on performance. The methodology for reporting these metrics varies from simple plus or minus signs to reporting actual performance scores and could be overwhelming to the average layperson.

NCQA reports accreditation status in one of its annual publications (the *State of Health Care Quality* report), available on the NCQA website. It also reports accreditation status in a publicly available data set (Quality Compass) both as ranked categories based on accreditation scores (excellent, commendable, accredited, provisional, and interim) and in the five major categories discussed earlier (Access and Service, Qualified Providers, Staying Healthy, Getting Better, and Living with Illness). Using NCQA data, *Consumers Union* publishes numeric and star plan rankings on its website.

The Cost of Accreditation Is Not Worth the Benefit
Issue

The concern that the cost of accreditation is not worth the benefit it provides is raised most frequently by those undergoing (and directly paying for) accreditation. However, purchasers and consumers who benefit from (as well as indirectly pay for) accreditation should see a net benefit. The costs of accreditation, both indirect (e.g., preparation, data collection, reports) and direct (e.g., the fee paid to be reviewed), can be considerable—especially when accreditation relies heavily on paper documentation of large quantities of data or on extensive on-site inspections. If purchasers or consumers do not use or require accreditation, providers may feel that accreditation is not a cost-effective use of their resources. If accreditation is required, concerns still exist about whether the standards reflect critical components of quality and safety and whether the evaluation methods are the most efficient means for determining compliance with those standards. Any quality improvement or regulatory process has associated costs, but given the high and rising costs of healthcare, investment in a form of accreditation that does not bring real value—either to providers through quality improvement or to those using the services through assurance of quality or choice—should be questioned.

Analysis and Response

In its traditional form, accreditation is a mechanism for enhancing improvement in the quality and safety of healthcare and for providing accountability of the entity to other stakeholders (e.g., patients, consumers, purchasers, insurers, regulators). Ultimately, those who pay for healthcare services and ask for accountability for those services must determine whether the benefits of accreditation exceed its costs. A healthcare organization may choose to undergo accreditation by an outside entity as a benchmark for its overall internal quality improvement processes, but this benefit may not be sufficient—if purchasers and consumers do not use the results—for the organization to maintain its accreditation. Some public purchasers (CMS and the majority of Medicaid programs), some regulators (more than half of all states), and many large private purchasers (mostly *Fortune* 500 companies) require accreditation of health plans as a precursor to contracting with them, but many health plans do not experience enough pressure to force them to become accredited. Likewise, most states and CMS accept (deem) hospital accreditation in lieu of government survey and certification, but they do not require accreditation of hospitals; a (free) state survey for licensure and Medicare certification is an option provided that the state agencies have adequate staffing to cover additional surveys. Surveys of consumers and private purchasers (specifically those selecting health plans) indicate a minimal understanding of the value or use of accreditation in decision making, which presents a mixed picture of how, in actual practice, the costs and benefits of accreditation are weighed.

However, given the ongoing concerns about the quality and safety of care in hospitals, organizations need some form of accountability. The value of the most common alternatives to accreditation (i.e., reliance on professionalism and voluntary quality improvement, government regulation, or contractually defined performance measures) in ensuring accountability is far from proven.

Some believe that government regulation may be more desirable than, or may be a replacement for, voluntary (or deemed) accreditation. However, regulation is fraught with political problems and frequently lags behind changes in healthcare. The history of healthcare licensure, state mandates, and other regulatory processes shows ample evidence of the limitations of regulation as a means of providing accountability. Regulation is often an adversarial process in which political power, rather than evidence-based analysis, determines the outcome. Regulation is also a slow legislative process and may quickly outdate in a fast-paced technological society. Conway and

Berwick (2011) outline the challenge of evidence-based standards and the process to keep them current in the CMS Conditions of Participation, which were last systematically updated in 1986. In late 2011, CMS proposed revisions to the Conditions of Participation in three major areas that affect morbidity, mortality, and costs: transitions from the hospital, patient-centered care, and quality improvement programs. The *Federal Register* (October 24, 2011) published proposed rules in response to the president's Executive Order 13563 ("Improving Regulation and Regulatory Review," January 18, 2011), which sought to reduce the regulatory burden currently placed on hospitals. The removal of unnecessary regulation was projected to save more than $900 million annually.

Evidence that the benefits of accreditation outweigh the costs is building. Longo and colleagues (2007) demonstrated that hospitals accredited by The Joint Commission showed significant improvement in patient safety system implementation over 18 months, while nonaccredited hospitals did not. Menachemi and colleagues (2008) examined common surgical procedures in ambulatory surgery centers in Florida and compared outcomes in centers accredited by AAAHC or The Joint Commission to outcomes in nonaccredited centers. While patients at centers accredited by The Joint Commission were less likely to be hospitalized after a colonoscopy, no other differences were found. Lutfiyya and colleagues (2009) compared accredited and nonaccredited rural critical access hospitals on four clinical core process measures and found better performance on 4 of 16 indicators at accredited hospitals. Schmaltz and colleagues (2011) evaluated changes in hospital performance between 2004 and 2008 for hospitals accredited by The Joint Commission and nonaccredited hospitals by leveraging publicly reported measures required by CMS. These authors concluded that accredited hospitals tended to have better baseline performance in 2004, had larger gains over time, and were significantly more likely to have high performance in 2008 on 13 of the 16 standardized clinical performance measures.

In addition, state and federal requirements may push organizations to become accredited. For example, because of substantial overlap in the list of performance measures between those required for accreditation and those included in the Medicare Stars Quality financial incentive program, in which higher-performing plans are not only compensated for performing better but are also presented to potential Medicare enrollees as "better" choices, investing in the accreditation process may become a natural choice for many Medicare HMOs and PPOs. Another example involves the state of Massachusetts, which has a robust program to cover the uninsured not eligible for Medicaid and is the model for the products offered on the federal and state exchanges. Insurers offering coverage through the program are required to report HEDIS performance measures, and as Song and colleagues (2011) demonstrated, as long as payment reform included incentives tied to HEDIS measures on quality, cost savings for a large number of insured individuals could be achieved at the same time that quality of care was improved for the insured members. Furthermore, participation in the federal and state exchange products created by the ACA requires insurers to seek eventual accreditation (NCQA 2014c).

Finally, accreditation can create an active dialogue between those being held accountable and those desiring the accountability. In addition, because legislative action is not required, accrediting bodies can adjust more quickly to changes in the scope, modes, and technologies of delivered services. Finally, a healthcare provider that seeks voluntary accreditation demonstrates a desire to take ownership of and responsibility for its performance rather than only to meet an outside party's requirements. Ultimately, these providers—not government agencies and accrediting bodies—control the quality and safety of care for the public.

Conclusion

This chapter discusses accreditation as an approach to addressing accountability in healthcare. Accreditation in its traditional form has, in some areas of healthcare, provided a successful approach to measuring and reporting accountability. Healthcare clearly needs enhanced accountability. This need demands a robust set of metrics and accountability at multiple levels of the healthcare system. The challenge is whether accreditation can evolve to meet the expanded demand for accountability across the continuum of care rather than within individual segments of the continuum. An expanded scope of accreditation can help to meet that challenge, but major barriers, such as CMS reimbursement models, first must be overcome for that expanded scope to meet its full potential.

Study Questions

1. Compare and contrast the use of licensure and accreditation in terms of accountability and quality improvement.
2. What role can or should accreditation play in the future, as the public availability of performance data increases?
3. What roles do the market, regulation, and professionalism play in defining and promoting the use of accreditation as a means of accountability across the continuum of care? How would the implementation of a single-payer, government-financed system affect

it (e.g., if Medicare coverage were extended to everyone living in the United States)?

4. If the ultimate goal is better health outcomes for individuals and populations, can measurement of health outcomes alone substitute for structure and process measures? Why or why not?

References

Center for Improvement in Healthcare (CIHQ). 2014. "Accreditation Standards for Acute Care Hospitals." Effective January. http://cihq.org/ah/dl/ CIHQ%20Acute%20Care%20Hospital%20Accreditation%20Standards%20 -%20Effective%20January%202014%20Rev.8.pdf.

Centers for Medicare & Medicaid Services (CMS). 2014. *State Operations Manual: Appendix A—Survey Protocol, Regulations and Interpretive Guidelines for Hospitals*. Rev. 99. Updated January 31. www.cms.gov/Regulations-and-Guidance/Guidance/Manuals/downloads/som107ap_a_hospitals.pdf.

———. 2013a. *CMS-Approved Accreditation Organization Contact Information.* Updated August 9. www.cms.gov/SurveyCertificationGenInfo/Downloads/ AOContactInformation.pdf.

———. 2013b. "Quality Care Finder." Accessed December 23. www.medicare.gov/ quality-care-finder/.

———. 2011. "Medicare Physician Group Practice Demonstration: Physicians Groups Continue to Improve Quality and Generate Savings Under Medicare Physician Pay-for-Performance Demonstration." Fact sheet. Issued July. www.cms. gov/Medicare/Demonstration-Projects/DemoProjectsEvalRpts/downloads/ PGP_Fact_Sheet.pdf.

Chassin, M., J. Loeb, S. Schmaltz, and R. Wachter. 2010. "Accountability Measures—Using Measurement to Promote Quality Improvement." *New England Journal of Medicine* 363 (7): 683–88.

Community Health Accreditation Program. 2014. "About CHAP." Accessed February 20. http://chapinc.org/AboutCHAP.

Conway, P., and D. Berwick. 2011. "Improving the Rules for Hospital Participation in Medicare and Medicaid." *Journal of the American Medical Association* 306 (20): 2256–57.

Cromwell, J., M. G. Trisolini, G. C. Pope, J. B. Mitchell, and L. M. Greenwald (eds.). 2011. *Pay for Performance in Health Care: Methods and Approaches.* Research Triangle Park, NC: RTI Press. www.rti.org/pubs/bk-0002-1103-mitchell. pdf.

Damberg, C. L. 2009. "Taking Stock of Pay-for-Performance: A Candid Assessment from the Front Lines." *Health Affairs* 28 (2): 517–25.

Det Norske Veritas (DNV). 2014. "Hospital Accreditation." Accessed February 20. http://dnvglhealthcare.com/accreditations/hospital-accreditation.

———. 2012. *National Integrated Accreditation for Healthcare Organizations (NIAHO): Interpretive Guidelines and Surveyor Guidance.* Version 10.1. Effective November 1.

Fung, V., J. A. Schmittdiel, B. Fireman, A. Meer, S. Thomas, N. Smider, J. Hsu, and J. V. Selby. 2010. "Meaningful Variation in Performance: A Systematic Literature Review." *Medical Care* 48 (2): 140–48.

Greenberg, E. L. 1998. "How Accreditation Could Strengthen Local Public Health: An Examination of Models from Managed Care and Insurance Regulators." *Journal of Public Health Management and Practice* 4 (4): 33–37.

Healthcare Facilities Accreditation Program (HFAP). 2014. "Accredited Facilities." Accessed February 20. www.hfap.org/AccreditedFacilities/index.aspx.

———. 2011. "Table of Contents." *Accreditation Requirements for Healthcare Facilities.* Chicago: HFAP.

Joint Commission. 2013a. "Facts About Hospital Accreditation." Posted December. www.jointcommission.org/assets/1/6/Hospital_Accreditation_8_26_13.pdf.

———. 2013b. "Home Care Accreditation Overview: A Snapshot of the Accreditation Process." www.jointcommission.org/assets/1/6/FINAL-OME_overview_guide_2012.pdf.

Longo, D., J. Hewett, G. Bin, S. Schubert, and R. Kiely. 2007. "Hospital Patient Safety: Characteristics of Best-Performing Hospitals." *Journal of Healthcare Management* 52 (3): 188–204.

Lutfiyya, M., A. Sikka, S. Mehta, and M. Lipsky. 2009. "Comparison of US Accredited and Non-Accredited Rural Critical Access Hospitals." *International Journal for Quality in Health Care* 21 (2): 112–18.

Menachemi, N., A. Chukmaitov, S. Brown, C. Saunders, and R. Brooks. 2008. "Quality of Care in Accredited and Nonaccredited Ambulatory Surgical Centers." *The Joint Commission Journal on Quality and Patient Safety* 34 (9): 546–51.

Merriam-Webster. 2014. "Accountability" (definition). Accessed February 20. www.merriam-webster.com/dictionary/accountability.

National Center for Health Statistics. 2012a. "FastStats: Ambulatory Care Use and Physician Visits." www.cdc.gov/nchs/fastats/docvisit.htm.

———. 2012b. "FastStats: Health Expenditures." www.cdc.gov/nchs/data/hus/hus12.pdf#113.

———. 2007a. "FastStats: Home Health Care." www.cdc.gov/nchs/fastats/homehealthcare.htm.

———. 2007b. "FastStats: Hospice Care." www.cdc.gov/nchs/fastats/hospicecare.htm.

National Committee for Quality Assurance (NCQA). 2014a. "Accountable Care Organization Accreditation." Accessed February 7. www.ncqa.org/Programs/Accreditation/AccountableCareOrganizationACO.aspx.

———. 2014b. "Healthcare Quality Report Cards." Accessed February 20. http:// reportcard.ncqa.org/portal/home.aspx.

———. 2014c. "NCQA Health Plan Accreditation." Accessed February 20. www. ncqa.org/Portals/0/Programs/Accreditation/HPA_FINAL_%202.14.13. pdf.

———. 2014d. "2014 NCQA Health Plan Accreditation Requirements: What Does NCQA Look for When Reviewing Organizations?" Accessed February 20. www.ncqa.org/Portals/0/Programs/Accreditation/2014%20NCQA%20 HP%20requirements%20and%20HEDIS%20Measures-2.pdf.

———. 2014e. *2014 Standards and Guidelines for the Accreditation of Health Plans.* www.ncqa.org/PublicationsProducts/AccreditationProducts/HealthPlan Publications.aspx.

Nicklin, W. 2013. *The Value and Impact of Health Care Accreditation: A Literature Review.* Updated October. www.accreditation.ca/sites/default/files/value-and-impact-en.pdf.

Schmaltz, S., S. Williams, M. Chassin, J. Loeb, and R. Wachter. 2011. "Hospital Performance Trends on National Quality Measures and the Association with Joint Commission Accreditation." *Journal of Hospital Medicine* 6 (8): 454–61.

Song, Z., D. G. Safran, B. E. Landon, Y. He, R. P. Ellis, R. E. Mechanic, M. P. Day, and M. E. Chernew. 2011. "Health Care Spending and Quality in Year 1 of the Alternative Quality Contract." *New England Journal of Medicine* 365 (10): 909–18.

URAC. 2013. "State Recognition of URAC Accreditation." Updated October. www. urac.org/wp-content/uploads/Overview_All_Recog.pdf.

US Department of Health & Human Services (HHS). 2014. "Medicare's Delivery System Reform Initiatives Achieve Significant Savings and Quality Improvements—Off to a Strong Start." Press release. Issued January 30. www.hhs. gov/news/press/2014pres/01/20140130a.html.

HOW PURCHASERS SELECT AND PAY FOR VALUE: THE MOVEMENT TO VALUE-BASED PURCHASING

François de Brantes

I n early 2012, the Congressional Budget Office (CBO) issued a report on several decades' worth of pilots and demonstrations by the Centers for Medicare & Medicaid Services (CMS), all aimed at improving the quality and affordability of healthcare in the United States (Nelson 2012b). The news was sobering and highly informative and can be summarized simply: Quality improves when physicians, nurses, and other clinicians take a high-touch approach; affordability improves when payment models are designed with built-in savings.

The simplicity of these findings underscores the complexity of reforming the US healthcare system. If reform were simple, the findings would suggest that successful strategies could have been implemented long ago to the great benefit of all. And yet they have not. Why?

Most US workers receive healthcare coverage through their employer. The employer, in turn, contracts with an administrator, either to purchase healthcare coverage on behalf of the employees or to administer the benefits that the employer pays for directly. Employees are therefore removed from many of the purchasing decisions. Employers themselves are removed from the actual function of healthcare delivery and from the payment for services because the third-party administrator organizes and manages those functions. Attempts to control the rise of healthcare costs, reflected in premiums paid to the third-party administrator or in medical claims paid by the employer, led to a succession of strategies that have, for the most part, failed to produce widespread effective results. They have, however, led to the introduction of value-based Medicare payment efforts, which should yield significant benefits. The evolution to today's value-based purchasing movement has gone through several prior phases.

Evolution of Value-Based Purchasing

The concept of value-based purchasing was imported into healthcare from industry and applied on the premise that plans would compete for employers' and employees' premium dollars by demonstrating greater effectiveness in caring for covered members and greater efficiency in paying for care services. The primary strategy to achieve efficiency was to consolidate the purchasing power of payers and health plan sponsors and obtain discounts from physicians, hospitals, and ancillary care providers. The primary strategy to achieve effectiveness was to standardize measures of quality across plans and create a common way of assessing plan quality. Efforts by the National Committee for Quality Assurance (NCQA), described in the previous chapter, helped create the methodology for assessing plan performance on effectiveness of care in a standard way.

Even before value-based purchasing at the plan level lost its ability to improve quality and control costs for the majority of Americans covered by health insurance, purchasers had started to understand that providers did not change their behaviors for one plan alone. They changed their behaviors for all plans. In fact, researchers observed little difference in the quality of care between managed care networks and non–managed care networks (McGlynn et al. 2003; Schuster, McGlynn, and Brook 1998; Wennberg 1999), especially as purchasers demanded that plans increase the size of their networks. With the expansion of networks came the reduction in relative purchasing power. Purchaser focus has, as a result, shifted from individual plan performance to individual provider performance, evidenced by the creation of the Leapfrog Group in 2000, Bridges to Excellence in 2003, and the Patient-Centered Primary Care Collaborative in 2006. With the release of the Institute of Medicine's report *Crossing the Quality Chasm* (IOM 2001), purchasers realized that serious gaps remained in the quality of care in the United States and that variations in quality at the individual provider level were significant. Reducing the variation and increasing the overall level of quality have become purchasing imperatives, especially in light of continued cost increases.

However, the movement from plan selection to provider selection was not a direct one. While many large employers worked together to form the organizations mentioned previously, many others focused almost exclusively on managing the demand for healthcare through employee-based interventions such as disease management and shared decision making. Many of these interventions, when tried by Medicare on a larger scale, have proven ineffective (Nelson 2012a).

The value-based purchasing movement has thus evolved from trying to get managed care organizations to compete for patients by delivering better value, to getting plan members to improve their personal healthcare consumption habits, to trying to affect provider behavior. Therein lies the reason that change has been so long in coming. Employers assumed that health plans that contract with providers would have an incentive to test payment models that would motivate the contracted providers to deliver higher-quality, more affordable care. However, health plans have barely innovated in the way they pay providers. Instead, the large employers in the United States have pushed for and piloted innovative payment models.

That activity, described in this chapter, has reached a new level thanks to the significant payment reform activities introduced by the Affordable Care Act (ACA). The ACA not only creates a burning platform for fee-for-service (FFS) payments but empowers the Center for Medicare & Medicaid Innovation (CMMI 2013), housed within CMS, to pilot new payment and delivery system models and to propagate those models throughout Medicare if they prove successful. The final pages of this chapter briefly touch on these innovations.

Background and Terminology

The payment systems that range between the two poles of FFS and capitation assign varying levels of financial risk to providers. The pole with the least risk is FFS, while the pole with the most risk is capitation. In FFS, physicians are neither responsible for the probability that a patient will require services nor at risk for the value of the service delivered. They bill a service to the payer, and if the service conforms to the payer's administrative requirements, the payer will pay the agreed-upon fee. The physician's only financial risk is that the cost of providing the service may be greater than the fee received. In capitation, the opposite is true. Providers are at risk both for the probability that a patient will require a service and for the cost (not necessarily the value) of delivering all the care the patient needs. These two forms of risk are called probability risk and technical risk.

Employers and, more recently, Medicare have experimented with programs that fit within the spectrum bounded by these poles (Exhibit 20.1):

- *FFS* entails a minimal amount of risk for the provider. FFS encourages physicians to provide more services, which can be useful when payers want to encourage use of services—for example, immunizations and screenings for certain diseases or conditions. Medicare, which is the largest payer in the United States, primarily pays physicians according to the FFS model.

- *Pay for performance* is the most prevalent method that attempts to counter the FFS model's tendency to reward the volume rather than the value of care by tying a portion of the payment to certain performance criteria. This chapter describes the work done by employers in this domain and lessons learned to date.

- *Upside-only bundles* group the services that center on a specific procedure, an acute medical event, or even a chronic condition. According to the CBO report, the most successful payment experiment undertaken by CMS as of early 2012 was the bundled payment demonstration of the early 1990s (Nelson 2012b). This form of payment does not lay probability risk on the provider, but it does entail technical risk because the provider is at risk for the frequency, mix, and costs of services produced within the defined bundle. Upside-only bundled payments are designed to insulate the providers against any downside risk but create the potential for financial gain if the actual costs of care are lower than the predefined budget for the bundle. This chapter describes the private-sector efforts to launch bundled payments in the United States.

- *Full-risk bundles*, in contrast to upside-only bundles, put the provider at full risk for any costs in excess of (or eligible for the full reward of any costs under) the defined price negotiated with the payer. This chapter also describes efforts related to this model.

- *Total cost of care shared-savings models* contain the costs associated with managing a defined population by picking a target rate of increase of the total costs of care; providers and payers share the savings realized through a lower-than-expected rate of increase. Many of these programs do not include penalties for going over budget and

EXHIBIT 20.1
Provider
Payment
Models in
Value-Based
Purchasing

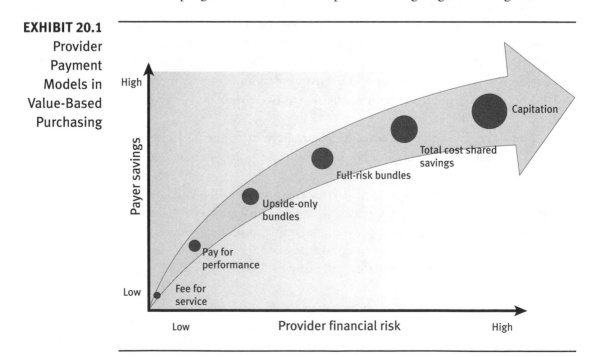

are based on a Medicare demonstration called the Physician Group Practice Demonstration, the results of which are summarized in the previously referenced CBO report (Nelson 2012b). In 2008–2009, several academic researchers launched a coordinated call for what they termed the *accountable care organization*, which is designed around the same principles as the Physician Group Practice Demonstration (Rittenhouse, Shortell, and Fisher 2009; Shortell and Casalino 2008). The ACA includes the implementation of this model in a formal pilot that launched in 2012.

- *Capitation* defines a specific budget for an entire patient population, and the providers are at full risk for all costs incurred above that budget. Even in its heyday in the mid-1990s, capitation was never widely adopted, principally because of the inherent financial risks assumed by the provider organizations. Further, many states require providers to file as insurance companies with state insurance regulators if they take on capitated payments for a patient population, thus increasing the administrative burden of such an approach.

Case Study: Bridges to Excellence: A Pay-for-Performance Model

In 2003 several large employers, including General Electric, Ford, Procter & Gamble, and UPS, launched Bridges to Excellence (BTE) to tie physician payments to the achievement of certain quality criteria. The concept was simple and continues to be implemented by employers and health plans throughout the United States (Health Care Incentives Improvement Institute 2013a). It asks physicians to demonstrate the quality of care delivered by submitting clinical data to an independent third-party evaluator. Physicians receive a financial reward per patient managed if their quality score exceeds a certain threshold. Like most pay-for-performance programs, BTE is an upside-only program. Physicians are never penalized; they are only rewarded on the basis of the premise that better quality care will lead to better financial outcomes. Since the program began, many variations have been launched, and much research has been published on the topic. The seminal work on designing a pay-for-performance program was done by Meredith Rosenthal and Adams Dudley (2007). In addition, several papers have been published on BTE and the lessons learned from its implementation. These lessons may be summarized as follows:

- *Avoid "tournament-style" programs* that retroactively rank providers in deciles or quartiles and distribute rewards based on that ranking. The primary drawback of this design is its uncertainty. A physician or a hospital could work hard to improve all year and never get a reward.

- *Measure what matters.* Outcome measures should be selected in careful consideration of the desired goal of the pay-for-performance program (de Brantes, Wickland, and Williams 2008). If the goal is to increase immunization rates, the measure should be immunization rates. If the goal is to achieve better outcomes for patients with chronic conditions, then blood pressure, cholesterol, and blood sugar levels may be appropriate measures.

- *Create meaningful incentives.* The research is clear. To pierce through the noise of FFS payment, a strong signal is needed. The greater the signal, the higher the response. De Brantes and D'Andrea (2009) studied the response of physician practices in several communities to the size of an offered bonus and found that response rises with the size of the bonus. Many pay-for-performance programs expect high response rates with paltry incentives, only to be disappointed.

- *Know that better-quality care can cost less.* This fundamental premise that led the BTE founders to launch the program was proven true (Rosenthal et al. 2008).

The lessons learned from BTE, as well as its seminal work in creating tools to measure systems in physician offices and the quality of care delivered to patients with certain chronic conditions, led to the design and implementation of incentive programs to reward patient-centered medical homes (PCMHs).

Patient-Centered Medical Homes

The PCMH concept is close to 50 years old. First introduced by the American Academy of Pediatrics, it was subsequently revised and adopted by a number of primary care specialty associations (e.g., the American Association of Family Physicians) as part of an overall effort in the early 2000s to address the future of family medicine (Robert Graham Center 2007). The observations were simple: The Medicare resource-based relative value scale (RBRVS) system had started to create significant distortions in the value of services, significantly favoring interventions to the detriment of evaluation and management. Medical school graduates were quick to respond to this shift, moving into specialties that provided far greater FFS billing opportunities, and the ranks of family practitioners started to significantly shrink.

The response to the report on the future of family medicine (Robert Graham Center 2007), in conjunction with the Institute of Medicine report

Crossing the Quality Chasm (IOM 2001) and the rising costs of healthcare, pointed policymakers, payers, and providers in the direction of shoring up primary care. IBM took a central role in launching the Patient-Centered Primary Care Collaborative (2013), which continues to serve as a general resource on the implementation of PCMH pilots across the United States.

The initial approach was to look at the design of primary care and its functions and figure out incentive or payment models that would suit the design and functions. This approach was evident in the proposal by Goroll and colleagues (2007) that soon became the rallying point for many field experiments. Goroll and colleagues calculated the cost of running a physician practice and then divided the needed revenue across a patient panel to arrive at a fixed payment per patient.

The path chosen was simple: First, design the form of the practice and its functions, and that design will lead to a financial incentive model. The challenge of such a path is that it does not provide incentives for the value of care delivered in these medical homes. Such incentives, if provided, would lead to innovation in primary care delivery regardless of the specific setting. In fact, a divide exists between researchers who propose specific forms of the delivery system—accountable care organizations and PCMHs—and those who propose specific incentives to drive care improvement, such as pay for performance, bundled payments, and shared savings. Interestingly, the ones focusing on the former are mostly from academia, whereas the ones focusing on the latter are mostly from the business community.

Some important early lessons have been learned about PCMHs:

- *It is very difficult to transform a traditional physician practice into the type of PCMH described and defined in the report on the future of family medicine.* Crabtree and colleagues (2010) describe the challenges encountered in a large national PCMH demonstration effort.
- *Evidence of financial impact is mixed.* Analyses suggest that pilot participants (those that were selected to participate in a PCMH pilot and are receiving an incentive for doing so) have better results than a random sample of physicians in the same community. Exhibit 20.2 shows that patients managed by PCMH pilot practices had fewer hospitalizations and shorter lengths of stay (resulting in fewer bed days) than patients managed by non-PCMH pilot practices. However, Exhibit 20.3 shows that practices designated as PCMHs by the NCQA that were not participating in a pilot did not obtain better results than other physicians in their community, whereas pilot participants did. The measures used in Exhibit 20.3 are the rates of potentially avoidable complications (PACs), which were approved in 2011 by the National Quality Forum as measures of comprehensive outcomes of care.

EXHIBIT 20.2
Bed Days per
Thousand
Patients

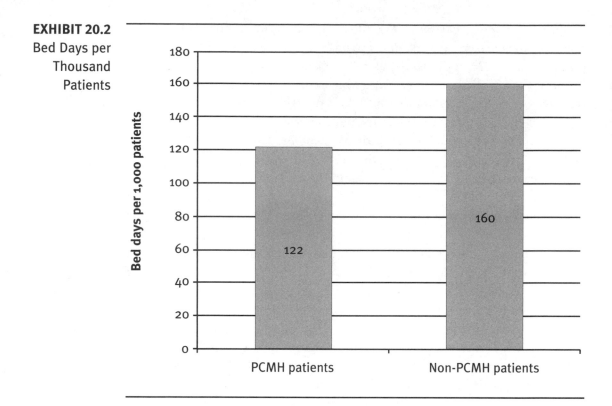

- *The search for a sustainable funding model for PCMH practices continues.* PCMH practices must fit into the larger context of a delivery system that associates a financial risk with its members' decisions on the type and frequency of services rendered. Therefore, health plans and physicians continue to explore incentives that would cause practices to transform in a manner consistent with the report on the future of family medicine while reducing the total medical spending associated with a population of patients. Options include

  - creating prospective budgets, especially for patients with chronic conditions, and assigning the financial risk to the practice for costs in excess of that budget;
  - defining a global cost per member per month for all patients based on historical trends and creating a mechanism to share gains with the practice on the basis of actual costs; and
  - establishing bonuses linked to a scorecard of cost and quality that are to be paid in addition to the routine FFS payments.

Pay for performance has natural limits because these programs simply attempt to counter the basic incentive of FFS, not to replace it. The following case study looks at the next rung on the ladder of value-based purchasing.

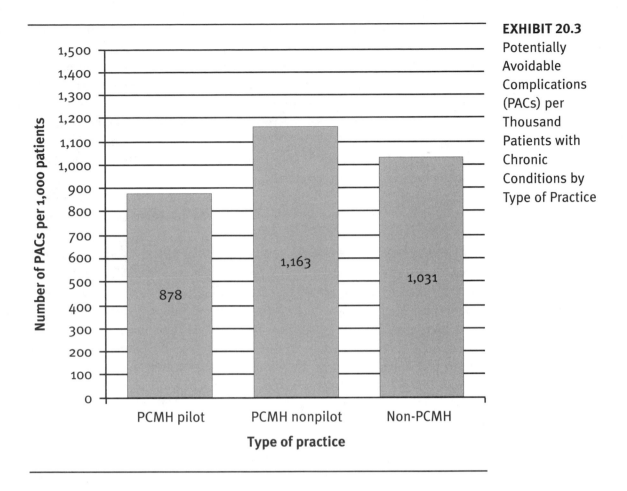

EXHIBIT 20.3
Potentially
Avoidable
Complications
(PACs) per
Thousand
Patients with
Chronic
Conditions by
Type of Practice

Case Study: PROMETHEUS Payment: A New Frontier in Value-Based Purchasing

In the mid-1990s, Medicare launched a demonstration project to pay hospitals and physicians a single fee for a bundle of services related to a cardiac bypass procedure. The CBO reported that this project was one of the more successful payment reform initiatives undertaken by CMS. Approximately ten years later, CMS launched a new demonstration called the Acute Care Episode Demonstration, which expanded on the first project but was still limited to bundling all inpatient-stay services for specific procedures.

After the launch of BTE, large employers realized that more fundamental payment reform would be needed to respond to the Institute of Medicine's reports on the quality of care in the United States and launched the Provider Payment Reform for Outcomes, Margins, Evidence, Transparency, Hassle-reduction, Excellence, Understandability, and Sustainability (PROMETHEUS) Payment effort. Following the same process used to create BTE, a design team composed of experts in healthcare economics, law, and delivery set about to create a new payment model that would appropriately and fairly shift financial risk to providers, making them responsible for the cost and quality of care delivered to patients for specific procedures, acute medical events, and chronic conditions.

The concepts and design were summarized in several papers (e.g., de Brantes, D'Andrea, and Rosenthal 2009) and served as a launchpad for actual implementations to pilot the model and evaluate it. The model has since been implemented in several communities across the United States, some of which have been and continue to be supported by charitable foundations; others are supported by private-sector payers (Health Care Incentives Improvement Institute 2013b).

One of the more important concepts was that providers, not the employer or payer, would be responsible for the cost of defects and waste. The main challenge in designing the PROMETHEUS Payment model was to impute the financial risk associated with care failures to providers, while limiting their probability risk as much as possible. Splitting these risks—performance and probability—would create more focus on providers to understand how to manage financial risk by reducing defects as opposed to managing financial risk by limiting the probability that a health event occurs, which providers are not particularly adept at doing. The PROMETHEUS Payment model was the first to quantify the cost of defects in episodes of chronic, procedural, and acute medical care. It named these defects PACs, which were subsequently endorsed by the National Quality Forum as measures of comprehensive outcomes of care. PACs became the foundation for the incentives in the PROMETHEUS Payment model because employers immediately grasped what they meant and understood the importance of reducing them to increase value in the delivery of medical care. When analyzed, PACs are converted into a dollar-denominated rate that represents the percentage of costs in any episode that can be attributed to PACs.

Exhibit 20.4 illustrates the variation in rates of PACs for patients with certain chronic conditions, from a large national database of commercially insured plan members. These data demonstrate the significant opportunity to reduce costs in the United States while improving the quality of care. Exhibit 20.5 illustrates the total costs in dollars consumed by PACs and the typical care for 21 patient conditions and procedures as measured in a regional health plan's commercial claims data set. Exhibit 20.6 represents the same data, aggregated across the episodes and expressed as a percentage of total costs.

For any employer, Exhibit 20.6 paints a clear and unambiguous picture: $1 of every $4 spent on certain episodes of chronic, procedural, and acute care is spent on PACs or defects in the care process. In a global economy in which firms that produce products compete for value and are severely punished when products fail, the contrast between what happens within those firms and what happens in healthcare delivery could not be starker. In response to these data, mainstream publications such as the *New York Times* (Chen 2009) and *Time* (Pickert 2009) started asking a simple question: Shouldn't healthcare services come with a warranty? That question is the driving force behind bundled payments. A bundled payment is a global fee for a specific medical event, condition, or procedure, and it includes an implicit warranty. If a patient is readmitted after being discharged following a total knee replacement surgery, the readmission costs are absorbed by the providers and not charged to the payer as an additional expense. If a patient with diabetes receives poor management and ends up repeatedly in the emergency department, those costs are absorbed by the providers and not charged separately to the payer. Bundled payments replicate, in effect, the dynamics that exist with most other purchases made by consumers or companies—the consumer negotiates or accepts the price up front, and if the product has a defect, the responsibility lies with the manufacturer, not the buyer. Furthermore, employers who had increasingly started to shift the cost of healthcare services to employees could use bundled prices as a mechanism to move market share from one provider to another on the basis of the price of the bundle. Several new consumer-directed tools such as Castlight (Castlight Health 2013) and Healthcare Blue Book (2013) are designed to provide consumable information to plan members, helping them understand the trade-offs in selecting different providers for a specific procedure.

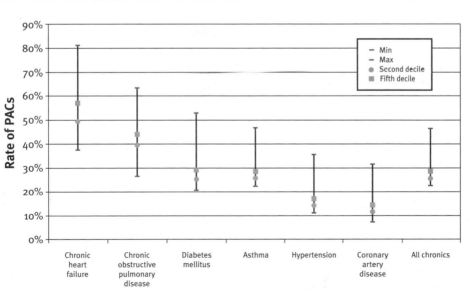

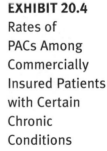

EXHIBIT 20.4
Rates of PACs Among Commercially Insured Patients with Certain Chronic Conditions

Source: Adapted from de Brantes, Rastogi, and Painter (2010).
Note: Each line represents the range, from minimum to maximum, of average PAC rates in different US states. The dot represents the PAC rate for the 20th percentile, and the square represents the PAC rate for the 50th percentile.

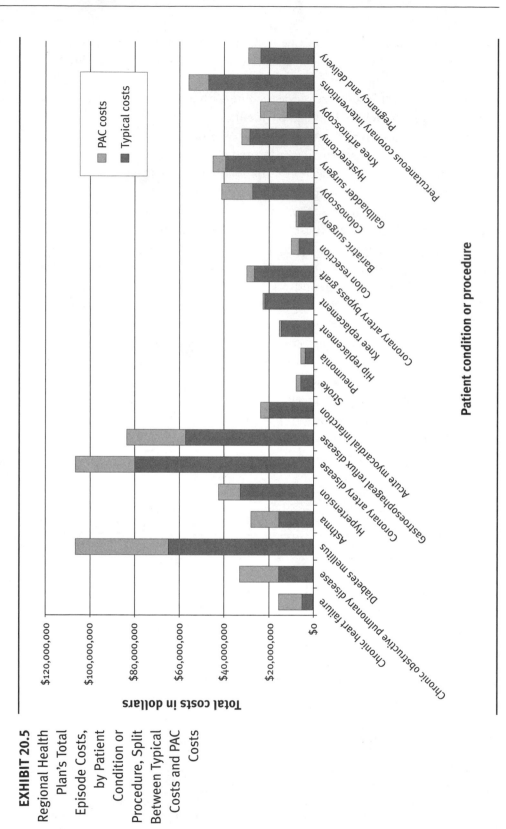

EXHIBIT 20.5
Regional Health
Plan's Total
Episode Costs,
by Patient
Condition or
Procedure, Split
Between Typical
Costs and PAC
Costs

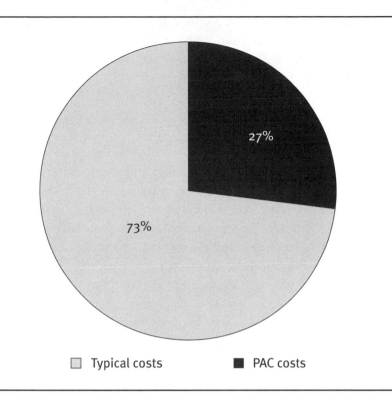

EXHIBIT 20.6
Regional Health Plan's Total Episode Costs Split Between PAC Costs and Typical Costs, Expressed as Percentage of Total

27%

73%

☐ Typical costs   ■ PAC costs

In 2008, the Robert Wood Johnson Foundation awarded a three-year grant to pilot the PROMETHEUS Payment model, to test the operational processes and determine how this type of bundled payment could be implemented on a larger scale in the United States. Three sites, each with a unique set of challenges, were selected and evaluated by a third party. That evaluation was published in late 2011 (Hussey, Ridgely, and Rosenthal 2011). Between 2008 and 2012, the model was launched at several other sites, some funded by other charitable foundations and some supported by regional health plans. In addition, the enactment of the ACA in 2010 changed the landscape, in particular by creating the CMMI and its push to launch payment reform initiatives.

Significant challenges to implementation remain, despite the promise to control costs, increase quality, and engage plan members in value-based purchasing. The combination of antiquated claims processing and member benefits systems, coupled with provider resistance to revenue contraction, creates a significant weight of inertia. Hussey, Ridgely, and Rosenthal (2011) summarized some of these challenges in their evaluation of the PROMETHEUS Payment model pilot sites. Despite those challenges, hundreds of provider organizations filed letters of intent with the CMMI as an initial step in applying to participate in that organization's bundled payment pilot. Furthermore, private-sector bundled payment initiatives have sprung up, including a statewide effort in California led by the Integrated Healthcare Association; an effort in Wisconsin led by an alliance of multiple stakeholders; and efforts in New Jersey, North Carolina, and South Carolina led by those states' Blue Cross and Blue Shield plans.

Conclusions and Key Lessons

Despite the challenges inherent in designing and implementing value-based payment models, the private sector—and in particular the leading employers in the United States—have paved the way for federal efforts to move away from basic FFS payments. Keys to success have stemmed from careful consideration of stakeholder needs and the desire to maintain a balanced and fair approach in shifting financial risk to providers.

Key principles of a successful design ensure that

- incentives meet provider needs (in particular, incentives have to be measurable, attainable, and meaningful);
- performance measures meet provider and purchaser needs, create a return on investment for purchasers, are achievable yet not easy, and are standard as opposed to custom; and
- operational structures to implement new payment models meet purchaser and plan needs, are relatively simple and easy for purchasers to implement, and keep the administrative burden on plans to a minimum.

Study Questions

1. What are the principal efforts led by employers since 2000 to usher in a new era in value-based purchasing?
2. Value-based payments are one side of a two-sided value-based purchasing coin. What is the other side, and why is it so essential to the long-term sustainability of the movement?
3. What forms of provider organizations are likely to develop in response to the different types of value-based payments being piloted?

References

Castlight Health. 2013. Accessed December 18. www.castlighthealth.com.
Center for Medicare & Medicaid Innovation (CMMI). 2013. Accessed December 18. www.innovations.cms.gov.

Chen, P. W. 2009. "Can Health Care Come with a Warranty?" *New York Times* June 25. www.nytimes.com/2009/06/25/health/25chen.html.

Crabtree, B. F., P. A. Nutting, W. L. Miller, K. C. Stange, E. E. Stewart, and C. R. Jaén. 2010. "Summary of the National Demonstration Project and Recommendations for the Patient-Centered Medical Home." *Annals of Family Medicine* 8 (Suppl. 1): S80–S90.

de Brantes, F. S., and G. D'Andrea. 2009. "Physicians Respond to Pay-for-Performance Incentives: Larger Incentives Yield Greater Participation." *American Journal of Managed Care* 15 (5): 305–10.

de Brantes, F. S., G. D'Andrea, and M. B. Rosenthal. 2009. "Should Health Care Come with a Warranty?" *Health Affairs* 28 (4): w678–w687.

de Brantes, F. S., A. Rastogi, and M. Painter. 2010. "Reducing Potentially Avoidable Complications in Patients with Chronic Diseases: The Prometheus Payment Approach." *Health Services Research* 45 (6): 1854–71.

de Brantes, F., P. Wickland, and J. Williams. 2008. "The Value of Ambulatory Care Measures: A Review of Clinical and Financial Impact from an Employer/Payer Perspective." *American Journal of Managed Care* 14 (6): 360–68.

Goroll, A. H., R. A. Berenson, S. C. Schoenbaum, and L. B. Gardner. 2007. "Fundamental Reform of Payment for Adult Primary Care: Comprehensive Payment for Comprehensive Care." *Journal of General Internal Medicine* 22 (3): 410–15.

Health Care Incentives Improvement Institute. 2013a. "Bridges to Excellence: Premise." Accessed December 18. www.hci3.org/what_is_bte/premise.

———. 2013b. "PROMETHEUS Implementations." Accessed December 18. www. hci3.org/implementations.

Healthcare Blue Book. 2013. Accessed December 18. http://healthcarebluebook. com.

Hussey, P. S., M. S. Ridgely, and M. B. Rosenthal. 2011. "The PROMETHEUS Bundled Payment Experiment: Slow Start Shows Problems in Implementing New Payment Models." *Health Affairs* 30 (11): 2116–24.

Institute of Medicine (IOM). 2001. *Crossing the Quality Chasm: A New Health System for the 21st Century.* Washington, DC: National Academies Press.

McGlynn, E. A., S. M. Asch, J. Adams, J. Keesey, J. Hicks, A. DeCristofaro, and E. A. Kerr. 2003. "The Quality of Health Care Delivered to Adults in the United States." *New England Journal of Medicine* 348 (26): 2635–45.

Nelson, L. 2012a. "Lessons from Medicare's Demonstration Projects on Disease Management and Care Coordination." Working paper 2012-01. Issued January 18. Washington, DC: Congressional Budget Office. www.cbo.gov/doc. cfm?index=12664.

———. 2012b. "Lessons from Medicare's Demonstration Projects on Value-Based Payment." Report. Issued January 18. Washington, DC: Congressional Budget Office. www.cbo.gov/publication/42925.

Patient-Centered Primary Care Collaborative. 2013. Accessed December 18. www. pcpcc.net.

Pickert, K. 2009. "Cutting Health-Care Costs by Putting Doctors on a Budget." *Time* (US) July 6. www.time.com/time/nation/article/0,8599,1908477,00.html.

Rittenhouse, D. R., S. M. Shortell, and E. S. Fisher. 2009. "Primary Care and Accountable Care—Two Essential Elements of Delivery-System Reform." *New England Journal of Medicine* 361 (24): 2301–3.

Robert Graham Center. 2007. *The Patient Centered Medical Home: History, Seven Core Features, Evidence and Transformational Change.* Washington, DC: Robert Graham Center. www.graham-center.org/online/graham/home/ publications/monographs-books/2007/rgcmo-medical-home.html.

Rosenthal, M. B., F. de Brantes, A. Sinaiko, M. Frankel, R. D. Robbins, and S. Young. 2008. "Bridges to Excellence—Recognizing High-Quality Care: Analysis of Physician Quality and Resource Use." *American Journal of Managed Care* 14 (10): 670–77.

Rosenthal, M. B., and R. A. Dudley. 2007. "Pay-for-Performance: Will the Latest Payment Trend Improve Care?" *Journal of the American Medical Association* 297 (7): 740–44.

Schuster, M. A., E. A. McGlynn, and R. Brook. 1998. "How Good Is the Quality of Healthcare in the United States?" *Milbank Quarterly* 76 (4): 517–63.

Shortell, S. M., and L. P. Casalino. 2008. "Health Care Reform Requires Accountable Care Systems." *Journal of the American Medical Association* 300 (1): 95–97.

Wennberg, J. A. 1999. "Understanding Geographic Variations in Health Care Delivery." *New England Journal of Medicine* 340 (1): 52–53.

TRANSFORMING THE HEALTHCARE SYSTEM FOR IMPROVED QUALITY

Steffanie Bristol and Maulik S. Joshi

Healthcare is in a time of great flux with many unknowns. These unknowns include how reimbursement systems will change in the private and public sectors; how electronic health records will affect the care delivery system; how regulation will support changing organizational structures and markets; and how market forces, such as increased public reporting and pay for performance, will affect patient outcomes across the healthcare system. A transformation of the healthcare system is taking place both financially and clinically, and the impact on healthcare quality is projected to be profound.

Transitioning from Volume-Based Care to Value-Based Care

The healthcare industry faces unprecedented pressures to transform and overcome foundational failings in both the short term and the long term. In contrast to other industries, the US healthcare delivery system pays for the volume of care rather than the value of care. Healthcare is on an unsustainable path that threatens the long-term fiscal stability of the nation. Annual US healthcare expenditures total $2.7 trillion, consume more than 17.3 percent of the gross domestic product (GDP), continue to outstrip inflation, and jeopardize the competitiveness of American businesses (Centers for Medicare & Medicaid Services [CMS] 2012). Intersecting environmental forces, such as the aging population, healthcare reform, subpar quality levels, and rising costs, will force the industry to move from volume-based to value-based care delivery.

Within the next decade, payment incentives will shift to reward the value of care rather than the quantity of care. Hospitals and health systems will need to adapt their core models of business and service delivery and move from the "first curve" (the current volume-based environment) to the "second curve" (the future value-based environment) (American Hospital

EXHIBIT 21.1
First Curve to
Second Curve

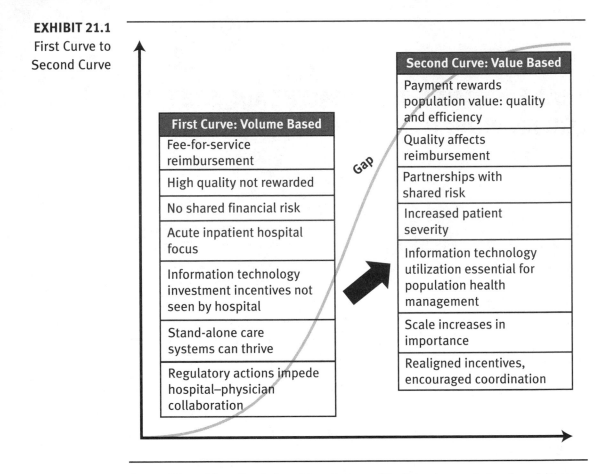

Source: Adapted from *Hospitals and Care Systems of the Future* by permission, Copyright 2011, American Hospital Association.

Association 2011, citing Ian Morrison's terminology). This transition is critical for hospitals' sustainability (Exhibit 21.1).

The transition from the first curve to the second curve is challenging and will require significant effort among providers. Each hospital or health system should complete an internal assessment to examine current capabilities and identify areas for improvement. Providers should also develop a transition plan to manage the evolving equilibrium and avoid taking on an unmanageable amount of change during a given period. Providers will need to carefully balance current market circumstances, such as how they are reimbursed for care, with the need to transition and prepare for the future.

To be successful, hospitals may use numerous key strategies, tactics, and measures. The American Hospital Association's (2011) Committee on Performance Improvement identified and prioritized four must-do strategies:

1. Align hospitals, physicians, and other providers across the continuum of care.

2. Utilize evidence-based practices to improve quality and patient safety.
3. Improve efficiency through productivity and financial management.
4. Develop integrated information systems.

A hospital's organizational culture will play a critical role in the successful implementation of strategies and initiatives to make the transformation from the first curve to the second curve. Hospitals must develop a culture of performance improvement, accountability, and high performance.

Providers should carefully track key metrics for each strategy to assess progress and guide future efforts (Exhibit 21.2). Furthermore, hospitals and health systems should work to achieve several core organizational competencies that will promote the delivery of high-performance, value-based care. These core competencies are aligned with the must-do strategies (indicated in boldface in Exhibit 21.3) and are integral to the successful achievement of these strategies.

Hospitals and health systems need to evaluate their internal capabilities as well as identify gaps and areas for improvement to make the transition from the first curve to the second curve. Careful tracking and continuous assessment and feedback will help providers manage emerging quality-of-care issues and implement the necessary changes to shift to the next age of healthcare delivery.

Emerging Quality-of-Care Issues

Numerous quality issues and innovations are rapidly spreading across the healthcare industry. The issues and innovations, which range from novel approaches to the way providers are reimbursed to a shift toward a population health focus, include

- reducing readmissions and improving the continuum of care;
- transitioning to population health;
- spreading improvement; and
- introducing innovative demonstrations and pilots: patient-centered medical homes (PCMHs), bundled payments, and accountable care organizations (ACOs).

Reducing Readmissions and Improving the Continuum of Care
Reducing hospital readmission rates poses a unique opportunity to improve the quality of care and reduce spending (Goodman, Fisher, and Chang 2011; Jencks, Williams, and Coleman 2009; Medicare Payment Advisory Commission [MedPAC] 2009). Approximately one-fifth of Medicare patients are

EXHIBIT 21.2
Key Metrics for Four Must-Do Strategies

Align Hospitals, Physicians, and Other Providers Across the Continuum of Care	Utilize Evidence-Based Practices to Improve Quality and Patient Safety	Improve Efficiency Through Productivity and Financial Management	Develop Integrated Information Systems
Number of aligned and engaged physicians	Effective measurement and management of care transitions	Expense per episode of care	Presence of an integrated data warehouse
Percentage of physician and provider contracts with quality and efficiency incentives aligned with ACO-type incentives	Management of utilization variation	Shared savings or financial gains from performance-based contracts	Lag time between analysis and availability of results
Availability of non-acute services	Preventable admissions, readmissions, ED visits, and mortality	Targeted cost-reduction goals	Understanding of population disease patterns
Distribution of shared savings/performance bonuses/gains to aligned physicians and clinicians	Reliable patient care processes	Management to Medicare margin	Use of health information across the continuum of care and community
Number of covered individuals for whom the provider is accountable for population health	Active patient engagement in design and improvement		Real-time information exchange
Number of providers in leadership			Active use of patient health records

Source: Adapted from *Hospitals and Care Systems of the Future* by permission, Copyright 2011, American Hospital Association.

Must-Do Strategies	Core Competencies
• **Clinician–hospital alignment** • **Quality and patient safety** • **Efficiency through productivity and financial management** • **Integrated information systems** • Integrated provider networks • Engaged employees and physicians • Strengthening finances • Payer–provider partnerships • Scenario-based planning • Population health improvement	• Design and implementation of patient-centered, integrated care • Creation of accountable governance and leadership • Strategic planning in an unstable environment • Internal and external collaboration • Financial stewardship and enterprise risk management • Engagement of employees' full potential • Utilization of electronic data for performance improvement

EXHIBIT 21.3
Must-Do
Strategies
and Core
Competencies

Source: Adapted from *Hospitals and Care Systems of the Future* by permission, Copyright 2011, American Hospital Association.

readmitted to the hospital within 30 days of initial discharge, costing Medicare an estimated $17.4 billion in 2004 (CMS 2007). About 90 percent of readmissions are estimated to be unplanned, leaving substantial room for improvement (Jencks, Williams, and Coleman 2009). As a result, improving performance on readmissions has come under intense scrutiny by policymakers and payers as a means to increase efficiency, value, and care coordination.

Planned readmissions represent good care and are typically part of the planned treatment course. Conversely, unplanned readmissions occur for reasons that include poorly coordinated care among multiple settings, misdiagnosis at initial hospitalization, premature discharge from the hospital, and inadequate discharge planning (Goodman, Fisher, and Chang 2011; MedPAC 2009). However, adequately distinguishing among different types of readmissions is difficult because readmissions may be planned or unplanned and may be related or unrelated to the initial hospitalization (Goodman, Fisher, and Chang 2011).

The best opportunity for quality improvements and financial savings at hospitals comes from reducing those readmissions within the hospital's control: readmissions that are preventable (unplanned) and predictable (related to the initial hospitalization). Thus, hospitals and health systems should focus on potentially preventable readmissions that the hospital may predict.

Hospital leaders should follow four steps to design an intervention strategy that best fits the hospital's unique circumstances (Osei-Anto et al. 2010):

1. *Examine the hospital's current rate of readmissions.* Compile data on readmission rates and trends to develop targeted strategies for reducing readmissions.

2. *Assess and prioritize improvement opportunities.* Once gaps are identified from the data analysis, health leaders need to prioritize their areas of focus, such as addressing specific patient populations, focusing on stages of care delivery, harnessing organizational strengths, or maximizing current priority areas and quality improvement initiatives.

3. *Develop an action plan of strategies to implement.* Synthesize foundational intervention strategies and involve key stakeholders in the action plan. Be certain to develop communication connections to improve the continuum of care and engage patients, families, and caregivers.

4. *Monitor the hospital's progress.* Review progress, redesign improvement efforts as needed, and realign the action plan to be in sync with the organization's current state.

Fortunately, hospitals may employ numerous strategies to reduce potentially preventable readmissions. These strategies involve different amounts of effort and organizational resources. Further, they have different levels of potential organizational value in addressing readmissions. Strategies that hospitals may employ fall into three major stages:

1. During hospitalization
2. At discharge
3. After discharge

Exhibit 21.4 outlines strategies to reduce readmissions for hospitals and health systems at each of the three stages.

Challenges to Measurement

The relationship between readmissions and quality is complex, and thus reliably measuring rates of readmission within the hospital's control poses multiple challenges.

First, the appropriateness of readmissions as a quality metric has been debated. Readmissions are largely driven by patient and community factors that are outside the hospital's control. Indeed, less than 30 percent of hospital readmissions are estimated to be preventable (van Walraven et al. 2011). Although hospitals should focus on preventing potentially avoidable readmissions, there is no consensus on how to adequately distinguish among different types of readmissions (Goodman, Fisher, and Chang 2011).

Second, current risk-adjustment methodology is imperfect and thus may unfairly rate a hospital's performance. A hospital's readmission rate is risk adjusted for patient factors such as age, gender, and comorbidity but excludes important patient factors such as socioeconomic status, race and ethnicity, social support structure, limited English proficiency, and dual

During Hospitalization	At Discharge	After Discharge
• Risk-screen patients and tailor care • Establish communication with primary care physician, family, and home care • Use teach-back* to educate patient about diagnosis and care • Use interdisciplinary or multidisciplinary clinical team • Coordinate patient care across multidisciplinary care team • Discuss end-of-life treatment wishes	• Implement comprehensive discharge planning • Educate patient and caregiver using teach-back* • Schedule and prepare for follow-up appointment • Help patient manage medications • Facilitate discharge to nursing homes with detailed discharge instructions and partnership with nursing home practitioners	• Promote patient self-management • Conduct patient home visit • Follow up with patients via telephone • Use personal health records to manage patient information • Establish community networks • Use telehealth in patient care

EXHIBIT 21.4
Readmission Reduction Strategies at Different Stages of Care

Source: Adapted with permission from Osei-Anto A, Joshi M, Audet AM, Berman A, Jencks S, *Health Care Leader Action Guide to Reduce Avoidable Readmissions*. Health Research & Educational Trust, Chicago, IL. January 2010.
*Teach-back is a teaching method in which a patient is asked to repeat back, in her own words, what she is supposed to know. It aims to confirm that the healthcare professional has explained what the patient should know in a manner the patient understands.

eligibility status, as well as the hospital's geographic region, mortality rates, and proportion of minority patients (Allaudeen et al. 2011; Epstein 2009; Jencks, Williams, and Coleman 2009; Joynt and Jha 2011; Joynt, Orav, and Jha 2011; Karliner et al. 2010; Lindenauer et al. 2010). If hospitals are not fairly rated, they may avoid taking complex and high-risk patients. Hospitals that disproportionately care for minority and poor patients are particularly at risk of being penalized because these institutions already face exacerbated resource and implementation challenges compared to other institutions.

Finally, attributing the readmission to the appropriate hospital is difficult because 20 to 40 percent of patients are readmitted to a different hospital than that of the index admission (Jencks, Williams, and Coleman 2009). In the absence of all-payer claims databases, providers are able to examine readmission drivers only within their institution. Consequently, providers may be penalized for readmissions that they are not responsible for and routinely lack access to adequate data to develop effective solutions.

Developing Community Connections

To reduce preventable readmissions, providers must take a community approach and develop connections with players across the care continuum.

Increasingly, while initial care may occur at the hospital, subsequent care is received at nursing homes, community health centers, or the patient's home. This pervasive fragmentation across the US healthcare delivery system creates a precarious situation. Providers must pay careful attention to care transitions and coordination among multiple sites of care.

Hospitals and health systems will need to partner with other providers as well as community groups. By developing partnerships, hospitals will be able to ensure continuity of care for their patients after discharge. Partners should share clinical information so that each provider in the care continuum understands the patient's status, previous medical treatment, and current needs. Further, hospitals may leverage community partners' key strengths that affect readmissions, such as promoting behavioral health, encouraging health literacy, and addressing cultural issues.

Transitioning to Population Health

The evolving healthcare environment requires providers to adopt a population health approach, one that manages health outcomes for a defined group of people rather than just an individual patient. The traditional health management model focuses on patients who are active seekers of healthcare services. However, this model will not be sustainable in the future. The delivery system will require a proactive approach to identifying, engaging, and addressing the needs of not only a growing number of healthcare users but also patients with increasingly complex health needs. Thus, shifting to a population health model that aims to improve the health of individual patients as well as larger communities is critical.

Forces Driving the Population Health Approach

One of the major forces driving the shift to a population health focus is the transition from volume-based care to value-based care. Over time, value-based care payment models will replace current payment models that reward providers for the volume of care provided. For example, the majority of ACOs incorporate a risk-sharing payment model, in which an ACO is held accountable for and is rated on the basis of the costs and quality of care provided to a defined population of patients, regardless of where the patients receive care. If the ACO achieves high performance on established cost and quality targets, it will receive a share of the savings realized from cost reductions and meeting targets. Achieving value-based care will require providers to collaborate with entities beyond their institution through a population health lens.

Additional market demands and external forces are driving the shift to a population health approach. Market demands include the aging population, the increasing rate of chronic diseases, population diversity, physician short-ages, and the increasing number of insured individuals. External forces include emerging performance standards and transparency, technological advances, shared-risk and shared-savings payment models, value-based reimbursement, and increased outpatient care. Furthermore, the Affordable Care Act (ACA) includes provisions that promote population health through incentives for prevention, quality and safety, and care coordination.

Determinant Factors

To achieve a population health focus and improve outcomes, providers must understand the interrelated factors that influence health. As described by the Health Research & Educational Trust (HRET 2012), numerous factors inside and outside the healthcare system affect population health. At the core of population health is the intersection between healthcare systems and external determinants that include societal, care delivery, and regulatory factors (Exhibit 21.5).

Mechanisms to Improve Population Health

As described by the HRET (2012, 4), improving population health hinges on the interaction among three distinct mechanisms: (1) increasing the prevalence of evidence-based preventive health services and preventive health behaviors, (2) improving care quality and patient safety, and (3) advancing care coordination across the healthcare continuum. These mechanisms influence three interrelated items within a defined population (HRET 2012, 4):

1. Health statuses and outcomes
2. Determinant factors
3. Interventions that modify determinant factors to improve outcomes

Fortunately, hospitals and individual providers are already pursuing initiatives to address these three mechanisms. Providers may leverage current programs to develop an effective population health strategy and track progress toward improving health outcomes. Initiatives may focus on small or large subgroups of patients, patients with particular chronic conditions, or the promotion of healthy behavior changes.

Population health cannot be achieved by a single organization. Instead, it requires systematic changes that are realized through a collaborative approach with entities outside the traditional healthcare spectrum, such as education systems, housing, welfare programs, recreation centers, and community organizations. These partners may be divided into two major types (HRET 2012):

EXHIBIT 21.5
Determinants
of Population
Health

Societal Factors Outside the Healthcare System	Care Delivery Inside the Healthcare System	Regulatory Environment
• Geographic location • Unemployment rate • Uninsured/under-insured rate • Median age • Sex • Race/ethnicity • Social network • Care-seeking behaviors • Health literacy • Patient choice • Morbidity rates • Transportation availability • Food safety • Healthful food availability • Housing conditions • Neighborhood violence • Open space and parks/recreation availability • Genetic inheritance • Disease prevalence • Income levels • Poverty rates	• Quality of care • Efficiency • Access • Physician training • Health information technology system availability • Distance to and number of providers • Provider supply • Physician mix • Payer contracts • Physician employment and payment structure • Disease management • Population subgroup disparity • Advanced technology availability • Care integration and coordination • Behavioral health availability • Cultural and linguistic access	• Medicare payment rates and policies • Medicare and Medicaid care delivery innovation • Certificate of need (CON) regulation • Medicaid/Children's Health Insurance Program (CHIP) policies • ACA implementation • Local coverage determination • Local, state, and federal laws

Source: Adapted with permission from *Managing Population Health: The Role of the Hospital*. Health Research & Educational Trust, Chicago: April 2012. Accessed at www.hpoe.org.

1. Partners with direct interaction with individual healthcare consumers
   a. Physicians and other clinicians
   b. Hospitals and health systems
   c. Post–acute care providers
   d. Government and commercial payers
   e. Employers
   f. Social and community services
2. Partners with indirect interaction with individual healthcare consumers
   a. Local, state, and federal policymakers
   b. Public health agencies

Even though value-based payment models are not yet widespread, providers should start developing systems and operational processes that connect stakeholders so that the systems and processes will be in place when these new reimbursement models become commonplace. Moving toward a population health approach will become increasingly important to ensure the long-term sustainability of providers and improve the quality of healthcare provided to all Americans.

Spreading Improvement

Spreading improvement is essential to overcoming the quality and patient safety shortcomings of the US healthcare system and transforming care delivery. The US healthcare system has experienced rapid growth in innovative techniques and processes that combat quality and patient safety failings. Substantial investments are being made at the organizational, local, state, and national levels. Innovations include using checklists for safe care, eradicating hospital-acquired infections, improving the work environment in hospital medical-surgical units, and instituting new payment models. Unfortunately, these successes frequently occur on a one-off basis, and a consistently lengthy lag time exists between when an innovation is proven to work and when it is adopted for widespread use.

Factors Affecting the Spread of Improvements

Moving to the next era of healthcare and achieving the six aims for improvement—care that is safe, timely, effective, efficient, equitable, and patient centered (Institute of Medicine 2001)—requires leveraging successes and investments. Effectively spreading improvement both within and across organizations in a reliable and consistent way is critical to accelerating progress. Four major types of factors affect the spread of improvements (Exhibit 21.6).

External environmental factors include financial considerations (e.g., will the effort make money?), legal issues (e.g., will the initiative cause a lawsuit?), regulatory factors (e.g., is the initiative likely to be required in the future?), societal views (e.g., will the initiative develop goodwill among patients?), and strategic priorities (e.g., is the initiative needed to stay in line with competitors?). *Initiative characteristics* include factors such as how easy the effort is for key stakeholders to understand and the strength of the evidence in support of the effort. Factors related to the *target audience for adoption* include how many people need to buy into the change, how many people will need to implement the change, and how the initiative will affect those directly affected by the change. *Internal organizational factors* include leadership buy-in, required resources, availability of needed skill sets, alignment with organizational culture, and degree of internal priority.

EXHIBIT 21.6
Factors
Affecting the
Spread of
Improvements

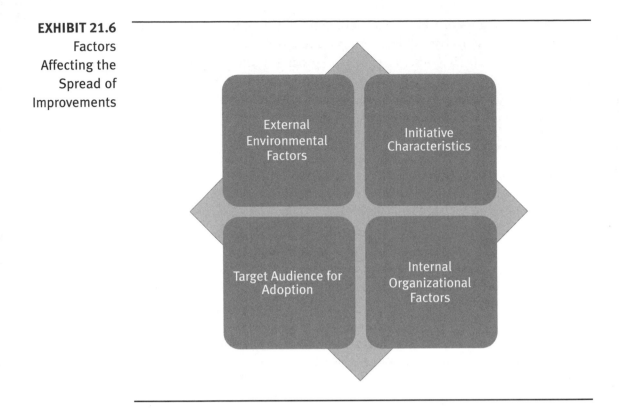

One Size Does Not Fit All

Each organization needs to develop its own best approach and strategic plan for spreading knowledge throughout the organization. No organization is just like another, and efforts must be individualized to be successful. For example, the Robert Wood Johnson Foundation's national Transforming Care at the Bedside program was tested at three major healthcare systems to identify strategies that could be used across organizations as well as challenges for large-scale spread. The evaluation found that the program was effectively replicated at all three healthcare systems. However, the hospitals took different approaches. The most obvious difference was in the management approach to implementation, where hospitals took either a top-down or bottom-up management approach (Pearson et al. 2008).

Strategies for Success

The Robert Wood Johnson Foundation also identified key factors for success that should be considered by organizations embarking on spreading improvements (Pearson et al. 2008):

- Have a designated spread organizer.
- Carefully select unit(s) for spread.
- Use off-site, multihospital meetings for sharing ideas, learning, and support.

- Designate nurse champions to promote innovations and spread improvements.
- Ensure ongoing communications.
- Focus on the role of the unit manager.
- Allocate resources (e.g., staff time) for staff to work on spreading improvements.
- Obtain clear and demonstrated senior leadership support.

Additional Considerations

Organizations also must develop metrics and measurable objectives to track progress and to identify areas for future development and refinement. Improvement requires continuous feedback and reevaluation, and measurement must continue after implementation. To further accelerate spread, organizers should incorporate a message that the innovation will evolve over time. Otherwise, if the spread is successful, the new practice may become so standardized that continuous improvement may meet resistance. The advancement of knowledge and learning is not a one-time event. Healthcare professionals must continue to learn from each other to reach the next era of healthcare.

Introducing Innovative Demonstrations and Pilots

The US healthcare delivery system requires transformational innovations across the industry to meet growing market and regulatory demands while simultaneously shifting toward value-based care. Until foundational changes are made to realign incentives toward value and care coordination, the ability to overcome cost and quality challenges will remain marginal. Emerging innovative models include new provider arrangements and payment models that aim to improve the delivery of care, drive better health outcomes, and lower costs.

The establishment of the CMS Innovation Center through the ACA further underscores the vitality of instilling transformational solutions across the healthcare industry. The CMS Innovation Center tests "innovative payment and service delivery models to reduce program expenditures . . . while preserving or enhancing the quality of care for those individuals who receive Medicare, Medicaid, or Children's Health Insurance Program (CHIP) benefits" (CMS 2013a). Such innovation solutions are critical to helping providers transition from the first curve to the second curve of care delivery. The CMS Innovation Center, provider groups, and private payers are increasingly focused on implementing new value-based models that are proven to drive change. Under these models, providers assume varying levels of risk and accountability for patient costs and outcomes. The models range from pay for performance (where providers receive financial incentives when they meet or exceed preestablished targets) to capitation (where providers receive a fixed amount of money per patient in advance to manage all patient care needs). Payment models in between these endpoints reflect a continuum of financial risk that includes methods such as bundling various services under one price or accepting upside or downside financial risk for care of a population. Prominent innovations underway include PCMHs, bundled payments, and ACOs.

Patient-Centered Medical Homes

PCMHs address the crux of health: primary care. Robust primary care is essential to a well-functioning healthcare delivery system. Yet, primary care has significant room for improvement in the United States. PCMHs are seen as a promising solution to bolster primary care and overcome its failings (Bitton, Martin, and Landon 2010; Fields, Leshen, and Patel 2010; Stange et al. 2010).

PCMHs have received wide support among policymakers and payers because of the model's potential to increase efficiency while improving quality of care. With the passage of the ACA and the projected increase in insured individuals, the stakes are high to transform primary care in the United States to deliver the quality and value of care that patients deserve. However, empirical data on the association between PCMHs and high-quality and lower-cost care are limited (Holmboe et al. 2010). New efforts to demonstrate the value of the model through research and evaluation are critical.

Primary care physicians are commonly the first point of contact for a patient. These physicians typically follow their patients over time, in contrast to specialists, who often provide care to a patient for a specific medical need over a defined period. Primary care physicians also regularly refer patients to specialists, yet communication and collaboration among physicians and sites of care are subpar.

PCMHs set clear standards that reflect elements necessary for high-quality, effective primary care (National Committee for Quality Assurance [NCQA] 2011). The model incorporates primary care and patient-centered care, performance-based payments, health information technology, and practice reengineering. Performance-based payments are a crucial component of the model and blend cost and clinical quality measures to foster improved efficiency and care outcomes (Merrell and Berenson 2010).

PCMHs are rapidly developing across the nation. In 2008, NCQA released standards for practices to achieve NCQA accreditation as a PCMH in response to the growing interest in PCMHs and the need for guidance. By the end of 2010, more than 7,600 clinicians and 1,500 practices received NCQA PCMH recognition (NCQA 2011). As of May 2012, 42 states, 3 federal initiatives, and more than 90 commercial health plans were experimenting with PCMHs (National Academy for State Health Policy 2013; Patient-Centered Primary Care Collaborative 2012; Rosenthal et al. 2012). Additionally, the CMS Innovation Center is conducting a PCMH demonstration, titled "Federally Qualified Health Center (FQHC) Advanced Primary Care Practice Demonstration," with more than 500 FQHCs participating (CMS 2013d).

A critical component of providing patient-centered care and achieving efficiency goals is improving coordination and the sharing of clinical data among providers. Practices must be able to track the care received by patients on-site and across settings. This requirement is particularly important and challenging for patients with chronic diseases. Health information technology and electronic health records are critical tools to help providers coordinate care. To maximize utility, these systems should share information across sites of care and use the data to achieve quality and cost goals.

Bundled Payments

The goal of bundled payments is to decrease fragmentation and incentivize collaboration among providers by linking reimbursements for multiple services received by a patient. Increased coordination is projected to decrease the total costs of an episode of care while improving quality.

A bundled payment is a single payment for healthcare services provided by two or more providers for a single episode of care or over a defined period (MedPAC 2008). Traditionally, different providers receive separate payments for the services they provide during a patient's course of treatment. In the traditional model, reimbursement is based on the services provided rather than on the quality and outcomes of the services. Thus, bundled payments incentivize providers to collaborate and improve the value of their services by sharing gains that are realized from more efficient care, which will likely require redesigned models and processes (Hackbarth, Reischauer, and Mutti 2008; Porter 2009).

Evidence indicates that bundled payments can be successful at increasing collaboration and alignment of traditionally siloed physicians and sites of care, such as a hospital, a nursing home, and a cardiologist for an elderly patient with congestive heart failure who underwent a coronary artery bypass graft after a heart attack (MedPAC 2008). The increased collaboration also holds the potential to improve a patient's experience of care and postdischarge recovery.

The CMS Innovation Center is currently testing four models within two bundled payment types that may be used to inform models implemented by other payers.

Payment Type 1: Retrospective Bundled Payments

In the retrospective bundled payment model, "CMS and providers would set a target payment amount for a defined episode of care" (CMS 2011). Providers, not CMS, will propose the target payment. Retrospective payments will be made at a negotiated rate under the fee-for-service system. Total payments will be compared to the target payment at the end of the episode of care.

Participating providers may then share the gains resulting from increased efficiency (CMS 2013c).

As outlined by the CMS Innovation Center, retrospective bundled payments include three models (CMS 2013c; see the following), which differ on the basis of the number of sites of care that are incorporated into the bundled payment. Higher model levels entail a greater risk for providers because they require increased collaboration among more sites of care, but they also have the potential to generate larger savings.

Model 1: Acute care hospital stay only

Model 2: Acute care hospital stay plus post–acute care for 30, 60, or 90 days after discharge

Model 3: Post–acute care only

Payment Type 2: Prospective Bundled Payments

Under the prospective bundled payment model (Model 4), a hospital receives one predetermined bundled payment for all services provided by the hospital, the physicians, and other practitioners during an inpatient stay. As described by CMS, "Physicians and other practitioners would submit 'no-pay' claims to Medicare and would be paid by the hospital out of the bundled payment" (CMS 2013c).

Bundled payments are a strategy to encourage providers to increase coordination and redesign care processes to be more efficient. They also aim to increase provider accountability, speed the adoption of evidence-based medicine, and promote an environment of change and innovation.

Accountable Care Organizations

ACOs are voluntary partnerships of providers who are accountable for a defined group of patients. ACOs aim to integrate and align providers across the care continuum by correcting misaligned incentives and eliminating barriers to coordination of care. ACOs will position providers to deliver more efficient and better-coordinated care while simultaneously slowing cost growth (Fisher, Staiger, et al. 2007; Fisher, McClellan, et al. 2009; MedPAC 2009).

Although the concept of ACOs stems from work completed more than 20 years ago (Welch 1989; Welch and Miller 1994), the term *ACO* was not introduced until 2006, when Dartmouth Atlas researcher Elliott Fisher and colleagues (2007, 2009) discussed the concept and MedPAC (2009) staff created potential ACOs across the United States on the basis of the retrospective utilization patterns of Medicare beneficiaries. In proposed ACO models, patients are assigned to an ACO on the basis of utilization of primary care services, and in most models, each physician is allowed to belong to one ACO. ACOs establish defined cost and quality targets that are risk adjusted on the basis of the ACO's attributed patient population.

A key component of ACOs is the incorporation of new payment models to drive value-based care. The most common payment approach is "shared savings." According to this approach, providers continue to receive fee-for-service payments. However, they qualify to share in any savings generated from cost reductions as well as from meeting performance or utilization targets. Other ACOs may elect to incorporate capitation or bundled payments for an episode of care that are negotiated between providers and payers in advance.

Providers face numerous challenges in the design and implementation of ACO models. These challenges include, but are not limited to, overcoming physician autonomy issues, dealing with patient leakage (care received from non-ACO providers), obtaining provider buy-in, sharing clinical data across sites of care, and overcoming legal barriers. Policymakers and ACO designers face additional challenges, such as determining a minimum number of eligible patients to maintain ACO stability, developing strategies to alleviate leakage, instituting the infrastructure support needed by rural and financially struggling providers, and managing potential financial losses.

Challenges

Furthermore, not all providers have the organizational, cultural, or structural capability to successfully become an ACO. Significant gaps exist between the majority of existing provider systems and the necessary structure to succeed as an ACO. Providers should complete an ACO readiness assessment that includes organizational, technical, and clinical competencies to gauge whether they should enter into ACO arrangements or identify areas for improvement to move toward becoming an ACO (Exhibit 21.7) (Goldsmith 2011).

Policymakers, providers, and payers have high hopes that the ACO model will be a key solution to overcome the pervasive fragmentation, poor coordination, and variable cost and quality performance across the healthcare delivery system. Interest in ACOs is burgeoning: Medicare has implemented three ACO programs (the Medicare Shared Savings Program,

---

- Leadership
- Organizational culture of teamwork
- Relationships with other providers
- Information technology infrastructure for population management and care coordination
- Infrastructure for monitoring, managing, and reporting quality
- Ability to manage financial risk
- Ability to receive and distribute payments or savings
- Resources for patient education and support

EXHIBIT 21.7
Required
Organizational
Competencies
for ACOs

Source: Adapted from *Accountable Care Organizations: AHA Research Synthesis Report* by permission, Copyright 2010, American Hospital Association.

Advance Payment Model, and Pioneer ACO Model), and commercial health plans (including Aetna, Cigna, UnitedHealthcare, and many Blues plans) are rapidly forming ACO partnerships (Aetna 2013; Bowman 2012; Cigna 2013; CMS 2013b; UnitedHealthcare 2012). Yet, whether ACOs will be successful in improving care for individual patients, promoting better health for populations, and fostering a more efficient approach to manage costs remains unclear.

Conclusion

A focus on healthcare quality permeates the transformation of the healthcare industry. As the industry moves from the first-curve business model resting on volume-based, fee-for-service medicine to a second-curve model promoting the value of healthcare services, quality is a major driver, a process, and an outcome of the ongoing system changes.

Initiatives that involve reducing avoidable readmissions, transitioning to population health management, spreading improvements, and testing and implementing new models of care and payment delivery—such as PCMHs and ACOs—serve as major examples of the evolving US healthcare system.

Study Questions

1. Provide examples of other industries in which business models have evolved from a first curve to a second curve.
2. Consider the six aims of quality set forth by the Institute of Medicine (2001) (care that is safe, effective, efficient, equitable, timely, and patient centered), and apply them to the issue of reducing readmissions. For example, for equitable care, how does reducing readmissions affect care across all race and ethnicity groups? How do care interventions to reduce readmissions vary for different patient groups? Identify two or three issues for each aim.
3. If one patient care unit in a hospital dramatically reduced the number of patient falls, how could the hospital support the spread of that improvement to other units?

References

Aetna. 2013. "Accountable Care Organizations: A Collaborative Model for Improving Health Care Quality." Accessed December 12. www.aetna.com/health-reform-connection/aetnas-vision/accountable-care-organizations.html.

Allaudeen, N., A. Vidyarthi, J. Maselli, and A. Auerbach. 2011. "Redefining Readmission Risk Factors for General Medicine Patients." *Journal of Hospital Medicine* 6 (2): 54–60.

American Hospital Association. 2011. *Hospitals and Care Systems of the Future*. A report from the AHA Committee on Performance Improvement. Published September. Chicago: American Hospital Association.

Bitton, A., C. Martin, and B. E. Landon. 2010. "A Nationwide Survey of Patient Centered Medical Home Demonstration Projects." *Journal of General Internal Medicine* 25 (6): 584–92.

Bowman, D. 2012. "Blues, UnitedHealth Launch IT Initiatives for ACOs, Cloud Computing." *FierceHealthIT*. Published February 14. www.fiercehealthit.com/story/blues-unitedhealth-launch-it-initiatives-acos-cloud-computing/2012-02-14.

Centers for Medicare & Medicaid Services. 2013a. Accessed December 12. "About the CMS Innovation Center." http://innovation.cms.gov/about/index.html.

———. 2013b. "Accountable Care Organizations (ACO)." Updated March 22. www.cms.gov/Medicare/Medicare-Fee-for-Service-Payment/ACO/index.html?redirect=/ACO/.

———. 2013c. "Bundled Payments for Care Improvement (BPCI) Initiative: General Information." Accessed December 12. http://innovations.cms.gov/initiatives/Bundled-Payments/index.html.

———. 2013d. "FQHC Advanced Primary Care Practice Demonstration." Accessed December 12. http://innovations.cms.gov/initiatives/fqhcs/index.html.

———. 2012. *National Health Expenditure Projections 2011–2021*. Baltimore, MD: Centers for Medicare & Medicaid Services. www.cms.gov/Research-Statistics-Data-and-Systems/Statistics-Trends-and-Reports/NationalHealthExpendData/Downloads/Proj2011PDF.pdf.

———. 2011. "Bundled Payments for Care Improvement Initiative." Published August 23. www.cms.gov/Newsroom/MediaReleaseDatabase/Fact-Sheets/2011-Fact-Sheets-Items/2011-08-23.html.

———. 2007. "Medicare & Medicaid Statistical Supplement: 2007 Edition." Baltimore, MD: Centers for Medicare & Medicaid Services. Accessed August 9, 2012. www.cms.hhs.gov/MedicareMedicaidStatSupp/downloads/2007Table5.1b.pdf.

Cigna. 2013. "Accountable Care Organizations (ACOs)." Accessed December 12. http://newsroom.cigna.com/KnowledgeCenter/ACO/.

Epstein, A. M. 2009. "Revisiting Readmissions—Changing the Incentives for Shared Accountability." *New England Journal of Medicine* 360 (14): 1457–59.

Fields, D., E. Leshen, and K. Patel. 2010. "Analysis & Commentary: Driving Quality Gains and Cost Savings Through Adoption of Medical Homes." *Health Affairs* 29 (5): 819–26.

Fisher, E. S., M. B. McClellan, J. Bertko, S. M. Lieberman, J. J. Lee, J. L. Lewis, and J. S. Skinner. 2009. "Fostering Accountable Health Care: Moving Forward in Medicare." *Health Affairs* 28 (2): w219–w231.

Fisher, E. S., D. O. Staiger, J. P. Bynum, and D. J. Gottlieb. 2007. "Creating Accountable Care Organizations: The Extended Hospital Medical Staff." *Health Affairs* 26 (1): w44–w57.

Goldsmith, J. 2011. "Accountable Care Organizations: The Case for Flexible Partnerships Between Health Plans and Providers." *Health Affairs* 30 (1): 32–40.

Goodman, D., E. S. Fisher, and C. Chang. 2011. *After Hospitalization: A Dartmouth Atlas Report on Post-Acute Care for Medicare Beneficiaries.* Hanover, NH: Dartmouth Institute for Health Policy and Clinical Practice.

Hackbarth, G., R. Reischauer, and A. Mutti. 2008. "Collective Accountability for Medical Care—Toward Bundled Medicare Payments." *New England Journal of Medicine* 359 (1): 3–5.

Health Research & Educational Trust (HRET). 2012. *Managing Population Health: The Role of the Hospital.* Chicago: Health Research & Educational Trust.

Holmboe, E. S., G. K. Arnold, W. Weng, and R. Lipner. 2010. "Current Yardsticks May Be Inadequate for Measuring Quality Improvements from the Medical Home." *Health Affairs* 29 (5): 859–66.

Institute of Medicine (IOM). 2001. *Crossing the Quality Chasm: A New Health System for the 21st Century.* Washington, DC: National Academies Press.

Jencks, S. F., M. V. Williams, and E. A. Coleman. 2009. "Rehospitalizations Among Patients in the Medicare Fee-for-Service Program." *New England Journal of Medicine* 360 (14): 1418–28.

Joynt, K. E., and A. K. Jha. 2011. "Who Has Higher Readmission Rates for Heart Failure, and Why? Implications for Efforts to Improve Care Using Financial Incentives." *Circulation: Cardiovascular Quality and Outcomes* 4 (1): 53–59.

Joynt, K. E., E. J. Orav, and A. K. Jha. 2011. "Thirty-Day Readmission Rates for Medicare Beneficiaries by Race and Site of Care." *Journal of the American Medical Association* 305 (7): 675–81.

Karliner, L. S., S. E. Kim, D. O. Meltzer, and A. D. Auerbach. 2010. "Influence of Language Barriers on Outcomes of Hospital Care for General Medicine Inpatients." *Journal of Hospital Medicine* 5 (5): 276–82.

Lindenauer, P. K., S. M. Bernheim, J. N. Grady, Z. Lin, Y. Wang, Y. Wang, A. R. Merrill, L. F. Han, M. T. Rapp, E. E. Drye, S. L. Normand, and H. M. Krumholz. 2010. "The Performance of US Hospitals as Reflected in Risk-Standardized 30-Day Mortality and Readmission Rates for Medicare Beneficiaries with Pneumonia." *Journal of Hospital Medicine* 5 (6): E12–E18.

Medicare Payment Advisory Commission (MedPAC). 2009. *Reforming America's Health Care Delivery System*. Washington, DC: MedPAC.

———. 2008. *Report to the Congress: Reforming the Delivery System*. Washington, DC: MedPAC. www.medpac.gov/documents/jun08_entirereport.pdf.

Merrell, K., and R. A. Berenson. 2010. "Structuring Payment for Medical Homes." *Health Affairs* 29 (5): 852–58.

National Academy for State Health Policy. 2013. "Medical Home and Patient-Centered Care." Accessed December 12. www.nashp.org/med-home-map.

National Committee for Quality Assurance (NCQA). 2011. *NCQA Patient-Centered Medical Home 2011*. www.ncqa.org/Portals/0/PCMH2011%20withCAHPS Insert.pdf.

Osei-Anto, A., M. Joshi, A. M. Audet, A. Berman, and S. Jencks. 2010. *Health Care Leader Action Guide to Reduce Avoidable Readmissions*. Chicago: Health Research & Educational Trust.

Patient-Centered Primary Care Collaborative. 2012. "Pilots and Demonstrations in the United States." www.pcpcc.org/resources.

Pearson, M. L., V. Upenieks, T. Yee, and J. Needleman. 2008. *Spreading Innovations in Health Care: Approaches for Disseminating Transforming Care at the Bedside*. Princeton, NJ: Robert Wood Johnson Foundation and Institute for Healthcare Improvement.

Porter, M. E. 2009. "A Strategy for Health Care Reform—Toward a Value-Based System." *New England Journal of Medicine* 361 (2): 109–12.

Rosenthal, M. B., M. K. Abrams, A. Bitton, and Patient-Centered Medical Home Evaluations' Collaborative. 2012. "Recommended Core Measures for Evaluating the Patient-Centered Medical Home: Cost, Utilization, and Clinical Quality." Data brief issued May 16. www.commonwealthfund.org/~/media/Files/Publications/Data%20Brief/2012/1601_Rosenthal_recommended_core_measures_PCMH_v2.pdf.

Stange, K. C., P. A. Nutting, W. L. Miller, C. R. Jaén, B. F. Crabtree, S. A. Flocke, and J. M. Gill. 2010. "Defining and Measuring the Patient-Centered Medical Home." *Journal of General Internal Medicine* 25 (6): 601–12.

UnitedHealthcare. 2012. "Value-Based Contracting and Accountable Care Organizations." www.uhc.com/united_for_reform_resource_center/health_reform_provisions/accountable_care_organizations/value_based_contracting_and_acos.htm.

van Walraven, C., C. Bennett, A. Jennings, P. C. Austin, and A. J. Forster. 2011. "Proportion of Hospital Readmissions Deemed Avoidable: A Systematic Review." *Canadian Medical Association Journal* 183 (7): E391–E402.

Welch, W. P. 1989. "Prospective Payment to Medical Staffs: A Proposal." *Health Affairs* 8 (1): 34–49.

Welch, W. P., and M. E. Miller. 1994. "Proposals to Control High-Cost Hospital Medical Staffs." *Health Affairs* 13 (4): 42–57.

INDEX

Note: Italicized page locators refer to figures; tables are indicated by *t.*

ABOUT THE EDITORS

Maulik S. Joshi, DrPH, MHSA, is president of the Health Research & Educational Trust (HRET) and senior vice president of research at the American Hospital Association (AHA). HRET conducts applied research in critical areas of the healthcare system and leads Hospitals in Pursuit of Excellence, AHA's strategy to accelerate performance improvement. In 2012, HRET received the Illinois Performance Excellence Bronze Award for Commitment to Excellence. Dr. Joshi also oversees AHA's Institute for Diversity in Health Management and the Association for Community Health Improvement.

Previously, Dr. Joshi served as senior advisor at the Agency for Healthcare Research and Quality; president and CEO of the Delmarva Foundation, which was an organizational recipient of the 2005 US Senate Productivity Award, based on the Malcolm Baldrige National Quality Award; vice president at the Institute for Healthcare Improvement; senior director of quality for the University of Pennsylvania Health System; and executive vice president for The HMO Group.

Dr. Joshi serves on the board of trustees of the Anne Arundel Health System, the board quality and patient safety committee of Catholic Health Partners, the health outcomes committee of Advocate Health Care, and the board of governors of the National Patient Safety Foundation. He is treasurer of the board of trustees of the Center for Advancing Health.

Dr. Joshi received his DrPH and MHSA from the University of Michigan and his BS in mathematics from Lafayette College. He is editor-in-chief of the *Journal for Healthcare Quality* and authored *Healthcare Transformation: A Guide for the Hospital Board Member* (CRC Press and AHA Press, 2009).

Elizabeth R. Ransom, MD, FACS, is the executive vice president and clinical leader for the nine-hospital north zone of Texas Health Resources (THR). She and the operations leader are jointly responsible for strategy, operations, finance, hospital management and leadership, and physician and board relations for the region with revenues of more than $1.8 billion. She focuses on collaborating with clinical partners, communities, employers, schools, religious organizations, physicians, and clinicians to create healthier lives for North Texans. This work continues THR's efforts to round out continuum-of-care capabilities and evolve into a fully integrated system of health that excels in physician-directed population health management.

Previously, Dr. Ransom served as chief quality officer at Texas Health Harris Methodist Hospital Southwest Fort Worth, where she was responsible for the quality improvement and safety program as well as oversight of medical staff affairs, pharmacy, patient safety and risk management, laboratory services, case management, and the environment of care. She also worked with the Texas Health Research & Education Institute on a strategic feasibility assessment of a coordinated graduate medical education initiative for THR.

Prior to joining THR, Dr. Ransom was the vice chair and chair-elect of the board of governors of the Henry Ford Medical Group. Additionally, she was the residency program director for the department of otolaryngology–head and neck surgery and chair of the credentials committee of the Henry Ford Health System. Dr. Ransom received her BSc in microbiology and immunology from McGill University in Montreal and her MD from Wayne State University School of Medicine in Detroit, Michigan. She completed her residency in otolaryngology–head and neck surgery at Henry Ford Hospital and was a senior staff physician there.

David B. Nash, MD, MBA, is the founding dean of the Jefferson School of Population Health, which provides innovative educational programming designed to develop healthcare leaders for the future. This appointment caps a 20-year tenure on the faculty of Thomas Jefferson University, where Dr. Nash is the Dr. Raymond C. and Doris N. Grandon Professor of Health Policy.

Dr. Nash has repeatedly been named to *Modern Healthcare*'s list of Most Powerful Persons in Healthcare, and his national activities cover a wide scope. He is on the VHA Center for Applied Healthcare Studies advisory board, and he is a member of the board of directors of the Population Health Alliance (formerly DMAA). He is a principal faculty member for quality-of-care programming for the American College of Physician Executives (ACPE) in Tampa, Florida, and is the developer of the ACPE Capstone Course on Quality.

Dr. Nash is a consultant to organizations in both the public and private sectors. He has chaired the technical advisory group of the Pennsylvania Health Care Cost Containment Council for more than a decade, and he is widely recognized as a pioneer in public reporting of outcomes. In December 2009 he was named to the board of directors of Humana Inc., one of the nation's largest publicly traded healthcare companies. He is on the board of Main Line Health, a four-hospital system in suburban Philadelphia. From 1998 to 2008, he served on the board of trustees of Catholic Health Partners in Cincinnati, Ohio, where he chaired the board committee on quality and safety.

Through publications, public appearances, his blog, and an online column on *MedPage Today*, Dr. Nash reaches more than 100,000 people every month. He has published more than 100 articles in major journals. He has edited 22 books, including *Connecting with the New Healthcare Consumer, The Quality Solution, Governance for Healthcare Providers, Population Health: Creating a Culture of Wellness,* and, most recently, *Demand Better.*

Dr. Nash received his BA in economics (Phi Beta Kappa) from Vassar College, his MD from the University of Rochester School of Medicine and Dentistry, and his MBA in health administration (with honors) from the Wharton School at the University of Pennsylvania. While at Penn, he was a Robert Wood Johnson Foundation Clinical Scholar and medical director of a nine-physician faculty group practice in general internal medicine.

Scott B. Ransom, DO, FACHE, FACS, FACOG, is a senior expert in the healthcare systems and services practice at McKinsey & Company, Inc. He advises hospitals, health systems, academic medical centers, universities, and other leading institutions on issues related to organizational transformation, restructuring, strategy development, physician integration, medical education, clinical and research operations, capability building, performance improvement, and academic affiliations.

Dr. Ransom has more than 20 years of operations and leadership experience, including appointments as president and CEO of an academic health science center with a multispecialty clinical enterprise, several research institutes, and schools in medicine, public health, pharmacy, biomedical sciences, and health professions; as senior vice president/chief quality officer of an eight-hospital healthcare system; and as hospital vice president for medical affairs. Dr. Ransom has been a faculty member of three universities, including the University of Michigan in Ann Arbor, where he was a tenured professor in obstetrics, gynecology, and health management and policy and director of the program for health improvement and leadership development. He has conducted research supported by National Institutes of Health and National Science Foundation funding and has authored more than 100 publications, including nine books, on topics related to healthcare management, quality, and women's health. He has delivered more than 4,000 babies as a practicing obstetrician.

Dr. Ransom is a Fellow of the American College of Healthcare Executives, the American College of Surgeons, and the American Congress of Obstetrics and Gynecologists. He is a Distinguished Fellow and a Past President of the American College of Physician Executives. He is board certified by the American Board of Obstetrics and Gynecology, the American Board of Medical Management, and the Certifying Commission in Medical Management.

Dr. Ransom received his MPH in clinical effectiveness from the Harvard University School of Public Health, his MBA from the University of Michigan Ross School of Business, and his medical degree from the Kansas City University of Medicine and Biosciences. He earned an undergraduate degree in chemistry at Pacific Lutheran University and is a graduate of the US Marine Corps Officer Candidates School.

ABOUT THE CONTRIBUTORS

Kimberly D. Acquaviva, PhD, MSW, is associate dean for faculty affairs and associate professor with tenure in the George Washington University School of Nursing in Washington, DC. Dr. Acquaviva holds a PhD in human sexuality education from the University of Pennsylvania Graduate School of Education, an MSW from the University of Pennsylvania School of Social Policy and Practice (formerly named the School of Social Work), and a BA in sociology from the University of Pennsylvania College of Arts and Sciences.

Al Al-Assaf, MD, MPH, CQA, is executive director of the American Institute for Healthcare Quality and Regents' Professor emeritus and professor emeritus of health administration and policy at the University of Oklahoma. An international consultant, he has advised organizations such as USAID, WHO, UNDP, and UNICEP—as well as many countries worldwide—on issues related to healthcare quality, including accreditation, performance measurement, and improvement. He has published 12 textbooks, authored more than 150 scientific publications, and given more than 300 national and international presentations. He is the recipient of more than 80 national and international awards and recognitions.

David J. Ballard, MD, PhD, MSPH, FACP, is chief quality officer of Baylor Scott & White Health (BSWH), the largest not-for-profit healthcare system in Texas. He is also president of the STEEEP Global Institute, whose mission is to leverage BSWH's experience and expertise to accelerate improved quality performance by healthcare delivery organizations worldwide. A board-certified internist, Mr. Ballard trained at the Mayo Graduate School of Medicine after completing degrees in chemistry, economics, epidemiology, and medicine at the University of North Carolina (UNC), where he was a Morehead Scholar. He received the AcademyHealth New Investigator Award in 1995, the Distinguished Alumnus Award of the UNC School of Medicine in 2008, and the *Health Services Research* John M. Eisenberg Article-of-the-Year Award in 2012. His book, *Achieving STEEEP Health Care*, was published in 2013.

Bettina Berman, RN, MPH, CPHQ, is the project director for quality improvement at the Jefferson School of Population Health, where she is responsible for the development, implementation, and evaluation of quality and safety initiatives for Jefferson University Physicians, the faculty practice plan at Thomas Jefferson University. Her background includes extensive experience in inpatient and outpatient quality measurement, including the implementation and evaluation of value-based strategies—topics on which she frequently lectures nationally. She has authored peer-reviewed papers on quality measurement and has coauthored book chapters on ambulatory quality measurement.

Donald M. Berwick, MD, MPP, is president emeritus and senior fellow at the Institute for Healthcare Improvement (IHI). Dr. Berwick was president and CEO of IHI for nearly 20 years. In July 2010, President Obama appointed him administrator of the Centers for Medicare & Medicaid Services, a position he held until December 2011. He was formerly clinical professor of pediatrics and healthcare policy at the Harvard Medical School and professor in the department of health policy and management at the Harvard School of Public Health. He has served as vice chair of the US Preventive Services Task Force, the first "independent member" of the American Hospital Association board of trustees, and chair of the National Advisory Council of the Agency for Healthcare Research and Quality. An elected member of the Institute of Medicine (IOM), Dr. Berwick served two terms on the IOM's governing council and was a member of the IOM's Board on Global Health. He served on President Clinton's Advisory Commission on Consumer Protection and Quality in the Healthcare Industry. He is a recipient of several awards and author of numerous articles and books, including *Curing Health Care* and *Escape Fire*.

François de Brantes, MS, MBA, is the executive director of the Health Care Incentives Improvement Institute. He holds an MS in finance and taxation from the University of Paris IX–Dauphine and an MBA from the Tuck School of Business at Dartmouth College. He has authored and coauthored many peer-reviewed papers and has published two books, including *The Incentive Cure*.

Steffanie J. Bristol, MPH, MBA, serves as a consultant with Accenture's health practice. Previously, she worked in healthcare services and solutions strategy at Medtronic, emerging markets product development at the Health Care Service Corporation, project management in the department of health policy and management at the Harvard School of Public Health, and health policy research at the Mongan Institute for Health Policy at Massachusetts

General Hospital. Ms. Bristol received her MBA and MPH from the University of Michigan and a BS in health science from Clemson University.

Diane Storer Brown, PhD, RN, CPHQ, FNAHQ, FAAN, is strategic leader for hospital accreditation programs for Kaiser Permanente–Northern California Region, a position involving accreditation leadership with 21 hospitals to ensure high-quality, safe patient care. As a founding leader, co-principal investigator, and senior scientist of the Collaborative Alliance for Nursing Outcomes, she has influenced regional, national, and international efforts to improve the quality of patient care, safety, and outcomes in acute care hospitals. Her research has focused on building capacity for nursing quality and safety measurement and translating emerging research findings to directly improve practice. She is a fellow of the National Association for Healthcare Quality and the American Academy of Nursing.

John Byrnes, MD, is the chief medical officer for Sisters of Charity of Leavenworth (SCL) Health System, a faith-based, nonprofit healthcare organization based in Denver, Colorado, with facilities in California, Colorado, Kansas, and Montana. Nationally recognized for his work in quality, safety, and outcome reporting, Dr. Byrnes has contributed to several books and regularly contributes to industry publications. He is a frequent speaker nationally and internationally. Prior to joining SCL Health System, Dr. Byrnes served as chief quality officer for Spectrum Health. He has held senior executive positions at some of the nation's leading healthcare systems, including Sharp HealthCare, Catholic Healthcare West, and Lovelace Health System, where he led the development of award-winning quality programs including the Lovelace Episodes of Care disease management program.

Susan Edgman-Levitan, PA, is executive director of the John D. Stoeckle Center for Primary Care Innovation at Massachusetts General Hospital (MGH), a lecturer in the department of medicine at MGH, and an associate in health policy at Harvard Medical School. Previously, she was the founding president of the Picker Institute. A constant advocate of understanding the patient's perspective on healthcare, she has been the co-principal investigator on the Harvard Consumer Assessment of Health Providers and Systems (CAHPS) study since 1995 and is the Institute for Healthcare Improvement Fellow for Patient and Family-Centered Care. She is an editor of *Through the Patient's Eyes* (a book on creating and sustaining patient-centered care) and *The CAHPS Improvement Guide*, and she has authored many papers and other publications on patient-centered care. She is a coauthor of the 2006 Institute of Medicine report *The Future of Drug Safety: Promoting and Protecting the Health of the Public.*

Briget da Graca, JD, MS, is a senior medical writer in the office of the chief quality officer at Baylor Scott & White Health in Dallas, Texas. She received her JD from Southern Methodist University.

Frances A. Griffin, RRT, MPA, is a registered respiratory therapist with a master's degree in public administration. Ms. Griffin has 20 years of hospital experience, including administrative oversight for quality, case management, and other related departments, and has been working on patient safety initiatives for more than 15 years. She has been on the faculty of the Institute for Healthcare Improvement (IHI) since 2000 and was a full-time staff member from 2002 to 2010. Her IHI roles included supporting patient safety and reliability content development, directing collaboratives and innovation projects, and serving as faculty for the 100,000 Lives and 5 Million Lives Campaigns. She is codeveloper of the IHI Global Trigger Tool and author of numerous articles related to patient safety and quality improvement in healthcare.

Linda S. Hanold, MHSA, CPHQ, is director of the department of quality measurement at The Joint Commission. In this capacity, she oversees the activities of the groups on performance measurement, performance measurement operations, and database management and statistical analysis. The work of these groups focuses largely on the identification, evaluation, testing, implementation, maintenance, and statistical analyses of standardized performance measures for use in accreditation and certification, public reporting, and hospital quality improvement efforts. Ms. Hanold is well published in the areas of performance measurement and data analysis and often serves as an invited speaker on these subjects.

Robert S. Hopkins III, MPH, PhD, is the former director of strategic development in the office of the chief quality officer at Baylor Scott & White Health in Dallas, Texas. After a career spanning a wide range of interests and experiences—from pilot and aircraft commander in the US Air Force to historian and adjunct lecturer at Creighton University in Omaha, Nebraska, and medical risk management consultant with LifeWings Partners, LLC, in Memphis, Tennessee—Mr. Hopkins retired in 2010.

Richard Jacoby, MD, is a clinical associate professor in the Jefferson School of Population Health and the director of ambulatory quality performance improvement for Jefferson University Physicians, a large, multispecialty clinical practice. Dr. Jacoby's interests in population health focus on elements that relate to clinical care and how it can be improved. His specific areas of interest include quality measurement, process reengineering, electronic health records, the use of evidence-based guidelines, and pay for performance and other reimbursement systems.

Jean E. Johnson, PhD, FAAN, is founding dean and professor of the School of Nursing at the George Washington University. Dr. Johnson received her PhD in health policy from the George Washington University, her MS in nursing as well as a geriatric nurse practitioner certificate from the University of Wisconsin–Madison, a BS in nursing from Texas Women's University, and a BA from the University of Illinois. She is a fellow of the American Academy of Nursing.

Richard G. Koss has, for more than 20 years, led Joint Commission initiatives to measure and analyze the organizational structures, processes, and outcomes associated with patient safety and healthcare quality. He has provided leadership and direction for professional research, statistical, and technical staff in efforts to identify and understand organizational and cultural factors related to improving patient care. He has published papers in a wide range of peer-reviewed journals, including the *New England Journal of Medicine*, the *Journal of the American Medical Association*, and the *International Journal for Quality in Health Care*.

Jerod M. Loeb, PhD, was executive vice president for research at The Joint Commission. During his 19 years there, he played a leadership role in identifying, evaluating, and implementing performance measures across the wide variety of Joint Commission accreditation and certification programs. In recognition of his efforts, he received the National Quality Forum and The Joint Commission's John M. Eisenberg Patient Safety and Quality Honorary Lifetime Achievement Award in 2012. Prior to his work at The Joint Commission, he was assistant vice president for science, technology, and public health at the American Medical Association. Dr. Loeb earned his PhD in cardiovascular physiology at the State University of New York–Downstate Medical Center in Brooklyn. He passed away in October 2013 after a two-year battle with cancer.

David Nicewander received his MS in biostatistics from the School of Public Health of the University of Illinois at Chicago. His 20 years of experience in healthcare analytics and research include 5 years as a statistician with the Centers for Medicare & Medicaid Services, where he was involved in national quality improvement projects targeting Medicare beneficiaries. He currently serves as director of analytics at Baylor Scott & White Health in Dallas, Texas, where he oversees analytic support provided to performance improvement and clinical effectiveness initiatives.

Kevin C. Park, MD, is the vice president of quality at Molina Healthcare, Inc., based in Long Beach, California. Molina Healthcare operates managed care organizations in more than ten states, focused on Medicaid, dual-eligible Medicare, and Marketplace members. Dr. Park has more than 16 years of experience working in healthcare and has specialized in quality. He graduated from Harvard Medical School and trained at Massachusetts General Hospital.

Michael D. Pugh, MPH, president of MdP Associates, LLC, has more than 30 years of CEO experience in hospitals, healthcare systems, managed care organizations, and consulting and healthcare services companies. He is a nationally known advisor and consultant to healthcare providers, payers, trade associations, technology companies, and government organizations. Mr. Pugh has served on the boards of the American Hospital Association (AHA), the AHA Health Forum, The Joint Commission, and the Colorado Hospital Association. He is a frequent speaker at regional and national conferences on leadership, governance, strategy, and quality. He is an adjunct professor at the University of Colorado Denver Business School and a senior faculty member of the Institute for Healthcare Improvement, where he currently serves as the vice chair of the leadership faculty. Mr. Pugh holds a BS and an MPH in healthcare administration from Tulane University in New Orleans, Louisiana, and is the author of multiple articles and book chapters on quality and governance.

James L. Reinertsen, MD, heads The Reinertsen Group, an independent consulting and teaching practice focused on improving the clinical quality performance of healthcare organizations. The winner of the 2011 John L. Eisenberg Individual Achievement Award, Dr. Reinertsen has an unusual combination of skills and experience. He practiced internal medicine and rheumatology for 20 years, was CEO of Park Nicollet Health Services in Minneapolis for 12 years, and was CEO of CareGroup, a six-hospital system in Boston, for 3 years. For 12 years, he was a senior fellow at the Institute for Healthcare Improvement (IHI), where he developed and delivered IHI's programs for boards, executives, and physician leaders. He was a founder and first chairman of Minnesota's Institute for Clinical Systems Improvement and is a former board member of the American Board of Internal Medicine, a former chairman of the board of the American Medical Group Association, and an honorary fellow of the English National Health Service's Institute for Innovation and Improvement. The author of more than 70 scholarly papers and the book *Ten Powerful Ideas for Patient Care Improvement*, Dr. Reinertsen is a graduate of St. Olaf College and Harvard Medical School.

Stephen Schmaltz, PhD, MPH, MS, is an associate director in the division of healthcare quality evaluation at The Joint Commission. In this position, he is responsible for performance measure data quality monitoring, reporting, and analysis; overseeing the development of core measure sampling and risk adjustment methodologies; providing statistical support to The Joint Commission's department of performance measurement in the development and testing of new performance measurement sets; and assisting in the development of grant proposals and manuscripts for publication. Prior to joining The Joint Commission, Dr. Schmaltz was a director of statistical analysis at Humana Inc. During his career in the performance measurement field, he has provided statistical consultation services for the design, data management, and analysis of quality, clinical, preventive, healthcare services, and outcomes studies occurring in academic, health insurance, and other healthcare research settings. Dr. Schmaltz received his BS, MPH, and PhD (biostatistics) degrees from the University of Michigan.

Jaan Sidorov, MD, MSHA, FACP, is principal of Sidorov Health Solutions Inc. in Harrisburg, Pennsylvania, and president of PMSLIC, the largest physician malpractice insurance company in Pennsylvania. Previously, he served as medical director of Geisinger Health Plan. He received his MD from Pennsylvania State University College of Medicine in Hershey and his MHSA from Marywood University in Scranton, Pennsylvania, and received additional training through the American Association of Health Plans certified managed care executive program. Of his numerous peer-reviewed publications, two were named "Best Article" by the Disease Management Association of America and one (on the electronic medical record) was listed as "most read" by *Health Affairs*. Dr. Sidorov is board certified in internal medicine and is a fellow of the American College of Physicians.

Quint Studer is founder of Studer Group. The outcomes-focused firm, which received the Malcolm Baldrige National Quality Award in 2010, implements evidence-based leadership systems that help organizations hardwire excellence through attaining and sustaining outstanding results. *Inc.* magazine named Mr. Studer its Master of Business, making him the only healthcare leader ever to have won this award, and *Modern Healthcare* has chosen him twice as one of the 100 Most Powerful People in Healthcare. Mr. Studer is the author of numerous books, including the *BusinessWeek* bestseller *Hardwiring Excellence*—one of the most-read leadership books ever written for healthcare, with more than 700,000 copies in circulation—and, most recently, *A Culture of High Performance: Achieving Higher Quality at a Lower Cost.*

Ferdinand Velasco, MD, FHIMSS, is senior vice president and chief health information officer of Texas Health Resources (THR), a large, nonprofit integrated healthcare delivery system in North Texas. In this role, Dr. Velasco provides clinical leadership for the implementation of the electronic health record and oversees the organization's clinical decision support, medical and nursing informatics, business intelligence, and data analytics functions across the continuum of care. In addition to his role at THR, he has chaired or served as a member of boards and committees of several national organizations, including the National Quality Forum and the Health Information Management Systems Society. Prior to joining THR, Dr. Velasco served as an assistant professor at the Weill Medical College of Cornell University and practiced as a cardiothoracic surgeon at New York–Presbyterian Hospital. He received his MD from the University of California, Los Angeles School of Medicine and a BS in biomedical sciences from the University of California, Riverside. He received his surgical training at the New York–Presbyterian Hospital.

Edward A. Walker, MD, MHA, is the Cheryl M. Scott / Group Health Cooperative Professor of Health Administration and professor of psychiatry and behavioral sciences at the University of Washington in Seattle. Dr. Walker is nationally recognized for his expertise in coaching and developing physicians and other senior healthcare leaders, improving quality measures, and leading change in medical institutions. A core faculty member of the American College of Physician Executives, he is also a seasoned physician executive and active clinician, bringing together expertise in clinical systems improvement and a clinically informed coaching style that has allowed him to assist physicians and senior executives in their journey of self-improvement and professional growth.

Kevin Warren, MHSM, is the deputy commissioner of the Texas State Veterans Homes and Cemeteries program with the Texas Veterans Land Board (VLB). Created through a partnership between the state of Texas and the US Department of Veterans Affairs, the state homes and cemeteries are owned and managed by the VLB. Previously, Mr. Warren was senior vice president and chief operating officer of TMF Health Quality Institute, the Texas quality improvement organization. Mr. Warren received an MHSM from the University of Mary Hardin–Baylor and is a Certified Professional in Healthcare Quality. He is a licensed nursing-home administrator and serves on the *Journal for Healthcare Quality* editorial board.

Valerie Weber, MD, MS, is founding chair of the department of clinical sciences at The Commonwealth Medical College. Previously, she served as division chief of general internal medicine (2000–2009) and vice chair of medicine (2007–2009) at Geisinger Health System. She served as president of the Association of Chiefs of General Internal Medicine (ACGIM) in 2007–2008 and is founding editor of *The Leadership Forum*, ACGIM's quarterly publication. Her scholarly interests include leadership and change management in quality improvement and the use of informatics to enable quality improvement. Dr. Weber received her MD from the University of Pennsylvania and her MS in healthcare management from the Harvard School of Public Health. She is certified by the American Board of Internal Medicine and continues to be engaged in clinical medicine. She has won multiple awards for patient satisfaction and, in 1999, won the University of Pennsylvania Health System Community Service Award.

Leon Wyszewianski, PhD, MHA, is associate professor in the department of health management and policy at the University of Michigan School of Public Health in Ann Arbor. His research and publications cover a broad spectrum of healthcare delivery and health policy topics. His major area of interest is quality of care. He received his PhD in medical care organization and his MHA from the University of Michigan.